Harald zur Hausen
Infections Causing
Human Cancer

Related Titles

Debatin, K.-M., Fulda, S. (eds.)

Apoptosis and Cancer Therapy 2 Vol.

From Cutting-edge Science to Novel Therapeutic Concepts

2006
ISBN 3-527-31237-4

Gospodarowicz

Prognostic Factors in Cancer, Second Edition

2006
ISBN 0–471–46373–6

Novartis

**Novartis Foundation Symposium 256 –
Cancer and Inflammation**

2004
ISBN 0–470–85673–4

Kaufmann, S. H. E. (ed.)

Novel Vaccination Strategies

2004
ISBN 3–527–30523–8

Stuhler, G., Walden, P. (eds.)

Cancer Immune Therapy

Current and Future Strategies

2002
ISBN 3–527–30441-X

Harald zur Hausen

Infections Causing Human Cancer

With a contribution of
James G. Fox, Timothy C. Wang
and Julie Parsonnet

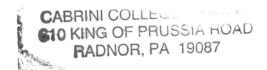

WILEY-VCH

WILEY-VCH Verlag GmbH & Co. KGaA

The Author

Prof. Dr. Harald zur Hausen
Deutsches Krebsforschungszentrum
Im Neuenheimer Feld 242
69120 Heidelberg
Germany

Cover illustration
Papilloma virus infection of cervical neo,
Wellcome Photo Library

■ All books published by Wiley-VCH are care-
fully produced. Nevertheless, authors, editors,
and publisher do not warrant the information
contained in these books, including this book,
to be free of errors. Readers are advised to
keep in mind that statements, data, illustrations, procedural details or other items may in-
advertently be inaccurate.

Library of Congress Card No.: applied for
**British Library Cataloguing-in-Publication
Data:** A catalogue record for this book is avail-
able from the British Library.
**Bibliographic information published by Die
Deutsche Bibliothek**
Die Deutsche Bibliothek lists this publication
in the Deutsche Nationalbibliografie; detailed
bibliographic data is available in the Internet
at http://dnb.ddb.de.

© 2006 WILEY-VCH Verlag GmbH & Co.
KGaA, Weinheim

Typesetting Druckhaus Götz GmbH,
Ludwigsburg
Printing betz-druck GmbH, Darmstadt
Binding Litges & Dopf Buchbinderei
GmbH, Heppenheim

Printed in the Federal Republic of Germany
Printed on acid-free paper

ISBN-13: 978–3-527–31056–2
ISBN-10: 3–527–31056–8

Table of Contents

Infections Causing Human Cancer. Harald zur Hausen
Copyright © 2006 WILEY-VCH Verlag GmbH & Co. KGaA, Weinheim
ISBN: 3-527-31056-8

Preface

For many years I have been tempted to write a comprehensive book on the role of infectious agents in human cancers. Progress has been particularly rapid in this field during the course of the past 25 years, and today we can convincingly report that approximately 20% of the global cancer incidence is initiated or promoted by infectious events. I had admired the task carried out by Ludwik Gross. Since his two-volume publication *Oncogenic Viruses* in 1961, with additional editions in 1970 and in 1983, a number of books have appeared on similar topics, virtually all of them authored by multiple scientists and some of them very heterogeneous in content and structure. For these reasons, I planned to write a book which attempted to develop a more unifying concept and a consistent structure for the individual chapters. Considering the overwhelming magnitude of data, I was sure that I could not undertake this task during my active period as scientific director of the German Cancer Research Center in Heidelberg, and so postponed this for "active retirement". Ultimately, I was pleased that I was able to persuade James Fox from Harvard University to contribute Chapter 10, on *Helicobacter*, as this would have been beyond my personal experience. He immediately consented and jointly with Timothy C. Wang and Julie Parsonnet delivered the chapter in time.

The book is not intended to cover the structure and molecular biology of the agents presented in great detail, but rather aims to concentrate on those aspects that link the respective agents to human oncogenesis. The book should introduce interested colleagues, clinicians, and students to the field, and help to analyze some of the developments that even 20 years ago attracted only minimal attention. Today, this research has culminated in the development of the first – and apparently successful – vaccines for the prevention of specific, common human cancers, cervical carcinomas, and liver cell cancer. Within the book we have tried to provide the readers with an extensive bibliography after each individual chapter, in order to permit further studies on the subject. However, even an attempt to select the most important papers in the field will almost inevitably miss some publications that our colleagues consider as very important. Consequently, I apologize in advance to all of those readers who feel that we did not cover their own or other research areas adequately.

Fortunately, the response on the part of my colleagues was friendly and generous, and they provided helpful suggestions and corrected some of my statements. I am particularly indebted to George and Eva Klein, Stockholm, for their many extremely helpful comments, to Bernhard Fleckenstein, Erlangen, and Georg Bornkamm, Munich, Vladimir Vonka, Prague, Nikolaus Müller-Lantzsch, Homburg, to Reinhard Kurth, Norbert Banner, and Georg Pauli, all Berlin, and to my Heidelberg colleagues, Frank Rösl, Rainer Schmidt, Lutz Gissmann and Henri-Jacques Delecluse. My secretary, Gudrun Küthe, competently and patiently checked the entire manuscript and corrected initial mistakes. Sherryl Sundell, the Managing Editor of the *International Journal of Cancer*, tried to correct at least some of the "Germanisms" in the language.

A special note of gratitude goes to my wife, Ethel-Michele de Villiers, who not only patiently tolerated two-and-a-half years of evenings and weekends devoted to reading and writing, but also actively contributed by discussing and modifying part of the text. Last, but not least, I would like to mention my granddaughters, Talisa and Johanna, who were to some extent neglected during this period. This is hopefully going to change now.

Harald zur Hausen
Heidelberg, April 2006

1
Historical Review

1.1
The Early Period (1898–1911)

On March 24, 1882 Robert Koch presented his famous lecture at the Physiological Society in Berlin, suggesting that tuberculosis is caused by a bacterium. It was probably this surprising discovery of the infectious etiology of tuberculosis – a disease which until then was not suspected to be caused by an infectious agent – that turned the interest of microbiologists at the end of the nineteenth century towards a possible infectious cause of other chronic conditions, among them cancer. Interestingly, at the turn of the past century, the first positive reports incriminated parasites, liver flukes and *Schistosoma* infections with specific human cancers: in 1900, Askanazy reported a link between *Opisthorchis felineus* infection and liver cancer in the former East Prussia. Only five years later, another report incriminated *Bilharzia* infections (schistosomiasis) in bladder cancer (Goebel, 1905). Goebel mentioned in his paper (without citation) that Griesinger and Bilharz, Zancarol, Kartulis, Harrison, Chaker, Rütimeyer, Scheube, Lortet and Vialleton, Brault and also Albarran had demonstrated previously that chronic schistosomiasis might eventually lead to the development of cancer. Possibly based on these findings, Johannes Fibiger in Denmark reported in the early 1920s the identification of a nematode, *Gangylonema neoplasticum* (initially named *Spiroptera carcinoma*), in rat tumors and drew far reaching conclusions from these investigations also for other types of cancer. For his studies, Fibiger was awarded the Nobel Prize in Medicine in 1926. Unfortunately, his results have not been confirmed by other groups, though an account of the developments leading to his award was published recently (Stolt et al., 2004). Subsequently, at least one other nematode, *Spirocerca lupi*, has been identified as causing esophageal granulomas in dogs, some of them converting into sarcomas (Bailey, 1963).

  In those years the evidence for a role of these parasites in human cancer was based exclusively on epidemiological observations and on the findings of clinical studies. Nevertheless – and based on numerous subsequent observations – a panel established in 1994 by the International Agency for Research on Cancer (IARC) in Lyon concluded that there exists sufficient evidence for a role of two parasites, *Schistosoma haematobium* and *Clonorchis viverrini*, in human cancers (IARC, 1994). The same report claimed that there is limited evidence for a carcinogenic function of *Schistosoma japonicum* and for the liver fluke *Clonorchis sinensis*.

Infections Causing Human Cancer. Harald zur Hausen
Copyright © 2006 WILEY-VCH Verlag GmbH & Co. KGaA, Weinheim
ISBN: 3-527-31056-8

The early reports of a link between parasitic infections and human cancers were even preceded by a study of M'Fadyan and Hobday in England. In 1898, these authors published details of the transmission of dog warts by papilloma filtrates known to retain all characterized bacteria identified to that time. Warts, of course, were not considered as "true" tumors, and therefore this publication received little attention. The existence of a "contagium fluidum", which passed filters that would retain all known microorganisms, had been established previously by Iwanowski in St. Petersburg in 1894, and also by Beyerinck in Amsterdam in 1898. Both M'Fadyan and Hobday and Iwanowsky successfully transmitted tobacco mosaic disease by cell-free extracts. In addition, Sanarelli in Montevideo in 1898 had recognized filterable agents as the cause of an acute proliferative disease, myxomatosis in rabbits.

Even in 1907, when Ciuffo in Rome conducted self-inoculation experiments with cell-free extracts from human warts and subsequently developed cutaneous warts at the inoculation site, this result barely created enthusiasm. One year later, in 1908, Ellermann and Bang in Copenhagen reported the cell-free transmission of chicken leukemia. The nature of leukemia and its relationship to malignant diseases were not known in those days. Thus, these experiments were not immediately recognized as the first successful transmission of a natural malignancy. However, this changed in 1911, when Peyton Rous at the Rockefeller Institute in New York demonstrated the cell-free transmission of a solid tumor – a chicken sarcoma – which was, undoubtedly, acknowledged as a malignant neoplasm. This was a first turning point in the public recognition of studies on the infectious origin of cancers.

1.2
Frustration and Successes (1912–1950)

Unfortunately, the following years failed to provide evidence for the applicability of the Rous data to human tumors, and even the cell-free transmission of many animal tumors to the same or to different species attempted during this period commonly resulted in frustration. In fact, more than 20 years passed before any further progress was recognized.

In 1932, Richard E. Shope at the Rockefeller Institute in Princeton noted fibromatous tumors in a wild cotton-tail rabbit. Shope could readily transmit these fibromas by cell-free extracts to either domestic or cotton-tail rabbits. Interestingly, this infection caused a partial cross-immunity against rabbit myxomatosis virus. Both conditions were later identified as being caused by members of the poxvirus family.

Only one year later (in 1933), Shope also discovered a filterable agent in cotton-tail rabbit papillomas; this induced papillomas when inoculated into the scarified skin. Shope partially characterized this virus and noted its remarkable heat stability as it was able to tolerated exposure at 65 C for 30 minutes. In 1934, Rous and Beard discovered that this infection also had malignant potential; this was especially noted in domestic rabbits, where many of the initial papillomas converted into squamous cell carcinomas. This conversion also occurred sporadically in its natural host, the cotton-tail rabbit, albeit at a lower rate (Syverton and Berry, 1935). During the following years, Rous and his coworkers continued to study this system, and investigated in particular the interaction of this virus infection with chemical carcinogens. Even after systemic application of the virus, they found a remarkable degree of synergism between infection and skin tarring or treatment of the skin with defined chemical carcinogens in carcinoma development (Rous and Kidd, 1938; Rous and Friedewald, 1944). In 1961, Ito and Evans showed that the carcinomas contained infectious papillomavirus DNA. Peyton Rous was conceptually far ahead of his time, his early studies having resulted in defining initiation as an early event in carcinogenesis, despite his not understanding the underlying mechanism. Finally, in 1966 – some 55 years after his seminal discovery in 1911 – Rous was awarded the Nobel Prize.

The 1930s were a relatively fruitful period for tumor virology: in 1936, Bittner described a "milk factor" which was transmissible from lactating mice to their offspring. The milk factor was first visualized in 1948 (Porter and Thompson), and Kinosita et al. (1953) characterized the virus in ultrathin sections by electron microscopy. The virus was later identified as a member of the retrovirus family, and its name was changed from Bittner factor or milk factor to mouse mammary tumorvirus (MMTV).

In 1938, Lucké reported a carcinoma of the kidney in the leopard frog (*Rana pipiens*), which was apparently caused by a transmissible virus. This tumor was known to be more prevalent in frogs during the cold season than in summer (McKinnel and McKinnel, 1968), and subsequently in 1956 Fawcett identified typical herpesvirus particles (now labeled as Lucké herpesvirus) in the tumors of winter frogs.

In 1907, an infectious chicken neurolymphomatosis had been recognized by the Hungarian veterinarian J. Marek, the condition subsequently being designated as Marek's disease. Some 20 years later, in 1926, Pappenheimer et al. recognized the neoplastic nature of this disease, while in 1969 Witter et al. identified the infectious agent as a member of the herpesvirus family. Thus, by the late 1960s two animal herpesviruses were being considered as etiological agents for malignant tumors in frogs and chickens.

Unfortunately, the promising studies of the 1930s were interrupted by the Second World War, and during the postwar period it took about 10 more years before any significant progress in this area re-emerged.

1.3
The Period from 1950 to 1965

Although numerous attempts had been made previously to identify an infectious etiology of at least some human tumors, the results had proved – until 1964 – to be rather disappointing. The involvement of parasites seemed true for some cancers outside of Europe and the United States, and appeared to represent an exotic curiosity. Even up to the early 1980s, most epidemiologists at best marginally considered a possible relationship between infections and cancer. Yet, the foundations for our present understanding of the specific function of tumorviruses were laid between 1950 and 1965.

In 1950 and 1951, Ludwik Gross in New York published the results of his pioneering studies on the transmission of murine leukemias following the inoculation of cell-free extracts into newborn mice. Gross had noticed that the susceptibility to cancer induction by viruses (later identified as members of the retrovirus family) depended largely on infections early in life. His studies in 1953 and 1955 resulted in the discovery of another cancer-inducing agent, later identified and described in more detail by Stewart et al. (1957) and designated polyomavirus.

In 1956 and 1957, Charlotte Friend isolated a virus which caused erythroblastosis in mice, and was able to pass it serially in weanling mice. This virus, which caused rapid enlargement of the spleen and liver and led to progressive anemia, was later identified as a member of the retrovirus family. In contrast to the earlier observations by Gross, Friend was also able to induce this proliferative condition in adult mice.

During the ensuing years, a number of additional retrovirus types were analyzed in other rodents, in chicken, cats, cattle, and even in nonhuman primates. Most frequently these infections were linked to leukemias or lymphomas in their respective hosts, and for these reasons many virologists suspected that human proliferative diseases of the hematopoietic system might also be caused by members of the same virus family.

Two other important observations were made during the early 1960s: (i) the discovery of a transforming and tumor-inducing small DNA virus, initially isolated from rhesus monkey kidney cells; and (ii) the identification of tumor-inducing properties of the widely spread human adenoviruses.

In 1960, Sweet and Hilleman described the simian vacuolating virus, labeled simian virus 40 or SV40, which was isolated from rhesus and cynomolgus monkey kidney cell culture material. One year later, Eddy et al. (1961) noted that the inoculation of rhesus monkey kidney extracts into newborn hamsters resulted after several months in invasively growing tumors. During the following year, this group identified the "oncogenic" substance as simian virus 40 (Eddy et al., 1962).

The tumors induced by SV40 failed to synthesize infectious virus, but did produce a virus-specific antigen, the Tumor- or T-antigen (Black et al., 1963a). Similar observations were made two years later for polyomavirus-induced tumors (Habel, 1965). Subsequently, T-antigen expression was also found in the early phase of lytic infection (Pope and Rowe, 1964; Rapp et al., 1964). The availability of a virus system which would readily transform a variety of tissue culture cells without virus production, permitted the development of novel experimental approaches aimed at understanding the molecular mechanisms of cancer. The persistence of integrated SV40 DNA in transformed cells added to the interest (Sambrook et al., 1968), and within a short time studies on cell transformation by SV40 became a favorite system of a large number of tumorvirologists. The subsequent isolation of two related DNA viruses directly from humans, namely BK virus (Gardner et al., 1971) and JC virus (Padgett et al., 1971), seemed to underline further the importance of this virus group as potential carcinogens.

The other important result obtained during this period was the identification of the oncogenic properties of virus infections that were widespread among the human population; these were the adenoviruses, which most frequently caused either respiratory or gastrointestinal symptoms upon infection. In 1962, Trentin and coworkers reported that adenovirus type 12 induced tumors when inoculated into newborn hamsters. These results were soon confirmed and extended by Huebner et al. (1962) for adenovirus type 18, by Girardi et al. (1964) for adenovirus type 7, and by Pereira et al. (1965) for adenovirus type 31. Huebner's group also demonstrated specific complement-fixing antigens in adenovirus-free hamster and rat tumors (Huebner et al., 1963).

Thus, by the mid-1960s several human pathogenic viruses had been identified which possessed oncogenic potential for newborn rodents. Although these viruses were also able to stimulate the permanent growth of tissue culture cells (immortalization), and left their footprints as T-antigens in every tumor cell, none of them transformed human cells or seemed to persist in human cancers. Nevertheless, this period stimulated a number of laboratories to search for viruses, or their footprints, in human tumors.

1.4
A First Human Tumorvirus?

In 1958, Dennis Burkitt, a British surgeon working in equatorial Africa, noted a specific childhood lymphoma that occurred only in specific geographic regions. As these regions coincided with areas of holoendemic malaria, Burkitt speculated that this tumor should have an infectious etiology, most likely vectored by an arthropod, possibly by a mosquito (1962). These initial observations by Burkitt stimulated interest among the scientific community, and consequently Pulvertaft (1964) in Western Nigeria and Epstein and Barr (1964) in Bristol, UK, began to develop tissue culture techniques for these tumors and to establish a number of lymphoblastoid lines. Epstein et al. (1964) noted herpesvirus-like particles in a small fraction of these cells, but in contrast to herpesviruses known at this time, they were unable to transfer the infection to other cell systems, embryonated chicken eggs, or to conventional laboratory animals. These authors concluded at an early stage that they had found a new member of the herpesvirus family which later, was named Epstein–Barr virus (EBV).

The subsequent development of an immunofluorescent test to detect viral antigens in virus-producing cells facilitated further studies (Henle and Henle, 1966). The availability of this test system resulted in the detection of highly elevated antibody titers against viral antigens in patients with Burkitt's lymphoma (Henle and Henle, 1966; Henle et al., 1969), and subsequently also in a second human cancer, in nasopharyngeal carcinomas (Old et al., 1966). In addition, these tests indicated that EBV must be widely spread among all human populations. In 1968, Henle's group identified EBV as the causative agent of infectious mononucleosis (Henle et al., 1968).

The first hints for an oncogenic potential of EBV originated from co-cultivation studies of lethally X-irradiated Burkitt's lymphoma tissue culture cells with umbilical cord lymphocytes (Henle et al., 1967). This resulted in the regular establishment of lymphoblastoid lines of cord blood origin, and was further underlined by the discovery of persisting EBV DNA in "virus-negative" Burkitt's lymphoma cells (zur Hausen and Schulte-Holthausen, 1970), as well as in primary biopsies from Burkitt's lymphomas and nasopharyngeal cancer (zur Hausen et al., 1970). The discovery of a complement-fixing specific nuclear antigen (Pope et al., 1969; Reedman and Klein, 1973), the induction of lymphoproliferative disease after inoculation of EBV into cotton-top marmosets (Shope et al., 1973) or owl monkeys (Epstein et al., 1973), and the identification of EBV persistence in epithelial nasopharyngeal carcinoma cells (Wolf et al., 1973) added to the evidence in this early phase.

Retrospectively, it is surprising that these exciting discoveries received relatively little attention from the scientific community. This was due in part to difficulties in understanding a role for a virus in cancer induction that is persistently present in the vast majority of all human populations. The remarkable geographic restriction of the incriminated human cancers, Burkitt's lymphoma and nasopharyngeal cancer, posed an additional problem. Another reason was that problems which arose during the 1970s created an atmosphere of general disbelief for an infectious etiology of human cancers.

1.5
The Difficult 1970s

The frequent identification of retroviruses from animal leukemias and lymphomas, as well as from some epithelial tumors, resulted in intensified efforts to identify members of this virus family which also corresponded with human malignancies. A number of reports were published during these years, claiming the isolation of C-type viruses from human leukemias or finding components of these viruses in the respective tumor cells. One series of reports characterized a virus isolated from acute myelogenous leukemia (Gallagher and Gallo, 1975; Gallagher et al., 1975; Teich et al., 1975). This virus proved to be closely related to – if not identical with – woolly monkey type C virus. In another set of experiments, DNA from several patients with leukemia was found to hybridize with 70% of RNA from baboon endogenous C RNA virus (BaEV), whereas DNA from normal human tissues hybridized only with 23% of BaEV-RNA (Reitz et al., 1976; Wong-Staal et al., 1976). Based on these data, the authors claimed the horizontal transmission of a BaEV-related virus among humans. In 1977, the same group (Aulakh and Gallo, 1977) reported sequences complementary to Rauscher murine leukemia virus in some patients with leukemia, Hodgkin's disease, and multiple myeloma. These sequences were not detected in non-neoplastic spleen and kidney biopsies from a patient without neoplasia. Thus, at the time these authors suggested that at least three types of type-C viral sequences were present among the human population.

The discovery of a viral RNA-dependent DNA polymerase, reverse transcriptase (which was postulated by Howard Temin in 1964, and demonstrated by Temin and Mizutani and by Baltimore in 1970), seemed to open a new experimental approach for the search of retroviruses in human tumors. Several reports were made on the detection of a high molecular-weight RNA associated with an RNA-instructed DNA polymerase in various human tumors, such as human leukemias (Gallo and Spiegelman, 1974), lymphomas (Spiegelman, 1975), human melanomas (Hehlmann et al., 1978) and human skin cancers (Balda et al., 1975). Unfortunately, none of these reports was later confirmed by other groups.

A third line of publications covered the possible presence of MMTV-like viruses in human breast cancer and milk. Electron microscopic investigations, as well as biochemical and biophysical analyses, suggested the presence of MMTV-like particles in human milk and malignant breast tumors (Moore 1974; Schlom et al., 1975). Particularly in the milk from women of the Parsee community in India, where there was a high incidence of breast cancer, polymerase and RNA studies provided early evidence for the existence of a MMTV-related virus in humans (Das et al., 1972). Although even controversial today, these reports still require confirmation.

It was the coincidence of these numerous reports during the 1970s (part of them presumably originating from inadvertent contaminations), and the inability of many other groups to confirm these findings that resulted in a widespread distrust and disbelief in a role of viruses in human cancers.

One other aspect added to the problems of tumor virology during the 1970s. In 1976, when Stehelin et al. reported the cellular origin of retroviral oncogenes, this had an immediate effect on tumorvirus research. Although modified cellular protooncogenes were clearly sufficient to stimulate cell growth and mediate cellular transformation, Knudson in 1971 proposed another class of genes – the tumor suppressor genes – based on his studies on retinoblastoma development. The failure of these genes is supposed to activate potential oncogenic functions within the affected cell. The identification and isolation of the retinoblastoma susceptibility gene Rb in 1986 and 1987, the demonstration of its modification in retinoblastomas and osteosarcomas (Friend et al., 1986; Lee et al., 1987), and the identification of a number of additional tumor suppressor genes paved the way for a new interpretation of cancer development. Accordingly, cancer development results from an interruption of the interplay of tumor suppressor genes and protooncogenes. This is usually mediated by mutations or loss of the suppressing alleles, or by activating mutations in oncogenes. This relatively simple and straightforward concept did not require any interaction with foreign, predominantly viral nucleic acids. In fact, it was only disturbing an otherwise clear-cut concept.

It was only consequent that, based on these considerations, a substantial number tumorvirologists turned to cell biology and the characterization of gene/gene interactions in normal and malignant cells.

1.6
The Re-Emergence of a Concept

Ten years later, the situation gradually started to change, due mainly to the contributions of three independent findings: (i) the discovery of a role of hepatitis B virus in liver cancer; (ii) the identification of a retrovirus in a rare form of human leukemia; and (iii) the characterization of novel types of papillomaviruses causing the second most frequent cancer in females, cancer of the cervix.

The history of the hepatitis B virus and its role in hepatocellular carcinoma (HCC) is not easily unraveled. As early as the 1950s, British and French pathologists in Africa noted the frequent coincidence of hepatitis infections and hepatocellular cancer (for a review, see Szmuness, 1978). In 1956, Payet et al. suggested directly that HCC is the consequence of chronic viral hepatitis. Further, some of the early epidemiological studies stressed a role for chronic hepatitis B infections in HCC development (Prince et al., 1970; Vogel et al., 1970; Denison et al., 1971; Sankalé et al., 1971; Teres et al., 1971; Nishioka et al., 1973; Trichopoulos et al., 1975; Larouzé et al., 1976). Clear-cut evidence of this was presented a few years later when, in a prospective study conducted in government employees in Taiwan, Beasley et al. (1981) noted an increase in relative risk by a factor of 103 for HCC of hepatitis B carriers in comparison to hepatitis B-negative individuals. This clearly emphasized an important role of hepatitis B in the development of liver cancer.

Although it is still unclear by which mechanism hepatitis B virus contributes to the emergence of liver cancer, vaccination studies performed today underline the importance of this infection for hepatocellular carcinomas (this will be discussed in Chapter 5, Section 5.3).

In 1980, the isolation of a human T-lymphotropic retrovirus (HTLV-1) was reported from a cutaneous T-cell lymphoma (Poiesz et al., 1980). The virus could be propagated in T-cell growth factor-stimulated lymphocytes. The factor, interleukin-2, was previously purified and characterized by the same group (Mier and Gallo, 1980). Japanese researchers later identified the same virus (Miyoshi et al., 1981), and linked this infection to adult T-cell leukemia, which is endemic in the coastal regions of Southern Japan (Hinuma et al., 1981). These findings were rapidly reproduced, and firmly established at least one member of the retrovirus family as the causative agent of a rare form of human leukemia. Today, the link is basically proven.

Studies on papillomaviruses have a long history, in part already described for the cotton-tail papillomavirus. Early studies on the cell-free transmission of bovine warts were initiated by Magelhaes in Brazil (1920) while later, in 1951, Olson and Cook showed that the transmission of these viruses to another species, horses, resulted in the induction of sarcoids. These invasively growing but nonmetastasizing tumors are also noted in domestic horses under natural conditions. The Olson group made another striking observation, namely the induction of bladder tumors in cattle by bovine papillomavirus (BPV) infection (Olson et al., 1959). Only four years later, two additional reports by Black et al. (1963 b) and Thomas and colleagues (1963) demonstrated the transforming activity of BPV preparations for bovine fetal and murine cells.

The analysis of human papillomatous lesions and their relationship to virus infections and carcinogenesis had a much slower start. Although the infectious etiology of human warts had been clearly established based on their cell-free transmission, they were mainly regarded as a cosmetic nuisance and not thought to be of any significant medical interest.

The gradual change of this view originated from the description of a syndrome first reported by Lewandowsky and Lutz in Basel, in 1922. These authors described an hereditary condition, characterized by an extensive verrucosis, epidermodysplasia verruciformis. In these patients, at sun-exposed sites such as the forehead, the face, and the backs of the hands and arms, some papillomatous lesions converted into squamous cell carcinomas. Lutz, in 1946, and subsequently Jablonska and Millewski in 1957, proved the viral etiology of these warts in autoinoculation experiments. It was mainly the merit of Stefania Jablonska to point out a potential role of the human papillomavirus (HPV) particles seen in these warts as causal factors for the subsequent development of squamous cell cancers of the skin (Jablonska et al., 1972). Working jointly with Gérard Orth, these groups successfully demonstrated the presence of novel types of papillomaviruses, most frequently HPV 5, within epidermodysplasia verruciformis lesions and within biopsies of squamous cell carcinomas of those patients. (Orth et al., 1978, 1979).

Although HPV 5 represents the first papillomavirus infection regularly detected in cutaneous squamous cell cancers of epidermodysplasia patients, the rarity of the syndrome, the difficulties in obtaining sufficient clinical materials for extensive studies, and the absence of tissue culture lines from these carcinomas were probably the reasons for a limited interest in this condition. Only in recent years has the study of cutaneous papillomavirus infections and their relationship to nonmelanoma skin cancer in immunosuppressed and immunocompetent patients received increasing attention.

Another track of papillomavirus research resulted in the identification of specific HPV types as causative agents for cancer of the cervix, other anogenital cancers, and a subset of oropharyngeal carcinomas. These investigations began with the search for a viral etiology of cancer of the cervix, but by the late 1960s and 1970s the results of serological studies had suggested a role for human herpes simplex virus type 2 (HSV 2) in this cancer (Rawls et al., 1968; Naib et al., 1969). The present author's group was unable to confirm these findings, and sought alternative viral candidates. A number of anecdotal reports on the malignant conversion of genital warts (condylomata acuminata), scattered among the medical literature of the preceding 100 years, attracted attention. Subsequently, a possible causal role of papillomavirus infections for cervical cancer was postulated, and initial attempts were begun to characterize the viral DNA in genital warts (zur Hausen et al., 1974, 1975; zur Hausen 1976, 1977). These and other studies had the early consequence of discovering the heterogeneity of the papillomavirus family (Gissmann and zur Hausen, 1976; Orth et al., 1977; Gissmann et al., 1977), presently counting close to 106 fully sequenced genotypes (de Villiers, 1994; also Personal communication). However, the eventual isolation of HPV DNA from genital warts, labeled as HPV 6 (Gissmann and zur Hausen, 1980), and from laryngeal papillomas (HPV 11) two years later (Gissmann et al., 1982), did not yield reproducibly positive data for these viruses in cervical cancer. Yet, the use of their DNA in hybridization experiments, performed under conditions of reduced stringency, permitted the subsequent cloning of HPV 16 (Dürst et al., 1983) and HPV 18 DNA (Boshart et al., 1984), the two papillomavirus types most frequently found in cervical cancer. This allowed further experiments to be conducted that would prove the role of these papillomaviruses in causing this malignancy (see Chapter 5).

The identification of three viral families with representative types that clearly cause cancers (including common carcinomas such as cancer of the cervix and liver) gradually resulted in an acceptance of infectious agents as important human carcinogens. The subsequent identification of additional infections clearly linked to other cancers further strengthened the role of infectious agents in human cancers. The hepatitis C virus was identified in 1989 (Choo et al., 1989), and initial reports on its relationship to a subset of hepatocellular carcinomas appeared in the same year (Bargiggia et al., 1989; Simonetti et al., 1989). Some earlier reports had been made, however, linking non-A, non-B hepatitis infections to liver cancer (Kiyosawa et al., 1982; Resnick et al., 1983; and others). Human herpesvirus type 8 was discovered in 1994 (Chang et al.) as being the most likely causative agent for Kaposi's sarcoma, while in 1989 (Forman et al., 1991; Nomura et al., 1991; Parsonnet et al., 1991) and 1993 (Wotherspoon et al.), *Helicobacter pylori*, as a bacterial infection, was added to the list of potential human carcinogens. Subsequently, a large number of additional HPV genotypes has been added, the pathogenic significance of which remains to be determined. The same is true for the recently discovered TT viruses; these clearly represent a new virus family, establishing probably life-long persistent infections in a high proportion of the human population.

Thus, today – more than 100 years after the first attempts to link infections to human cancer, and after more than 80 years of mainly frustrating experimentation – infections causing cancer emerge as a major factor in human carcinogenesis. This mode of research leads to new approaches towards cancer diagnosis and treatment, and – most importantly – of cancer prevention.

References

Askanazy, M. Über Infektion des Menschen mit *Distomum felineum (sibiricum)* in Ostpreussen und ihren Zusammenhang mit Leberkrebs. *Centr. Bakt. Orig.* 28: 491–502, **1900**.

Aulakh, G.S. and Gallo, R.C. Rauscher-leukemia-virus-related sequences in human DNA: presence in some tissues of some patients with hematopoietic neoplasias and absence in DNA from other tissues. *Proc. Natl. Acad. Sci. USA* 74: 353–357, **1977**.

Bailey, W.S. Parasites and cancer: sarcoma in dogs associated with *Spirocerca lupi*. *Ann. N.Y. Acad. Sci.* 108: 890–923, **1963**.

Balda, B.R., Hehlmann, R., Cho, J.R., and Spiegelman, S. Oncornavirus-like particles in human skin cancers. *Proc. Natl. Acad. Sci. USA* 72: 3697–3700, **1975**.

Baltimore, D. RNA-dependent DNA polymerase in virions of RNA tumour viruses. *Nature* 226: 1209–1211, **1970**.

Bargiggia, S., Piva, A., Sangiovanni, A., and Donato, F. [Primary carcinoma of the liver and hepatitis C virus in Italy. A prospective study in patients with cirrhosis] *Medicina (Firenze)* 9: 424–426, **1989**.

Beasley, R.P., Hwang, L.Y. Lin, C.-C., and Chien, C.-S. Hepatocellular carcinoma and hepatitis B virus. A prospective study of 22707 men in Taiwan. *Lancet* II: 1129–1133, **1981**.

Beyerinck, M.W. Über ein Contagium vivum fluidum als Ursache der Fleckenkrankheit der Tabakblätter. *Verhandl. Konink. Akad. Wetenschappen te Amsterdam* 6: 3–22, **1898**.

Bittner, J.J. Some possible effects of nursing on the mammary gland tumor incidence in mice. *Science* 84: 162, **1936**.

Black, P.H., Rowe, W.P., Turner, H.C., and Huebner, R.J. A specific complement-fixing antigen present in SV40 tumor and transformed cells. *Proc. Natl. Acad. Sci. USA* 50: 1148–1156, **1963a**.

Black, P.H., Hartley, J.W., Rowe, W.P., and Huebner, R.J. Transformation of bovine tissue culture cells by bovine papilloma virus. *Nature* 199: 1016–1018, **1963b**.

Boshart, M., Gissmann, L., Ikenberg, H., Kleinheinz, A., Scheurlen, W., and zur Hausen, H. A new type of papillomavirus DNA, its presence in genital cancer and in cell lines derived from genital cancer. *EMBO J.* 3: 1151–1157, **1984** .

Burkitt, D. A sarcoma involving the jaws in African children. *Br. J. Surg.* 46: 218–223, **1958**.

Burkitt, D. A children's cancer dependent on climatic factors. *Nature* 194: 232–234, **1962**.

Chang, Y., Cesarman, E., Pessin, M.S., Lee, F., Culpepper, J., Knowles, D.M., and Moore, P.S. Identification of herpesvirus-like DNA sequences in AIDS-associated Kaposi's sarcoma. *Science* 266: 1865–1869, **1994**.

Choo, Q.L., Kuo, G., Weiner, A.J., Overby, L.R., Bradley, D.W., and Houghton, M. Isolation of a cDNA clone derived from a blood-borne non-A, non-B viral hepatitis genome. *Science* 244: 359–362, **1989**.

Ciuffo, G. Innesto positive con filtrato di verruca vulgare. *Giorn. Ital. Mal. Venereol.* 48:12, **1907**.

Das, M.R., Vaidya, A.B., Sirsat, S. M., and Moore, D.H. Polymerase and RNA studies on milk virions from women of the Parsi community. *J. Natl. Cancer Inst.* 48: 1191–1196, **1972**.

Denison, E.K., Peters, R.L., and Reynolds, T.B. Familial hepatoma with hepatitis-associated antigen. *Ann. Intern. Med.* 74: 391–394, **1971**.

de Villiers, E.-M. Human pathogenic papillomaviruses: an update. *Curr. Top. Microbiol. Immunol.* 186: 1–12, **1994**.

Dürst, M., Gissmann, L., Ikenberg, H., and zur Hausen, H. A papillomavirus DNA from a cervical carcinoma and its prevalence in cancer biopsy samples from different geographic regions. *Proc. Natl. Acad. Sci. USA* 80: 3812–3815, **1983** .

Eddy, B.E., Borman, G.S., Berkeley, W.H., and Young, R.D. Tumors induced in hamsters by injection of rhesus monkey kidney cell extracts. *Proc. Soc. Exp. Biol. Med.* 107: 191–197, **1961**.

Eddy, B.E., Borman, G.S., Grubbs, G.E., and Young, R.D. Identification of the oncogenic substance in rhesus monkey kidney cell cultures as Simian Virus 40. *Virology* 17: 65–75, **1962**.

Epstein, M.A. and Barr, Y.M. Cultivation in vitro of human lymphoblasts from Burkitt's malignant lymphoma. *Lancet* 1: 252–253, **1964**.

Epstein, M.A., Achong, B.G., and Barr, Y.M. Virus particles in cultured lymphoblasts from Burkitt's lymphoma. *Lancet* 1: 702–703, **1964**.

Epstein, M.A., Hunt, R.D., and Rabin, H. Pilot experiments with EB virus in owl monkeys (*Aotus trivirgatus*) I. Reticuloproliferative disease in an inoculated animal. *Int. J. Cancer* 12: 309–318, **1973**.

Fawcett, D.W. Electron microscope observations on intracellular virus-like particles associated with the cells of the Lucke renal adenocarcinoma. *J. Biophys. Biochem. Cytol.* 2(6): 725–741, **1956**.

Forman, D., Newell, D.G., Fullerton, F., Yarnell, J.W., Stacey, A.R., Wald, N., and Sitas, F. Association between infection with *Helicobacter pylori* and risk of gastric cancer: evidence from a prospective investigation. *Br. Med. J* . 302: 1302–1305, **1991**

Friend, C. The isolation of a virus causing a malignant disease of the hematopoietic system in adult Swiss mice (Abstract). *Proc. Am. Ass. Cancer Res.* 2: 106, **1956**.

Friend, C. Cell-free transmission in adult Swiss mice of a disease having the character of a leukemia. *J. Exp. Med.* 105: 307–318, **1957**.

Friend, S. H., Bernards, R., Rogelj, S., Weinberg, R.A., Rapaport, J.M., Albert, D.M., and Dryja, T.P. A human DNA segment with properties of the gene that predisposes to retinoblastoma and osteosarcoma. *Nature* 323: 643–646, **1986**.

Gallagher, R.E. and Gallo, R.C. Type C RNA tumor virus isolated from cultured human acute myelogenous leukemia cells. *Science* 187: 350–353, **1975**.

Gallagher, R.E., Salahuddin, S. Z., Hall, W.T., McCredie, K.W., and Gallo, R.C. Growth and differentiation in culture of leukemic leukocytes from a patient with acute myelogenous leukemia and re-identification of type-C virus. *Proc. Natl. Acad. Sci. USA* 72: 4137–4141, **1975**.

Gallo, R.C. and Spiegelman, S. Letter: Reverse transcriptase in acute leukaemia. *Lancet* 1: 1117–1178, **1974**.

Gardner, S. D., Field, A.M., Coleman, D.V., and Hulme, B. New human papovavirus (B.K.) isolated from urine after renal transplantation. *Lancet* 1: 1253–1257, **1971**.

Girardi, A.J., Hilleman, M.R., and Zwickey, R.E. Tests in hamsters for oncogenic quality of ordinary viruses including adenovirus type 7. *Proc. Soc. Exp. Biol. Med.* 115: 1141–1150, **1964**.

Gissmann, L. and zur Hausen, H. Human papilloma virus DNA: physical mapping and genetic heterogeneity. *Proc. Natl. Acad. Sci. USA* 73: 1310–1313, **1976**.

Gissmann, L. and zur Hausen, H. Partial characterization of viral DNA from human genital warts (condylomata acuminata). *Int. J. Cancer* 25: 605–609, **1980**.

Gissmann, L. Pfister, H., and zur Hausen, H. Human papilloma viruses (HPV): Characterization of four different isolates. *Virology* 76: 569–580. **1977**.

Gissmann, L., Diehl, V., Schultz-Coulon, H.J., and zur Hausen, H. Molecular cloning and characterization of human papillomavirus DNA derived from a laryngeal papilloma. *J. Virol.* 44: 393–400, **1982**.

Goebel, C. Über die bei Bilharziakrankheit vorkommenden Blasentumoren mit besonderer Berücksichtigung des Carcinoms. *Zeitschr. Krebsforsch.* 3: 369–513, **1905**.

Gross, L. Susceptibility of newborn mice of an otherwise resistant strain to inoculation with leukemia. *Proc. Soc. Exp. Biol. Med.* 73: 246–248, **1950**.

Gross, L. "Spontaneous" leukemia developing in C3 H mice following inoculation in infancy, with AK-leukemic extracts. *Proc. Soc. Exp. Biol. Med.* 76: 27–32, **1951**.

Gross, L. A filterable agent, recovered from Ak-leukemic extracts, causing salivary gland carcinomas in C3 H mice. *Proc. Soc. Exp. Biol. Med.* 83: 414–421, **1953**.

Gross, L. Induction of parotid carcinomas and/or subcutaneous sarcomas in C3 H mice with normal C3 H organ extracts. *Proc. Soc. Exp. Biol. Med.* 88: 362–368, **1955**.

Habel, K. Specific complement-fixing antigens in polyoma tumors and transformed cells. *Virology* 25: 55–61, **1965**.

Hehlmann, R., Balda, B.R., and Spiegelman, S. Murine and human melanomas containing a high molecular weight RNA associated with an RNA-instructed DNA polymerase. *Int. J. Dermatol.* 17: 115–122, **1978**.

Henle, G. and Henle, W. Immunofluorescence in cells derived from Burkitt's lymphoma. *J. Bacteriol.* 91: 1248–1256, **1966**.

Henle, W., Diehl, V., Kohn, G., zur Hausen, H., and Henle, G. Herpes-type virus and chromosome marker in normal leukocytes after growth with irradiated Burkitt cells. *Science* 157: 1064–1065, **1967**.

Henle, G., Henle, W., and Diehl, V. Relation of Burkitt's tumor-associated herpes-type virus to infectious mononucleosis. *Proc. Natl. Acad. Sci. USA* 59: 94–101, **1968**.

Henle, G., Henle, W., Clifford, P., Diehl, V., Kafuko, G.W., Kirya, B.G., Klein, G., Morrow, R.H., Munube, G.M.R., Pike, P., Tukei, P.M., and Ziegler, J.L. Antibodies to Epstein-Barr virus in Burkitt's lymphoma and control groups. *J. Natl. Cancer Inst.* 43: 1147–1157, **1969**.

Hinuma, Y., Nagata, K., Hanaoka, M., Nakai, M., Matsumoto, T., Kinoshita, K.I., Shirakawa, S., and Mioshi, I. Adult T-cell leukemia: antigen in an ATL cell line and detection of antibodies to the antigen in human sera. *Proc. Natl. Acad. Sci. USA* 78: 6476–6480, **1981**.

Huebner, R.J., Rowe, W.P., and Lane, W.T. Oncogenic effects in hamsters of human adenoviruses 12 and 18. *Proc. Natl. Acad. Sci. USA* 48: 2051–2058, **1962**.

Huebner, R.J., Rowe, W.P., Turner, H.C., and Lane, W.T. Specific adenovirus complement-fixing antigens in virus-free hamster and rat tumors. *Proc. Natl. Acad. Sci. USA* 50: 379–389, **1963**.

IARC Monographs on the Evaluation of Carcinogenic Risks to Humans. Volume 61. Schistosomes, Liver flukes and *Helicobacter pylori*. IARC, Lyon, **1994**.

Ito, Y. and Evans, C.A. Induction of tumors in domestic rabbits with nucleic acid preparations from partially purified Shope papilloma virus and from extracts of the papillomas of domestic and cotton tail rabbits. *J. Exp. Med.* 114: 485–491, **1961**.

Iwanowski, D. Über die Mosaikkrankheit der Tabakpflanze. *Bull. Acad. Imp. Sci., St. Petersburg* 3: 67–70, **1894**

Jablonska, S. and Milewski, B. Zur Kenntnis der Epidermodysplasia verruciformis Lewandowsky-Lutz. *Dermatologica* 115: 1–22, **1957**.

Jablonska, S., Dabrowski, J., and Jakubowicz, K. Epidermodysplasia verruciformis as a model in studies on the role of papovaviruses in oncogenesis. *Cancer Res.* 32: 583–589, **1972**.

Kinosita, R., Erickson, J.O., Armen, DS. M., Dolch, M.E., and Ward, J.P. Electron microscope study of mouse mammary carcinoma tissue. *Exp. Cell Res.* 4: 353–4361, **1953**.

Knudson, A.G. Mutation and cancer: statistical study of retinoblastoma. *Proc. Natl. Acad. Sci. USA* 68: 820–823, **1971**.

Koch, R. Die Aetiologie der Tuberkulose. Nach einem in der Physiologischen Gesellschaft zu Berlin am 24. März 1882 gehaltenen Vortrage. *Berl. Klin. Wochenschr.* 19: 1990, **1882**.

Kiyosawa, K., Akahane, Y., Nagata, A., Koike, Y., and Furuta, S. The significance of blood transfusion in non-A, non-B chronic liver disease in Japan. *Vox Sang.* 43: 45–52, **1982**.

Larouzé, B., Saimot, G., Lustbader, E.D., London, W.T., Werner, B.G., and Payet, M., Host responses to hepatitis-B infection in patients with primary hepatic carcinomas and their families: A case-control study in Senegal, West Africa. *Lancet* 2: 534–538, **1976**.

Lee, W.-H., Bookstein, R., Hong, F., Young, L.-J., Shew, J.-Y., and Lee, E.Y. Human retinoblastoma susceptibility gene: cloning, identification and sequence. *Science* 235: 1394–1399, **1987**.

Lewandowsky, F. and Lutz, W. Ein Fall einer bisher nicht beschriebenen Hauterkrankung (Epidermodysplasia verruciformis). *Arch. Dermatol. Syph. (Berlin)* 141: 193–203, **1922**.

Lutz, W. A propos de l'epidermodysplasie verruciforme. *Dermatologica* 92, 30–43, **1946**.

Magelhaes – Verruga dos bovideos. *Brasil-Medico* 34: 430–431, **1920**.

Marek, J. Multiple Nervenentzündung (Polyneuritis) bei Hühnern. *Deutsche Tierärztl. Wochenschr.* 15: 417–421, **1907**.

McKinnell, R.G. and McKinnell, B.K. Seasonal fluctuation of frog renal adenocarcinoma. Prevalence in natural populations. *Cancer Res.* 28(3): 440–444, **1968**.

M'Fadyan, J. and Hobday, F. Note on the experimental "transmission of warts in the dog". *J. Comp. Pathol. Ther.* 11: 341–344, **1898**.

Mier, J.W. and Gallo, R.C. Purification and some characteristics of human T-cell growth factor from phytohemagglutinin stimulated lymphocyte conditioned media. *Proc. Natl. Acad. Sci. USA* 77: 6134–6138, **1980**.

Miyoshi, I., Kubonishi, I., Yoshimoto, S., Akagi, T., Ohtsuki, Y., Shiraishi, Y., Nagato, K., and Hinuma, Y. Type C virus particles in a cord T-cell line derived by co-cultivating normal human cord leukocytes and human leukaemic T cells. *Nature* 294: 770–771, **1981**.

Moore, D.H. Evidence in favor of the existence of human breast cancer virus. *Cancer Res.* 34: 2322–2329, **1974**.

Naib, Z.M., Nahmias, A.J., Josey, W.E., and Kramer, J.H. Genital herpetic infection. Association with cervical dysplasia and carcinoma. *Cancer* 23: 940–945, **1969**.

Nishioka, K., Hirayama, T., Sekine, T., Okochi, K., Mayumi, M., Jueilow, S., Chen-Hui, L., and Tong-Min, L. Australia antigen and hepatocellular carcinoma. *GANN Monogr.* *Cancer Res.* 14: 167–175, **1973**.

Nomura, A., Stemmermann, G.N., Chyou, P.H., Kato, I., Perez-Perez, G.I., and Blaser, M.J. *Helicobacter pylori* infection and gastric carcinoma among Japanese Americans in Hawaii. *N. Engl. J. Med.* 325: 1132–1136, **1991** .

Old, L.J., Boyse, E.A., Oettgen, H.F., De Harven, E., Geering, G., Williamson, B., and Clifford, P. Precipitating antibody in human serum to an antigen present in cultured Burkitt's lymphoma cells. *Proc. Natl. Acad. Sci. USA* 56: 1699–1705, **1966**.

Olson, C. and Cook, R.H. Cutaneous sarcoma-like lesions of the horse caused by the agent of bovine papilloma. *Proc. Soc. Exp. Biol. Med.* 77: 281–284, **1951**.

Olson, C., Pamukcu, A.M., Brobst, D.F., Kowalczyk, T., Satter, E.J., and Price, J.M. A urinary bladder tumor induced by a bovine cutaneous papilloma agent. *Cancer Res.* 19: 779–782, **1959**.

Orth, G., Favre, M., and Croissant, O. Characterization of a new type of human papillomavirus that causes skin warts. *J. Virol.* 24: 108–120, **1977**.

Orth, G., Jablonska, S., Favre, M., Jarzabek-Chorzelska, M., and Rzesa, G. Characterization of two new types of human papillomaviruses from lesions of epidermodysplasia verruciformis. *Proc. Natl. Acad. Sci. USA* 75: 1537–1541, **1978**.

Orth, G., Jablonska, S., Jarzabek-Chorzelska, M., Obalek, S., Rzesa, G., Favre, M., and Croissant, O. Characteristics of the lesions and risk of malignant conversion associated with the type of the human papillomavirus involved in epidermodysplasia verruciformis. *Cancer Res.* 39: 1074–1082, **1979**.

Padgett, B.L., Walker, D.L., Zu Rhein, G.M., Eckroade, R.J., and Dessel, B.H. Cultivation of papova-like virus from human brain with progressive multifocal leukencephalopathy. *Lancet* 1: 1257–1260, **1971**.

Pappenheimer, A.M., Dunn, L.C., and Cone, V. A study of fowl paralysis (neuro-lymphomatosis gallinarum). *Storrs Agric. Exp. Station Bull.* 143: 185–290, **1926**.

Parsonnet, J., Friedman, G.D., Vandersteen, D.P., Chang, Y., Vogelman, J.H., Orentreich, N., and Sibley, R.K. *Helicobacter pylori* infection and the risk of gastric carcinoma. *N. Engl. J. Med.* 325: 1127–1131, **1991**.

Payet, M., Camain, R., and Pene, P. Primary cancer of the liver. Critical study of 240 patients. *Rev. Int. Hepatol.* 6: 1–86, **1956**.

Pereira, M.S., Pereira, H.G., and Clarke, S. K.R. Human adenovirus type 31. A new serotype with oncogenic properties. *Lancet* 1: 21–23, **1965**.

Poiesz, B.J., Ruscetti, F.W., Gazdar, A.F., Bunn, P.A., Minna, J.D., and Gallo, R.C. Detection and isolation of type C retrovirus particles from fresh and cultured lymphocytes of a patient with cutaneous T-cell lymphoma. *Proc. Natl. Acad. Sci. USA* 77: 7415–7419, **1980**.

Pope, J.H. and Rowe, W.P. Detection of specific antigen in SV40-transformed cells by immunofluorescence. *J. Exp. Med.* 120: 121–127, **1964**.

Pope, J.H., Horne, M.K., and Wetters, E.J. Significance of a complement-fixing antigen associated with herpes-like virus and detected in the Raji cell line. *Nature* 222: 186–187, **1969**.

Porter, K.R. and Thompson, H.P. A particulate body associated with epithelial cells cultured from mammary carcinoma of mice of a milk factor strain. *J. Exp. Med.* 88: 15–24, **1948**.

Prince, A.M., Leblanc, L., Krohn, K., Masseyeff, R. and Alpert, M.E. SH antigen and chronic liver disease. *Lancet* 2: 717–718, **1970**.

Pulvertaft, R.J.V. Cytology of Burkitt's tumour (African lymphoma). *Lancet* 1: 238–240, **1964**.

Rapp, F., Kitahara, T., Butel, J.S., and Melnick, J.L. Synthesis of SV40 tumor antigen during replication of simian papovavirus (SV40). *Proc. Natl. Acad. Sci. USA* 52: 1138–1142, **1964**.

Rawls, W.E., Tompkins, W.A., Figueroa, M.E., and Melnick, J.L. Herpesvirus type 2: association with carcinoma of the cervix. *Science* 161: 1255–1256, **1968**.

Reedman, B.M. and Klein, G. Cellular localization of Epstein-Barr virus (EBV)-associated complement-fixing antigen in producer and nonproducer lymphoblastoid cell lines. *Int. J. Cancer* 11: 499–520, **1973**.

Reitz, M.S., Miller, N.R., Wong-Staal, F.. Gallagher, G.E., Gallo, R.C., and Gillespie, D.H. Primate type-C virus nucleic acid sequences (woolly monkey and baboon types) in tissues from a patient with acute myelogenous leukemia and in viruses isolated from cultured cells of the same patient. *Proc. Natl. Acad. Sci. USA* 73: 2113–2117, **1976**.

Resnick, R.H., Stone, K., and Antonioli, D. Primary hepatocellular carcinoma following non-A, non-B posttransfusion hepatitis. *Dig. Dis. Sci.* 28: 908–911, **1983**.

Rous, P. A sarcoma of the fowl transmissible by agent separable from tumor cells. *J. Exp. Med.* 13: 397–411, **1911**.

Rous, P. and Beard, J.W. Carcinomatous changes in virus-induced papillomas of the skin of the rabbit. *Proc. Soc. Exp. Biol. Med.* 32: 578–580, **1934**.

Rous, P. and Kidd, J. G. The carcinogenic effect of a papillomavirus on the tarred skin of rabbits. I. Description of the phenomenon. *J. Exp. Med.* 67: 399–422, **1938**.

Rous, P. and Friedewald, W.F. The effect of chemical carcinogens on virus-induced rabbit papillomas. *J. Exp. Med.* 79: 511–537, **1944**.

Sambrook, J., Westphal, H., Srinivasan, P.R., and Dulbecco, R. The integrated state of viral DNA in SV40-transformed cells. *Proc. Natl. Acad. Sci. USA* 60: 1288–1295, **1968**.

Sanarelli, G. Das myxomatogene Virus: Beitrag zum Studium der Krankheitserreger ausserhalb des Sichtbaren. *Centralbl. f. Bakt. Abt. I,* 23: 865–873, **1898**.

Sankalé, M., Seck, I., Linhard, J., Thaim, A.-A., Wane, A.-B., Diebolt, G., and Poll-Gouater, A. L'antigène Australie au cours de la cirrhose et du cancer primitive du foie chez l'Africain de Dakar. *Bull. Soc. Med. Afr. Noire Lang. Fr.*16: 167–171, **1971**.

Schlom, J., Michalides, R., Colcher, D., Feldman, S., and Spiegelman, S. Evidence for an RNA tumor virus in human milk. *Bibl. Haematol.* 40: 471–482, **1975**.

Shope, R.E. A filtrable virus causing tumor-like condition in rabbits and its relationship to virus myxomatosum. *J. Exp. Med.* 56: 803–822, **1932**.

Shope, R.E. Infectious papillomatosis of rabbits. *J. Exp. Med.* 58: 607–624, **1933**.

Shope, T., Dechairo, D., and Miller, G. Malignant lymphoma in cottontop marmosets after inoculation with Epstein–Barr virus. *Proc. Natl. Acad. Sci. USA* 70: 2487–2491, **1973**.

Simonetti, R.G., Cottone, M., Craxi, A., Pagliaro, L., Rapicetta, M., Chionne, P., and Constantino, A. Prevalence of antibodies to hepatitis C virus in hepatocellular carcinoma. *Lancet* 2: 1338, **1989**.

Spiegelman, S. Evidence for viruses in human neoplasias. *Haematologia* 60: 339–372, **1975**.

Stehelin, D., Varmus, H.ED., Bishop, J.M. and Vogt, P.K. DNA related to the transforming gene(s) of avian sarcoma viruses is present in normal avian DNA. *Nature* 260: 170–173, **1976**.

Stewart, S. E., Eddy, B.E., Gochenour, A.M., Borgese, M.G., and Grubbs, G.E. The induction of neoplasms with a substance released from mouse tumors by tissue culture. *Virology* 3: 380–400, **1957**.

Stolt, C.-M., Klein, G., and Jansson, A.T.R. An analysis of the wrong Nobel Prize – Johannes Fibiger, 1926: a study in the Nobel Archives. *Adv. Cancer Res.* pp. 1–12, **2004**.

Sweet, B.H. and Hilleman, M.R. The vacuolating virus, SV 40. *Proc. Soc. Exp. Biol. Med.* 105: 420–427, **1960**.

Syverton, J.T. and Berry, G.P. Carcinoma in the cottontail rabbit following spontaneous virus papilloma (Shope). *Proc. Soc. Exp. Biol. Med.* 33: 399–400, **1935**.

Szmuness, W. Hepatocellular carcinoma and the hepatitis B virus: evidence for a causal association. *Prog. Med. Virol.* 24: 40–69, **1978**.

Teich, N.M., Weiss, R.A., Salahuddin, S. Z., Gallagher, R.E. Gillespie, D.H., and Gallo, R.C. Infective transmission and characterisation of a C-type virus released by cultured human myeloid leukaemia cells. *Nature* 256: 551–555, **1975**.

Temin, H.M. Nature of provirus of Rous sarcoma. *Nat. Cancer Inst. Monograph 17, Avian Tumor Viruses,* pp. 557–570, **1964**.

Temin, H.M. and Mizutani, S. RNA-dependent DNA polymerase in virions of Rous sarcoma virus. *Nature* 226: 1211–1213, **1970**.

Teres, J., Guardia, J., Bruguera, M., and Rodes, J. Hepatitis-associated antigen and hepatocellular carcinoma. *Lancet* 2: 215, **1971**.

Thomas, M., Levy, J.-P., Tanzer, J., Boiron, M., and Bernard, J. Transformation in vitro de cellules de peau de veau embryonnaire sous l'action d'extraits acellulaires de papillomes bovins. *C. R. Hebd. Seances Acad. Sci.* 257: 2155–2158, **1963**.

Trentin, J.J., Yabe, Y., and Taylor, G. The quest for human cancer viruses. *Science* 137: 835–841, **1962**.

Trichopoulos, D., Violaki, M., Sparros, L., and Xirouchaki, E. Epidemiology of hepatitis B and primary hepatic carcinoma. *Lancet* 2: 1038–1039, **1975**.

Vogel, C.L., Anthony, P.P., Mody, N., and Barker, L.F. Hepatitis-associated antigen in Ugandan patients with hepatocellular carcinoma. *Lancet* 2: 621–624, **1970**.

Witter R.L., Burgoyne, G.H., and Solomon, J.J. Evidence for a herpesvirus as an etiologic agent of Marek's disease. *Avian Dis.* 13: 171–185, **1969**.

Wolf, H., zur Hausen, H., and Becker, V. EB-viral genomes in epithelial nasopharyngeal carcinoma cells. *Nature New Biol.* 244: 245–247, **1973**.

Wong-Staal, F., Gillespie, D., and Gallo, R.C. Proviral sequences of baboon endogenous type C RNA virus in DNA of human leukaemic tissues. *Nature* 262: 190–195, **1976**.

Wotherspoon, A.C., Doglioni, C., Diss, T.C., Pan, L., Moschini, A., de Boni, M., and Isaacson, P.G. Regression of primary low-grade B-cell gastric lymphoma of mucosa-associated lymphoid tissue type after eradication of *Helicobacter pylori*. *Lancet* 342: 575–577, **1993**.

zur Hausen, H. Condylomata acuminata and human genital cancer. *Cancer Res.* 36: 794, **1976**.

zur Hausen, H. Human papilloma viruses and their possible role in squamous cell carcinomas. *Curr. Top. Microbiol. Immunol.* 78: 1–30, **1977**.

zur Hausen, H. and Schulte-Holthausen, H. Presence of EB virus nucleic acid homology in a "virus-free" line of Burkitt tumour cells. *Nature* 227: 245–247, **1970**.

zur Hausen, H., Schulte-Holthausen H., Klein, G., Henle, W., Henle, G., Clifford, P., and Santesson, L. EBV DNA in biopsies of Burkitt tumours and anaplastic carcinomas of the nasopharynx. *Nature* 228: 1056–1058, **1970**.

zur Hausen, H., Meinhof, W., Scheiber, W., and Bornkamm, G.W. Attempts to detect virus-specific DNA sequences in human tumors: I. Nucleic acid hybridizations with complementary RNA of human wart virus. *Int. J. Cancer* 13: 650–656, **1974**.

zur Hausen, H., Gissmann, L., Steiner, W. Dippold, W., and Dregger, J. Human papilloma viruses and cancer. *Bibl. Haematol.*, Clemensen, J. and Yohn, D.S. (Eds.) 43: 569–571, **1975**.

2
The Quest for Causality

Whenever human cancers are analyzed for the presence of viruses, depending upon on the method used for detection, a number of different agents may be identified. The sensitivity of the polymerase chain reaction (PCR) in particular permits the discovery even of very small concentrations of DNA or RNA of infectious agents. In the majority of cancers caused by viral infections the viral DNA is present in very small copy numbers, usually less than one DNA copy per 10 tumor cells. For instance, it is possible to detect human cytomegalovirus (CMV), human herpesvirus (HHV) type 6 (HHV 6), Epstein–Barr virus (EBV) and even herpes simplex virus type 1 (HSV-1) DNA in a broad spectrum of different tumors, and even more so a larger number of TT virus genotypes (de Villiers et al., 2002). Similarly, several reports have claimed the presence of polyomavirus types, BK, JC and SV40 virus in human cancer biopsies (for a review, see Gazdar et al., 2002). However, it is unclear whether these agents are causally involved in the development of those cancers.

In several types of human cancer, including nasopharyngeal carcinoma, cancer of the cervix, specific B-cell lymphomas and Kaposi's sarcoma, the discovery of virus-specific DNA was taken as a first clear-cut hint for a viral etiology. In almost all of these systems every individual tumor cell frequently contained multiple copies of viral DNA. In addition, this viral DNA was present in a clonal form, implying its presence at early onset of malignant proliferation. Although in all these systems additional data later on confirmed a close link of these infections to the malignant outcome, it remains unclear as to whether the presence of low copy numbers (e.g., < 1 in 10 tumor cells) excludes causality.

Evidently, there is a need to define causality here against a background of multiple genetic changes, apparently underlying the vast majority of human cancers, and the stepwise progression to malignant proliferation commonly over a period of several decades. During the last decades of the nineteenth century, Robert Koch developed his postulates based on straightforward observations in bacterial infections: he established methods to cultivate bacteria on semisolid media, to purify them from other, contaminating microorganisms, and to use the purified types to induce specific clinical symptoms in laboratory animals. Koch was able to re-cultivate the agent from the sick animal and to re-induce the disease in further experimentation (Koch, 1881). His beautiful documentation of the causal role of specific bacteria in causing *anthrax*, *diphtheria*, *cholera* and *tuberculosis*, respectively, underlined the validity of his postulates. For decades, these served as baseline to link infectious agents to human and animal diseases. The question remains, however, as to whether they are applicable to establish a causal role of infectious agents in human cancers.

Clearly, the answer to this question is "no". One major problem is the long latency period between the primary infection and the eventual emergence of cancer, frequently covering periods of several decades. In addition, most of these agents are widely spread among the human population, yet, only a fraction of infected individuals develops cancer – a fact which suggests the presence of additional events affecting the infected cell prior to malignant conversion. Tumorviruses frequently integrate their DNA into the host cell genome. The viral genome is commonly modified in the process of integration, often revealing deletions or mutations. Thus, no infectious progeny can be produced, even if the viral DNA were to be excised from the host cell genome. The detection of persisting viral DNA usually relies on hybridization procedures or PCR technology. An isolation of the infectious agent in the sense of Koch's postulates is regularly impossible. In some of these infections, however, viral DNA can be recovered that, upon transfection into suitable host cells or laboratory animals, induces cell transformation or tumors, respectively. To some extent this fulfills the criteria raised by Robert Koch.

Nonetheless, the major difficulty arises from the fact that different tumor-inducing infectious agents perform this function using different mechanisms. Increasing evidence exists that several infections that result eventually in cancer development act indirectly and do not require the persistence of the microbial genome. In all likelihood, this is the case for *Helicobacter pylori* infections which lead, after a long time of persistence, to gastric cancer or to gastric lymphoma. The same is true for parasitic infections such as schistosomiasis or liver flukes. Human immunodeficiency viruses (HIV) provoke a severe immunodeficiency with a drastically enhanced risk for B-cell lymphomas or Kaposi's sarcoma. Herpesvirus infections may lead to an amplification of persisting other DNA viral genomes (polyoma-type and papillomaviruses), and thus contribute indirectly to an enhanced gene expression of the latter. As yet, it remains unclear as to whether hepatitis B or C genome persistence and gene expression is necessary for liver cancer proliferation. Finally, an increasing number of virus infections are being discovered that prevent apoptosis in persistently infected cells, enabling these cells to continue proliferation even under conditions of extensive genome damage.

Evans and Mueller summarized their view in establishing causality neatly in 1990, by concentrating specifically on oncogenic viruses, as follows:

- The long incubation or induction period between initial infection with the putative virus and the cancer(s) with which it is associated.
- The common and ubiquitous nature of most candidate viruses and the rarity of the cancer with which they are associated.
- The initial infection with the candidate virus is often subclinical, so that the time of infection can not be established by clinical features.

- The need for co-factors in most virus-related cancers.
- The causes of cancer may vary in different geographic areas or by age.
- Different virus strains may have different oncogenic potential.
- The human host plays a critical role in susceptibility to cancer, especially the age at the time of infection, the genetic characteristics, and the status of the immune system.
- Cancers result from a complex and multistage process, in which a virus may play a role at different points in pathogenesis in association with alterations in the host's immune system, oncogenes, chromosomal translocations, and a variety of events at the molecular level.
- The inability to reproduce many human cancers in experimental animals with the putative virus.
- The recognition that a virus, toxin, chemical, altered gene, or other causal factor may all be capable of initiating or promoting the processes that result in a cancer with the same histological features.

These considerations clearly demonstrate the difficulties in establishing uniform criteria to define causality in cancer induction by infections. A number of attempts have been made to solve this dilemma. Bradford Hill, for example (1965), attempted to develop criteria to define environmental causes of disease, based on strength of association, consistency, specificity, temporality, biological gradient, plausibility, coherence, experimental evidence, and analogy. As stressed by Vonka (2000), Hill was convinced that none of his "nine viewpoints" would "...bring indisputable evidence for or against the cause and effect hypothesis and none can be required as a *sine qua non*". In 1990, Evans and Mueller based their criteria for an etiological relationship between virus infection and tumor development more on immunological aspects, in part influenced by a previous publication by Rivers (1937). They subdivided their "...guidelines for relating a putative virus to human cancers" into an epidemiological and virological part. For epidemiological evidence, they summarized four points:

- The geographic distribution of infection with the virus should be similar to that of the tumor with which it is associated when adjusted for the age of infection and the presence of co-factors known to be important in tumor development.
- The presence of the viral marker (high antibody titers or antigenemia) should be higher in cases than in matched controls in the same geographic setting, as shown in case-control studies.
- The viral marker should precede the tumor, and a significantly higher incidence of the tumor should follow in persons with the marker than in those without it.
- Prevention of infection with the virus (vaccination) or control of the host's response to it (such as delaying the time of infection) should decrease the incidence of the tumor.

The following three requirements should be provided on the virological side:
- The virus should be able to transform human cells *in vitro* into malignant ones.
- The viral genome or DNA should be demonstrated in tumor cells and not in normal cells.
- The virus should be able to induce the tumor in a susceptible experimental animal and neutralization of the virus prior to injection should prevent development of the tumor.

The considerations by Evans and Mueller were also influenced by a relatively large set of seroepidemiological data obtained up to that period on a role of EBV in human tumors (see Chapter 5, Section 5.11). As it turned out, however, elevated antibody titers against EBV antigens are not limited to EBV-linked cancer patients, but are also found under conditions of T-cell immunosuppression.

Interestingly, successful vaccination against the incriminated agent to prevent the respective tumors – an argument that should strongly support causality – seems not to have been considered before 1990 in various publications. Yet, although prevention of cancer development after vaccination with the suspected agent or its eradication seems to argue strongly for causality, on a second glance it is also highly questionable. For example, holoendemic malaria seems to be a contributing factor to the development of Burkitt's lymphoma in equatorial Africa (Kafuko et al., 1969; Kafuko and Burkitt, 1970). It is possible that malaria eradication in endemic areas for Burkitt's lymphoma will drastically reduce the rate of these cancers. However, it will only prove that malaria is indeed an important contributing factor for this malignancy – the "causation" seems to rely on other infections. The same accounts for the role of HIV infections in B-cell lymphomas and Kaposi's sarcoma. It is likely that successful vaccination or antiviral treatment of HIV infections will result in a drastic reduction of Kaposi's sarcoma and immunoblastoma. Although HIV is a contributing factor, it is not the cause of those sarcomas. It is known today that prolonged immunosuppression paves the way for a tumorigenic function of another herpesvirus infection, HHV type 8 (HHV-8), which seems to be the primary cause of Kaposi's sarcoma or EBV, which causes immunoblastomas.

Clearly, this is an extremely complex issue. Present knowledge of basic mechanisms of viral oncogenesis may, however, provide some encouragement to attempt a new definition. In order to escape from the previously described difficulties, there is a need to develop different criteria for those agents which induce cancer by direct interaction, which require persistence and possibly continued expression of the respective genome, and for those which contribute indirectly to tumorigenesis.

2.1
Infectious Agents as Direct Carcinogens

Infectious direct carcinogens are most readily defined among small DNA-containing viruses. In particular, the transformation of human cells by papilloma- and polyoma-type viruses is regularly accompanied by persistence of the whole genome or specific parts of it, by transcriptional activity of derived viral gene products, and by the expression of specific viral "early" proteins (viral oncoproteins). The use of temperature-sensitive mutants in the case of polyoma-type viruses (Butel et al., 1975; Brugge and Butel, 1975) showed that the transformed phenotype depends on the functioning of viral T-antigens. The results of these experiments reveal that the function of viral oncogenes is necessary for maintaining the transformed state of the respective cells. In the case of cervical carcinoma cells, harboring high risk papillomavirus DNA, the malignant phenotype can be reversed by blocking the expression or function of viral E6 and E7 genes (Storey et al., 1991; von Knebel Doeberitz et al., 1992, 1994; Shillitoe and Steele, 1992; Tan and Ting, 1995). Cervical cancer represents the first case where molecular techniques directly prove a necessary role of viral proteins for the maintenance of the malignant phenotype. However, *necessary* does not mean *sufficient* and, as discussed later, viral oncogene expression is not sufficient for cell transformation, as additional modifications of the host cell genome are required in order to develop invasive growth properties. Yet, the expression of viral oncogenes is clearly an essential and determining factor for continued cell proliferation. The availability of epidemiological studies demonstrating that the incriminated virus infection represents a significant risk factor for the respective cancer type strongly underlines causality further.

Based on these considerations, it is not too difficult to define criteria for a causal role in direct carcinogenesis by infectious agents (zur Hausen, 1991):

- the regular presence of the genome or parts of it of the infectious agent in every cancer cell;
- transfection of this nucleic acid into tissue culture cells or suitable laboratory animals should result in cell immortalization or tumor induction, respectively;
- excision of this nucleic acid from transfected cells or inhibition of its function should lead to a reversion of the immortalized or malignant phenotype of cells carrying the respective genome or parts of it;
- epidemiological case/control and prospective studies should identify the agent as a major risk factor for the respective tumor type.

The prevention of such cancers by specific immunization against this agent here would, of course, further underline causality.

If an attempt is made to identify agents which fit this definition, then three groups of viral infections can be labeled as direct carcinogens:

- Viruses expressing specific oncogenes which are necessary for the transformed phenotype (examples are "high-risk" human papillomaviruses, Epstein-Barr virus, human herpesvirus type 8, and human T-lymphotropic retrovirus).
- Viruses with acquired cellular oncogenes ("acute" transforming retroviruses, e.g., Rous sarcoma virus and others).

- Viruses which, when inserted into specific cellular chromosomal sites, activate cellular oncogenes and mediate transformation of the infected cells (e.g., mouse mammary tumor virus).

At this stage only members of the first group have been identified as carcinogens for humans, though clearly only one part of the spectrum of infectious agents engaged in carcinogenesis is covered by this definition. A leukemia of cattle caused in Mediterranean and East African countries by protozoon infections with *Theileria parva* and *Theileria annulata*, requires a special consideration. Here, the production of an epidermal growth factor-like protein by the parasite seems to be sufficient for induction of the disease. Successful treatment of the parasite also cures the leukemia. The mechanism by which these parasites cause leukemia still fits into the definition of direct carcinogenesis. The continuous presence of the protozoon is required for maintaining the malignant phenotype. However, different criteria must be developed to characterize other infectious carcinogens.

2.2
Infectious Agents as Indirect Carcinogens

At present, several possible mechanisms can be defined by which infectious agents may contribute to the development of specific carcinomas or lymphomas in humans. The most obvious one is the induction of immunosuppression. The pronounced immunosuppression caused by HIV infections in a number of patients results in the development of tumors that are commonly rejected in immunocompetent individuals due to their T-cell antigenicity. These tumors are mainly caused by persistent EBV infections (B-cell lymphoblastomas) and by infections with HHV-8. Whereas EBV and HHV-8 act as direct carcinogens under conditions of immunosuppression, HIV contributes indirectly to carcinogenesis, via immunosuppression. Successful treatment or prevention of the HIV infection would also prevent at least the vast majority of these EBV- or HHV-8-induced malignant proliferations, in spite of the fact that the latter are the direct cause and essential factors for the respective carcinogenesis.

Another example for indirect carcinogenesis is the prevention of apoptosis by cutaneous papillomavirus infections, as well as by a number of other viruses (see Chapter 5). Cells which are persistently infected with these viruses and acquire genetic damage due to physical or chemical factors may survive under conditions which otherwise would result in apoptotic cell death. The accumulation of mutational events within these cells may occasionally result in a loss of growth control and eventually lead to cancer development. Squamous cell carcinomas of the skin are suspected to be caused by this mechanism (Jackson et al., 2000, 2002).

There exist several other (most likely indirect) modes by which infectious agents may contribute to carcinogenesis: parasites and bacteria induce cancer by relatively poorly defined mechanisms. Chronic inflammation, increased development of oxygen radicals, the production of carcinogenic metabolites, as well as growth-stimulating factors excreted by these parasites are suspected as being the prime drivers for the eventual development of cancer in the infected tissues (see Chapters 10 and 11). At this stage, persistence of the inducing agents is no longer required.

A number of additional modes for indirect carcinogenesis by infectious agents can be envisaged, among which the induction of amplification of persisting polyoma- or papillomavirus genomes by herpesvirus infection (Schlehofer et al., 1983; Schmitt et al., 1989) deserves attention. At present, the evidence for this is based only on laboratory observations, while the clinical significance remains undetermined. Mutations and chromosomal rearrangements of host cell DNA induced by various viruses (e.g., vaccinia, adenoviruses, herpesviruses), even under conditions of abortive infections, could occasionally contribute to the development of cancer. In addition, there exists the possibility that some persisting virus infections may introduce long-lasting chromosomal instability into the infected cells that may again, in rare instances, result in invasive growth properties of the affected cell.

Thus, carcinogenesis mediated by infectious agents by an indirect mode is clearly complex. It is extremely difficult to define clear-cut criteria for identifying and characterizing these agents, though in somewhat vague terms the following criteria may act as a baseline:
- clinical observations, experimental and animal studies should point to a role of the respective agents as co-carcinogenic factors;
- epidemiological studies should identify these infections as risk factors for cancer development;
- vaccination against or successful treatment of the respective infection should provide significant protection against cancers suspected to be co-induced by these infections.

Thus, while there remains a very soft definition of indirect carcinogenesis by infectious agents, it seems nonetheless useful to some extent. The previously used term of "hit and run" mechanisms characterizes the existing situation very poorly: neither under conditions of immunosuppression by HIV, nor in cases of chronic bacterial or parasitic infections is cancer development necessarily accompanied by any loss of the contributing agent. Hence, the term "indirect carcinogen" appears to describe the existing situation more appropriately.

2.2.1
Induction of Chromosomal Aberrations

The induction of chromosomal aberrations may represent a specific indirect effect by which infectious agents could contribute to human cancers. Alterations of human chromosomes by virus infections have been noted for DNA and RNA viruses, among them adenovirus, HSV, varicella virus, EBV, human CMV, and polyomaviruses (for reviews, see Nichols, 1970; Stich and Yohn, 1970; Harnden, 1974; Fortunato and Spector, 2003). Most of the observed changes represent random modifications such as chromatid breaks, translocations, chromosome pulverization, coiling deficiencies and persistent overcondensation, though specific chromosomal abnormalities have been noted for three viruses (Table 2.1).

Table 2.1 Viruses inducing specific modifications of human chromosomes.

Virus	Type of change	Localization of modification	Reference(s)
Adenovirus type 12	chromatid break	1p36 1q21 1q42–43 17q21–22	zur Hausen (1967) McDougall (1971)
Herpes simplex virus	chromatid break	1p32 1q32 3p21	Mincheva et al. (1984)
	uncoiling of pericentric regions	1 9 16	Peat and Stanley (1986)
Humanic cytome-galovirus	chromatid break	1q21 1q42	Fortunato et al. (2000)

The first report on specific chromosomal changes induced by a virus infection was made in 1967 (zur Hausen, 1967). Subsequently, specific changes were also reported for HSV infections (Mincheva et al., 1984) and human CMV (Fortunato et al., 2000). The localization of these changes is shown in Table 2.1.

It is striking that adenovirus type 12 and human CMV appear to affect the same region at two loci on chromosome 1. The region of 1q42 harbors a putative tumor suppressor gene (Li et al., 1995), the *ADPRT* gene involved in DNA repair and replication (Baumgartner et al., 1992), and the 5S rRNA locus (Sorensen et al., 1991). The region 1q21 again contains among others a putative tumor suppressor gene (Bieche et al., 1995) and a family of snRNA pseudogenes, apparently not transcribed as stable RNA (Lindgren et al., 1985 a, 1985 b; Lund, 1988). The two additional sites of adenovirus type 12-induced changes seem to code for small structural RNAs and consist of tandemly arranged sequences (Durnam et al., 1988; Lund, 1988). The adenovirus E1B 55 000 protein which blocks p53-dependent and p53-independent apoptosis emerges as the necessary protein to induce specific changes on chromosomes 17q21–22 and 1p36 (Schramayr et al., 1990). In HSV infections the *ICP4* gene seems to be required for induction of the chromosomal modifications (Chenet-Monte et al., 1986; Johnson et al., 1992). According to Fortunato et al. (2000), CMV-induced chromosomal changes do not require cellular DNA synthesis.

It is presently unproven whether the described chromosomal aberrations play a role in human oncogenesis. Adenovirus type 12 is a potent carcinogen when inoculated into newborn hamsters and mice. The induction of chromosomal changes may contribute to viral carcinogenesis by mutating host cell genes that may interfere with viral oncogene expression or function.

No convincing evidence exists for a role of HSV and for human CMV in the etiology of specific human cancers. These viruses, however, have been reported to transform rodent cells; indeed, CMV has even been claimed to immortalize specific human cells (see Chapter 4, Sections 4.1.1 and 4.2.1, respectively). The modification of host cell chromosomes may be important, especially in rodent cell transformation.

References

Baumgartner, M., Schneider, R., Auer, B., Herzog, H., Schweiger, M., and Hirsch-Kauffmann, M. Fluorescence *in situ* mapping of the human nuclear NAD+ ADP-ribosyltransferase gene (ADPRT) and two secondary sites to human chromosomal bands 1q42, 13q34, and 14q24. *Cytogenet. Cell. Genet.* 61: 172–174, **1992**.

Bieche, I., Champeme, M.H., and Lidereau, R. Loss and gain of distinct regions of chromosome 1 q in primary breast cancer. *Clin. Cancer Res.* 1: 123–127, **1995**.

Brugge, J.S. and Butel, J.S. Role of simian virus 40 gene A function in maintenance of transformation. *J. Virol.* 15: 619–635, **1975**.

Butel, J.S., Brugge, J.S. and Noonan, C.A. Transformation of primate and rodent cells by temperature-sensitive mutants of SV40. *Cold Spring Harbor Symp. Quant. Biol.* 39 Pt 1: 25–36, **1975**.

Chenet-Monte, C., Mohammad, F., Celluzi, C.M., Schaffer, P.A., and Farber, F.E. Herpes simplex virus gene products involved in the induction of chromosomal aberrations. *Virus Res.* 6: 245–260, **1986**.

de Villiers, E.-M., Schmidt, R., Delius, H., and zur Hausen, H. Heterogeneity of TT virus-related sequences isolated from human tumour biopsies. *J. Mol. Med.* 80: 44–50, **2002**.

Durnam, D.M., Menninger, J.C., Chandler, S. H., Smith, P.P. and McDougall, J.K. A fragile site in the human U2 small nuclear RNA gene cluster is revealed by adenovirus type 12 infection. *Mol. Cell. Biol.* 8: 1863–1867, **1988**.

Evans, A.S. and Mueller, N.E. Viruses and cancer. Causal associations. *Ann. Epidemiol.* 1: 71–92, **1990**.

Fortunato, E.A. and Spector, D.H. Viral induction of site-specific chromosome damage. *Rev. Med. Virol.* 13: 21–37, **2003**.

Fortunato, E.A., Dell'Aquila, M.L., and Spector, D.H. Specific chromosome 1 breaks induced by human cytomegalovirus. *Proc. Natl. Acad. Sci. USA* 97: 853–858, **2000**.

Gazdar, A.F., Butel, J.S., and Carbone, M. SV40 and human tumours: myth, association or causality? *Nature Rev. Cancer* 2: 957–964, **2002**.

Harnden, D.G. Viruses, chromosomes and tumors: the interaction between viruses and chromosomes. In: German, J. (Ed.), *Chromosomes and Cancer*, John Wiley & Sons, New York, pp. 151–191, **1974**.

Hill, A.B. The environment and disease: association or causation? *Proc. R. Soc. Med.* 58: 295–300, **1965**.

Jackson, S., Harwood, C., Thomas, M., Banks, L., and Storey, A. Role of Bak in UV-induced apoptosis in skin cancer and abrogation by HPV E6 proteins. *Genes Dev.* 14:, 3065–3073, **2000**.

Jackson, S., Ghali, L., Harwood, C., and Storey, A. Reduced apoptotic levels in squamous but not basal cell carcinomas correlates with detection of cutaneous human papillomavirus. *Br. J. Cancer* 87: 319–323, **2002**.

Johnson, P.A., Miyanohara, A., Levine, F., Cahill, T., and Friedmann, T. Cytotoxicity of a replication-defective mutant of herpes simplex virus type 1. *J. Virol.* 66: 2952–2965, **1992**.

Kafuko, G.W. and Burkitt, D. Burkitt's lymphoma and malaria. *Int. J. Cancer* 6: 1–9, **1970**.

Kafuko, G.W., Baingana, N., Knight, E.M., and Tibemanya, J. Association of Burkitt's tumour and holoendemic malaria in West Nile District, Uganda: malaria as a possible aetiologic factor. *East Afr. Med. J.* 46: 414–436, **1969**.

Koch, R. Zur Untersuchung von pathogenen Organismen. *Mitt. Kaiserl. Gesundheitsamt Berlin* 1: 1–48, **1881**.

Li, Y.S., Ramsay, D.A., Fan, Y.S., Armstrong, R.F., and Del Maestro, R.F.D. Cytogenetic evidence that a tumor suppressor gene in the long arm of chromosome 1 contributes to glioma growth. *Cancer Genet. Cytogenet.* 84: 46–50, **1995**.

Lindgren, V., Ares, M., Weiner, A.M., and Francke, U. Human genes for U2 small nuclear RNA map to a major adenovirus 12 modification site on chromosome 17. *Nature* 314: 115–116, **1985**a.

Lindgren, V., Bernstein, L.B., Weiner, A.M., and Francke, U. Human U1 small nuclear RNA pseudogenes do not map to the site of the U1 genes in 1p36 but are clustered in 1q12-q22. *Mol. Cell. Biol.* 5: 2172–2180, **1985**b.

Lund, E. Heterogeneity of human U1 snRNAs. *Nucleic Acids Res.* 16: 5813–5826, **1988**.

McDougall, J.K. Adenovirus-induced chromosome aberrations in human cells. *J. Gen. Virol.* 12: 43–51, **1971**.

Mincheva, A., Dundarov, S., and Bradvarova, I. Effect of herpes simplex virus strains on human fibroblast and lymphocyte chromosomes and the localization of chromosomal aberrations. *Acta Virol.* 28: 97–106, **1984**.

Nichols, W.W. Virus-induced chromosome abnormalities. *Annu. Rev. Microbiol.* 24: 479–500, **1970**.

Peat, D.S. and Stanley, M.A. Chromosome damage induced by herpes simplex virus type 1 in early infection. *J. Gen. Virol.* 67: 2273–2277, **1986**.

Rivers, T.M. Viruses and Koch's postulates. *J. Bacteriol.* 33: 1–12, **1937**.

Schlehofer, J.R., Gissmann, L., Matz, B., and zur Hausen, H. Herpes simplex virus induced amplification of SV40 sequences in transformed Chinese hamster embryo cells. *Int. J. Cancer* 32: 99–103, **1983**

Schmitt, J., Schlehofer, J.R., Mergener, K., Gissmann, L., and zur Hausen, H. Amplification of bovine papillomavirus DNA by N-methyl-N'-nitro-N-nitrosoguanidine, ultraviolet-irradiation, or infection with herpes simplex virus. *Virology* 172: 73–81, **1989**.

Schramayr, S. , Caporossi, D., Mak, I., Jelinek, T., and Bacchetti, S. Chromosomal damage induced by human adenovirus type 12 requires expression of the E1B 55-kilodalton viral protein. *J. Virol.* 64: 2090–2095, **1990** .

Shillitoe, E.J. and Steele, C. Inhibition of the transformed phenotype of carcinoma cells that contain human papillomavirus. *Ann. N.Y. Acad. Sci.* 660: 286–287, **1992**.

Sorensen, P.D., Lomholt, B., Frederiksen, S., and Tommerup, N. Fine mapping of human 5S rRNA genes to chromosome 1q42.11–1q42.13. *Cytogenet. Cell. Genet.* 57: 26–29, **1991**.

Stich, H.F., and Yohn, D.S. Viruses and chromosomes. *Progr. Med. Virol.* 12: 78–127, **1970**.

Storey, A., Oates, D., Banks, L., Crawford, L., and Crook, T. Anti-sense phosphorothioate oligonucleotides have both specific and non-specific effects on cells containing human papillomavirus type 16. *Nucleic Acids Res.* 19: 4109–4114, **1991**.

Tan, T.M. and Ting, R.C. In vitro and in vivo inhibition of human papillomavirus type 16 E6 and E7 genes. *Cancer Res.* 55: 4599–4605, **1995**.

Vonka, V. Causality in medicine: the case of tumours and viruses. *Philos. Trans. R. Soc. Lond. B. Biol. Sci.* 355: 1831–1841, **2000**.

von Knebel Doeberitz, M., Rittmüller, C., zur Hausen, H. and Dürst, M. Inhibition of tumorigenicity of cervical cancer cells in nude mice by HPV E6-E7 anti-sense RNA. *Int. J. Cancer* 51: 831–834, **1992**.

von Knebel Doeberitz, M., Rittmüller, C., Aengeneyndt, F., Jansen-Dürr, P., and Spitkovsky, D. Reversible repression of papillomavirus oncogene expression in cervical carcinoma cells: consequences for the phenotype and E6-p53 and E7-pRB interactions. *J. Virol.* 68: 2811–2821, **1994**.

zur Hausen, H. Induction of specific chromosomal aberrations by adenovirus type 12 in human embryonic kidney cells. *J. Virol.* 1: 1174–1185, **1967**.

zur Hausen, H. Papillomavirus host cell interactions in the pathogenesis of anogenital cancers. In: Brugge, J., Curran, T., Harlow, E., and McCormick, F. (Eds.), *Origins of Cancer: A Comprehensive Review*. Cold Spring Harbor Laboratory Press, pp. 685–705, **1991**.

3
Tumors Linked to Infections: Some General Aspects

3.1
Tumor Types Linked to Infections

The spectrum of tumors linked to infectious events reveals a remarkable diversity. Leukemias and lymphomas were the original prime suspects and, indeed, the relationship of Epstein–Barr virus (EBV) to Burkitt's lymphoma and to immunoblastic lymphomas, and the role of human T-lymphotropic retrovirus to adult T-cell leukemia seemed to confirm the preferential role of infectious events in the etiology of proliferative diseases of the hematopoietic system. Yet, almost simultaneously two important epithelial cancers emerged as being caused by infections, namely hepatocellular carcinoma and cancer of the cervix. The subsequent discovery of a relationship between gastric cancer and *Helicobacter pylori* and, to a more limited degree also with EBV, linked another important epithelial tumor system to infectious causes. The tumor types presently linked to, or associated, with infections are listed in Table 3.1.

Table 3.1 Tumor types presently linked to infections

Tumor type	Infectious cause
B-cell lymphomas in immunocompromised patients (ca. 50%) and in a subset of T-cell lymphomas	EBV
Burkitt's lymphomas	
Nasopharyngeal cancer	
Hodgkin's disease (30–40%)	
Gastric cancer (~10%)	
Cancer of the cervix, anal and perianal cancers	various HPV types
Vulvar, penile and vaginal cancers	
Oropharyngeal cancers (ca. 25%)	
Specific squamous cell carcinomas of the skin	
Hepatocellular carcinomas	HBV and HCV

Infections Causing Human Cancer. Harald zur Hausen
Copyright © 2006 WILEY-VCH Verlag GmbH & Co. KGaA, Weinheim
ISBN: 3-527-31056-8

Table 3.1 (Continued)

Tumor type	Infectious cause
Adult T-cell leukemia (ATL)	HTLV-1
Seminomas?	Endogenous human retroviruses
Kaposi's sarcoma	HHV-8
Gastric cancer, gastric lymphoma	**Helicobacter pylori**
Bladder cancer (Rectal cancer)	**Schistosoma haematobium, (japonicum, mansoni)**
Cholangiocarcinoma	**Opisthorchis viverrini and felineus, Clonorchis sinensis, (Helicobacter bilis?)**

There exist a number of other cancers (these will be discussed subsequently) which may have an infectious etiology. In particular, not only leukemias and lymphomas but also epithelial cancers linked to inflammatory events (e.g., cancer of the prostate) deserve attention. In addition, for seminomas a role of specific endogenous retroviruses has been postulated. The analysis of a potential role of these viruses for various human tumors remains to be intensified.

3.2
Global Contributions of Infections to Human Cancers

An estimation of the global contribution of infections to human cancers depends on the information received from regional cancer registries. A first estimation taking into account contributions of major viral infections linked to human cancers [EBV, human papillomaviruses (HPV), hepatitis B virus] was published in 1986 (zur Hausen). This was based on a previous publication of Parkin et al. (1984), according to whom approximately 15% of human cancers were linked to viral infections. The subsequent identification of the involvement of *H. pylori* in human gastric cancers resulted in an upgrading of this percentage (Parkin et al., 2002). In the calculation by Parkin and his colleagues, the participation of high-risk papillomavirus infections in oropharyngeal cancers was substantially underestimated. The majority of studies conducted came to the conclusion that approximately 25% of these cancers were linked to papillomavirus infections. In addition, Parkin's estimates did not include approximately 10% of gastric cancers which are presently linked to EBV infections. Thus, the estimates in Figures 3.1 and 3.2 are derived from the published data of Parkin et al., but contain some modifications.

By including cancers at all genital sites linked to HPV infections (ca. 90% of perianal and anal cancers, and ca. 50% of penile and vulvar cancers, vaginal cancers), adult T-cell leukemia, Kaposi's sarcoma and cancers caused by parasitic infections,

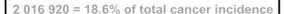

2 016 920 = 18.6% of total cancer incidence

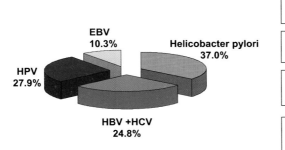

EBV
10.3%

Helicobacter pylori
37.0%

HPV
27.9%

HBV +HCV
24.8%

25% of cancers of the oral cavity
68 572 (HPV)

Cancer of the cervix
493 243 (HPV)

Hepatocellular carcinoma 80%
500 930 (HBV, HCV)

Gastric cancer 80%
747 150 (Helicobacter pylori)

Gastric cancer 10%
93 3937 (EBV)

Nasopharyngeal carcinoma
80 043 (EBV)

Non-Hodgkin's lymphoma 10%
30 057 (EBV)

Hodgkin's lymphoma 30%
18 694 (EBV)

This graph ignores
- anal and perianal cancers (HPV)
- vulvar, vaginal and penile cancers (HPV)
- adult T cell leukemia
- Kaposi's sarcomas and prim. effusion lymphomas
- cancers linked to parasitic infections

Fig. 3.1 Estimation of the annual contribution of Epstein–Barr virus, human papillomaviruses, hepatitis B and C viruses and *Helicobacter pylori* to global cancer incidence. (Modified from: Parkin et al., Global Cancer Statistics, 2002.)

slightly more than 20% of the global cancer incidence should presently be due to infectious events.

There exist remarkable differences between males and females in the incidence of cancers linked to infections: high-risk HPV infections are the main contributers to cancers in females, due to the high rate of cervical cancers worldwide (Fig. 3.2). In males, the role of this infection is relatively small, but *H. pylori* plays the main role in gastric cancer, which is still one of the most frequent cancers globally.

The geographic distribution of cancers linked to infections differs substantially between developed and developing parts of the world (Fig. 3.3).

In particular, sub-Saharan Africa is most severely affected by these types of cancer. Australia, North America and Central and Western Europe reveal the lowest percentages of infection-linked cancers.

Females: estimated annual global cancer incidence due to the 5 most frequent infections linked to cancer 1 006 544 = 19.9% of total cancer incidence in females	Males: estimated annual global cancer incidence due to the 5 most frequent infections linked to cancer 1 025 524 = 17.7% of total cancer incidence in males

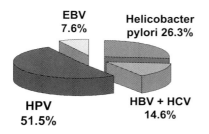

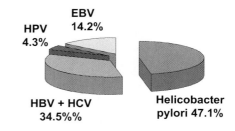

Fig. 3.2 Estimation of the annual contribution of Epstein–Barr virus, human papillomaviruses, hepatitis B and C viruses and *H. pylori* to global cancer incidence in females and males.

3.3
Host Interactions with Potentially Carcinogenic Infections: The CIF Concept

An early postulation of the loss of a cellular control of persisting tumorviruses resulted from: (i) the long latency periods elapsing between primary infection and subsequent tumor emergence; (ii) the observed synergism between physical and chemical mutagens and oncogenic viruses (reviewed by Casto and DiPaolo, 1973); (iii) the obvious stepwise progression to malignant growth; and (iv) the growing knowledge of monoclonal tumor development, even of those cancers associated with viral infections (zur Hausen, 1977). These observations formed the background for suspecting the existence of a cellular interference factor (CIF), the allelic deletion of which could explain most of the previously mentioned observations.

Subsequent developments clearly indicated that a single interference factor could not be responsible for a growing number of observations linked to persistent tumorvirus infections and for the protection against malignant proliferations of persistently infected cells (zur Hausen, 1994). This resulted in an extension of the hypothesis to a cellular interference factor cascade (CIF-cascade). Today, there exists ample evidence for the existence of at least three protective signaling cascades, providing custody to prevent malignant conversion of those virus-infected cells.

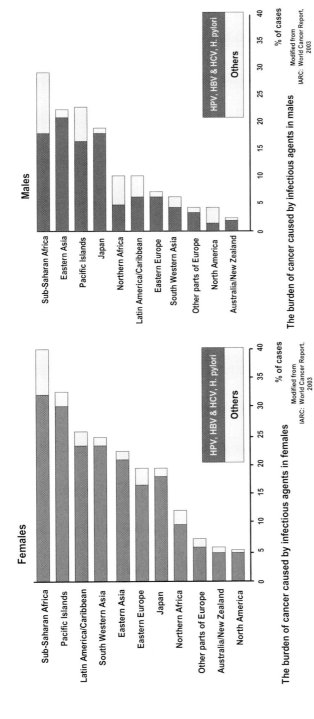

Fig. 3.3 Geographic differences in the annual incidence of cancers linked to infection in males and females. (Modified from World Cancer Report, Stewart, B.W. and Kleihues, P. (Eds.), Lyon, France: IARC Press, 2003.)

3.3.1
The CIF-I Cascade

Immunosuppression substantially increases the risk for malignant tumors linked to infectious events. This accounts in particular for EBV-associated lymphomas, human herpesvirus type 8-linked Kaposi's sarcomas and high-risk human papillomavirus (HPV)-caused intraepithelial neoplasias at cervical, anogenital and oral sites (see Chapters 4.3.1, 4.4.1 and 5.4, respectively). Clearly, in immunocompetent individuals malignant progression of persistently infected tissues is at least in part controlled and prevented by immune functions of the host. Most or all of the viruses mentioned here are able to suppress specific acquired or innate immune functions (in case of herpes group viruses, frequently the HLA class I and II presentation [Walev et al., 1992; Brander et al., 2000; Neumann et al., 2003; reviewed in Schust et al., 1999]. E5 functions of HPV down-regulate MHC class I molecules [Cartin and Alonso, 2003; Ashrafi et al., 2005]. Expression of HPV 16 E5 also perturbs MHC class II antigen maturation [Zhang et al., 2003], and hepatitis B and C viruses block interferon expression [Twu and Schloemer, 1989; Foster et al., 1991; Fernandez et al., 2003; Breiman et al., 2005; Zhang et al., 2005]). Although this suppression may facilitate long-term viral genome persistence, it is not sufficient to result in premalignant or malignant proliferations. Clearly, additional modifications must take place that enable the viral genome-carrying cells to continue growth.

In EBV infections at least three different events may interfere with immune functions and lead to malignant proliferations:

1. A general suppression of cell-mediated immune functions, as occurs in organ allograft recipients treated with immunosuppressive drugs or in HIV-infected patients. Apparently, the mere immunosuppression is still not sufficient for the outgrowth of EBV genome-carrying B cells, as indicated by a prolonged period of immunosuppression prior to the onset of lymphomatous growth and the common monoclonality of the arising lymphomas (Levine et al., 1992; Kimura et al., 2001). It is therefore highly likely that additional genetic or epigenetic modifications must take place before the appearance of continuously proliferating cells.

2. A modification in Xq25 of the SAP-gene in the X-chromosome-linked lymphoproliferative disease, as a hereditary disorder disturbing the immunological control of persistently EBV-infected cells (see Chapter 4).

3. The c-myc translocation, altering the EBV transcriptional regulation (Pajic et al., 2000) and resulting in a defect of c-myc to promote apoptosis due to a failure to induce the BH3-only protein Bim (a member of the B-cell lymphoma 3 [Bcl-2] family) and effectively to inhibit Bcl-2 (Hemann et al., 2005).

In high-risk papillomavirus-infected cells modifications in the antigen-presentation system appear to occur more randomly, yet, more than 95 % of HPV-positive cervical cancers (in which the E5 gene is commonly deleted) reveal defects in the HLA class I presentation system (for a review, see Stern, 2005). Related observations, which here mainly affect the innate immune system, have also been reported for hepatitis C (see Chapter 7 and Jinushi et al., 2004).

Thus, either adaptive immunity or its auxiliary systems including innate immune functions need to gain specific defects, probably to ensure a state of long-term persistence. This is shown schematically in Figure 3.4.

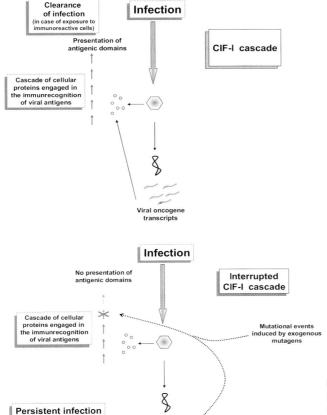

Fig. 3.4 Schematic outlines of the CIF-I cascades whose failure abolish or reduce immune recognition of viral genomes facilitating genome persistence.

3.3.2
The CIF-II Cascade

An intracellular control of viral oncogene functions was postulated during the late 1970 s (zur Hausen, 1977). This was in part based on the observation that a number of human and other primate viruses (BK, JC, several types of human pathogenic adenoviruses, SV40) possess oncogenes which efficiently induce malignant tumors if inoculated into newborn rodents (mice, hamsters, rats), but fail to be tumorigenic in their native hosts. Clearly, this effect is not due to the immune competence of the human host, since until now tumors linked to these infections have neither been detected in immunosuppressed allograft recipients, nor in HIV-infected persons. Since BK and JC polyoma-type viruses can be reactivated under conditions of immunosuppression without subsequent tumor induction, it is apparently not an immune function that negatively controls the oncogenic potential of these viruses. Thus, it is likely that an intracellular control developed during the course of human evolution protects our species against the potentially deleterious effects of these infections.

This concept is nicely supported by somatic cell fusion experiments conducted either with SV40- or HPV 16-immortalized cell lines. Somatic cell hybridization of different clones of such cells with each other frequently results in complementation to senescence with complete loss of their proliferative capacity in spite of ongoing viral oncoprotein synthesis (Pereira-Smith and Smith, 1981; Whitaker et al., 1992; Chen et al., 1993; Seagon and Dürst, 1994). In the absence of immunological interference and of contacts with other cell compartments and in presence of viral oncogene expression, this clearly points to an intracellular control of viral oncogene function. Senescence seems to be the consequence of complementation of different mutated genes in the respective cell fusion partners. This is outlined schematically in Figure 3.5.

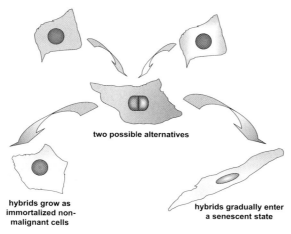

two possible alternatives

hybrids grow as immortalized non-malignant cells

hybrids gradually enter a senescent state

Fig. 3.5 Schematic outline of somatic cell hybridization between two cell clones expressing the same viral oncogene. Some combinations comple-

Thus, apparently several different genes suppress the viral oncogene function, possibly within the same signaling cascade.

Cyclin-dependent kinase inhibitors are proteins relatively clearly identified in suppressing functions of high-risk papillomaviral oncogenes (see Chapter 5). In particular, p16^{INK4} negatively interferes with the E6 function, whereas some evidence points to an important role of p14^{ARF} in blocking E7 functions. Mutagenic events, in part induced by functions of the viral oncogenes, in part also triggered by exogenous mutagens or epigenetic modifications, result in the interruption of the CIF-II cascade. This is outlined schematically in Figure 3.6.

CIF-II functions thus prevent the development of premalignant lesions in latently papillomavirus- and probably also polyomavirus-infected cells. It seems that polyomavirus and adenovirus infections in their respective natural hosts are commonly – but not uniformly (e.g., polyomavirus infection in mice) – controlled by more than one intracellular signaling cascade, probably as an adaptive response of the host during the course of evolution. On the other hand, this type of control may be absent in virus-linked tumors emerging after a relatively short incubation period, such as EBV-linked immunoblastic lymphomas, Kaposi's sarcoma and the endemic form of Burkitt's lymphoma. The highly specialized cells (B cells and endothelial cells) from which these tumors originate seem to have lost this control mechanism, possibly as consequence of their degree of differentiation.

3.3.3
The CIF-III Cascade

Evidence for a third signaling pathway negatively interfering with the transcription of viral oncogenes originated from studies on a paracrine transcriptional control of high-risk HPV infections (see also Chapter 5). Human keratinocytes immortalized by HPV 16 actively transcribe the viral oncogenes E6 and E7 under tissue culture conditions (Bosch et al., 1990; Dürst et al., 1991, 1992; Stoler et al., 1992). Following

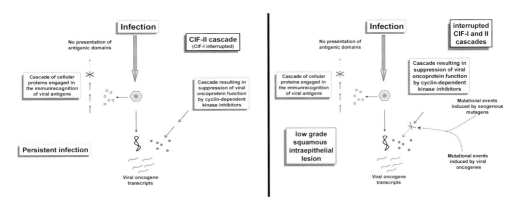

Fig. 3.6 Schematic outlines of the CIF-II cascades which interfere with the function of viral oncogenes.

xenotransplantation of these cells into nude mice, however, cell growth ceases and transcription of viral DNA is drastically reduced. In contrast to HPV-containing malignant cells, HPV-immortalized cells fail to form tumors under these conditions and persist for long periods of time as small nodules. Malignant cells commonly grow as xenotransplant and do not reveal any inhibition of viral oncogene transcription.

The existence of a paracrine transcriptional control exerted by cell compartments surrounding the immortalized cells in xenotransplants was further supported by experiments revealing the inhibition of HPV transcription in non-malignant HeLa-fibroblast hybrids by the addition of activated macrophages (Rösl et al., 1994) and subsequently also by tumor necrosis factor (TNF)-α (Delvenne et al., 1995; Vieira et al., 1996; Soto et al., 1999). The mechanism of this inhibition was partially clarified: TNF-α caused a modification of the transcription factor AP-1 within the HPV promoter, modifying pre-existing jun/jun dimers to jun/Fra-1 heterodimers (Soto et al., 1999, 2000). Malignant HeLa cells, containing HPV 18 DNA, reveal at the same site c-jun/c-fos heterodimers. Overexpression of c-fos in immortalized cells results in malignant conversion of those cells in a single step (Soto et al., 1999; Prusty and Das, 2005). Recent data point to a dysregulation of c-fos expression in malignant cells due to the absence of c-fos repression by the negative regulator Net (van Riggelen et al., 2005). A scheme depicting the interruption of this third regulatory cascade is shown in Figure 3.7.

It is likely that similar regulatory mechanisms exist in other viral systems which may lead to malignant transformation of human cells. Cells immortalized by EBV also fail to form tumors after xenotransplantation into nude mice. Similarly, hybrids between EBV-positive Burkitt's lymphoma cells and lymphoblastoid cells from the same donor are non-tumorigenic, in spite of the tumorigenic properties of the parental Burkitt's lymphoma line (Wolf et al., 1990; Jox et al., 1998). After an initial period of growth they regularly undergo apoptosis (Figs. 3.8 and 3.9). The underlying mechanism is presently not understood, but it is likely that the apoptotic events are triggered by the surrounding cellular environment.

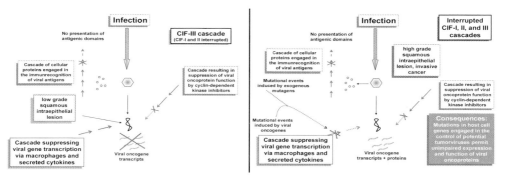

Fig. 3.7 A third regulatory cascade (CIF-III) suppressing the transcription of HPV oncogenes in immortalized cells (left) and its interruption in malignant proliferations (right).

A similar situation seems to exist for HTLV-1 immortalized cells (for reviews, see Ambinder, 1990; Suzuki and Yoshida, 1997), although no detailed mechanistic studies are available.

It should be noted that a large number of studies have shown in the past that immortalization of a variety of cell types by animal viruses (e.g., SV40, polyoma, adenoviruses) does not result in a tumorigenic phenotype (Asselin and Bastin, 1985; Pontén, 1985; Steinberg and Defendi, 1983). Similarly, some human viruses immortalizing animal cells (e.g., BK or JC polyomaviruses, adenoviruses types 12, 18, 31) do not induce a malignant phenotype under these conditions (Casto, 1968; Wright et al., 1976).

In stark contrast to these observations, the inoculation of certain tumor viruses into evolutionarily not too distantly related species (e.g., herpesvirus saimiri, herpesvirus ateles and EBV virus into cotton-top marmosets) may result in the acute development of leukemias and lymphomas. Apparently, adaptive mechanisms interfering with these infections do not exist in those species which are not infected by these viruses under natural conditions. This points to an interesting correlation between the length of the latency period between primary infection and subsequent tumor development and the existence of cellular interfering factors. The absence of

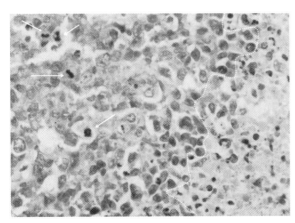

Fig. 3.8 Epstein–Barr virus-immortalized cells may initially grow rapidly after xenotransplantation into nude mice. After several days a central necrosis becomes visible and the tumors regress completely. The figure shows a tumor in regression. The white line reveals a relatively sharp demarcation of still actively proliferating cells (left side, arrows depict cells in mitosis) and progressive apoptosis (right side).

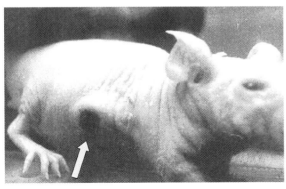

Fig. 3.9 Regressing tumor of Figure 3.8, revealing a typical central necrosis. (Illustration courtesy of Jürgen Wolf, Cologne.)

the latter seems to result in immediate cell proliferation and tumor formation, their partial absence or reduced function abbreviates the latency period. Latency periods of 20 years and more probably underline long periods of co-evolution between the virus and the human host.

References

Ambinder, R.F. Human lymphotropic viruses associated with lymphoid malignancy: Epstein-Barr and HTLV-1. *Hematol. Oncol. Clin. North Am.* 4: 821–833, **1990**.

Ashrafi, G.H., Haghshenas, M.R., Marchetti, B., O'Brien, P.M., and Campo, M.S. E5 protein of human papillomavirus type 16 selectively downregulates surface HLA class I. *Int. J. Cancer* 113: 276–283, **2005**.

Asselin, C. and Bastin, M. Sequences from polyomavirus and simian virus 40 large T genes capable of immortalizing primary rat embryo fibroblasts. *J. Virol.* 56: 958–968, **1985**.

Bosch, F., Schwarz, E., Boukamp, P., Fusenig, N.E., Bartsch, D., and zur Hausen, H. Suppression in vivo of human papillomavirus type 18 E6-E7 gene expression in nontumorigenic HeLa-fibroblast hybrid cells. *J. Virol.* 64: 4743–4754, **1990**.

Brander, C., Suscovich, T., Lee, Y., Nguyen, P.T., O'Connor, P., Seebach, J., Jones, M.G., van Gorder, M., Walker, B.D., and Scadden, D.T. Impaired CTL recognition of cells latently infected with Kaposi's sarcoma-associated herpesvirus. *J. Immunol.* 165: 2077–2083, **2000**.

Breiman, A., Grandvaux, N., Lin, R., Ottone, C., Akira, S., Yoneyama, M., Fujita, T., Hiscott, J., and Meurs, E.F. Inhibition of RIG-1-dependent signaling to the interferon pathway during hepatitis C virus expression and restoration of signaling by IKKε. *J. Virol.* 79: 3969–3978, **2005**.

Cartin, W. and Alonso, A. The human papillomavirus HPV 2 a E5 protein localizes to the Golgi apparatus and modulates signal transduction. *Virology* 314: 572–579, **2003**.

Casto, B.C. Adenovirus transformation of hamster embryo cells. *J. Virol.* 2: 376–383, **1968**.

Casto, B.C. and DiPaolo, J.A. Viruses, chemicals and cancer. *Prog. Med. Virol.* 16: 1–47, **1973**.

Chen, T.M., Pecoraro, G., and Defendi, V. Genetic analysis of in vitro progression of human papillomavirus-transfected human cervical cells. *Cancer Res.* 53: 1167–1171, **1993**.

Delvenne, P., al-Saleh, W., Gilles, C., Thiry, A., and Boniver, J. Inhibition of growth of normal and human papillomavirus-transformed keratinocytes in monolayer and organotypic cultures by interferon- and tumor necrosis factor-α. *Am. J. Pathol.* 146: 589–598, **1995**.

Dürst, M., Bosch, F.X., Glitz, D., Schneider, A., and zur Hausen, H. Inverse relationship between human papillomavirus (HPV) type 16 early gene expression and cell differentiation in nude mouse epithelial cysts and tumors induced by HPV-positive human cell lines. *J. Virol.* 65: 796–804, **1991**.

Dürst, M., Glitz, D., Schneider, A., and zur Hausen, H. Human papillomavirus type 16 (HPV16) gene expression and DNA replication in cervical neoplasia: analysis by in situ hybridization. *Virology* 189: 132–140, **1992**.

Fernandez, M., Quiroga, J.A., and Carreno, V. Hepatitis B virus downregulates the human interferon-inducible MxA promoter through direct interaction of pre-core/core proteins. *J. Gen. Virol.* 84: 2073–2082, **2003**.

Foster, G.R., Ackrill, A.M., Goldin, R.D., Kerr, I.M., Thomas, H.C., and Stark, G.R. Expression of the terminal protein region of hepatitis B virus inhibits cellular responses to interferons α and γ and double-stranded RNA. *Proc. Natl. Acad. Sci. USA* 88: 2888–2892, **1991**.

Hemann, M.T., Bric, A., Teruya-Feldstein, J., Herbst, A., Nilsson, J.A., Cordon-Cardo, C., Cleveland, J.L., Tanseya, W.P., and Lowe, S.W. Evasion of the p53 tumour surveillance network by tumour-derived myc mutants. *Nature* 436: 807–811, **2005**.

Jinushi, M., Takehara, T., Tatsumi, T., Kanto, T., Miyagi, T., Suzuki, T., Kanazawa, Y., Hiramatsu, N., and Hayashi, N. Negative regulation of NK cell activities by inhibitory receptor CD94/NKG2 A leads to altered NK cell-induced modulation of dendritic cell functions in chronic hepatitis C virus infection. *J. Immunol.* 173: 6072–6081, **2004**.

Jox, A., Taquia, E., Vockerodt, M., Draube, A., Pawlita, M., Möller, P., Bullerdiek, J., Diehl, V., and Wolf, J. Stable non-tumorigenic phenotype of somatic cell hybrids between malignant Burkitt's lymphoma cells and autologous EBV-immortalized B cells despite induction of chromosomal breakage and loss. *Cancer Res.* 58: 4930–4939, **1998**.

Kimura, H., Hoshino, Y., Kanegane, H., Tsuge, I., Okamura, T., Kawa, K., and Morishima, T. Clinical and virological characteristics of chronic active Epstein-Barr virus infection. *Blood* 98: 280–286, **2001**.

Levine, A.M., Shibata, D., Sullivan-Halley, J., Nathwani, B., Brynes, R., Slovak, M.L., Mahterian, S., Riley, C.L., Weiss, L., Levine, P.H., et al. Epidemiological and biological study of acquired immunodeficiency syndrome-related lymphoma in the County of Los Angeles: preliminary results. *Cancer Res.* 52 (Suppl. 19): 5482 s–5484 s, **1992**.

Neumann, R., Eis-Hubinger, A.M., and Koch, N. Herpes simplex virus type 1 targets the MHC class II processing pathway for immune evasion. *J. Immunol.* 171: 3075–3083, **2003**.

Pajic, A., Spitkovsky, D., Christoph, B., Kempkes, B., Schuhmacher, M., Staege, M.S., Brielmeier, M., Ellwart, J., Kohlhuber, F., Bornkamm, G.W., Polack, A., and Eick, D. Cell cycle activation by c-myc in a Burkitt lymphoma model cell line. *Int. J. Cancer* 87: 787–793, **2000**.

Parkin, D.M., Stjernswärd, J., and Muir, C.S. Estimates of the worldwide frequency of twelve major human cancers. *Bull. World Health Org.* 62: 163–182, **1984**.

Parkin, D.M., Bray, F., Ferlay, J., and Pisani, P. Global cancer statistics, 2002. *CA Cancer J. Clin.* 55: 74–108, **2002**.

Pereira-Smith, O.M. and Smith, J.R. Expression of SV40 T antigen in finite life span hybrids of normal and SV40-transformed fibroblasts. *Somatic Cell. Genet.* 7: 411–421, **1981**.

Pontén, J. Life span and 'immortalization' of mammalian cells. *IARC Sci Publ.* 58: 171–179, **1985**.

Prusty, B.K. and Das, B.C. Constitutive activation of transcription factor AP-1 in cervical cancer and suppression of human papillomavirus (HPV) transcription and AP-1 activity in HeLa cells by curcumin. *Int. J. Cancer* 113: 951–960, **2005**.

Rösl, F., Lengert, M., Albrecht, J., Kleine, K., Zawatzky, R., Schraven, B., and zur Hausen, H. Differential regulation of the JE gene encoding the monocyte chemoattractant protein (MCP-1) in cervical carcinoma cells and derived hybrids. *J. Virol.* 68: 2142–2150, **1994**.

Schust, D.J., Tortorella, D., and Ploegh, H.L. HLA-G and HLA-C at the feto-maternal interface: lessons learned from pathogenic viruses. *Semin. Cancer Biol.* 9: 37–46, **1999**.

Seagon S. and Dürst, M. Genetic analysis of an in vitro model system for human papillomavirus type 16-associated tumorigenesis. *Cancer Res.* 54: 5593–5598, **1994**.

Soto, U., Das, B.C., Lengert, M., Finzer, P., zur Hausen, H., and Rösl, F. Conversion of HPV 18 positive non-tumorigenic HeLa-fibroblast hybrids to invasive growth involves loss of TNF-α mediated repression of viral transcription and modification of the AP-1 transcription complex. *Oncogene* 18: 3187–3198, **1999**.

Soto, U., Denk, C., Finzer, P., Hutter, K.J., zur Hausen, H., and Rösl, F. Genetic complementation to non-tumorigenicity in cervical carcinoma cells correlates with alterations in AP-1 composition. *Int. J. Cancer* 86: 811–817, **2000**.

Steinberg, M.L. and Defendi, V. Transformation and immortalization of human keratinocytes by SV40. *J. Invest. Dermatol.* 81: 131 s–136 s, **1983**.

Stern, P.L. Immune control of human papillomavirus (HPV) associated anogenital disease and potential for vaccination. *J. Clin. Virol.* 32: S72–S82, **2005**.

Stoler, M.H., Rhodes, C.R., Whitbeck, A., Wolinsky, S.M., Chow, L.T., and Broker, T.R. Human papillomavirus type 16 and 18 gene expression in cervical neoplasias. *Hum. Pathol.* 23: 117–128, **1992**.

Suzuki, T. and Yoshida, M. HTLV-1 Tax protein interacts with cyclin-dependent kinase inhibitor p16 Ink4a and counteracts its inhibitory activity to CDK4. *Leukemia* 11 Suppl 3 : 14–16, **1997**.

Twu, J.S. and Schloemer, R.H. Transcription of the human â interferon gene is inhibited by hepatitis B virus. *J. Virol.* 63: 3065–3071, **1989**.

van Riggelen, J., Buchwalter, G., Soto, U., De-Castro Arce, J., zur Hausen, H., Wasylyk, B., and Rösl, F. Loss of net as repressor leads to constitutive increased c-fos transcription in cervical cancer cells. *J. Biol. Chem.* 280: 3286–3294, **2005**.

Vieira, K.B., Goldstein, D.J., and Villa, L.L. Tumor necrosis factor α interferes with the cell cycle of normal and papillomavirus-immortalized human keratinocytes. *Cancer Res.* 56: 2452–2457, **1996**.

Walev, I., Kunkel, J., Schwaeble, W., Weise, K., and Falke, D. Relationship between HLA I surface expression and different cytopathic effects produced after herpes simplex virus infection in vitro. *Arch. Virol.* 126: 303–311, **1992** .

Whitaker, N.J., Kidston, E.L., and Reddel, R.R. Finite life span of hybrids formed of different Simian virus 40-immortalized human cell lines. *J. Virol.* 66: 1202–1206, **1992**.

Wolf, J., Pawlita, M., Bullerdiek, J., and zur Hausen, H. Suppression of the malignant phenotype in somatic cell hybrids between Burkitt's lymphoma cells and Epstein-Barr virus-immortalized lymphoblastoid cells despite deregulated c-myc expression. *Cancer Res.* 50: 3095–3100, **1990**.

Wright, P.J., Bernhardt, G., Major, E.O., and di Mayorca, G. Comparison of the serology, transforming ability, and polypeptide composition of human papovaviruses isolated from urine. *J. Virol.* 17: 762–775, **1976**.

Zhang, B., Li, P., Brahmi, Z., Dunn, K.W., Blum, J.S. , and Roman, A. The E5 protein of human papillomavirus type 16 perturbs MHC class II maturation in human foreskin keratinocytes treated with interferon-α. *Virology* 310: 100–108, **2003**.

Zhang, T., Lin, R.T., Li, Y., Douglas, S. D., Maxcey, C., Ho, C., Lai, J.P., Wang, Y.J., Wan, Q., and Ho, W.Z. Hepatitis C virus inhibits intracellular interferon α expression in human hepatic cell lines. *Hepatology* 42: 819–827, **2005**.

zur Hausen, H. Cell-virus gene balance hypothesis of carcinogenesis. *Behring Inst. Mitt.* 61: 23–30, **1977**.

zur Hausen, H. Intracellular surveillance of persisting viral infections. Human genital cancer results from deficient cellular control of papillomavirus gene expression. *Lancet* 2: 489–491, **1986**.

zur Hausen, H. Disrupted dichotomous control of human papillomavirus infection in cancer of the cervix. *Lancet* 343: 955–957, **1994**.

4
Herpesviruses and Oncogenesis

There are presently eight members of the herpesvirus group known as human pathogens: herpes simplex viruses type 1 and 2 (also known as HSV-1 and HSV-2 or HHV-1 and HHV-2); varicella-zoster virus (VZV or HHV-3); Epstein–Barr virus (EBV or HHV-4); human cytomegalovirus (CMV or HHV-5); human herpesvirus 6 (HHV-6); human herpesvirus 7 (HHV-7); and Kaposi sarcoma-associated herpesvirus or human herpesvirus type 8 (KSHV or HHV-8). The virion contains a core with linear double-stranded DNA, varying in size between 120 and 230 kbp, an icosahedral capsid of about 100–110 nm in diameter with 162 capsomeres. The capsid is surrounded by an envelope containing viral glycoproteins on its surface.

Herpesviruses are found in a large number of different species, and almost 100 herpesviruses have at least been partially characterized (Roizman, 1996). Virtually all of these types contain linear DNA with terminal repeat sequences, some of them juxtaposed internally. All of these viruses share the property of persisting in a latent state in specific types of cells. The cell type harboring persisting viruses of this family differs according to the virus type. In the state of latency and prior to viral DNA replication in productive infections, the DNA circularizes.

The current classification subdivides the herpesvirus family into three subfamilies. This subdivision is based on DNA sequence homology, similarities in genomic sequence arrangements and the relatedness of viral proteins:

- Alphaherpesvirinae: These are characterized by a variable host range and the establishment of latent infections in sensory neuronal cells. Human representatives of this group are HSV-1 and -2 and the VZV.
- Betaherspevirinae: These reveal a rather restricted host range, a slow reproductive cycle, and remain latent preferentially in salivary gland cells, cells of the hematopoietic system, kidneys and some other tissues. Human representatives of this group are CMV and HHV types 6 and 7.
- Gammaherpesvirinae: Viruses in this group specifically infect B and T lymphocytes, where they result either in lytic or latent infections. Some are also able to infect epithelial, fibroblastic and endothelial cells. This subfamily contains two genera, the *Lym-*

Infections Causing Human Cancer. Harald zur Hausen
Copyright © 2006 WILEY-VCH Verlag GmbH & Co. KGaA, Weinheim
ISBN: 3-527-31056-8

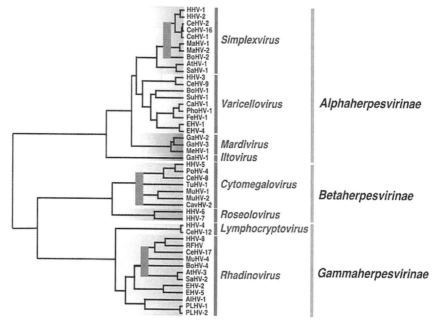

Fig. 4.1 Phylogenetic tree of the herpesvirus family. (Reprinted from VIRUS TAXONOMY, Eighth Report of the International Committee on Taxonomy of Viruses, Vol 1, Fauquet, C.M., Mayo, M.A., Maniloff, J., Desselberger, U. and Ball, L.A. (Eds.), Part II – The Double Stranded DNA Viruses, Herpesviridae, 211. Copyright 2005, with permission from Elsevier.)

phocryptoviruses (e.g., EBV) and the *Rhadinoviruses* (e.g., HHV type 8).

Whereas EBV and HHV type 8 were linked immediately after their discovery with human malignancies, a role of other members of this family remains uncertain until today. Human herpesviruses induce mutations in host cell DNA (Schlehofer and zur Hausen, 1982). Even under conditions of abortive infections these virus infections effectively amplify persisting genomes of small DNA tumorviruses (e.g., polyoma-type and papillomavirus genomes) (Schlehofer et al., 1983; Matz et al., 1984; Schmitt et al., 1989; Heilbronn and zur Hausen, 1989; Heilbronn et al., 1990). Human CMV even permits the replication of the human JC polyomavirus co-transfected into CMV-infected human fibroblasts (Heilbronn et al., 1993). This may represent an indirect mode by which these infections could contribute to human carcinogenesis, although epidemiological evidence for their contribution under *in-vivo* conditions is still missing.

Besides human pathogenic herpesviruses, a number of animal representatives of this group are known to represent potent carcinogens, either in their natural species of infection or upon inoculation into related species. *Marek virus* of chickens induces an infectious neurolymphomatosis in chickens, while the *Lucke frog herpesvirus* emerges as the responsible agent for kidney carcinomas in American leopard frogs. It is interesting to note that Marek's herpesvirus may incorporate complete genomes of avian retroviruses, such as the chicken reticuloendotheliosis virus, into its own DNA under natural as well as under experimental conditions (Isfort et al., 1992; Jones et al., 1993; Witter et al., 1997; Davidson and Borenshtain, 2001). *Herpesvirus saimiri* and *herpesvirus ateles*, which persistently infect their natural hosts, are potent leukemogenic agents in related species and induce acute leukemias and lymphomas there. A large number of species have been identified harboring EBV-related herpesviruses.

All these observations stress the importance of members of this virus family as important carcinogens or as potential candidates for human carcinogenicity.

References

Davidson, I. and Borenshtain, R. In vivo events of retroviral long terminal repeat integration into Marek's disease virus in commercial poultry: detection of chimeric molecules as a marker. *Avian Dis.* 45: 102–121, **2001**.

Heilbronn, R. and zur Hausen, H. A subset of herpes simplex virus replication genes induces DNA amplification within the host cell genome. *J. Virol.* 63: 3683–3692, **1989**.

Heilbronn, R., Weller, S. and zur Hausen, H. Herpes simplex virus type 1 mutants for origin binding protein induce DNA amplification in the absence of viral replication. *Virology* 179, 478–481, **1990**.

Heilbronn, R. Albrecht, I., Stephan, S., Bürkle, A., and zur Hausen, H. Human cytomegalovirus induces JC virus DNA replication in human fibroblasts. *Proc. Natl. Acad. Sci. USA* 90: 11 406–11 410, **1993**.

Isfort, R., Jones, D., Kost, R., Witter, R., and Kung, H.J. Retrovirus insertion into herpesvirus in vitro and in vivo. *Proc. Natl. Acad. Sci. USA* 89: 991–995, **1992**.

Jones, D., Isfort, R., Witter, R., Kost, R., and Kung, H.J. Retroviral insertions into a herpesvirus are clustered at the junctions of the short repeat and short unique sequences. *Proc. Natl. Acad. Sci. USA* 90: 3855–3859, **1993**.

Matz, B., Schlehofer, J.R., and zur Hausen. H. Identification of a gene function of herpes simplex virus type 1 essential for amplification of simian virus 40 DNA sequences in transformed hamster cells. *Virology* 134: 328–337, **1984** .

Roizman, B. Herpesviridae. In: Fields, B.N., Knipe, D.M., Howley, P.M. (Eds.), *Fields Virology*, Third edition, Chapter 71, pp. 2221–2230, **1996**.

Schlehofer, J.R. and zur Hausen, H. Induction of mutations within the host cell genome by partially inactivated herpes simplex virus type 1. *Virology* 122: 471–475, **1982**.

Schlehofer, J.R., Gissmann, L., Matz, B., and zur Hausen, H. Herpes simplex virus induced amplification of SV40 sequences in transformed Chinese hamster cells. *Int. J. Cancer* 32: 99–103, **1983**.

Schmitt, J., Schlehofer, J.R., Mergener, K. Gissmann, L., and zur Hausen, H. Amplification of bovine papillomavirus DNA by N-methyl-N'-nitro-N-nitrosoguanidine, ultraviolet-irradiation, or infection with herpes simplex virus. *Virology* 172: 73–81, **1989**.

Witter, R.L., Li, D., Jones, D., Lee, L.F., and Kung, H.J. Retroviral insertional mutagenesis of a herpesvirus: a Marek's disease virus mutant attenuated for oncogenicity but not for immunosuppression or in vivo replication. *Avian Dis.* 41: 407–421, **1997**.

4.1
Alphaherpesvirinae

4.1.1
Herpes Simplex Viruses Types 1 and 2

Herpes simplex virus infections are very common and affect a high percentage of all human populations. In 1962, Schneweiss identified two different serotypes, subsequently confirmed by Nahmias and Dowdle (1968). Whereas HSV-1 is found predominantly in oropharyngeal infections, HSV-2 has a strong predilection for anogenital sites. Both types of viruses cause a large number of different clinical symptoms. Their molecular biology, as well as clinical aspects of herpetic infections, have been described extensively elsewhere (Roizman, 1996; Whitley, 1996).

In 1968 and 1969, the first reports appeared on increased antibody levels against HSV-2 antigens in women with cervical cancer (Rawls et al., 1968; Naib et al., 1969). Studies confirming these findings were published one year later (Nahmias et al., 1970; Rawls and Kaufman, 1970). These studies initiated a burst of activities which attempted to link herpetic infections to human cancers, particularly to cancer of the cervix. Reports appeared identifying virus-specific antigens as markers for cervical cancer (e.g., Aurelian et al., 1977, 1983; MacNab et al., 1980; Gupta et al., 1981). Fifteen years after the first report by Naib et al., a large-scale prospective study conducted in the former Czechoslovakia failed to provide serological evidence in support of a role of HSV in cervical cancer (Vonka et al., 1984 a,b). At approximately the same time, specific types of human papillomaviruses (HPV) were incriminated as the main cause of cervical cancer (Dürst et al., 1983; Boshart et al., 1984; Schwarz et al., 1985). The combined effect of these publications was most likely the prime reason for a reduced interest in seroepidemiological studies analyzing the relationship between HSV infections and anogenital cancer. Very recently, however, two further large-scale seroepidemiological studies have been published, one linking HSV-2 seropositivity with an increased risk of cervical squamous cell carcinoma (relative risk [RR] 2.19) and of adeno- or adenosquamous cell carcinoma (RR 3.37) after adjustment of potential confounders (Smith et al., 2002). A follow-up of a cohort of 550 000 women in Scandinavia (Lehtinen et al., 2002) arrived at an opposite result: after adjustment for smoking and HPV infections, the relative risks for HSV-2 were 1.0 and 0.7, respectively, and even in a meta-analysis the relative risk for HSV-2 was 0.9. Thus, seroepidemiological evidence for a role of HSV-2 in cervical cancer remains inconclusive.

Additional experimental studies, however, seemed to support a possible role of HSV in human cancers. These originated in part from reports of HSV DNA or RNA persistence in cervical cancer cells: in 1972, Frenkel et al., and in 1973 Roizman and Frenkel, identified a fragment of HSV-2 in one cervical cancer biopsy and also analyzed transcripts of this DNA. Two other groups reported similar findings: initially, HSV RNA was detected in premalignant cervical cells only (McDougall et al., 1980), but subsequently RNA and HSV protein was found in tumors of the uterine cervix (McDougall et al., 1982), the RNA representing limited regions of the viral genome.

Four years later, the same group reported the occasional detection of HSV and HPV DNA and RNA within the same tumor (McDougall et al., 1986).

These data require cautious interpretation: several studies noted regions of homology between HSV and mammalian (including human) DNA (Peden et al., 1982; Puga et al., 1982; Jones et al., 1985; Gomez-Marquez et al., 1985). Although most of the homologies were located within the long and short inverted repeat regions, an additional one was noted near the center of the long unique region. Hybridization occurred even at relatively stringent conditions (Peden et al., 1982). The *in-situ* hybridization labeling not only of cervical carcinoma cells, but also of apparent macrophages by the HSV-specific probe (McDougall et al., 1982), could suggest a homology with cellular RNA expressed preferentially in proliferating cells and activated macrophages. In addition, other reports failed to confirm the presence of HSV-2 DNA in cervical cancer cells (zur Hausen et al., 1974; zur Hausen, 1976).

Another puzzling aspect originates from *in-vitro* transformation studies of rodent cells with partially inactivated HSV DNA or with DNA fragments of these viruses. Duff and Rapp (1971, 1973) reported initially oncogenic transformation of hamster embryo cell after exposure to partially inactivated HSV-2 or HSV-1. A number of additional reports followed which revealed the transformation also of murine and rat cells, in part by fragments of HSV DNA (for a review, see Minson, 1984). In one of these studies persistence of HSV-2 DNA sequences was noted in transformed hamster cells (Galloway et al., 1980), corresponding to a sequence also found in some cervical cancers (McDougall et al., 1984).

Overall, three distinct transforming regions have been identified: in HSV-1 DNA the fragment BglII (map units 0.31–0.42), the HSV-2 fragment BglII N (map units 0.58–0.63) and the HSV-2 BglII C fragment (reviewed in Di Luca et al., 1995). Although the BglII N fragment contains the information of at least five polypeptides (Galloway et al., 1982), subsequent publications by the same group stated that the transforming part of this fragment may not specify a viral polypeptide (Galloway et al., 1984). An insertion sequence-like structure was incriminated as the possible transformant. As a consequence of these observations, a "hit-and-run" mechanism was postulated for HSV oncogenesis (Skinner, 1976; Galloway and McDougall, 1983).

In-vitro transformation studies could represent a strong correlate to seroepidemiology and nucleic acid hybridization studies. It is somewhat unfortunate, however, that human cells proved to be refractory to cell immortalization by HSV DNA fragments or by partially inactivated virus particles. In rodent cells, spontaneous transformation is a relatively frequent event which may be enhanced by nonspecific exposures, such as DNA transfection. The activation of endogenous retroviruses by HSV or its DNA fragments (Hampar et al., 1976; Boyd et al., 1978, 1980) may further complicate the interpretation of transformation studies in rodent cells. The activation of murine type C viruses is not limited to transformed murine cells, but occurs also in nontransformed cells (Hampar et al., 1977). Even in human cells, endogenous HERV-K and HERV-W retrovirus long terminal repeats (LTRs) become activated by HSV infection (Kwun et al., 2002; Lee et al., 2003). HSV infection also results in activation of the LTR of human immunodeficiency virus (HIV) (Gendelman et al., 1986;

Mosca et al., 1987), which seems to result from an interaction between HIV Tat and Rex and the HSV US11 protein (Popik and Pitha, 1994; Schaerer-Uthurralt et al., 1998). Thus, the reported transformation of cells by HSV may have resulted from specific retrovirus insertion after their activation by the HSV infection.

In addition, there exists a remarkable paucity of further transformation studies during the past two decades, when compared to the 1970s and the early 1980s. Thus, the evidence for a role of HSV infections in human cancers remains inconclusive.

Some other experimental approaches still could point to an indirect role of HSV infections in carcinogenesis: HSV infection actively induces chromosomal aberrations in infected host cells, even under conditions of an abortive infection (Hampar and Ellison, 1961; Boiron et al., 1966; Waubke et al., 1968; O'Neill and Miles, 1969). This points to a potential mutagenic activity of these virus infections. Direct proof for a mutagenic effect of HSV infections originated from a number of different experiments: Schlehofer and zur Hausen (1982) and Pilon et al. (1986) showed that partially UV-inactivated HSV or HSV-2 infecting nonpermissive cells induced mutations within host cell DNA. Clarke and Clements (1991) revealed that mutagenesis occurring after infection with HSV types 1 or 2 does not require virus replication. Shillitoe et al. (1986) and Das and colleagues (1994) induced mutations in a bacterial assay with the cloned Bam HI G fragment of HSV type 1, and showed that the UL 26 gene, expressed with a different carboxy terminus early in infection, codes for a mutagenic peptide. Brandt et al. (1987) induced mutations within the HGPRT gene by transfection with fragments of HSV-2 DNA.

Another interesting possibility by which HSV infection may contribute to cell transformation is the ability of these viruses to amplify genomes of persisting small DNA tumorviruses even under conditions of abortive infection. Initially, Sara Lavi (1981) showed the amplification of persisting SV40 DNA in Chinese hamster cells after treatment of these cells with chemical carcinogens. The mutagenic activity of HSV infections for host cell DNA prompted similar experiments after HSV infection of SV40-transformed cells (Schlehofer et al., 1983), resulting also in the amplification of persisting SV40 genomes. It was subsequently shown that the HSV DNA polymerase is an essential component for this amplification (Matz et al., 1984). Amplification is not limited to polyoma-type viruses, but has also been noted in HSV-infected papillomavirus-positive cells (Brandt et al., 1987; Schmitt et al., 1989; Hara et al., 1997).

The induction of chromosomal aberrations, of mutations in host cell DNA, and the amplification of other DNA tumorvirus genomes after infection with HSV could all contribute (as an indirect mode) to human carcinogenesis. Unfortunately, epidemiological support for such a role is still very weak and hardly convincing. Thus, as there exists no evidence that HSV-1 or -2 do act as direct carcinogens, even their role as indirect carcinogenic factors remains to be established.

4.1.2
Varicella-Zoster Virus

Varicella-zoster virus is the etiological agent of chickenpox, an acute infectious disease, resulting in life-long persistence of viral DNA in the dorsal root ganglia. Reactivation of the virus may occur under conditions of long-lasting stress or immunosuppression, resulting in typical localized zoster eruptions. Patients at high risk for zoster eruptions are AIDS patients, organ allograft recipients, patients with malignant hematopoietic disorders, and those receiving chemotherapy (for a review, see Arvin, 1996). The zoster lesions produce infectious virus and may give rise to new chickenpox epidemics among nonexposed children. A detailed account of the molecular biology and clinical features of VZV infections is provided elsewhere (Cohen and Straus, 1996; Arvin, 1996).

Data relating VZV infections to human malignant tumors are scarce, and based on a few studies on the transformation of rodent cells and the biochemical transformation of mammalian cells. In 1980, Gelb et al. reported the oncogenic transformation of primary hamster embryo cells after infection with VZV. Inoculation of these cells into inbred hamsters resulted in aggressively growing fibrosarcomas. The tumor-bearing hamsters developed antibodies to VZV antigens. In a later study, Gelb and Dohner (1984) state that transformation of cells by VZV is a very rare event, and one that may require a recent clinical isolate. Transformed hamster cell lines did not retain VZV DNA.

Transformation to thymidine kinase expression of mouse L-cells lacking the enzyme thymidine kinase (Ltk⁻) by VZV infection was reported by Yamanishi et al. (1981). The transformed cells showed almost the same growth rate as the parental Ltk⁻ cells. The converted clones revealed, however, a nuclear VZV-specific antigen and their tk-activity was neutralized by hyperimmune serum against VZV.

Altogether, the available publications presently provide no evidence for a role of VZV infection in the causation of human malignancies.

References

Arvin, A.M. Varicella-zoster virus. In: Fields, B.N., Knipe, P.M. and Howley, P.M. (Eds.), *Fields Virology*, Third Edition, Lippincott-Raven Publishers, Philadelphia, vol. 2: 2547–2585, **1996**.

Aurelian, L., Strnad, B.C., and Smith, M.F. Immunodiagnostic potential of a virus-coded, tumor-associated antigen (AG-4) in cervical cancer. *Cancer* 39: 1834–1849, **1977**.

Aurelian, L., Smith, C.C., Klacsman, K.T., Gupta, P.K., and Frost, J.K. Expression and cellular compartmentalization of a herpes simplex virus type 2 protein (ICP 10) in productively infected and cervical tumor cells. *Cancer Invest.* 1: 301–313, **1983**.

Boiron, M., Tanzer, J., Thomas, M., and Hampe, A. Early diffuse chromosome alterations in monkey kidney cells infected in vitro with herpes simplex virus. *Nature* 209: 737–738, **1966**.

Boshart, M., Gissmann, L., Ikenberg, H., Kleinheinz, A., Scheurlen, W., and zur Hausen, H. A new type of papillomavirus DNA, its presence in genital cancer biopsies and in cell lines derived from genital cancer. *EMBO J.* 3: 1151–1157, **1984**.

Boyd, A.L., Derge, J.G., and Hampar, B. Activation of endogenous type C virus in BALB/c mouse cells by herpesvirus DNA. *Proc. Natl. Acad. Sci. USA* 75: 4558–4562. **1978**.

Boyd, A.L., Enquist, L., Van de Woude, G.F., and Hampar, B. Activation of mouse retrovirus by herpes simplex virus type 1 cloned DNA fragments. *Virology* 103: 228–231, **1980**.

Brandt, C.R., Buonagouro, F.M., McDougall, J.K., and Galloway, D.A. Plasmid mediated mutagenesis of a cellular gene in transfected eukaryotic cells. *Nucleic Acids Res.* 15: 561–573, **1987**.

Brandt, C.R., McDougall, J.K., and Galloway, D.A. Synergistic interactions between human papilloma virus type-18 sequences, herpes simplex virus infection and chemical carcinogen treatment. In: Steinberg, B.M., Brandsma, J.L., and Taichman, L.B. (Eds.), *Papillomaviruses, Cancer Cells*. Cold Spring Harbor Laboratory Press, New York, Vol. 5, pp. 179–186, **1987**.

Clarke, P. and Clements, J.B. Mutagenesis occurring following infection with herpes simplex virus does not require virus replication. *Virology* 182: 597–606, **1991**.

Cohen, J.I. and Straus, S. E. Varicella-zoster virus and its replication. In: Fields, B.N., Knipe, P.M. and Howley, P.M. (Eds.), *Fields Virology*, Third Edition, Lippincott-Raven Publishers, Philadelphia, vol. 2: 2525–2545, **1996**.

Das, C.M., Zhang, S., and Shillitoe, E.J. Expression of the mutagenic peptide of herpes simplex virus type 1 in virus-infected cells. *Virus Res.* 34: 97–114, **1994**.

Di Luca, D., Caselli, E., and Cassai, E. Herpes simplex virus as a cooperating agent in human genital carcinogenesis. In: Barbanti-Brodano, G., Bendinelli, M., and Friedman, H. (Eds.), *DNA Tumor Viruses: Oncogenic Mechanisms*. Plenum Press New York, London, pp. 281–293, **1995**.

Duff, R. and Rapp, F. Oncogenic transformation of hamster cells after exposure to herpes simplex virus type 2. *Nat. New Biol.* 233: 48–50, **1971**.

Duff, R. and Rapp, F. Oncogenic transformation of hamster embryo cells after exposure to inactivated herpes simplex virus type 1. *J. Virol.* 12: 209–217, **1973**.

Dürst, M. Gissmann, L., Ikenberg, H., and zur Hausen, H. A papillomavirus DNA from a cervical carcinoma and its prevalence in cancer biopsy samples from different geographic regions. *Proc. Natl. Acad. Sci. USA* 80: 3812–3815, **1983** .

Frenkel, N., Roizman, B., Cassai, E., and Nahmias, A. A DNA fragment of Herpes simplex 2 and its transcription in human cervical cancer tissue. *Proc. Natl. Acad. Sci. USA* 69: 3784–3789, **1972**.

Galloway, D.A. and McDougall, J.K. The oncogenic potential of herpes simplex viruses: evidence for a 'hit-and-run' mechanism. *Nature* 302: 21–24, **1983**.

Galloway, D.A., Copple, C.D., and McDougall, J.K. Analysis of viral DNA sequences in hamster cells transformed by herpes simplex virus type 2. *Proc. Natl. Acad. Sci. USA* 77: 880–884, **1980**.

Galloway, D.A., Goldstein, L.C., and Lewis, J.B. Identification of proteins encoded by a fragment of herpes simplex virus type 2 DNA that has transforming activity. *J. Virol.* 42: 530–537, **1982**.

Galloway, D.A., Nelson, J.A., and McDougall, J.K. Small fragments of herpesvirus DNA with transforming activity contain insertion sequence-like structures. *Proc. Natl. Acad. Sci. USA* 81: 4636–4740, **1984**.

Gelb, L.D., Huang, J.J., and Wellinghoff, W.J. Varicella-zoster virus transformation of hamster embryo cells. *J. Gen. Virol.* 51: 171–177, **1980**.

Gelb, L.D. and Dohner, D. Varicella-zoster virus-induced transformation of mammalian cells in vitro. *J. Invest. Dermatol.* 83 (1 Suppl.): 77s–81s, **1984**.

Gendelman, H.E., Phelps, W., Feigenbaum, L., Ostrove, J.M., Adachi, A., Howley, P.M., Khoury, G., Ginsberg, H.S., and Martin, M.A. Trans-activation of the human immunodeficiency virus long terminal repeat sequence by DNA viruses. *Proc. Natl. Acad. Sci. USA* 83: 9759–9763, **1986**.

Gomez-Marquez, J., Puga, A., and Notkins, A.L. Regions of the terminal repetitions of the herpes simplex virus type 1 genome. Relationship to immunoglobulin switch-like DNA sequences. *J. Biol. Chem.* 260: 3490–3495, **1985**.

Gupta, P.K., Aurelian, L., Frost, J.K., Carpenter, J.M., Klacsmann, K.T., Rosenhein, N.B., and Tyrer, H.W. Herpesvirus antigens as markers for cervical cancer. *Gynecol. Oncol.* 12: S232–258, **1981**.

Hampar, B. and Ellison, S. A. Chromosomal aberrations induced by an animal virus. *Nature* 192: 145–147, **1961**.

Hampar, B., Aaronson, S. A., Derge, J.G., Chakrabarty, M., Showalter, S. D., and Dunn, C.Y. Activation of an endogenous mouse type C virus by ultraviolet-irradiated herpes simplex virus types 1 and 2. *Proc. Natl. Acad. Sci. USA* 73: 646–650, **1976**.

Hampar, B., Hatanaka, M., Aulakh, G., Derge, J.G., Lee, L., and Showalter, S. Type C virus activation in "nontransformed" mouse cells by UV-irradiated herpes simplex virus. *Virology* 76: 876–881, **1977**.

Hara, Y., Kimoto, T., Okuno, Y., and Minekawa, Y. Effect of herpes simplex virus on the DNA of human papillomavirus 18. *J. Med. Virol.* 53: 4–12. **1997**.

Jones, T.R., Parks, C.L., Spector, D.J., and Hyman, R.W. Hybridization of herpes simplex virus DNA and human ribosomal DNA and RNA. *Virology* 144: 384–397, **1985**.

Kwun, H.J., Han, H.J., Lee, W.J., Kim, H.S., and Jang, K.L. Transactivation of the human endogenous retrovirus K long terminal repeat by herpes simplex virus type 1 immediate early protein 0. *Virus Res.* 86: 93–100, **2002**.

Lavi, S. Carcinogen-mediated amplification of viral DNA sequences in simian virus 40-transformed Chinese hamster embryo cells. *Proc. Natl. Acad. Sci. USA* 78: 6144–6148, **1981**.

Lee, W.J., Kwun, H.J., Kim, H.S., and Jang, K.L. Activation of human endogenous retrovirus W long terminal repeat by herpes simplex virus type 1 immediate early protein 1. *Mol. Cells* 15: 75–80, **2003**.

Lehtinen, M., Koskela, P., Jellum, E., Bloigu, A., Anttila, T., Hallmans, G., Luukkaala, T., Thoresen, S., Youngman, L., Dillner, J., and Hakama, M. Herpes simplex virus and risk of cervical cancer: a longitudinal, nested case-control study in the Nordic countries. *Am. J. Epidemiol.* 156: 687–692, **2002**.

MacNab, J.C.M., Visser, L., Jamieson, A.T., and Hay, J. Specific viral antigens in rat cells transformed by herpes simplex virus type 2 and in rat tumors induced by inoculation of transformed cells. *Cancer Res.* 40: 2074–2079, **1980** .

Matz, B., Schlehofer, J.R., and zur Hausen, H. Identification of a gene function of herpes simplex virus type 1 essential for amplification of simian virus 40 DNA sequences in transformed hamster cells. *Virology* 134: 328–337, **1984** .

McDougall, J.K., Galloway, D.A., and Fenoglio, C.M. Cervical carcinoma: detection of herpes simplex RNA in cells undergoing neoplastic change. *Int. J. Cancer* 25: 1–8, **1980**.

McDougall, J.K., Crum, C.P., Fenoglio, C.M., Goldstein, L.C., and Galloway, D.A. Herpesvirus-specific RNA and protein in carcinoma of the uterine cervix. *Proc. Natl. Acad. Sci. USA* 79: 3853–3857, **1982**.

McDougall, J.K., Nelson, J.A., Myerson, D., Beckmann, A.M., and Galloway, D.A. HSV, CMV, and HPV in human neoplasia. *J. Invest. Dermatol.* 83 (1 Suppl.): 72s–76s, **1984**.

McDougall, J.K., Myerson, D., and Beckmann, A.M. Detection of viral DNA and RNA by in situ hybridization. *J. Histochem. Cytochem.* 34: 33–38, **1986**.

Minson, A.C. Cell transformation and oncogenesis by herpes simplex virus and human cytomegalovirus. *Cancer Surv.* 3: 91–111, **1984**.

Mosca, J.D., Bednarik, D.P., Raj, N.B., Rosen, C.A., Sodroski, J.G., Haseltine, W.A., Hayward, G.S., and Pitha, P.M. Activation of human immunodeficiency virus by herpesvirus infection: identification of a region within the long terminal repeat that responds to a trans-acting factor encoded by herpes simplex virus 1. *Proc. Natl. Acad. Sci. USA* 84: 7408–7412, **1987**.

Nahmias, A.J., and Dowdle, W.R. Antigenic and biologic differences in herpesvirus hominis. *Prog. Med. Virol.* 10: 110–159, **1968**.

Nahmias, A.J., Josey, W.E., Naib, Z.M., Luce, C.F., and Guest, B.A. Antibodies to Herpesvirus hominis types 1 and 2 in humans. II. Women with cervical cancer. *Am. J. Epidemiol.* 91: 547–552, **1970**.

Naib, Z.M., Nahmias, A.J., Josey, W.E., and Kramer, J.H. Genital herpetic infections. Association with cervical dysplasia and carcinoma. *Cancer* 23: 940–945, **1969**.

O'Neill, F.J. and Miles, C.P. Chromosome changes in human cells induced by herpes simplex, types 1 and 2. *Nature* 223: 851–852, **1969**.

Peden, K., Mounts, P., and Hayward, G.S. Homology between mammalian cell DNA sequences and human herpesvirus genomes detected by a hybridization procedure with high complexity probe. *Cell* 31: 71–80, **1982**.

Pilon, L., Langelier, Y., and Royal, A. Herpes simplex virus type 2 mutagenesis: characterization of mutants induced at the hprt locus of non-permissive XC cells. *Mol. Cell. Biol.* 6: 2977–2983, **1986**.

Popik, W. and Pitha, P.M. The presence of tat protein or tumor necrosis factor α is critical for herpes simplex virus type 1-induced expression of human immunodeficiency virus type 1. *J. Virol.* 68: 1324–1333, **1994**.

Puga, A., Cantin, E.M., and Notkins, A.L. Homology between murine and human cellular DNA sequences and the terminal repetition of the S component of herpes simplex virus type 1 DNA. *Cell* 31: 81–87, **1982**.

Rawls, W.E. and Kaufman, R.H. Herpesvirus and other factors related to the genesis of cervical cancer. *Clin. Obstet. Gynecol.* 13: 857–872, **1970**.

Rawls, W.E., Tompkins, W.A., Figueroa, M.E., and Melnick, J.L. Herpesvirus type 2: association with cancer of the cervix. *Science* 161: 1255–1256, **1968**.

Roizman, B. Herpesviridae. In: Fields, B.N., Knipe, P.M. and Howley, P.M. (Eds.), *Fields Virology*, Third Edition. Lippincott-Raven Publishers, Philadelphia, vol. 2: 2221–2295, **1996**.

Roizman, B. and Frenkel, N. The transcription and state of herpes simplex virus DNA in productive infection and in human cervical cancer tissue. *Cancer Res.* 33: 1402–1416, **1973**.

Schaerer-Uthurralt, N., Erard, M., Kindbeiter, K., Madjar, J.Y., and Diaz, J.J. Distinct domains in herpes simplex virus type 1 US11 protein mediate post-transcriptional transactivation of human T-lymphotropic virus type I envelope gylcoprotein gene expression and specific binding to the Rex responsive element. *J. Gen. Virol.* 79: 1593–1602, **1998**.

Schlehofer, J.R. and zur Hausen, H. Induction of mutations within the host cell genome by partially inactivated herpes simplex virus type 1. *Virology* 122: 471–475, **1982**.

Schlehofer, J.R., Gissmann, L., Matz, B., and zur Hausen, H. Herpes simplex virus induced amplification of SV40 sequences in transformed Chinese hamster embryo cells. *Int. J. Cancer* 32: 99–103, **1983**.

Schmitt, J., Mergener, K., Gissmann, L., Schlehofer, J.R., and zur Hausen, H. Amplification of bovine papillomavirus DNA by N-methyl-N'-nitro-N-nitrosoguanidine, ultraviolet-irradiation, or infection with herpes simplex virus. *Virology* 172: 73–81, **1989**.

Schneweis, K.E. Serologische Untersuchungen zur Typendifferenzierung des Herpesvirus hominis. *Z. Immun. Exp. Ther.* 124: 337–341, **1962**.

Schwarz, E.. Freese, U.K., Gissmann, L., Mayer, W., Roggenbuck, B., Stremlau, A., and zur Hausen. H. Structure and transcription of human papillomavirus sequences in cervical carcinoma cells. *Nature* 314: 111–114, **1985**.

Shillitoe, E.J., Matney, T.S., and Conley, A.J. Induction of mutations in bacteria by a fragment of DNA from herpes simplex virus type 1. *Virus Res.* 6: 181–191, **1986**.

Skinner, G.R. Transformation of primary hamster fibroblasts by type 2 simplex virus: evidence for a hit and run mechanism. *Br. J. Exp. Pathol.* 57: 361–376, **1976**.

Smith, J.S., Herrero, R., Bosetti, C., Munoz, N., Bosch, F.X., Eluf-Neto, J., Castellsague, X., Meijer, C.J., Van den Brule, A.J., Franceschi, S., Ashley, R. and International Agency for Research on Cancer (IARC) Multicentric Cervical Cancer Study Group. Herpes simplex virus-2 as a human papillomavirus cofactor in the etiology of invasive cervical cancer. *J. Natl. Cancer Inst.* 94: 1604–1613, **2002**.

Vonka, V., Kanka, J., Jelinek, J., Subrt, I., Suchanek, A., Havrankova, A., Vachal, M., Hirsch, I., Domorazkova, A., Zavadova, H., et al. Prospective study on the relationship between cervical neoplasia and herpes simplex type-2 virus. I. Epidemiological characteristics. *Int. J. Cancer* 33: 49–60, **1984a**.

Vonka, V., Kanka, J,., Hirsch, I., Zavadova, H., Krcmar, M., Suchankova, A., Rezakova, D., Broucek, J., Press, M., Domorazkova, E., Svoboda, B., Havrankova, A., and Jelinek, J. Prospective study on the relationship between cervical neoplasia and herpes simplex type-2. II Herpes simplex virus type-2 antibody presence in sera taken at enrollment. *Int. J. Cancer* 33: 61–66, **1984b**.

Waubke, R., zur Hausen, H., and Henle, W. Chromosomal and autoradiographic studies of cells infected with herpes simplex virus. *J. Virol.* 2: 1047–1054, **1968**.

Whitley, R.J. Herpes simplex viruses. In: Fields, B.N., Knipe, P.M. and Howley, P.M. (Eds.), *Fields Virology*, Third Edition, Lippincott-Raven Publishers, Philadelphia, vol. 2: 2297–2343, **1996**.

Yamanishi, K., Matsunaga, Y., Ogino, T., and Lopetegui, P. Biochemical transformation of mouse cells by varicella-zoster virus. *J. Gen. Virol.* 56: 421–430, **1981**.

zur Hausen, H. DNA viruses in human cancer: biochemical approaches. *Cancer Res.* 36: 414–416, **1976**.

zur Hausen, H., Schulte-Holthausen, H., Wolf, H., Dörries, K., and Egger, H. Attempts to detect virus-specific DNA in human tumors: II. Nucleic acid hybridizations with complementary RNA of human herpes group viruses. *Int. J. Cancer* 13: 657–664, **1974**.

4.2
Betaherpesvirinae

4.2.1
Human Cytomegalovirus

Human CMV infects the majority of individuals in all human populations, results commonly in a latent infection, and is responsible for a large number of different clinical symptoms. Serological and molecular studies have attempted to link this infection to cervical carcinoma, to adenocarcinomas of the prostate and colon, and to Kaposi's sarcoma (reviewed in Doniger et al., 1999; Harkins et al., 2002; Samanta et al., 2003). These studies either yielded conflicting results or were based on individual reports. Detailed descriptions of its molecular biology and of the clinical symptoms caused by this infection have been published elsewhere (Mocarski, 1996; Britt and Alford, 1996).

Human CMV shares at least three properties with HSV infections: it induces chromosomal aberrations (Lüleci et al., 1980; AbuBakar et al., 1988; Deng et al., 1992) and amplifies the persisting DNA of polyoma-type viruses, SV40 (Pari and St. Jeor, 1990a,b) and human JC virus (Heilbronn et al., 1993), permitting replication of JC DNA in otherwise nonpermissive human fibroblasts. The enhancement of bovine papillomavirus (BPV)-induced transformation of NIH 3 T3 cells by co-infection with human CMV (Goldstein et al., 1987) seems to follow a different pattern, since amplification of BPV DNA was not noted in these experiments. Induction of specific chromosomal aberrations by human CMV has also been reported (Fortunato et al., 2000). The induction of host cell DNA synthesis by human CMV (St Jeor et al., 1978) seems to result in a subsequent block in cell cycle progression and cell division, mediated by the immediate early protein 86 (Murphy et al., 2000). Although the biological behavior of betaherpesvirinae differs substantially from that of HSV, transforming properties have also been reported for human CMV and HHV-6 infections. As another common property, similar to HSV, CMV and HHV type 6 also act as helper viruses for adeno-associated virus (McPherson et al., 1985).

Based on their data on transformation of hamster embryo cells by ultraviolet (UV)-irradiated HSV, Rapp and his colleagues initiated similar experiments with human CMV. In 1973, Albrecht and Rapp reported malignant transformation of hamster embryo fibroblasts following exposure to UV-irradiated human CMV. Induction of cellular DNA synthesis and increased mitotic activity was enhanced by irradiation with UV-light of the virus prior to infection (Albrecht et al., 1976). Three years later, the same group published the oncogenic transformation of human embryo lung cells by human CMV strain Mj (Geder et al., 1976). Here, the persistent infection of human embryonic lung fibroblasts with a genital isolate of CMV resulted in transformed human cells inducing progressively growing tumors in weanling athymic nude mice. The cells expressed virus-specific antigens, although at that time a potential contamination with transforming anogenital papillomavirus types could not be ruled out. An additional report claimed the transformation of human embryonic lung cells by additional CMV strains, BT1757 and Towne (Huang et al., 1986). A cell line obtained from human prostate cancer reacted positively with CMV-immune sera in indirect immunofluorescence (Geder et al., 1977). There was, however, no direct evidence that this cell line resulted from the exposure to human CMV. One of the transformation studies of human cells by CMV was subsequently clouded by the isolation of *infectious bovine rhinotracheitis virus* (IBRV) from the transformed human embryo lung fibroblasts (Geder et al., 1979). This virus apparently induced permanent growth upon infection of a primary human kidney cell culture. The apparent demonstration of intracellular immunofluorescent antigens specific for CMV resulted in the speculation that CMV might be involved in the development of prostatic neoplasia (Geder and Rapp, 1980). A CMV-induced transformation of human endothelial cells was reported by Smiley et al. (1988); CMV transformed these cells to anchorage-independent growth, persistently producing infectious CMV particles. Dog embryo kidney cells were also transformed by human CMV infection (Yelle et al., 1990). These cells are nonpermissive for this virus and, after infection, showed an unlimited division potential, and were poorly tumorigenic in mice.

Several additional reports stress a potential role of CMV in human cell proliferation: the cellular proto-oncogenes *fos, jun* and *myc* are transcriptionally transactivated by CMV infection (Boldogh et al., 1991). The prevention of apoptosis, mediated by viral immediate-early genes, may point to a role in indirect carcinogenesis (Zhu et al., 1995). The immediate-early genes IE 72 and IE 86 cooperate with adenovirus E1A in the transformation of baby rat kidney cells (Shen et al., 1997). Physical interaction of IE 86 with p53 has been noted without affecting p53-mediated cell cycle growth arrest (Bonin and McDougall, 1997). A similar interaction has been observed with pRb (Sommer et al., 1994; Fortunato et al., 1997).

In several studies the characterization of a transforming fragment of the human CMV genome was reported. Nelson et al. (1982) defined a 2.9-kilobase fragment between map units 0.123 and 0.14 on the prototype molecule of the CMV AD169 strain as transforming segment for NIH 3 T3 cells. This fragment was not retained within the transformed cells. The region was designated as "morphological transforming region I" (*mtr* I). A different fragment was identified by Clanton et al. (1983). By using a different CMV strain (Towne), their *Xba*I-E fragment immortalized primary diploid Syrian hamster cells and transformed established NIH 3 T3 cells. A sub-clone containing the 3.0 kbp *Xba*I-*Bam*HI EM fragment with efficient transforming activity was labeled as *mtr* II. A further characterization of the transforming part of the *Xba*I-E fragment published by *Clanton et al.*, revealed a small, potentially spliced open reading frame (ORF) which possessed some of the signals involved in eukaryotic gene expression (Kouzarides et al., 1983). Jariwalla et al. (1989) reported that the terminal fragments (EJ [designated as *mtr* III] and EM) of the XbaI-E segment of human CMV can independently induce tumorigenic conversion of immortalized Rat-2 cells. Both fragments cooperated in tumorigenic conversion, inducing foci at a tenfold higher frequency than the individual fragments. The transformants commonly retained the *mtr* II sequences, frequently in multiple copies, whereas *mtr* III or *mtr* I did not persist (el-Beik et al., 1986). The genomic organization of human CMV is outlined in Figure 4.2.

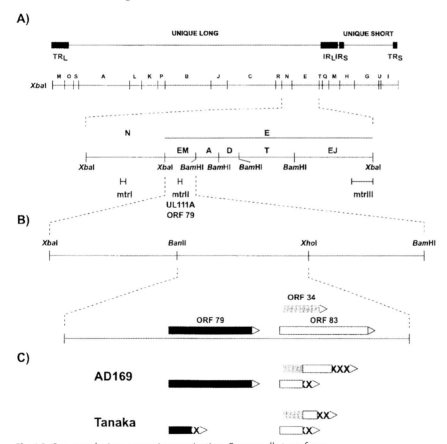

Fig. 4.2 Cytomegalovirus genomic organization. Supposedly transforming regions are indicated in the lower panel in black. (Doniger et al., 1999. With permission.)

The persistence of the *mtr* II region in immortalized and transformed cells promoted additional interest in these sequences. The transforming activity was further localized to a 980-bp subfragment with three ORFs with a coding capacity of 79, 83 and 34 amino acids (Razzaque et al., 1988). In the 5' terminus of the ORFs several regulatory elements and transcription initiation signals were located, in addition to six copies of the heptanucleotide sequence GGTG(A/G)TC. This motif has similarity to the SV40 enhancer core consensus sequence. All three putative proteins were observed 24 h after infection with CMV. Interruption of the *mtr* II ORF resulted in loss of transforming activity (Inamdar et al., 1992), strongly suggesting a direct involvement of these proteins in transformation and virtually excluding promoter insertion as mechanism for the observed transforming activity. Mutational analyses conducted by Thompson et al. (1994) pointed to a specific role of ORF 79 for the transforming activity of *mtr* II. An additional report (Muralidhar et al., 1996) claimed an interaction of mtr II protein with p53. mtr II also inhibited p53-activated transcription in transient transfection assays, as well as in transformed cells. In stably *mtr* II-transformed NIH 3 T3 cells the level of p53 was ten- to twenty-fold higher than in parental cells.

Based on these data, it is extremely difficult to assess a potential role for CMV in human carcinogenesis. Clearly, specific genes of this virus have transforming potential for rodent cells. The data on immortalization of human cells are not yet fully convincing and require further confirmation. The ubiquity of this infection, and its frequent persistence in normal and neoplastic tissues, makes it difficult to analyze any potential tumorigenicity. The situation might be reminiscent of infections with oncogenic human adenovirus types where, in spite of efficient tumor induction in rodents, no evidence for a role in human cancers has been obtained. Clearly, this field requires that further studies be conducted since, at present, there exists no convincing evidence for a direct role of CMV in human cancer, though an indirect contribution cannot be excluded.

4.2.2
Human Herpesvirus Type 6

Human herpesvirus type 6 (HHV-6) was initially named human B-lymphotropic virus (HBLV) and identified by Salahuddin et al. (1986) from patients with lymphoproliferative disorders or from HIV-positive individuals. This virus grows well in phytohemagglutinin-stimulated umbilical cord blood lymphocytes and T-cell lines, and requires interleukin (IL)-2 addition for efficient propagation (Black et al., 1989; Frenkel et al., 1990). HHV-6 is a ubiquitous virus which infects children at a young age, persisting subsequently and being found in at least 90% of all adults (Segondy et al., 1992; Portolani et al., 1993). It causes exanthema subitum and roseola ("sixth disease") in approximately 30% of infected children. Two subgroups of HHV-6 have been identified, namely HHV-6A and HHV-6B; these have an overall nucleotide identity of 90% (Dominguez et al., 1999), with a most divergent region in direct repeats (DR) and the right end of the unique region with 85% and 72% nucleotide sequence identity, respectively. A novel homologue of HHV-6B was isolated from chimpanzees, with about 95 % sequence homology at the nucleotide and amino acid levels (Lacoste et al., 2005). Recent studies have demonstrated a difference in the biological behavior of both subgroups: whereas HHV-6B virus depletes predominantly CD4[+] T cells, HHV-6A virus infection results in a depletion of both, CD4[+] and CD8[+] T cells (Grivel et al., 2003). HHV-6 has been suggested as a cofactor in HIV infections, as both viruses infect CD4 human T cells and accelerate the cytopathic effect (Lusso et al., 1989).

The original isolation of this virus from various malignant lymphatic disorders raised the suspicion of a possible etiologic involvement of this infection in those conditions. Indeed, especially in some lymphoproliferative disorders, increased antibody titers against HHV-6 antigens were demonstrated. Elevated HHV-6 titers were noted in acute myeloid leukemia (AML), Hodgkin's disease and low-grade non-Hodgkin lymphomas (NHL) (Clark et al., 1990), and in myelodysplasia and chronic myeloproliferative diseases (Krueger et al., 1994). For AML this was also reported by Gentile et al. (1999). Another study reported elevated titers in lymphoma, multiple myeloma and leukemia patients, but not in patients with solid tumors (Carricart et al., 2002). In children with acute lymphoblastic and myeloid leukemia, an elevated level of IgA antibodies against HHV-6 was noted (Salonen et al., 2002). In Hodgkin's disease, Alexander et al. (1995) showed a significant difference in geometric mean titers between Reed–Sternberg cell EBV-positive cases (mean titer 11.5) and those with Reed–Sternberg cell EBV-negative patients (mean titer 73.7), compared to a value in healthy individuals of 20.5. In another study, the pre-treatment sera of Hodgkin patients did not reveal significantly different antibody titers when compared to controls; however, the titers increased during the course of follow-up of patients who relapsed, but decreased significantly over time in patients who did not (Levine et al., 1992). In contrast to the demonstration of EBV latent membrane antigens in Reed–Sternberg cells of EBV-positive Hodgkin biopsies, HHV-6 antigens or viral DNA were not demonstrated in Reed–Sternberg cells of HHV-6 positive biopsies. Rather, they were restricted to macrophages and surrounding follicular cells (Maeda et al., 1993; Valente et al., 1996).

A number of studies reported an elevated level of positivity for HHV-6 DNA in patient materials from acute myeloid leukemias, NHL and Hodgkin's disease (Fillet et al., 1995; Valente et al., 1996; Pan et al., 1998; Schmidt et al., 2000; Hermouet et al., 2003). It is noteworthy that in some of these as well as in other studies, reactive lymph nodes were also found frequently to be positive for HHV-6 DNA (Borisch et al., 1991; Sumiyoshi et al., 1993; Valente et al., 1996). There exist additional reports of HHV-6 in lymphoproliferative disorders, particularly in AIDS-related lymphomas, contrasting the rarity of HHV-6 in HHV-8 positive primary effusion lymphomas (Asou et al., 2000). In addition, HHV-6 DNA has been noted in ocular lymphomas (Daibata et al., 2000), in B- and T-cell lymphomas (Ohyashiki et al., 1999), and in T-cell acute lymphoblastic leukemia (Luka et al., 1991). One report claims that HHV-6-positive Hodgkin biopsies are exclusively of the nodular sclerosis subtype of Hodgkin's disease (Collot et al., 2002). With regard to solid tumors, two reports have revealed the presence of HHV-6 DNA in some nasopharyngeal carcinoma tissue (Kositanont et al., 1993; Chen et al., 1999).

In our own studies (E.-M. de Villiers and H. zur Hausen, unpublished results), by using herpes consensus primers covering predominantly the herpes DNA polymerase region, we noted a relatively high percentage of positive bladder cancers (~10%), of gastric cancers (~12%), lung and rectum cancers (~15%), esophageal cancers (~20%), and of cancers of the colon (~28%). Biopsies from several other tumors were negative in this test series. The data obtained are shown in Figure 4.3.

It should be of substantial interest that HHV-6 infection trans-activates high-risk HPV gene expression in HPV-immortalized or malignant HPV-containing cervical carcinoma cell lines (Chen et al., 1994), and also trans-activates the HIV promoter (Horvat et al., 1989). A few reports describe an oncogenic potential of HHV-6. Full-length HHV-6 DNA or subgenomic clones transformed NIH 3 T3 cells to colony formation and tumorigenicity (Razzaque, 1990; Thompson et al., 1994). Neoplastic transformation was also recorded in immortalized human epidermal keratinocyte lines after transfection with subgenomic fragments of HHV-6 (Razzaque et al., 1993). The transforming region was localized by Kashanchi et al. (1997) to ORF-1 (DR-7) in the *Sal*I-*Hind*III subfragment of HHV-6 DNA. Western blot analysis confirmed the expression of ORF-1 in transformed NIH 3 T3 cells which produced fibrosarcomas in athymic nude mice. ORF-1 sequences were detected in five of 12 lymph nodes from patients with angioimmunoblastic lymphadenopathy, but rarely in tumor tissue. The protein coded for by ORF-1 (pORF-1) binds p53 (Kashanchi et al., 1997). ORF-1 is able to transactivate the minimal HIV-1 promoter (Kashanchi et al., 1994). In addition to the reported transforming activities, HHV-6A was shown to

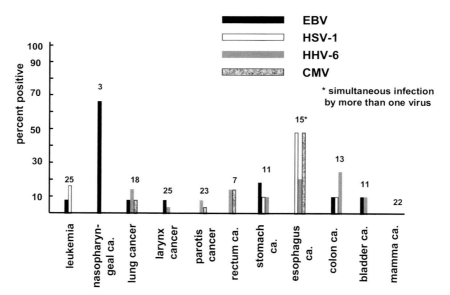

Fig. 4.3 Detection of various human herpes-group viruses in human tumor biopsies. The numbers at the top of the columns indicate the total number of biopsy materials tested from the respective tumor type. (E.-M. de Villiers and H. zur Hausen, unpublished data.)

contain a 1473-bp transformation suppressor gene that inhibits the transformation of NIH 3 T3 cells by H-ras and transcription of H-ras and HIV-1 promoters in transient transfection experiments (Araujo et al., 1997). This gene also down-regulates the BPV p89 and the HPV type 16 p97 promoter. Figure 16 shows The organization of the HHV-6 genome is illustrated in Figure 4.4.

Under certain conditions, HHV-6 appears able to integrate stably into host cell chromosomal DNA. Luppi et al. (1993) and Torelli et al. (1995) described the integration of HHV-6 sequences into the telomeric region of chromosome 17 in peripheral blood cells of individual cases of one Hodgkin lymphoma (among 55 cases investigated), one NHL (among 64 cases), and in one patient with multiple sclerosis (31 cases studied). A detailed analysis revealed chromosome band 17p13.3 as the integration site (Morris et al., 1999). It is interesting to note that HHV-6 DNA has been found integrated into various chromosomal sites, in a case of a woman with HHV-6 infected Burkitt's lymphoma in chromosome 22 q13 (Daibata et al., 1999). An EBV-negative, HHV-6-positive cell line was established from this Burkitt's lymphoma (Daibata et al., 1998a). The asymptomatic husband of this patient also carried HHV-6 DNA integrated into chromosome 1q44 of peripheral blood mononuclear cells.

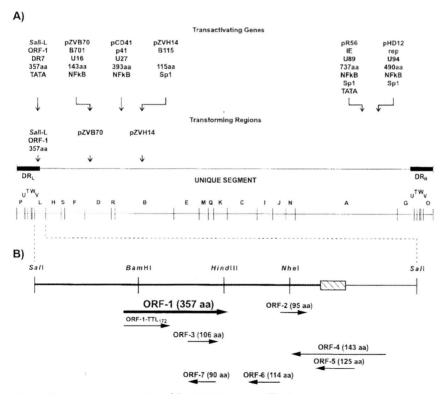

Fig. 4.4 Schematic representation of the HHV-6 genome. (Doniger et al., 1999. With permission.)

Their daughter had HHV-6 DNA in both chromosomes, 22q13 and 1q44. Another B- and T-cell line was established from a patient with acute lymphocytic leukemia after transformation with EBV or *herpesvirus saimiri*, respectively. Both cell lines contained integrated HHV-6 sequences, located in the long arm of chromosome 1q44 (Daibata et al., 1998 b). A summary of these results is provided in Table 4.1.

In 1991, Thomson and colleagues described the presence of the adeno-associated virus (AAV) type 2 *rep* gene within the HHV-6 genome. This gene is required for AAV-2 replication, and trans-regulates homologous and heterologous gene expression. It is also responsible for the AAV-mediated inhibition of cell transformation. The HHV-6 linked *rep* gene complements the replication of *rep*-deficient AAV-2 genomes and activates the LTR of HIV in fibroblast cell lines but not in T cells (Thomson et al., 1994). This contrasts the function of the native AAV-2 *rep* which inhibits the HIV LTR both, HIV LTR activity in fibroblasts and T cells. Thus, the properties of HHV-6 *rep* and AAV-2 *rep* are related, but not identical.

The rep sequence is found at the right end of the HHV-6 genome and is present in the A and B variants of HHV-6. Although 13 of the 17 ORFs at this right end differ in the amino acid composition derived from these ORF by more than 10%, the rep region differs by only 2.4% (Dominguez et al., 1999). This seems to point to an important function of this gene. In another investigation, HHV-6A and HHV-6B isolates differed in the *rep* gene by only 3.5% and 2.5% in nucleotide and amino acid sequence, respectively (Rapp et al., 2000). Seventeen clinical and geographical disparate isolates of HHV-6A differed in this region by between 0.2% and 0.6%, while 13 HHV-6B isolates were identical. Transcripts of this gene were present at low abundance (~10 copies per cell 3 days after infection). Mori et al. (2000) demonstrated three transcripts of the HHV-6 rep gene of 9.0, 5.0, and 2.7 kb, where the 2.7-kb transcript was most abundant. HHV-6 rep binds to the human TATA-binding protein

Table 4.1 Reports on the integration of HHV-6 DANN into host cell chromosomes

Human material	Chromosomal localization	Reference(s)
M. Hodgkin (peripheral blood lymphocytes – PBL)	17 p13.3	Luppi et al. (1993)
Non-Hodgkin lymphoma (PBL)	17 p13.3	Morris et al. (1999)
Multiple sclerosis (PBL)	17 p13.3	
Burkitt's lymphoma[a]	22 q13	Daibata et al. (1999)
Asymptomatic PBL[a]	1 q44	Daibata et al. (1998 a)
Asymptomatic PBL[b]	1 q44 and 22q13	Daibata et al. (1998 a)
Lymphocytic leukemia B- and T-cell line[c]	1 q44	Daibata et al. (1998 b)

[a] Wife and husband.
[b] Daughter of both.
[c] EBV-transformed B-cell line and Herpesvirus saimiri-transformed T-cell line.

through its N-terminal region. In Western blot analysis, an anti-rep monoclonal antibody recognized a 56-kDa polypeptide (Dhepakson et al., 2002). The same authors also demonstrated a binding activity of this protein to single-stranded DNA.

It seems that the role of the *rep* gene (U94) in HHV-6 relates to viral DNA persistence and to maintenance of the latent state. In HHV-6 infected lymphoid cell lines this gene was stably expressed in the absence of viral DNA replication (Rotola et al., 1998).

Overall, published data on cell transformation by HHV-6 are persuasive, but not fully convincing, and further studies are required in this respect. Nevertheless, the number of positive reports of HHV-6 DNA in a certain percentage of myeloid leukemias, NHL, and in Hodgkin's disease may point to a potential role of this virus in these malignancies. It should be noted that HHV-6, similar to HSV infections, is able to up-regulate HIV-1 expression by inducing the LTR activity of the latter virus (Ensoli et al., 1989; Campbell et al., 1991; Garzino-Demo et al., 1996). Under specific conditions of infection (e.g., of dendritic cells) however, HHV-6 may even suppress HIV replication (Carrigan et al., 1990; Asada et al., 1999). Conversely, the tat gene of HIV may enhance replication of HHV-6 (Sieczkowski et al., 1995). Until now, no reports have been published analyzing the potential activation of human endogenous retroviruses by HHV-6. It is interesting to note that HHV-6 replication – particularly in the leukemic HSB cell line – results in HHV-6 particles with the frequent attachment of exosome-like particles (Fig. 4.5). The nature of the latter has not yet been identified.

Although HHV-6 has frequently been noted in reactive lymph nodes, it seems interesting that this has rarely been found and incriminated in specific inflammatory conditions, such as morbus Crohn or polyarthritis. Except for efficiently transforming gamma-herpesviruses, however, it is presently very difficult to assess the role of other herpesvirus subfamilies, including herpes simplex and human CMV and VZV in human cancers.

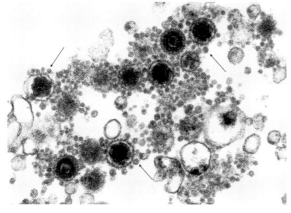

Fig. 4.5 HHV-6 particles with exosome-like particles attached.

References

AbuBakar, S., Au, W.W., Legator, M.S., and Albrecht, T. Induction of chromosome aberrations and mitotic arrest by cytomegalovirus in human cells. *Environ. Mol. Mutagen.* 12: 409–420, **1988**.

Albrecht, T., Nachtigal, M., St Jeor, S. C., and Rapp, F. Induction of cellular DNA synthesis and increased mitotic activity in Syrian hamster embryo cells abortively infected with human cytomegalovirus. *J. Gen. Virol.* 30: 167–177, **1976**.

Albrecht, T. and Rapp, F. Malignant transformation of hamster embryo fibroblasts following exposure to ultraviolet-irradiated human cytomegalovirus. *Virology* 55: 53–61, **1973**.

Alexander, F.E., Daniel, C.P., Armstrong, A.A., Clark, D.A., Onions, D.E., Cartwright, R.A., and Jarrett, R.F. Case clustering, Epstein–Barr virus Reed–Sternberg cell status and herpes virus serology in Hodgkin's disease: results of a case-control study. *Eur. J. Cancer* 31 A: 1479–1486, **1995**.

Araujo, J.C., Doniger, J., Stöppler, H., Sadaie, M.R., and Rosenthal, L.J. Cell lines containing and expressing the human herpesvirus 6A ts gene are protected from both H-ras and BPV-1 transformation. *Oncogene* 14: 937–943, **1997** .

Asada, H., Klaus-Kovtun, V., Golding, H., Katz, S. I., and Blauvelt, A. Human herpesvirus 6 infects dendritic cells and suppresses human immunodeficiency virus type 1 replication in coinfected cultures. *J. Virol.* 73: 4019–4028, **1999** .

Asou, H., Tasaka, T., Said, J.W., Daibata, M., Kamada, N., and Koeffler, H.P. Co-infection of HHV-6 and HHV-8 is rare in primary effusion lymphoma. *Leukemia Res.* 24: 59–61, **2000**.

Black, J.B., Sanderlin, K.C., Goldsmith, C.S., Gary, H.E., Lopez, C., and Pellett, P.E. Growth properties of human herpesvirus-6 strain Z29. *J. Virol. Methods* 26: 133–145, **1989**.

Boldogh, I., AbuBakar, S., Deng, C.Z., and Albrecht, T. Transcriptional activation of cellular oncogenes *fos, jun,* and *myc* by human cytomegalovirus. *J. Virol.* 65: 1568–1571, **1991**.

Bonin, L.R. and McDougall, J.K. Human cytomegalovirus IE2 86-kilodalton protein binds p53 but does not abrogate G1 checkpoint function. *J. Virol.* 71: 5861–5870, **1997**.

Borisch, B., Ellinger, K., Neipel, F., Fleckenstein, B., Kirchner, T., Ott, M.M., and Müller-Hermelink, H.K. Lymphadenitis and lymphoproliferative lesions associated with the human herpes virus-6 (HHV-6). *Virchows Arch. B Cell. Pathol. Incl. Mol. Pathol.* 61: 179–187, **1991**.

Britt, W.J. and Alford, C.A. Cytomegalovirus. In: Fields, B.N., Knipe, P.M. and Howley, P.M. (Eds.), *Fields Virology*, Third Edition, Lippincott-Raven Publishers, Philadelphia, vol. 2: 2493–2523, **1996**.

Campbell, M.E., McCorkindale, S., Everett, R.D., and Onions, D.E. Activation of gene expression by human herpesvirus 6 is reported gene-dependent. *J. Gen. Virol.* 72: 1123–1130, **1991**.

Carricart, S. E., Bustos, D.A., Grutadauria, S. L., Nates, S. V., Garcia, J.J., Yacci, M.R., Gendelman, H., and Pavan, J.V. [Human herpesvirus-6 circulation in healthy adults and oncologic patients] *Article in Spanish. Medicina (B. Aires)* 62: 9–12, **2002**.

Carrigan, D.R., Knox, K.K., and Tapper, M.A. Suppression of human immunodeficiency virus type 1 replication by human herpesvirus-6. *J. Infect. Dis.* 162: 844–851, **1990**.

Chen, X., Jian, S., and Wang, H. [The study on clinical significance of human herpesvirus 6 infection of NPC tissue] *Article in Chinese. Zhonghua Shi Yan He Lin Chuang Bing Du Xue Za Zhi.* 13: 262–265, **1999**.

Chen, M., Popescu, N., Woodworth, C., Berneman, Z., Corbellino, M., Lusso, P., Ablashi, D.V., and DiPaolo, J.A. Human herpesvirus 6 infects cervical epithelial cells and transactivates human papillomavirus gene expression. *J. Virol.* 68: 1173–1178, **1994**.

Clanton, D.J., Jariwalla, R.J., Kress, C., and Rosenthal, L.J. Neoplastic transformation by a cloned human cytomegalovirus DNA fragment uniquely homologous to one of the transforming regions of herpes simplex virus type 2. *Proc. Natl. Acad. Sci. USA* 80: 3826–3830, **1983**.

Clark, D.A., Alexander, F.E., McKinney, P.A., Roberts, B.E., O'Brian, C., Jarrett, R.F., Cartwright, R.A., and Onions, D.E. The seroepidemiology of human herpesvirus-6 (HHV-6) from a case-control study of leukaemia and lymphoma. *Int. J. Cancer* 45: 829–833, **1990**.

Collot, S., Petit, B., Bordessoule, D., Alain, S., Touati, M., Denis, F., and Ranger-Rogez, S. Real-time PCR for quantification of human herpesvirus 6 DNA from lymph nodes and saliva. *J. Clin. Microbiol.* 40: 2445–2451, **2002**.

Daibata, M., Komatsu, T., and Taguchi, H. Human herpesviruses in primary ocular lymphoma. *Leuk. Lymphoma* 37: 361–365, **2000**.

Daibata, M., Taguchi, T., Nemoto, Y., Taguchi, H. and Miyoshi, I. Inheritance of chromo-somally integrated human herpesvirus 6 DNA. *Blood,* 94: 1545–1549, **1999**.

Daibata, M., Taguchi, T., Kubononishi, I., Taguchi, H., and Miyoshi, I. Lymphoblas-toid cell lines with integrated human her-pesvirus type 6. *J. Hum. Virol.* 1: 475–481, **1998 b**.

Daibata, M., Taguchi, T., Taguchi, H. and Miyoshi, I. Integration of human her-pesvirus 6 in a Burkitt's lymphoma cell line. *Br. J. Haematol.* 102: 1307–1313, **1998 a**.

Deng, C., AbuBakar, S., Fons, M.P., Boldogh, I., and Albrecht, T. Modulation of the frequency of human cytomegalovirus-induced chromosome aberrations by camptothecin. *Virology* 189: 397–401, **1992**.

Dhepakson, P., Mori, Y., Jiang, Y.B., Huang, H.L., Akkapaiboon, P., Okuno, T., and Yamanashi, K. Human herpesvirus-6 rep/U94 gene product has single-stranded DNA-binding activity. *J. Gen. Virol.* 83: 847–854, **2002**.

Dominguez, G., Dambaugh, T.R., Stamey, F.R., Dewhurst, S., Inoue, N., and Pellett, P.E. Human herpesvirus 6 B genome sequence: coding content and comparison with human herpesvirus 6 A. *J. Virol.* 73: 8040–8052, **1999** .

Doniger, J., Muralidhar, S., and Rosenthal, L.J. Human cytomegalovirus and human herpesvirus 6 genes that transform and transactivate. *Clin. Microbiol. Rev.* 12: 367–382, **1999**.

el-Beik, T., Razzaque, A., Jariwalla, R., Cihlar, R.L., and Rosenthal, L.J. Multiple trans-forming regions of human cytome-galovirus DNA. *J. Virol.* 60: 645–652, **1986**.

Ensoli, B., Lusso, P., Schachter, F., Josephs, S. F., Rappaport, J., Negro, F., Gallo, R.C., and Wong-Staal, F. Human herpes virus-6 increases HIV-1 expression in co-infected T cells via nuclear factors binding to the HIV-1 enhancer. *EMBO J.* 8: 3019–3027, **1989**.

Fillet, A.M., Raphael, M., Visse, B., Audouin, J., Poirel, L., and Agut, H. Controlled study of human herpesvirus 6 detection in acquired immunodeficiency syndrome-associated non-Hodgkin's lymphoma. The French Study Group for HIV-Associated Tumors. *J. Med. Virol.* 45: 106–112, **1995**.

Fortunato, E.A., Dell'Aquila, M.L., and Spec-tor, D.H. Specific chromosome 1 breaks induced by human cytomegalovirus. *Proc. Natl. Acad. Sci. USA* 97: 853–858, **2000**.

Fortunato, E.A., Sommer, M.H., Yoder, K., and Spector, H.D. Identification of domains within the human cytome-galovirus major immediate-early 86-kilo-dalton-protein and the retinoblastoma pro-tein required for physical and functional interaction with each other. *J. Virol.* 71: 8176–8185, **1997**.

Frenkel, N., Schirmer, E.C., Katsafanas, G., and June, C.H. T-cell activation is required for efficient replication of human her-pesvirus 6. *J. Virol.* 64: 4598–4602, **1990**.

Garzino-Demo, A., Chen, M., Lusso, P., Ber-neman, Z., and DiPaolo, J.A. Enhance-ment of TAT-induced transactivation of the HIV-1 LTR by two genomic fragments of HIV-6. *J. Med. Virol.* 50: 20–24, **1996**.

Geder, K.M., Lausch, R., O'Neill, F., and Rapp, F. Oncogenic transformation of human embryo lung cells by human cytomegalovirus. *Science* 192: 1134–1137, **1976**.

Geder, L. and Rapp, F. Herpesviruses and prostate carcinogenesis. *Arch. Androl.* 4: 71–78, **1980**.

Geder, L., Lidda, R.L., Kreider, J.W., Sanford, E.J., and Rapp, F. Properties of human epithelioid cells established in vitro by a herpesvirus [IBRV(HMC)] isolated from cytomegalovirus-transformed human cells. *J. Natl. Cancer Inst.* 63: 1313–1321, **1979**.

Geder, L., Sanford, E.J., Rohner, T.J., and Rapp, F. Cytomegalovirus and cancer of the prostate: in vitro transformation of human cells. *Cancer Treat. Rep.* 61: 139–146, **1977**.

Gentile, G., Mele, A., Ragona, G., Faggioni, A., Zompetta, C., Tosti, M.E., Visani, G., Castelli, G., Pulsoni, A., Monarca, B., Martino, P., and Mandelli, F. Human herpesvirus-6 seroprevalence and leukaemias: a case-control study. GINEMA (Gruppo Italiano Malattie Ematologiche dell' Adulto). *Br. J. Cancer* 80: 1103–1106, **1999**.

Goldstein, S. C., Byrne, J.C., and Rabson, A.S. Human cytomegalovirus (HCMV) enhances bovine papilloma virus (BPV) transformation in vitro. *J. Med. Virol.* 23: 157–164, **1987**.

Grivel, J.-C., Santoro, F., Chen, S., Fagá, G., Malnati, M.S., Ito, Y., Margolis, L., and Lusso, P. Pathogenic effects of human herpesvirus 6 in human lymphoid tissue ex vivo. *J. Virol.* 77: 8280–8289, **2003**.

Harkins, L., Volk, A.L., Samanta, M., Mikolaenko, I., Britt, W.J., Bland, K.I., and Cobbs, C.S. Specific localisation of human cytomegalovirus nucleic acids and proteins in human colorectal cancer. *Lancet* 360: 1557–1563, **2002**.

Heilbronn, R. Albrecht, I., Stephan, S., Bürkle, A., and zur Hausen, H. Human cytomegalovirus induces JC virus replication in human fibroblasts. *Proc. Natl. Acad. Sci. USA* 90: 11406–11410, **1993**.

Hermouet, S., Sutton, C.A., Rose, T.M., Greenblatt R.J., Corre, I., Garand, R., Neves, A.M. Bataille, R., and Casey, J.W. Qualitative and quantitative analysis of human herpesviruses in chronic and acute B cell lymphocytic leukaemia and in multiple myeloma. *Leukemia* 17: 185–195, **2003**.

Horvat, R.T., Wood, C., and Balachandran, N. Transactivation of human immunodeficiency virus promoter by human herpesvirus 6. *J. Virol.* 63: 970–973, **1989**.

Huang, E., Davis, M.G., Baskar, J.F., and Huong, S. Molecular epidemiology and oncogenicity of human cytomegalovirus. In: Harris, C.C. (Ed.), *Biochemical and Molecular Epidemiology of Cancer.* Allan R. Liss, Inc. New York, NY, pp. 323–344, **1986**.

Inamdar, A., Thompson, J., Kashanchi, F., Doniger, J., Brady, J.N., and Rosenthal, L.J. Identification of two promoters within human cytomegalovirus morphologic transforming region II. *Intervirology* 34: 146–153, **1992**.

Jariwalla, R.J., Razzaque, A., Lawson, S., and Rosenthal, L.J. Tumor progression mediated by two cooperating DNA segments of human cytomegalovirus. *J. Virol.* 63: 425–428, **1989**.

Kashanchi, F., Araujo, J.C., Doniger, J., Muralidhar, S., Khleif, S., Mendelson, E., Thompson, J., Azumi, N., Brady, J.N., Luppi, M., Torelli, G., and Rosenthal, L.J. Human herpesvirus 6 (HHV-6) ORF-1 transactivating gene exhibits malignant transforming activity and its protein binds to p53. *Oncogene* 14; 359–367, **1997**.

Kashanchi, F., Thompson, J., Sadaie, M.R., Doniger, J., Duvall, J., Brady, J.N., and Rosenthal, L.J. Transcriptional activation of minimal HIV-1 promoter by ORF-1 protein expressed from the SalI-L fragment of human herpesvirus 6. *Virology* 201: 95–106, **1994**.

Kositanont, U., Kondo, K., Chongkolwatana, C., Metheetrairut, C., Puthavathana, P., Chantarakul, N., Wasi, C., and Yamanishi, K. Detection of Epstein–Barr virus DNA and HHV-6 DNA in tissue biopsies from patients with nasopharyngeal carcinoma by polymerase chain reaction. *Southeast Asian J. Trop. Med. Public Health* 24: 455–460, **1993**.

Kouzarides, T., Bankier, A.T., and Barrell, B.G. Nucleotide sequence of the transforming region of human cytomegalovirus. *Mol. Biol. Med.* 1: 47–58. **1983**.

Krueger, G.R., Kudlimay, D., Ramon, A., Klueppelberg, U., and Schumacher. K. Demonstration of active and latent Epstein–Barr virus and human herpesvirus-6 infections in bone marrow cells of patients with myelodysplasia and chronic myeloproliferative diseases. *In Vivo* 8: 533–542, **1994**.

Lacoste, V., Verschoor, E.J., Nerrienet, E., and Gessain, A. A novel homologue of human herpesvirus 6 in chimpanzees. *J. Gen. Virol.* 86: 2135–2140, **2005**.

Levine, P.H., Ebbesen, P., Ablashi, D.V., Saxinger, W.C., Nordentoft, A., and Connelly, R.R. Antibodies to human herpes virus 6 and clinical course in patients with Hodgkin's disease. *Int. J. Cancer* 51: 53–57, **1992**.

Luka, J., Pirruccello, S. J., and Kersey, J.H. HHV-6 genome in T-cell acute lymphoblastic leukaemia. *Lancet* 338: 1277–1278, **1991**.

Lüleci, G., Sakizli, M., and Günalp, A. Selective chromosomal damage caused by human cytomegalovirus. *Acta Virol.* 24: 341–345, **1980**.

Luppi, M., Marasca, R., Barozzi, P., Ferrari, S., Ceccherini-Nelli, L., Batoni, G., Merelli, E., and Torelli, G. Three cases of human herpesvirus-6 latent infection: integration of viral genome in peripheral blood mononuclear cell DNA. *J. Med. Virol.* 40: 44–52, **1993**.

Lusso, P., Ensoli, B., Markham, P.D., Ablashi, D.V., Salahuddin, S. Z., Tschachler, E., Wong-Staal, F., and Gallo, R.C. Productive dual infection of human CD4 + T lymphocytes by HIV-1 and HHV-6. *Nature* 337: 370–373, **1989**.

Maeda, A., Sata, T., Enzan, H., Tanaka, K., Wakiguchi, H., Kurashige, T., Yamanishi, K., and Kurata, T. The evidence of human herpesvirus 6 infection in the lymph nodes of Hodgkin's disease. *Virchows Arch. A Pathol. Anat. Histopathol.* 423: 71–75, **1993**.

McPherson, R.A., Rosenthal, L.J., and Rose, J.A. Human cytomegalovirus completely helps adeno-associated virus replication. *Virology* 147: 217–222, **1985**.

Mocarski, E.S., Jr. Cytomegaloviruses and their replication. In: Fields, B.N., Knipe, P.M. and Howley, P.M. (Eds.), *Fields Virology*, Third Edition, Lippincott-Raven Publishers, Philadelphia, vol. 2: 2447–2492, **1996**.

Mori, Y., Dhepakson, P., Shimamoto, T., Ueda, K., Gomi, Y., Tani, H., Matsuura, Y., and Yamanishi, K. Expression of human herpesvirus 6 B rep within infected cells and binding of its gene product to the TATA-binding protein in vitro and in vivo. *J. Virol.* 74: 6096–6104, **2000**.

Morris, C., Luppi, M., McDonald, M., Barozzi, P., and Torelli, G. Fine mapping of an apparently targeted latent human herpesvirus type 6 integration site in chromosome band 17 p13.3. *J. Med. Virol.* 58: 69–75, **1999**.

Muralidhar, S., Doniger, J., Mendelson, E., Araujo, J.C., Kashanchi, F., Azumi, N., Brady, J.N., and Rosenthal, L.J. Human cytomegalovirus mtrII oncoprotein binds to p53 and down-regulates p53-activated transcription. *J. Virol.* 70: 8691–8700, **1996**.

Murphy, E.A., Streblow, D.N., Nelson, J.A., and Stinski, M.F. The human cytomegalovirus IE86 protein can block cell cycle progression after inducing transition into the S phase of permissive cells. *J. Virol.* 74: 7108–7118, **2000**.

Nelson, J.A., Fleckenstein, B., Galloway, D.A., and McDougall, J.K. Transformation of NIH 3 T3 cells with cloned fragments of human cytomegalovirus strain AD169. *J. Virol.* 43: 83–91, **1982**.

Ohyashiki, J.H., Abe, K., Ojima, T., Wang, P., Zhou, C.F., Suzuki, A., Ohyashiki, K., and Yamamoto, K. Quantification of human herpesvirus 6 in healthy volunteers and patients with lymphoproliferative disorders by PCR-ELISA. *Leukemia Res.* 23: 625–630, **1999**.

Pan, F., Lu, H., and Fan, H. [Detection of type 6 human herpesvirus (HHV-6) specific DNA sequences in lymphoma tissues by PCR] *Article in Chinese*. *Zhonghua Zhong liu Za Zhi* 20: 196–198, **1998**.

Pari, G.S. and St Jeor, S. C. Effect of human cytomegalovirus on replication of SV40 origin and the expression of T antigen. *Virology* 177: 824–828, **1990 a**.

Pari, G.S. and St Jeor, S. C. Human cytomegalovirus major intermediate early gene product can induce SV40 DNA replication in human embryonic lung cells. *Virology* 179: 785–794, **1990 b**.

Portolani, M., Cermelli, C., Moroni, A., Bertolani, M.F., Di Luca, D., Cassai, E., and Sabbatini, A.M. Human herpesvirus-6 infections in infants admitted to hospital. *J. Med. Virol.* 39: 146–151, **1993**.

Rapp, J.C., Krug, L.T., Inoue, N., Dambaugh, T.R., and Pellett, P.E. U94, the human herpesvirus 6 homolog of the parvovirus nonstructural gene, is highly conserved among isolates and is expressed at low mRNA levels as a spliced transcript. *Virology* 268: 504–516, **2000**.

Razzaque, A. Oncogenic potential of human herpesvirus-6 DNA. *Oncogene* 5: 1365–1370, **1990**.

Razzaque, A., Jahan, N., McWeeney, D., Jariwalla, R.J., Jones, C., Brady, J., and Rosenthal, L.J. Localization and DNA sequence analysis of the transforming domain (mtr II) of human cytomegalovirus. *Proc. Natl. Acad. Sci. USA* 85: 5709–5713, **1988**.

Razzaque, A., Williams, O., Wang, J., and Rhim, J.S. Neoplastic transformation of immortalized human epidermal keratinocytes by two HHV-6 DNA clones. *Virology* 195: 113–120, **1993**.

Rotola, A., Ravaioli, T., Gonelli, A., Dewhurst, S., Cassai, E., and Di Luca, D. U94 of human herpesvirus 6 is expressed in latently infected peripheral blood mononuclear cells and blocks viral gene expression in transformed lymphocytes in culture. *Proc. Natl. Acad. Sci. USA* 95: 13 911–13 916, **1998**.

Salahuddin, S. Z., Ablashi, D.V., Markham, P.D., Josephs, S. F., Sturzenegger, S., Kaplan, M., Halligan, G., Biberfeld, P., Wong-Staal, F., Krammarsky, B. et al. Isolation of a new virus, HBLV, in patients with lymphoproliferative disorders. *Science* 234: 596–601, **1986**.

Salonen, M.J., Siimes, M.A., Salonen, E.M., Vaheri, A., and Koskiniemi, M. Antibody status to HHV-6 in children with leukaemia. *Leukemia* 16: 716–719, **2002**.

Samanta, M., Harkins, L., Klemm, K., Britt, W.J., and Cobbs, C.S. High prevalence of human cytomegalovirus in prostatic intraepithelial neoplasia and prostatic carcinoma. *J. Urol.* 170: 998–1002, **2003**.

Schmidt, C.A., Oettle, H., Peng, R., Binder, T., Wilborn, F., Huhn, D., Siegert, W., and Herbst, H. Presence of human β- and γ-herpes virus DNA in Hodgkin's disease. *Leukemia Res.* 24: 865–870, **2000**.

Segondy, M., Astruc, J., Atoui, N., Echenne, B., Robert, C., and Agut, H. Herpesvirus 6 infection in young children. *N. Engl. J. Med.* 327: 1099–1100, **1992**.

Shen, Y., Zhu, H., and Shenk, T. Human cytomegalovirus IE1 and IE2 proteins are mutagenic and mediate "hit-and-run" oncogenic transformation in cooperation with adenovirus E1A proteins. *Proc. Natl. Acad. Sci. USA* 94: 3341–3345, **1997**.

Sieczkowski, L., Chandran, B., and Wood, C. The human immunodeficiency virus tat gene enhances replication of human herpesvirus-6. *Virology* 211: 544–553, **1995**.

Smiley, M.L., Mar, E.C., and Huang, E.S. Cytomegalovirus infection and viral-induced transformation of human endothelial cells. *J. Med. Virol.* 25: 213–226, **1988**.

Sommer, M.H., Scully, A.L., and Spector, D.H. Transactivation by the human cytomegalovirus IE2 86-kilodalton protein requires a domain that binds to both the TATA-box binding protein and the retinoblastoma protein. *J. Virol.* 68: 6223–6231, **1994**.

St. Jeor, S. C., Hernandez, L., and Tocci, M. Cell DNA induction by human cytomegalovirus. *IARC Sci. Publ.* 24: 373–379, **1978**.

Sumiyoshi, Y., Kikuchi, M., Ohshima, K., Takeshita, M., Eizuru, Y., and Minamishima, Y. Analysis of human herpesvirus-6 genomes in lymphoid malignancy in Japan. *J. Clin. Pathol.* 46: 1137–1138, **1993**.

Thompson, J., Choudhury, S., Kashanchi, F., Doniger, J., Berneman, Z., Frenkel, N." and Rosenthal, L.J. A transforming fragment within the direct repeat region of human herpesvirus type 6 that transactivates HIV-1. *Oncogene* 9: 1167–1175, **1994**.

Thompson, J., Doniger, J., and Rosenthal, L.J. A 79 amino acid oncogene is responsible for human cytomegalovirus mtrII induced malignant transformation. *Arch. Virol.* 136: 161–172, **1994**.

Thomson, B.J., Efstathiou, S. and Honess, R.W. Acquisition of the human adeno-associated virus type-2 rep gene by human herpesvirus type-6. *Nature* 351: 78–80, **1991**.

Thomson, B.J., Weindler, F.W., Gray, D., Schwaab, V., and Heilbronn, R. Human herpesvirus 6 (HHV-6) is a helper virus for adeno-associated virus type 2 (AAV-2) and the AAV-2 rep gene homologue in HHV-6 can mediate AAV-2 DNA replication and regulate gene expression. *Virology* 204: 304–311, **1994**.

Torelli, G., Barozzi, P., Marasca, R., Cocconcelli, P., Merelli, E., Checcerini-Nelli, L., Ferrari, S., and Luppi, M. Targeted integration of human herpesvirus 6 in the p arm of chromosome 17 of human peripheral blood mononuclear cells in vivo. *J. Med. Virol.* 46: 178–188, **1995**.

Valente, G., Secchiero, P., Lusso, P., Abete, M.C., Jemma, C., Reato, G., Kerim, S., Gallo, R.C., and Palestro, G. Human herpesvirus 6 and Epstein–Barr virus in Hodgkin's disease: a controlled study by polymerase chain reaction and in situ hybridization. *Am. J. Pathol.* 149: 1501–1510, **1996**.

Yelle, J., Lussier, G., Pramatarova, A., and
  Hamelin, C. Low tumorigenicity of canine
  cells transformed by the human cytomegalovirus. *Biol. Cell* 70: 9–18, **1990**.

Zhu, H., Shen, Y., and Shenk, T. Human
  cytomegalovirus IE1 and IE2 proteins
  block apoptosis. *J. Virol.* 69: 7960–7970,
  1995.

4.3
Gammaherpesvirinae (Lymphocryptoviruses)

4.3.1
Epstein–Barr Virus

The Epstein–Barr virus (EBV) was initially seen by electron microscopy in lymphatic tissue culture cells derived from Burkitt's lymphoma (Epstein et al., 1964). The viral structure is illustrated in Figure 4.6. The virus could not be transmitted to other tissue cultures or common laboratory animals, nor did it infect the chorioallantoic membrane of embryonated chicken eggs. The development of an indirect immuno-fluorescence test to detect EBV-specific antigens (Henle and Henle, 1966) and the identification of the fluorescent cells as EBV-producing cells (zur Hausen et al., 1967), permitted an early approach to study the seroepidemiology of this infection. Within a short time it became clear that EBV represents a new member of the herpesvirus family, that infections with EBV are ubiquitous (Henle et al., 1969), and that close to 90% of the population became infected during childhood or adolescence. Two types of human cancers were detected initially with high antibody titers against EBV antigens, namely Burkitt's lymphoma (Henle et al., 1969) and nasopharyngeal cancer (Old et al., 1966; de Schryver et al., 1969). Shortly thereafter, EBV was recognized as the causative agent of infectious mononucleosis (Henle et al., 1968). The subsequent development of an immunofluorescence test to detect early EBV-induced antigens (Henle et al., 1970, 1971) showed again the specificity of a highly elevated immune response against EBV in patients with Burkitt's lymphoma or nasopharyngeal carcinoma. Electron micrographs showing EBV particles are shown in Figure 4.6.

Three other developments occurred during the late 1960s and early 1970s: a first biological function of EBV infections was identified in 1967 and 1968 (Henle et al., 1967; Pope et al., 1968), when these groups each revealed immortalizing activity of EBV-producing lethally X-irradiated Burkitt's lymphoma cells for human lymphocyte preparations in co-cultivation experiments or of cell-free filtrates from an EBV-producing leukemic cell line. In addition, zur Hausen and Schulte-Holthausen (1970) demonstrated persistence of EBV DNA in a "virus-free" cell line, Raji, of Burkitt's lymphoma origin. Shortly thereafter, the same group demonstrated EBV DNA in biopsies from Burkitt's lymphoma and from nasopharyngeal carcinomas (zur Hausen et al., 1970). Three years later, it was shown that EBV persists not only in cells of lymphatic origin, but also in epithelial nasopharyngeal carcinoma cells (Wolf et al., 1973). Viral DNA persistence in Burkitt's lymphomas was soon confirmed by Nonoyama and Pagano (1973), and in epithelial cells of nasopharyngeal carcinomas by Klein et al. (1974).

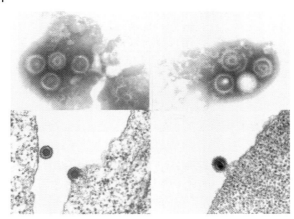

Fig. 4.6 Epstein–Barr virus particles seen in negative contrast staining (upper panel) and budding from the cell surface (lower panel). (Illustration courtesy of Birgit Hub, Heidelberg.)

Two other developments marked this period: the identification of a complement-fixing antigen in latently EBV-infected cells (Pope et al., 1969), and its demonstration by anticomplement immunofluorescence tests (Reedman and Klein, 1973). The other important step was the induction of lymphoproliferative disease resembling malignant lymphoma in cotton-top marmosets (Shope et al., 1973) and in owl monkeys (Epstein et al., 1973). At this time, the evidence was firm that EBV represents a HHV infection with carcinogenic potential, though the etiologic role for Burkitt's lymphomas and nasopharyngeal carcinomas remained questionable.

Today, this virus infection has been linked with several human malignancies, including B-cell lymphomas in immunocompromised patients, the endemic form of Burkitt's lymphomas, nasopharyngeal cancer, a subset of Hodgkin's lymphoma, with nasal natural killer (NK)/T-cell lymphomas, and with approximately 10% of gastric cancers. Data pertinent to EBV oncogenicity will be outlined in the following sections, while for a detailed account of the molecular biology of EBV infections the reader is referred to the reviews of Kieff (1996) and Rickinson and Kieff (1996).

4.3.1.1 Characterization of the Virus, and its Biological Properties

The complete nucleotide sequence of the double-stranded genome of EBV was initially determined for one specific EBV isolate (B95–8) with 172 282 base pairs (Baer et al., 1984), and subsequently for another EBV strain from nasopharyngeal carcinoma with 171 656 base pairs (bp) (Zeng et al., 2005). Among different isolates, the nucleotide sequence varies between 168 000 and 184 000 bp, and encodes more than 85 genes. Terminal repeat regions and an internal region of repeats of 3072 bp divide the genome into a short and a long unique region containing most of the genetic information (Cheung and Kieff, 1982). Upon latent infection of cells, the linear EBV genome circularizes with characteristic numbers of terminal repeats preserved from the parental genome.

Two subtypes of EBV have been identified (EBV-1 and EBV-2); these differ in genes coding for nuclear proteins EBNA-LP, -2, -3 A, -3 B, and -3 C, with differences in the predicted amino acid sequence of between 28 % and 47 % (Dambaugh et al., 1984; Adldinger et al., 1985; Sample et al., 1990). They also differ in their transforming activity; EBV-2 transforms B lymphocytes less efficiently than EBV-1, apparently due to the different amino acid composition of EBNA 2 (Rickinson et al., 1987; Cohen et al., 1989). There exists no clear-cut evidence for differences between the two EBV subtypes in pathogenicity, although about 85 % of nasopharyngeal carcinomas from Taiwan contain EBV-1 (Shu et al., 1992).

Although EBV was initially recognized as a B lymphotropic virus, it became clear recently that the virus can also infect epithelial cells, probably depending upon the production of specific glycoproteins, gHgL (Borza and Hutt-Fletcher, 1998; Borza et al., 2004) or gp 110 (Neuhierl et al., 2002). In most of the earlier publications in which the cell tropism of EBV was studied, viral preparations derived from the B95–8 line were used. This line resulted from EBV infection of marmoset leukocytes and produced spontaneously relatively high concentrations of EBV (Miller et al., 1972). EBV derived from these cells barely expresses gp110 (Gong et al., 1987), whereas EBV derived from some other lines, such as MA-BA (originating from a nasopharyngeal carcinoma patient) and Akata (originating from a Japanese Burkitt's lymphoma), produce high quantities of this protein and do infect epithelial cells (Neuhierl et al., 2002).

4.3.1.2 **EBV Gene Products in Latent Infection**

EBV gene products synthesized in latent infection are of particular interest in relation to the oncogenic properties of this virus. A number of gene products have been characterized which are expressed in specific tumors or in nontransformed, latently infected cells. Some of these share structural and functional homologies with cellular gene products, or interfere with the function of the latter. The nuclear EBNA-1 protein is consistently expressed. This is a sequence-specific DNA-binding phosphoprotein that fulfills a central role in the episomal maintenance of the EBV genome and is required for its DNA replication (Middleton and Sugden, 1994). At least in Burkitt's lymphoma cells it is a survival factor and prevents apoptosis (Kennedy et al., 2003). A role is also suggested for this protein in malignant transformation, by directing its expression to B cells of transgenic mice, where this results in B-cell lymphomas (Wilson et al., 1996).

EBNA-1 binds to the origin of replication within the EBV plasmid which contains two distinct EBNA-1 binding sites (Rawlins et al., 1985; Reisman et al., 1985; Jones et al., 1989; Ambinder et al., 1990). The EBNA-1 binding elements are located in a family of repeats and the dyad symmetry binding elements (Wysokenski and Yates, 1989). They contain multiple EBNA-1 binding sites each of 18 bp. The binding of EBNA-1 to the plasmid origin of replication may initiate viral DNA replication, with the additional aid of host cell enzymes (Frappier et al., 1994). The EBV origin of replication contains both, the initiation and termination sites of viral plasmid DNA replication (Gahn and Schildkraut, 1989). The EBNA-1 protein is divided into amino-and carboxy-terminal domains by a glycine-glycine-alanine repeat sequence, which varies in size for different EBV strains. This repeat domain acts as a cis inhibitor of MHC class I-restricted presentation, and blocks antigen processing in the ubiquitin/proteasome pathway (Levitskaya et al., 1995). EBNA-1 interacts and suppresses functions of the suppressor of metastasis and cell migration, Nm23-H1 (Murakami et al., 2005).

EBV deprived of EBNA-1 is able to induce B-cell proliferation, albeit with a 10 000-fold lower frequency than wild-type virus (Humme et al., 2003). Expression of dominant-negative derivatives of EBNA-1 decreases the survival of EBV virus-positive cells (Kennedy et al., 2003), this inhibition being due to the induction of apoptosis. Thus, EBNA-1 apparently prevents apoptosis in EBV-positive cells. Tumor induction by EBNA-1 in transgenic mice has been reported in these animals (Wilson et al., 1996), and EBNA-1 also appears to cooperate with myc in lymphomagenesis (Drotar et al., 2003). EBNA-1 transgenic mouse lymphocytes induce *BLC-xL* and *RAG* genes and reveal an enhanced response to IL-2 (Tsimbouri et al., 2002). Another study failed to confirm these data (Kang et al., 2005), though this may of course depend on the genetic background of the mouse strains used. Even in the negative study an increased level of pulmonary adenomas was noted in EBNA-1 transgenic lineages. The structure of the EBV genome is depicted in Figure 4.7.

EBNA-2 is a nuclear protein which plays a critical role in lymphatic cell immortalization, and also acts as a transcriptional coactivator. It regulates the expression of a number of viral and cellular genes (Ambinder et al., 1990). Deletion of the EBNA-2 gene covering also the last two exons of EBNA-LP in the transformation-defective

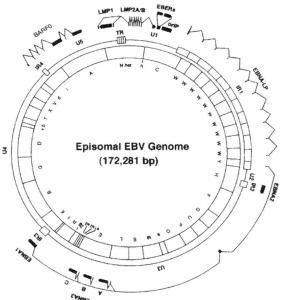

Fig. 4.7 The genome organization of the Epstein-Barr virus. (Reprinted from SEMINARS IN CANCER BIOLOGY, Vol 7, Issue 4, Osato, T. and Imai, S. Epstein-Barr virus and gastric carcinoma, 175–182. Copyright 1996, with permission from Elsevier.)

P3 HR-1 line initially revealed an important role for EBNA-2 in cell immortalization (Rabson et al., 1982; King et al., 1982). The correct location of the deletion was determined in the same year (Bornkamm et al., 1982). The reintroduction of EBNA-2 into this viral DNA resulted in restoration of the transforming properties, and emphasized the role of EBNA-2 in immortalization (Hammerschmidt and Sugden, 1989). EBNA-2 trans-activates a number of cellular genes, among them CD 23, CD 21, and *c-frg* (Wang et al., 1987 a; Cordier et al., 1990; Knutson, 1990). EBNA-2 abolishes the repression mediated by a protein complex including the DNA-binding Jκ-recombination binding protein (RBP-jκ) (Henkel et al., 1994; Grossman et al., 1994; Zimber-Strobl et al., 1994; Hsieh et al., 1995), and functionally replaces the intracellular region of Notch (Sakai et al., 1998). Conversely, Notch 1 IC partially replaces EBNA-2 function in EBNA-2 estrogen-dependent EBV-immortalized B cells (Gordadze et al., 2001). EBNA-2 also regulates the expression of other latency-associated EBV genes, namely LMP-1 and LMP-2 (Wang et al., 1987 b; Abbot et al., 1990; Fahraeus et al., 1990; Wang et al., 1990; Zimber-Strobl et al., 1990).

4.3.1.2.1 **LMP-1**

LMP-1 functions as a constitutively activated member of the tumor necrosis factor (TNF) receptor superfamily. This leads to the activation of several signaling pathways, including the NFκB transcription factor pathway, the MAP kinase cascade, the JAK/STAT, and the PI3 K/Akt pathways (Gires et al., 1999; Dawson et al., 2003; Young and Murray, 2003). This results in the up-regulation of anti-apoptotic proteins (e.g., BCL2 and A20) and the stimulation of cytokine production (Laherty et al., 1992; Eliopoulos et al., 1997, 1999). Although, with the exception of Burkitt's lymphomas, LMP-1 is expressed in most EBV-linked tumors, only 20–60% of nasopharyngeal cancers unequivocally are LMP-1 positive (Fahraeus et al., 1988; Niedobitek et al., 1992). LMP-1 induces several cellular chemokines, as for instance the interferon-γ-inducible protein 10 (IP-10) (Vockerodt et al., 2005) or CCL/RANTES (Uchihara et al., 2005). In addition, the two members of the inhibitor of differentiation (Id) family, Id1 and Id3, were also induced by expression of LMP-1 in C33 A and Rat-1 cells (Everly et al., 2004). A high level of LMP-1 expression can be induced by the ectopic expression of Rta, an immediate-early protein of EBV, initiating the lytic cycle (Chang et al., 2004). The expression of Rta is induced during the course of terminal differentiation of plasma cells (Laichalk and Thorley-Lawson, 2005).

4.3.1.2.2 **LMP-2 A**

LMP-2 A modulates the NFκB pathway (Stewart et al., 2004), and is consistently expressed in nasopharyngeal carcinomas. In tonsillar epithelial cells, LMP-2 A expression causes them to become migratory and invasive, and also enhances integrin-α-6 (ITGα6) expression (Pegtel et al., 2005). LMP-2 A is not essential for transformation of B lymphocytes (Tierney et al., 1994), but it interferes with B-cell receptor signaling (Dykstra et al., 2001). In primary B cells, the initiation of B-cell receptor signaling results in the activation of *Src* family protein tyrosine kinases and in the binding of *Syk* protein tyrosine kinases to the immunoreceptor tyrosine-based activation motifs (ITAM) present in the B-cell receptor (Kurosaki, 1999; Benschop and Cambier, 1999). LMP-2 A shares some of these properties, but renders B cells unresponsive to stimulation by B-cell receptor and prevents the reactivation of EBV virus from latency following surface immunoglobulin crosslinking (Miller, C.L. et al., 1994). LMP-2 A inhibits the autocrine secretion of IL-6, which seems to result from its property of negatively modulating the expression of NFκB (Stewart et al., 2004). In epithelial cells, the expression of LMP-2 A as well as LMP-2 B is associated with an increased capacity of the cells to spread and migrate on extracellular matrix (Allen et al., 2005).

The cellular transcription factor NF-κB seems to play a central role in all EBV-associated tumors. It fulfills several functions in these conditions, besides inhibiting the lytic replication of gammaherpesviruses (Brown et al., 2003): it is constitutively activated by LMP-1 (Eliopoulos et al., 2003; Thornburg et al., 2003), its activity is required for the deregulation of the rearranged c-myc expression in Burkitt's lymphoma cells by activating the immunoglobulin heavy chain enhancer (Ji et al., 1994; Kanda et al., 2000). Finally, its expression regulates the anti-apoptotic activity mediated by LMP-1 (Devergne et al., 1998; D'Souza et al., 2004).

4.3.1.2.3 **LMP-2 B**

The LMP-2 B and LMP-1 promoters are separated by 200 bp, and act bidirectionally. The function of LMP-2 B has been relatively poorly analyzed. It has been reported that mutations in either LMP-1 or LMP-2 do not affect the immortalizing activity for EBV in human lymphocytes, nor do they modify the growth properties of the immortalized cells in tissue culture (Kim and Yates, 1993; Longnecker et al., 1993). A more recent publication, however, documents that the LMP-2 A gene is important for efficient B-cell immortalization (Brielmeier et al., 1996).

Besides EBNA-1, EBNA-2, LMP-1 and LMP-2 A and -2 B, at least eight additional EBV genes are active in latent infection. Two of these code for small non-polyadenylated RNAs, EBER 1 and EBER 2, while four others code for EBNA 3 A, 3 B, 3 C, and LP. The EBNA 3 A, 3 B and 3 C genes are tandemly placed within the EBV genome. Their RNAs initiate at the CP or Wp EBNA promoters and represent the least abundant EBNA mRNAs. They accumulate in the nuclei and localize in clumps sparing the nucleoli (Hennessy et al., 1983, 1986; Kallin et al., 1986; Petti and Kieff, 1988; Petti et al., 1990). EBNA 3 C can up-regulate CD21 mRNA and LMP-1 expression (Wang et al., 1990; Allday et al., 1993). EBNA 3 A and EBNA-3 C are essential for B-cell immortalization (Tomkinson et al., 1993), and EBNA 3 C cooperates with RAS in rodent fibroblast transformation (Parker et al., 1996). EBNA 3 B has been reported to bind retinoblastoma and p53 proteins (Szekely et al., 1993), and may thus play an important additional role in transformation events.

EBNA LP, besides EBNA 2, represents the first viral protein expressed in B-lymphocyte infection (Alfieri et al., 1991). It is a nuclear protein which is partly spread through the nucleus, and partly concentrated in small nuclear granules

(Wang et al., 1987 a; Petti et al., 1990). It seems to cooperate with EBNA-2 in cell immortalization (Hammerschmidt and Sugden, 1989; Mannick et al., 1991). A recent study shows that the EBNA LP protein binds p14 ARF, a nucleolar protein that regulates the p53 pathway. In addition, it binds the v-fos transformation effector FTE (FTe-1/S3 a) which enhances v-fos-mediated cellular transformation (Kashuba et al., 2005). EBV-induced B-cell transformation leads to the up-regulation of FTe/S3 a.

4.3.1.2.4 **EBER 1 and EBER 2**

Recently, an important role of the commonly abundant EBER transcripts was reported which remain, however, untranslated (Takada and Nanbo, 2001). These authors postulated a key role for those transcripts in maintaining the malignant phenotype of Burkitt's lymphoma cells. According to their results, the EBERs confer clonability in soft agarose, tumorigenicity in nude mice, and resistance to interferon-α-induced apoptosis (Nanbo et al., 2002). EBER also confers resistance to apoptosis mediated through Fas by blocking the PKR pathway (Nanbo et al., 2005). In addition, EBER transcripts induce transcription of IL-10, acting as an autocrine growth factor in Burkitt's lymphomas (Takada and Nanbo, 2001). The putative secondary structure of EBER-1 and Eber-2 was published by Rosa et al. (1981) (see Fig. 4.8).

Other abundantly expressed RNA is transcribed from the *Bam*H1 region of the EBV genome. This family of spliced transcripts is commonly designated as *Bam*H1 A rightward transcripts (BARTs). They are expressed in all EBV latency programs whose TATA-less promoter regions reveal different expression patterns in epithelial and B cells (Chen et al., 2005). They contain ORFs, although no BART-pro-

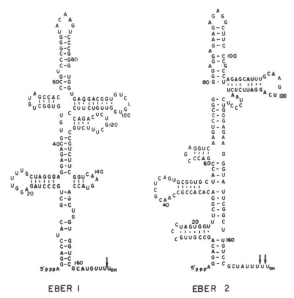

EBER I

EBER 2

Fig. 4.8 Putative structure of EBER transcripts. (Rosa et al., 1981. With permission.)

tein has yet been identified (Karran et al., 1992; Smith et al., 2000). Recently, *micro RNAs* originating from the intronic regions of the *BART* gene, were detected in all latent stages which seem to target regulators of cell proliferation and apoptosis, B-cell-specific chemokines and cytokines, transcriptional regulators and components of signal transduction pathways (Pfeffer et al., 2004). Three other regions coding for microRNAs were discovered in the BHRF1 (*Bam*H1 fragment H rightward open reading frame 1) gene. These three other regions appear to be preferentially active in lytic infections.

An additional transcript from the *Bam*H1 A region is represented by *BARF-1*, encoding a 31-kDa protein, mainly found in nasopharyngeal and EBV-positive gastric carcinomas (Decaussin et al., 2000; zur Hausen et al., 2000). *BARF-1* shares some homology with human colony-stimulating factor 1 receptor, and is able to transform rodent fibroblasts and simian primary epithelial cells (Sheng et al., 2001). Another transcript from this region, *BARF-0*, codes for a 279-amino acid protein. It interacts with cellular Notch and epithelin and mediates their proteasome-dependent degradation (Thornburg et al., 2004).

Several viral proteins share some homology with cellular genes, and some of these are expressed in lytic infections. Thus, the BCRF-1 protein reveals an 84% homology with human IL-10 (Vieira et al., 1991). The latter is known as an activation factor for B-cell proliferation (Miyazaki et al., 1993). Another EBV protein (BDLF2) which has been detected in oral hairy leukoplakia shares some homology with human cyclin B1 (Hayes et al., 1999). BHRF-1 shows a limited degree of homology with BCL-2 (Henderson et al., 1993). In addition, BARF-1 reveals some homology with intracellular adhesion molecule 1 and with the human colony-stimulating factor 1 receptor (Strockbine et al., 1998). It seems likely that further structural and even more functional homologies will be discovered in the future, permitting the persistent EBV to interfere specifically with host cell signaling pathways.

4.3.1.3 Transforming Properties of EBV and Tumor Induction in Animals

Since the initial studies by Henle and colleagues (1967) on the transformation of human lymphocytes by co-cultivation with X-irradiated EBV-producing Burkitt's lymphoma cells and by cell-free filtrates of EBV-positive cells (Pope et al., 1968), the transforming properties of EBV have been intensively investigated. The virus is extremely effective in immortalizing B lymphocytes. Since most human adults carry latently infected B cells in their peripheral blood, outgrowth of these cells can be readily achieved, particularly by depleting or inactivating accompanying T cells (von Knebel Doeberitz et al., 1983).

Interestingly, a number of different EBV-coded proteins possess immortalizing properties, at least for specific cell types. Immortalized B lymphoblasts express the six EBV nuclear antigens (EBNA 1, 2, 3 A, 3 B, 3 C and LP) and also three latent membrane proteins (LMP-1, -2 A and -2 B). In addition, small, non-polyadenylated RNAs, EBER-1 and EBER-2 are abundantly expressed. A list of EBV latency-associated proteins and their partly putative functions is provided in Table 4.2.

Table 4.2 Gene products of Epstein-Barr virus expressed in
viral latency[a]

Gene	Protein or RNA function	Engaged in immortalization
EBNA-1	Transcriptional regulation of other EBNAs maintenance and replication of EBV episomes	Survival factor for EBV-positive BLs, B-cell lymphomas in transgenic mice
EBNA-2	Interaction with RBP-Jκ, activation of LMP-1 and LMP-2A and the cellular gene CD23	Essential component for B-cell immortalization
EBNA-3A EBNA-3C	Disruption of cell cycle checkpoints Cooperation with RAS	Essential for B-cell immortalization. EBNA-3C with Ras transforms rodent cells
EBNA-3B	Interaction with RB2/p130 and p53	Interruption of checkpoint control
EBNA-LP	Interacts with EBNA-2	Mediates efficient transformation of B-cells
LMP-1	Activation of several cellular pathways and of anti-apoptotic proteins and cytokines	Main transforming protein of EBV, a "classic" oncogene
LMP-2A	Drives proliferation and survival of B-cells receptor (BCR)	Non-essential for immortalization
LMP-2B	Similar functions as LMP-2A (?)	Non-essential for immortalization
EBER-1 EBER-2	May inhibit ds-stranded RNA – activated Protein kinase (PKR), induce interleukin-10, inhibit apoptosis	Increase tumorigenicity of BL-cell lines
BART	RNA of unknown function	No evidence
BARF-1	31 kDa protein, shares homology with human colony-stimulating factor 1	Expressed in nasopharyngeal and gastric cancers

[a] Modified from *Young and Rickinson (2004)*.

EBNA-1, EBNA-2, EBNA-3 A, EBNA3 C, and LMP-1 emerge as essential components for the immortalization of B lymphoblasts. The amino-terminal domains of EBNA-3A, 3B, and 3C interact with RBP-Jκ (Robertson et al., 1996). For EBNAs 3A and 3C, it has been shown that these proteins repress RBP-Jκ-EBNA-2-activated transcription by inhibiting the binding of RBP-Jκ to DNA (Waltzer et al., 1996). In addition, EBNA-3C binds Nm23-H1, a known suppressor of cell migration and metastasis, and up-regulates metallomatrix proteinase-9 (MMP-9) (Kuppers et al., 2005). EBNA 3 C also mediates coactivation of the LMP-1 promoter with EBNA-2 (Lin et al., 2002). A number of additional interactions of these EBNAs with cellular proteins have been described (Rosendorff et al., 2004).

Although the immortalization of B lymphoblasts by EBV is remarkably efficient, the cloning of immortalized cells is relatively difficult. It appears that several of the EBV-infected and growth-stimulated lymphoblasts go into crisis (Counter et al.,

1994; Sugimoto et al., 1999). Those which survive stabilize relatively short telomeres and retain telomerase activity in later passages. The genetic background of the lymphocyte donor appears to affect the frequency of immortalizing events (Sugimoto et al., 2004). During the early stages most of the immortalized lines are diploid and nontumorigenic when inoculated into nude mice; chromosomal rearrangements may occur during later passages.

Early experimental proof for a tumorigenic function of EBV was obtained after inoculation of EBV into cotton-top tamarins (*Sanguinus oedipus*) (Shope et al., 1973) and owl monkeys (*Aotus trivirgatus*) (Epstein et al., 1973). These animals develop a lethal lymphoproliferative disorder resembling immunoblastic lymphoma in humans. The tumors are either mono- or oligoclonal (Zhang et al., 1993). The proliferating cells express EBNA-1, EBNA-2, and EBNA-LP, as well as LMP-1 (Young et al., 1989), and EBV-containing cell lines are readily established from diseased animals. Occasionally, even latent EBV infection without lymphoma development was noted in a cotton-top tamarin (Niedobitek et al., 1994). A poorly defined mononucleosis-like syndrome has been reported after EBV infection of the common marmoset (*Callithrix jaccus*) (Wedderburn et al., 1984).

Another animal model which works surprisingly well results from human B- and T- cell-reconstituted severe combined immunodeficient (SCID) mice. If the human lymphocytes originate from EBV-positive donors, the animals frequently develop a B-cell lymphoproliferative disease within 8–16 weeks (Mosier et al., 1988). This model represents a convenient system to analyze therapeutic interferences with these lymphoproliferations.

Virtually all Old World monkeys and nonhuman primates harbor species-specific EBV-like agents as natural persisting infections. They all reveal extensive regions of homology with human EBV. To date, 30 different lymphocryptoviruses have been detected in nonhuman primates by using a panherpesvirus PCR assay (Ehlers et al., 2003). Although no obvious pathogenicity has been observed in these infections, immunosuppression induced by simian immunodeficiency virus (SIV) in cynomolgus monkeys (*Macaca fascicularis*) results in these animals in the development of immunoblastic B-cell lymphomas, driven by a species-specific EBV-related herpesvirus (Feichtinger et al., 1992; Schatzl et al., 1993).

It is interesting to note that EBV infection apparently trans-activates the human endogenous retrovirus HERV-K18 (Sutkowski et al., 2001). The *env* gene of the latter possesses superantigen activity.

4.3.1.4 Various Stages of Epstein–Barr Viral Latency

Shortly after the first identification of viral gene products in latent infection, it was recognized that the expression pattern of viral DNA in EBV-immortalized lines is different from that of Burkitt's lymphoma cells and other EBV-positive tumor types (Rowe et al., 1987). Three different latency patterns emerged from this and additional studies.

- Latency pattern I was first analyzed in Burkitt's lymphoma cells (Rooney et al., 1986; Rowe, D. et al., 1986; Rowe, M. et al., 1987; Kerr et al., 1992). This stage is characterized by the expression of EBNA-1, EBER and BARF RNA. While the Cp/Wp promoters are silenced, the downstream promoter FQp is activated, initiating the transcription of EBNA-1 mRNA with a unique splice structure (Schaefer et al., 1991; Sample et al., 1991). The expression of LMP transcripts is abrogated; this gene expression pattern seems to be specific for Burkitt's lymphoma cells. Body cavity lymphomas, carrying HHV type 8 and EBV genomes also express the EBV type I pattern (see Section 4.4.1).
- Latency pattern II was recognized in the following EBV-positive tumor types: nasopharyngeal carcinoma, Hodgkin's disease, gastric cancer and T-cell lymphomas (Contreras-Brodin et al., 1991; Kerr et al., 1992). Here again, the EBER and *Bam*H1 RNAs are expressed, the Cp/Wp promoters are silenced, and FQp is activated as in the previous latency pattern. In contrast to the latter, however, LMP promoters are activated, resulting in the expression of LMP-1 and also in several biopsies of LMP-2 A and/or LMP-2 B (Kerr et al., 1992).
- The expression of viral latency genes in EBV-immortalized lymphoblastoid cells and in immunoblastic lymphomas has been described as latency pattern III. Here, all genes listed in Table 4.3 are expressed.

There seems to exist a fourth latency pattern, here tentatively labeled as latency 0: it has been demonstrated that EBV persists in resting memory B cells in the blood (Babcock et al., 1998; Joseph et al., 2000). It has also been anticipated that the latently EBV-infected cells would produce solely EBNA-1 which would not be recognized by cytotoxic T cells (Levitskaya et al., 1995). Recently, however, evidence has been pres-

Table 4.3 Various stages of Epstein-Barr virus latency[a]

Pattern	Cell type	Mode of expression
I	Burkitt's lymphoma	EBNA-1, EBER-RNA, BART-RNA Cp/Wp promoter silenced, Qp promoter activated
II	NPC, gastric cancer, HD, T-cell lymphomas	EBNA-1, EBER-RNA, BART-RNA Cp/Wp promoter silenced, Qp promoter activated. LMP-1, in several biopsies also LMP-2 A and LMP 2 B
III	Immunoblastic lymphoma	EBNAs 1, 2, 3 A, 3 B, 3 C, EBNA-LP, LMP-1, 2 A, 2 B Cp/Wp promoter active EBER and BART RNA, BARF
0	Resting memory cells (Hochberg et al. 2004)	EBNA-1 only during cell division (Laichalk and Thorley-Lawson, 2005)

[a] Modified from *Young and Rickinson (2004)*.

76 4 *Herpesviruses and Oncogenesis*

ented for a virtual null expression of EBV genes in resting memory cells (Hochberg et al., 2004). These cells start to produce EBNA-1 if stimulated for cell division. Since the dividing cells seem to produce solely EBNA-1, this led to the speculation that Burkitt's lymphoma (see below) originates from memory B cells but differs from them because of the constitutive expression of EBNA-1. According to the same research group, cell differentiation into plasma cells also regulates the switch from viral latency to a replicative cycle of the virus (Laichalk and Thorley-Lawson, 2005).

4.3.1.5 EBV in Infectious Mononucleosis

Epstein–Barr virus has been identified as the causative agent of infectious mononucleosis (Henle et al., 1968), a self-limiting lymphoproliferative disease, developing as the consequence of hyperproliferation of EBV-containing B cells and a reactive T-cell response. The primary infection frequently occurs during the first years of life (Henle et al., 1969 b; Lang et al., 1977), and is often not noticed by the infected person. Particularly in young adults, previously growing up in a hygienically protected environment, the primary EBV infection more regularly leads to sometimes severe symptoms of infectious mononucleosis. The transmission occurs in most cases orally via the saliva. This resulted in the original name for infectious mononucleosis as *college* or *kissing disease* (Hoagland, 1955). Cell-free virus is detectable in the throat washings and saliva of acute infectious mononucleosis patients, and there exist indications that initial rounds of viral replication occur in epithelial cells lining the tongue, the nasopharynx and the parotid duct (Chang and Golden, 1971; Gerber et al., 1972; Morgan et al., 1979; Sixbey et al., 1984; Wolf et al., 1984). Subsequently, in a still asymptomatic phase, the virus colonizes the B-lymphoid system, before a later dominating reactive T-cell response results in the typical clinical symptoms. The state of infected B lymphoblasts corresponds to EBV latency state III and thus seems to correspond to *in-vitro* EBV-immortalized B cells (Tierney et al., 1994).

The immunological responses to EBV infection in patients with infectious mononucleosis or in symptom-free carriers have been described extensively (Henle and Henle, 1979), and are only briefly recorded here: an early transient IgM-response against viral capsid antigen (VCA) is quickly followed by IgG antibodies to VCA which persist in most cases for lifetime. Similarly neutralizing antibodies persist. Antibodies against early antigens (EA) are frequently noted in the symptom phase and either disappear later or persist at a low level The development of EBNA-2 and in particular of EBNA-1 antibodies follows at a somewhat later stage, and commonly results in their life-long persistence. Cytotoxic T lymphocyte levels are high during the acute phase of infectious mononucleosis and remain at a lower level in the asymptomatic carrier state.

The primary infection with EBV results in a carrier state for the patient's life time and in a low level of continuous virus secretion into the saliva. This explains the remarkable success of this virus in infecting more than 90% of the world population. The high global prevalence of this infection has caused substantial problems in explaining its role in malignant diseases, specifically in view of the wide variation in geographic endemicity of some of the EBV-linked cancers.

4.3.1.6 EBV in X-Chromosome-Linked Lymphoproliferative Disease

The X-linked lymphoproliferative (XLP) syndrome can be characterized as a rare inherited immunodeficiency, initially described by Purtilo et al. (1975) as an inappropriate response to EBV infection. The disease typically affects young boys, and results in a fulminant EBV-caused infectious mononucleosis with usually fatal outcome, malignant B-cell lymphomas, and dysgammaglobulinemia. More than 70% of these patients die before the age of 10 years (Seemayer et al., 1995). In individuals not infected by EBV, other lymphoproliferative disorders, such as malignant lymphomas and lymphoid vasculitis are noted (Morra et al., 2001a).

In 1998, three groups identified a mutated gene in XLP (Coffey et al., 1998; Nichols et al., 1998; Sayos et al., 1998). This gene maps to the X chromosome at Xq25, receiving initially three different designations (*SAP, SH2D1A, DSHP*), and is presently labeled as *SAP* (signaling lymphocytic activation molecule [*SLAM*]-associated protein). It contains four exons coding for a protein of 128 amino acids. Its expression is mainly restricted to T and NK cells. Memory B cells also seem to express SAP (Feldhahn et al., 2002). A wide range of different mutations within the *SAP* gene is observed in XLP patients (Morra et al., 2001a). Some of these cause premature stops, others result in reduced stability of the SAP protein, and still others affect the *SAP* function. Although those mutations are clearly linked to the XLP-phenotype with a family history of more than one case, approximately 30–50% of XLP patients do not reveal detectable *SAP* mutations (Latour and Veilette, 2003). These are commonly patients with no family history of XLP (Sumegi et al., 2000).

SAP contains a single SH2 domain with a 28-amino acid tail (Morra et al., 2001b) which binds to tyrosine 327 of SLAM after previous phosphorylation (Li et al., 2003). SAP expression emerges as an absolute requirement for SLAM-triggered protein tyrosine phosphorylation events in T cells (Latour et al., 2001). This function reflects the specific capacity of SAP to recruit and activate the src-related protein tyrosine kinase FynT. This interaction is critical for further signaling by SLAM and its modulation of cytokine production. For a detailed description of the events involved, the reader is referred to reviews by Latour and Veilette (2003) or Engel et al. (2003).

The failing function of the SAP/SLAM complex or its absence emerges as a reason for the inability of the immune system to cope with EBV-immortalized cells or cells potentially modified by other as yet putative agents engaged in lymphomagenesis. Thus, XLP represents a beautiful example where molecular biology and immunology clarified at least an important part of the underlying cause of a serious lymphoproliferative condition, triggered in many cases by EBV infections.

4.3.1.7 EBV in Immunoblastic Lymphoma

Non-Hodgkin lymphoma (NHL), besides lung cancers and melanomas, represents the fastest rising malignancies in most parts of the Western world. In the United States, they account for approximately 4% of all cancers (Vose et al., 2002). The overall incidence is about 50% higher for males than for females. The incidence rates in whites are about 35 % higher than in blacks. In children, NHLs account for 10.9 % of childhood cancers in the United States (Linet et al., 1999).

NHL are particularly frequent under conditions of immunosuppression: in patients receiving immunosuppressive drugs after undergoing organ or bone marrow allografting the relative risk is increased 30- to 50-fold (Young, 1989; Hoover, 1992). In HIV-infected patients the risk is even more than 100-fold higher than that of the general population (Beral et al., 1991). NHL is the most frequent malignancy in persons with Wiskott–Aldrich syndrome, ataxia teleangiectasia, XLP syndrome and combined immunodeficiencies (Filipovich et al., 1992; Vose et al., 2002). With the recent developments of HIV-antiviral therapy and increasing CD4+ T-cell counts, the frequency of immunoblastic lymphomas decreased substantially, whereas the rate of Burkitt and Burkitt-like lymphomas with Ig/myc translocations remained constant (G. Klein, personal communication).

With the exception of Burkitt's lymphomas, spontaneously arising lymphomas in immunocompetent individuals are commonly EBV-negative. In immunosuppressed patients, however, the situation is remarkably different: the majority of arising NHLs is of B-cell origin, contains EBV genomes, and reveals most often the latency III expression pattern of EBV gene expression (Young et al., 1989). In the early phase of immunosuppression, EBV infection or reactivation leads to a polyclonal expansion, while additional genetic changes acquired subsequently (in particular of the BCL-6 locus) result in the emergence of clonal proliferations (Cesarman et al., 1998; Knowles, 1998). Thus, at least in the early phase these tumors seem to represent an *in-vivo* counterpart to EBV-immortalized cells *in vitro*. This renders it likely that in these EBV-positive B-cell lymphomas the failing immunosurveillance permits the proliferation of EBV-transformed B lymphoblasts and implies that EBV is the driving force (direct carcinogen) for the malignant phenotype of these lymphomas. This is further underlined by the observation that reconstitution of the immune system frequently results in lymphoma regression (O'Reilly et al., 1998). Usually, EBV-negative forms of post-transplant lymphomas appear later than EBV-positive tumors, originate mainly from T cells, and grow more aggressively (Dotti et al., 2000; Nelson et al., 2000). Central nervous system lymphomas, which are seen especially in highly immunosuppressed AIDS patients, are almost uniformly EBV-positive (Cesarman and Mesri, 1999; Young and Rickinson, 2004). However, these lesions have virtually disappeared since the introduction of antiviral therapy.

4.3.1.8 EBV in Burkitt's Lymphoma

Burkitt's lymphoma (BL) was originally described by Dennis Burkitt (1958, 1962) as an endemic lymphoma in equatorial Africa, frequently affecting the jaw of children aged 5 to 12 years. The peculiar endemic pattern of this tumor led Burkitt to the initial speculation that this tumor may be caused by an arthropod-borne virus (1962). Subsequently, he and others suspected that holoendemic infections with the malaria parasite *Plasmodium falciparum* may contribute to the lymphoma development (summarized in Magrath, 1990). The discovery of EBV particles initially in tissue culture cells derived from this tumor (Epstein et al., 1964), and subsequently also EBV DNA by molecular hybridization directly in tumor biopsies (zur Hausen et al., 1970), may be considered as the starting point for human tumor virology.

Today, endemic as well as sporadic forms of BL have been described, combining a group of somewhat heterogeneous B-cell lymphomas of germinal center origin, classified as small, non-cleaved-cell lymphomas which respond well to chemotherapeutic interference (Harris et al., 1994; Magrath et al., 1996). One central feature of almost all of these lymphomas is a chromosomal translocation, initially discovered by Manolov and Manolova (1972) that dysregulates the expression of c-myc (Dalla-Favera et al., 1982; Taub et al., 1982). This dysregulation was an early postulate of G. Klein (1979), who inferred this from chromosomal analyses of murine T-cell leukemia cells. Within the same year, Klein and his coworkers demonstrated a reciprocal 8;14 translocation in EBV-negative B-cell acute lymphocytic leukemia with Burkitt-type cells (Mitelman et al., 1979).

The c-myc translocation occurs in the vast majority of all clinical forms of BL: the endemic form, predominantly found in equatorial Africa and also in New Guinea, the relatively rare sporadic form arising in all regions of the world, frequently in adolescents and young adults, and the human immunodeficiency-associated form of Burkitt's lymphoma (Hecht and Aster, 2000). It uniformly involves the c-*myc* locus on chromosome 8q24 and results in most cases in a reciprocal translocation from chromosome 14 at q32. Less frequently, the q11 locus on chromosome 22 and the p12 locus on chromosome 2 are involved. In each of these cases expression of the c-myc gene becomes controlled by elements regulating immunoglobulin genes. Their enhancer elements bind B-cell-specific factors which may activate transcription located up to 500 kb away (Hecht and Aster, 2000). The breakpoints on chromosomes 14, 22, and 2 are within or in the immediate neighborhood of the IgH, Igλ or Igκ genes, respectively. A schematic outline of these recombinations is shown in Figure 4.9.

It is interesting to note – and possibly also of pathognomonic significance – that the breakpoints in endemic and sporadic BL frequently differ. In the endemic form the breakpoints are found in some distance 5' to the first c-myc exon (in some cases more than 100 kb upstream). The breakpoint on chromosome 14 is located in the IgH joining regions (Joos et al., 1992). In sporadic BL, the breakpoints are regularly found within exons 1 and 2 of the c-myc gene on chromosome 8 and within the IgH Sμ switch region on chromosome 14 (Pellicci et al., 1986; Neri et al., 1988; Shiramizu et al., 1991; Gutierrez et al., 1992; Yano et al., 1993). In the variant recombination, the breakpoints occur on chromosomes 2 or 22 of the κ and λ constant regions, respectively. In these cases the breakpoints on chromosome 8 occur at variable distances downstream of c-*myc* (Magrath, 1990; Gerbitz et al., 1999). Although immunoglobulin gene rearrangements are clearly engaged in these recombinations, the mechanism causing c-myc breaks is unknown. Conflicting data exist on the role of activation-induced cytidine deaminase (AID) for the induction of c-myc/IgH translocations (Ramiro et al., 2004; Unniraman et al., 2004). There exist no regions of homology between these breakpoints and sites of the V(D)J or switch recombinase recognition sequences (Hecht and Aster, 2000). A recent speculation

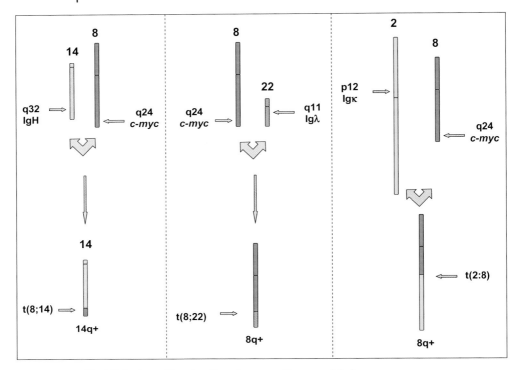

Fig. 4.9 Reciprocal translocation of c-*myc* and immunoglobulin genes.

postulates that specific persistent infections with TT-like viruses may contribute to these recombinations by inducing specific recombinations (zur Hausen and de Villiers, 2005).

C-myc translocations are not limited to BLs. They occur occasionally in large B-cell lymphomas (Sigaux et al., 1984; Thangevelu et al., 1990), lymphoblastic lymphoma (Slavutsky et al., 1996), in a subset of very aggressive follicular lymphomas (Thangevelu et al., 1990; Akasaka et al., 2000), and in late stages of multiple myelomas (Sawyer at al., 1995; Shou et al., 2000). Occasionally, however, lymphoma-associated translocations have also been detected in B cells from normal individuals (Limpens et al., 1995). Since constitutive c-myc activation drives cells into apoptosis, they may however be rescued by EBV infection or by high levels of B-cell stimulatory cytokines, as are found in malaria- or HIV-infected persons (G. Klein, personal communication).

The role of EBV in BL is not easily explained. Viral DNA persists in the EBV-positive tumors commonly at multiple copies per tumor cells (zur Hausen and Schulte-Holthausen, 1970; zur Hausen et al., 1970; Nonoyama and Pagano, 1973). Although most of the genomes persist as circular episomes, some Burkitt-derived cell lines also contain integrated copies (Lawrence et al., 1988; Delecluse et al., 1993; Takakuwa et al., 2004). The expression pattern represents the classical stage latency I with the sole expression of EBNA-1 and EBER and BARF RNA. Although EBNA-1 is immunologically not silent and its expression results in specific antibody production and specific CD4⁺ T cells, it is not processed to appropriate HLA class I-associated target peptides, due to the glycine-alanine repeat-dependent processing defect (Lee et al., 2004). Interestingly, myc overexpression imposes a non-immunogenic phenotype on EBV-infected B cells (Staege et al., 2002).

There exist reasons to assume that the virus plays an important role in EBV-positive tumors: the presence of monoclonal viral episomes suggests that EBV infection preceded the proliferation of the precursor B cells (Neri et al., 1991); viral DNA is present in slightly more than 90% of endemic tumors, but in only about 15% of sporadic BLs. In BLs arising under immunosuppression the percentage seems to be slightly higher than in other sporadic cases (Subar et al., 1988). Recent evidence suggests that EBV infection, at least in tumor-derived cell lines investigated thus far, determines the malignant phenotype of the respective cells. Sublines of the Akata line, originating from a Japanese patient with Burkitt's lymphoma, lost their EBV genomes and concomitantly became non-tumorigenic after inoculation into nude mice (Shimizu et al., 1994). Reinfection with EBV restores the malignant growth properties of these cells (Komano et al., 1998). Even the sole transfection of these cells with BARF-1 conferred tumorigenicity to Akata cells again (Sheng et al., 2003). In another set of experiments, Kennedy et al. (2003) demonstrated that EBV provides a survival factor for the EBV-positive cells. Here in particular EBNA-1 was shown as a protective factor against apoptosis. There seems to exist an interesting difference between EBV-positive and EBV-negative BLs concerning reactive oxygen signaling. EBV-positive BLs express high levels of mitogen-activated protein kinase and reactive oxygen species (ROS), whereby ROS directly regulate NF-κB stimulation, whereas EBV-negative tumors do not show elevated levels of ROS (Cerimele et al., 2005).

Additional arguments can be raised from studies which reveal a synergistic interplay between the rearranged c-myc and EBV: human lymphoblasts immortalized *in vitro* by EBV become tumorigenic upon transfection with a rearranged myc gene (Lombardi et al., 1987). The introduction of an activated c-myc gene into an EBV-immortalized line in which EBNA-2 expression was estrogen-dependent, induced continuous proliferation even without expression of EBNA-2 and LMP-1 (Polack et al., 1996). Specific mutants of c-myc retain their ability to stimulate cell proliferation and activate p53, but are defective in promoting apoptosis, as they fail to induce the BH3-only protein Bim and effectively inhibit Bcl2 (Hemann et al., 2005). Thus, mutant myc proteins selectively disable a p53-independent pathway to enable tumor cells to evade p53 functions.

A number of additional genetic changes have been noted in BLs: p53 mutations occur in approximately 30% of these lesions (Gaidano et al., 1991; Ichikawa et al., 1993; Schoch et al., 1995), and it was suggested that this represents a late effect during lymphoma progression (Cherney et al., 1997). Some of the BL lines expressing wt p53 reveal p14ARF deletions or show HDM2 overexpression (Lindstrom et al., 2001; Capoulade et al., 1998). Silencing of the p73 gene has been reported in 30% of BLs (Corn et al., 1999). The retinoblastoma-related gene RB2/p130 is also frequently mutated in endemic BL (Cinti et al., 2000a,b). The Rb pathway is also frequently inactivated in BLs by epigenetic modifications of Rb or p16^{INK4}.

Transcriptional silencing in BLs affects the cellular gene coding for the death-associated protein (DAP) kinase (Katzenellenbogen et al., 1999), enabling the generation of death signals by interferon γ, tumor necrosis factor and Fas (Levy-Strumpf et al., 1998; Cohen et al., 1999). The BCL-6 gene is also involved in translocations and mutations in 30–50% of BLs (Capello et al., 1997, 2000). In addition, chromosome 6q abnormalities occur at high frequency in this type of tumor (Parsa et al., 1994).

EBV infection of EBV-negative subclones of the Akata BL cell line (Komano et al., 1998) and two other pairs of initially EBV-positive lines with EBV-negative subclones induces a cellular transcript of the T-cell leukemia I (*TCL-1*) oncogene (Kiss et al., 2003). Although expression of the *TCL-1* gene is normally restricted to very early thymocytes (Teitell et al., 1999; Narducci et al., 2000), biopsies from both endemic and sporadic cases of BL are commonly positive, irrespective of the presence of EBV genomes. It is speculated that other yet undefined events lead to TCL-1 induction in EBV-negative sporadic BL cases (Bell and Rickinson, 2003).

In conclusion, the obvious cooperation between rearranged c-myc and EBV in malignant transformation, the dependence of the malignant phenotype of EBV-negative subclones of previously EBV-positive BL cells on EBV reinfection, and the demonstration of an anti-apoptotic function of EBNA-1, are results that stress the important role of EBV infection in EBV-positive BLs in the endemic regions for this disease. A number of important questions, however, remain completely open:

- What determines the geographic restriction of the endemic form of BL?
- Which cofactors contribute to regional differences in tumor incidence?
- Why do endemic and sporadic cases of BL differ in c-myc breakpoints?
- Is there another viral factor involved in the etiology of EBV-negative BLs?

There are no clear-cut answers to any of these questions. Although the geographic restriction of the endemic form of BL has frequently been attributed to the induction of B-cell proliferation by holoendemic infections with the malaria parasite *P. falciparum* (Rowe et al., 1987), there exist regions in India, in Cambodia, Malaysia, and Indonesia with a comparatively high rate of *P. falciparum* transmission but a low rate of BL (Sharma et al., 2004). Clearly, immunosuppression in organ transplant recipients – and even more so in AIDS patients – represents a risk factor for BL development. It does, however, neither explain the endemic cases nor the sporadic cases arising without recognizable immunosuppression. Attempts have been made to explain the different c-myc breakpoints by different stages of maturation between germinal center pre-B cells in early childhood in endemic regions in comparison to adolescents and young adults most frequently affected by sporadic BL (Hecht and Aster, 2000). Yet, the reasons for modifying specifically the c-myc gene at different sites in endemic and sporadic BLs remain unexplained. It also remains an open question as to whether additional infectious agents contribute in particular to the EBV-negative cases of BL. A recent hypothesis attempted to explain at least several of these open questions (zur Hausen and de Villiers, 2005). According to this view, latent infections with specific types of TT-like viruses contribute to chromosomal translocations. The geographic prevalence of the endemic form of BL would be due to such virus types with predominance in the equatorial BL tumor belt and a preference for affecting the upstream region of the c-*myc* gene.

Although BL represents the first human malignant tumor, harboring (at least in endemic regions) a latent tumor virus in every tumor cell, it represents a tumor system in which 40 years of intensive research did not provide any clear-cut answers to the quest for causality.

4.3.1.9 EBV in Nasopharyngeal Carcinoma

In 1966, Old and colleagues reported immunoprecipitation studies revealing a specific reactivity of sera from patients with nasopharyngeal carcinoma (NPC) against an antigen present in BL cells. Immunofluorescent tests developed to detect EBV antigens in BL cells subsequently confirmed the high reactivity of NPC sera against EBV antigens (Henle and Henle, 1969). One year later, EBV DNA was detected in NPC cancer biopsies by nucleic acid hybridization (zur Hausen et al., 1970). Original assumptions that the viral genomes may reside within the infiltrating lymphocytes were refuted three years later (Wolf et al., 1973; Klein et al., 1974). EBV DNA persisted usually in multiple copies within the epithelial tumor cells. The link between EBV infection and NPC was further strengthened by the demonstration of high IgG and IgA antibody titers not only against VCAs, but also against viral EAs (Henle and Henle, 1976).

The histological classification of NPC depends on the degree of differentiation. According to the WHO classification, three types can be distinguished: (i) a keratinizing squamous cell carcinoma (type 1); (ii) a non-keratinizing carcinoma (type 2); and (iii) the undifferentiated carcinoma (type 3) (Shanmugaratnam, 1978). The latter type is also designated as lymphoepithelioma or Schmincke tumor. Serological studies in particular linked types 2 and 3 to EBV infections, but less so type 1. The presence of EBV DNA in type 1 tumors remains somewhat controversial: one study consistently found EBV DNA in these tumors (Raab-Traub et al., 1987), while another failed to detect EBV DNA within the differentiated form (Niedobitek et al., 1991). By analyzing NPC cases from Europe, our group consistently was unable to detect EBV DNA in a small percentage of NPC biopsies (H. zur Hausen, unpublished results; E.-M. de Villiers and H. zur Hausen; unpublished results). In our view, the situation seems reminiscent of EBV in BLs with some EBV-negative cases, even in areas of high tumor incidence.

4.3.1.9.1 Epidemiology and Risk Factors

Nasopharyngeal carcinoma shows a peculiar geographic distribution, reaching particularly high levels among Cantonese males in Southern China with 20–30 cases per 100 000 population (Yu et al., 1986). The incidence is also high in Hong Kong

(21.4), in Singapore (16.3), among Hawaiian Chinese (10.7), in Hanoi, Vietnam (10.4) and in Manila, Philippines (7.2) (Parkin et al., 2002). Outside of Asia a higher incidence is reported for the Northwest Territories of Canada (9.2), for Californian Chinese (7.6), Algeria (2.7) and Uganda (1.8) in Africa, and in Europe for Malta (2.6). In most other parts of the world the incidence is below 1 per 100 000 inhabitants.

Initially, it was proposed that the consumption of Cantonese-style salted fish is a possible risk factor for the increased incidence of NPC in this area (Ho, 1972). In subsequent studies, salted fish specimens were shown to be low in volatile nitrosamines and in bacterial mutagenicity (Tannenbaum et al., 1985), although exposure to nitrite yielded substantial quantities of nitrosamines and mutagenic activity. A few additional preserved foods (fermented fish sauce, salted shrimp paste, moldy bean curd and preserved plum) were reported as risk factors, independent of salted fish exposure (Yu and Henderson, 1987; Yu et al., 1989). Although very suggestive, the accurate role of dietary factors in the etiology of NPC remains unclear, especially in their interaction with persisting EBV infections.

An interesting hypothesis was put forward by Ito and colleagues (1983 a). Based on the observation that tumor promoters of the diterpene ester type efficiently activate the lytic cycle of persisting herpes-type viruses (zur Hausen et al., 1979), these authors investigated the EBV activation by tung oil from the Chinese tung oil tree, *Aleuritis fordii* (Ito et al., 1983 b). One of the main constituents of this oil, 12-*O*-hexadecanoyl-16-hydrophorbol-13-acetate (HHPA), retained its EBV-inducing activity even after treatment for 2 h at 120 °C (Yanase and Ito, 1984). Soil samples collected under tung oil trees which are frequently planted in high-risk areas for NPC, revealed the EBV-inducing activity (Ito et al., 1983 c). Ito and colleagues speculated that the regular activation of EBV after exposure to tung oil might represent one contributing factor to the geographic clustering of NPC in Southern China.

The frequency of NPC incidence in specific Chinese and among Innuit populations suggested, at an early stage, the involvement of genetic factors in the occurrence of this disease. Indeed, it seems that two specific HLA haplotypes HLA-A2 Bw46 and A19 B17 increase the risk for NPC by two- to four-fold (Chan et al., 1983). Two other alleles, HLA-A11 and B13, reveal a protective effect. This seems to indicate that genes closely linked to the HLA locus, but not necessarily identical with HLA, seem to influence susceptibility to NPC (Lu et al., 1990). According to a more recent publication, among Taiwanese Chinese the extended haplotype HLA-A*3303-B*5801/2-DRB1*0301-DQB1*β201/2-DPB1*0401 was associated with a statistically significantly decreased risk for NPC (OR = 0.24, 95 % CI = 1.1 to 6.4) (Hildesheim et al., 2002).

It remains presently very difficult to assess the relevance of these published observations in order to pinpoint modifications of specific genes as factors in NPC development. More direct information may originate from the analysis of individual genes or specific chromosomal changes in cancer tissue from NPC patients. Studies in Tunisia revealed a polymorphism of the stress protein HSP70–2 gene as a susceptibility risk factor for NPC (Jalbout et al., 2003). A polymorphism of a gene *CYP2 E1* (a cytochrome p450), the product of which is involved in the activation of nitrosamines into reactive intermediates, has also been shown to be associated with an increased risk for NPC (Hildesheim et al., 1997). This led to an investigation of polymorphisms in genes involved in DNA repair (Cho et al., 2003), and the subsequent identification of high-risk polymorphisms for the genes *hOGG1* (codon 326) and *XRCC1* (codon 280) which, in combination with *CYP2 E1*, resulted in a drastically increased OR of 25 (95% CI = 3.5–177).

Chromosomal aberrations specific for NPC have been described for several chromosomal sites: non-random changes were observed in chromosomes 1, 3p, 3q, 5q, 9p, 11q, 12, 13q, 14q, and X (for a review, see Lo and Huang, 2002). The inactivation of tumor suppressor genes on 3p, 9p, 11q, 13q, 14q, and 16q and alterations in oncogenes on chromosomes 8 and 12 seem to be particularly important for NPC development. The most frequent change involves a deletion in chromosome 3p. A most interesting candidate region seems to locate at 3p21.3. The critical target here appears to be an isoform of the *RASSF1* gene, *RASSF1A* (Lo et al., 2001). Epigenetic inactivation of this gene has also been noted in small-cell lung cancer, non-small-cell lung cancer, breast cancer, and in renal carcinoma (Dammann et al., 2000; Burbee et al., 2001; Dreijerink et al., 2001). Other loci frequently modified in NPC involved the gene coding for the fragile histidine triad protein (FHIT) on chromosome 3p14.2, and the gene coding for the retinoic acid receptor β 2 (for a review, see Lo and Huang, 2002). On chromosome 9p, modifications involve the site 9p21 containing the genes for the cyclin-dependent kinase inhibitors p14^{ARF}, p15^{INK4B} and p16^{INK4A} (Lo et al., 1995). Transfer of normal chromosome 11 suppressed the malignant phenotype of NPC cells (Cheng et al., 2002). Here, it is likely that the TSLC1 gene located at 11q23 plays a significant role (see Lo and Huang, 2002). Genes located in other chromosomal regions have thus far not been precisely identified. Inactivation of the genes discussed here is frequently mediated via promoter methylation.

4.3.1.9.2 **EBV Genome Persistence and Gene Activity in NPC Cells**

As in BL cells, the EBV genome circularizes after infection of nasopharyngeal cells and persists in this state in NPC. In some tumors, however, integration of viral DNA occurs (Kripalani-Joshi and Law, 1994). The structure of the viral termini serves as a marker of clonal cellular proliferation (Raab-Traub and Flynn, 1986). Indeed, the identical number of terminal structures within one individual tumor permits the conclusion that EBV-infection preceded the development of malignant outgrowth and suggests a role of the viral infection within this process. *In-situ* hybridization and Northern blots permitted the detection of EBNA-1, LMP-1 and LMP-2, and EBER RNA transcription in tumor biopsy material (Yeung et al., 1993; Raab-Traub et al., 1983; Wu et al., 1991). Approximately 60% of EBV-positive NPC biopsies were LMP-1-positive (Fahraeus et al., 1988), while other studies found only in part of the tumors evidence for LMP-1 protein expression (Young et al., 1988; Niedobitek et al., 1992), whereas LMP-2 protein has not been discovered within the tumor tissue, although NPC patients reveal increased antibody titers to this protein (Frech et al., 1993). This latter finding, as well as the variable detectability of LMP-1 protein in NPC materials, suggests that very low levels of these proteins are probably expressed in all NPC tumors. LMP-2 A seems to influence the migratory pattern of epithelial cells and induces an invasive phenotype by activating the integrin-α-6 gene expression (Pegtel et al., 2005).

NPC cells commonly express the EBV latency pattern II. EBNA 1 expression is constantly observed in these cells, a situation reminiscent of Burkitt's lymphomas. EBNA 2 and all EBNA 3s are absent. In both types of tumors the promoter in BAM HI F/Q is used for EBNA 1 transcription, leaving all other EBNAs unexpressed (Sample et al., 1990, 1991; Smith and Griffin, 1992). In spite of the regulation of the LMP-1 promoter by EBNA 2 and EBNA-LP, in epithelial cells LMP-1 is expressed from a larger mRNA (Gilligan et al., 1990 a,b). The initiation starts from a promoter regulated by SP1 and STAT3 which is constitutively active in NPC (Sadler and Raab-Traub, 1995; Chen et al., 2001). LMP-1 induces the cyclooxygenase-2 in nasopharyngeal carcinoma cells, and this seems to result in an increased vascular endothelial growth factor production (Murono et al., 2001). Thus, LMP-1 may play a role in angiogenesis in NPC.

EBER RNA is consistently expressed in NPC cells. It was recently reported that EBER is responsible in nasopharyngeal carcinoma-derived cell lines for the induction of insulin-like growth factor 1, and that this may directly affect the pathogenesis of NPC (Iwakiri et al., 2005). There exists however, a remarkable heterogeneity in EBER-RNA expression within the same NPC biopsies (Fig. 4.10). The EBER-negative cells have not yet been analyzed for the presence of EBV DNA.

Interestingly, another group of abundant and consistent transcripts exists in NPC tumors: three mRNAs can be detected in Northern blots mapping at the 3'-end of the

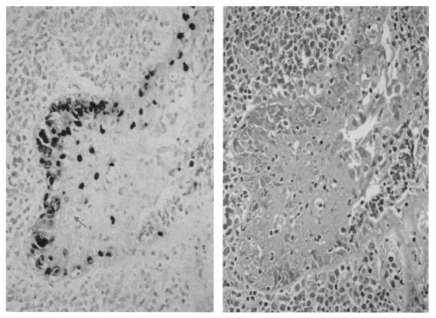

Fig.4.10 EBER-RNA expression in a nasopharyngeal carcinoma biopsy.
(Illustration courtesy of Kwok Wai Lo, Hong Kong.)

BAM H1 A rightward frame 0 (BARF0). They originate from an alternate splicing of seven exons forming several ORFs (Sadler and Raab-Traub, 1995). Although protein translation of the BARF transcripts has not been demonstrated, some experiments point to a possible interaction of specific BARF transcripts and their *in-vitro*-derived proteins with Notch family proteins, resulting in Notch protein degradation and translocation of unprocessed Notch into the nucleus (Kusano, 2001). In the EBNA2-negative line P3 HR-1, expression of one of the BARF ORFs results in the induction of LMP-1 (Kusano and Raab-Traub, 2001).

4.3.1.9.3 EBV Strain Variation and NPC

The peculiar geographic pattern of NPC incidence suggested at an early stage that different EBV strains, prevalent in endemic areas for NPC, may play a significant role. Although two genotypically different EBV strains have been identified (EBV types 1 and 2), no stringent relationship between infection by these types and NPC has been uncovered. The two types are almost identical, except for differences in EBNA-LP, -2, -3A, -3B and -3C proteins, ranging between 16% and 47% (Dambaugh et al., 1984; Adldinger et al., 1985; Sample et al., 1990). A polymorphism was, however, noted within the LMP-1 gene (Hu et al., 1991). LMP-1 gene polymorphisms were found quite consistently in Chinese populations and Alaskan Innuits (Miller et al., 1994; Sung et al., 1998). In addition, differences in an 11-amino acid repeat element of LMP-1 were noted, in some strains with a 5-amino acid insertion (Miller et al., 1994), yet a disease-specific association remains questionable. It is interesting to note that some LMP-1 variants isolated from NPC possessed an increased ability to activate NF-κB (Miller et al., 1998; Johnson et al., 1998).

4.3.1.9.4 EBV in Premalignant Lesions of NPC

Few studies have attempted to identify the presence of EBV DNA in premalignant lesions of NPC. This is due mainly to the difficulties in identifying these lesions and in obtaining sufficient material for a detailed analysis. Whereas one study describes the consistent presence of EBV in all precursor cells of nasopharyngeal cancer (Pathmanathan et al., 1995), another study had difficulties in discovering EBV in early lesions, although the virus was present in all late stages studied (Yeung et al., 1993). This leaves the question open, as to whether EBV infection is a relatively late event in possibly genetically premodified epithelial cells of the nasopharynx (as discussed for EBV-linked gastric cancer), or not. It also permits the speculation that EBV might play a key role as a malignizing factor in an already pre-damaged cellular environment.

   In conclusion, the consistency of association of EBV, at least with the undifferentiated histological type of NPC, the presence of viral DNA in all tumor cells of a virus-positive nasopharyngeal carcinoma, the specific pattern of virus antigen expression, and the monoclonal pattern of virus persistence, point strongly to a role of EBV in the causation of these tumors. Despite vast geographic differences in NPC incidence, EBV-positive tumors occur everywhere in the world.

Many questions regarding the role of EBV in NPC remain unanswered, however:

- Present observations on local risk factors, genetic predisposition, and EBV strain variation do not fully explain the wide variations in the incidence of NPCs.
- It is not clear at which stage of proliferation (normal cell, early precursor lesion or late precursor lesion) EBV enters the scene. Although it is well established that EBV can infect epithelial cells, there exists the possibility that late-stage precursors become more readily infected than early stages.
- It is unclear which type of host cell genetic modifications interact with EBV during the course of malignant conversion, and to what extent the environment contributes to the development of these modifications.
- The existence of EBV-negative NPCs requires further studies. The lesions may arise from specific host cell modifications in regulatory pathways, but potentially other viruses might also be involved.

These and other questions need to be answered before EBV can be considered as the major contributing factor for the causation of NPC and as a direct carcinogen for nasopharyngeal cancers.

4.3.1.10 EBV in Hodgkin's Disease

The suspicion that Hodgkin's disease (HD) is caused by an infection reaches back for more than 70 years (for a review, see Kaplan, 1980) with, initially, environmental factors being implied as risk factors for this condition (Fraumeni and Li, 1969; Dörken, 1975). Dörken suggested a possible relationship of HD with exposure to pets and farm animals, and this resulted in the speculation that HD might represent a zoonosis. Hodgkin-like disease has been occasionally noted in domestic animals, particularly in cats (Maeda et al., 1993; Blomme et al., 1999; Walton and Hendrick, 2001). Several studies have pointed to a higher prevalence of this condition in rural residences, in agricultural occupations, and among woodworkers (Milham and Hesser, 1967; Acheson, 1967; McCunney, 1999). The peculiar age distribution of HD suggested the delayed exposure to a common infectious agent (Gutensohn and Cole, 1980). Males are more frequently affected than females, with the male:female gender ratio ranging between 1.2 and 2.0

Initial studies to detect EBV DNA in biopsy material from patients with HD failed due to the insensitivity of the method used at that time (zur Hausen et al., 1970; Nonoyama et al., 1974). Several serological studies performed at the same time in various laboratories revealed elevated antibody titers of HD patients against Epstein–Barr viral capsid and early antigens (Johannsson et al., 1970; Levine et al., 1971; Henle and Henle, 1973; Henderson et al., 1973; Hesse et al., 1973). The data were partially obscured by reports from some of the same groups, describing elevated antibody titers directed also against other members of the herpesvirus group.

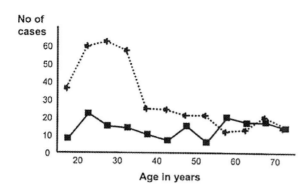

No of cases

Fig. 4.11 Age distribution of Hodgkin's disease in Scotland and the North of England, 1994–119, by EBV status (solid line) EBV-associated cases (dashed line) non-EBV-associated cases. (Jarrett, 2002. With permission.)

Subsequent epidemiological studies demonstrated a two- to four-fold increased risk for HD within the first three years following infectious mononucleosis (Rosdahl et al., 1974; Munoz et al., 1978). Direct evidence for a role of EBV in at least a proportion of HD patients originated from the detection of monoclonal viral genomes in several biopsies by Southern blotting and terminal repeat analysis and the subsequent demonstration of EBV persistence within the Hodgkin Reed–Sternberg cells by in-situ hybridization (Anagnostopoulos et al., 1989; Weiss et al., 1987, 1989). A number of subsequent studies confirmed these results. Based on the differentiation of Hodgkin types according to the Rye classification (Lukes et al., 1966), there exist substantial differences in EBV positivity for the four histological types of classical HD (Fig. 4.11): the lymphocytes-predominant subtype is rarely linked to EBV infections, the nodular sclerosing type in 10–30% is EBV-positive, whereas lymphocyte-depleted and mixed cellularity types are 80–90% EBV-positive (Pallesen et al., 1993; Jarrett, 2002).

It is of interest to note that in Western Europe and the United States the nodular sclerosis and lymphocyte-predominant types prevail, occurring mainly in late adolescence or in young adults. In contrast, in economically less developed parts of the world early childhood cases are more common, revealing predominantly the mixed cellularity histology (Correa and O'Conor, 1971; Macfarlane et al., 1995; Glaser and Jarrett, 1996). The Rye classification of HD is depicted in Table 4.4.

Table 4.4 The Rye classification of different histologies in Hodgkin's disease

Histological classification	Epstein-Barr virus-positive* [%]
Lymphocyte predominance	Rare
Nodular sclerosis	10–30
Mixed cellularity	80–90
Lymphocyte depletion	80–90

* The EBV-negative types prevail in Europe and in the United States.

In addition to these four forms of classical HD, a nodular lymphocyte-predominant form of Hodgkin's lymphoma has been described with clonal immunoglobulin gene rearrangements and ongoing mutations. This defines a mutating germinal center clone with antigen-selection properties as a possible precursor of lymphocytic and histiocytic cells (Küppers et al., 1994; Braeuninger et al., 1997; Marafioti et al., 1997). In spite of functional immunoglobulin rearrangements, Hodgkin and Reed–Sternberg cells are defective in immunoglobulin transcription (Marafioti et al., 2000). This is in part due to destructive mutations within the rearranged molecules (Kanzler et al., 1996; Marafioti et al., 2000), in part to the failure of transcription factors to bind to the mutated promoter (Jox et al., 1999; Theil et al., 2001), and also to the absence of immunoglobulin-specific transcription factors (Re et al., 2001; Stein et al., 2001; Torlakovic et al., 2001).

4.3.1.10.1 **EBV Genome Persistence and Gene Expression**

Hodgkin's lymphoma is characterized by the appearance of Reed–Sternberg cells, large binucleated or polynucleated cells. They are surrounded by a reactive infiltrate of T cells, histiocytes, eosinophils and plasma cells (reviewed in Thomas et al., 2004). The cellular origin of Reed–Sternberg cells was clarified by micromanipulation of single cells from Hodgkin biopsies (Küppers et al., 1994). The clonal rearrangement of immunoglobulin genes and somatic mutations within these genes characterized them as germinal center or post-germinal center B cells (Kanzler et al., 1996). Occasionally, clonal T-cell receptor rearrangements were noted, pointing to the T-cell origin of some HD cases (Müschen et al., 2000; Seitz et al., 2000).

In EBV-positive Reed–Sternberg cells the pattern of EBV genome expression is restricted and corresponds to the latency pattern II. The cells express EBNA1, LMP-1, -2A and -2B proteins and EBER RNAs (reviewed in Rickinson and Kieff, 1996). Expression of LMP-1 is unusually strong in EBV-positive Reed–Sternberg cells (Herbst et al., 1991; Pallesen et al., 1991). In EBV-positive, as well as in EBV-negative cases, expression of members of the tumor necrosis factor receptor superfamily CD30, CD40, and CD95 is observed in a high proportion (Kim et al., 2003). The expression of LMP-1 seems to mimic a constitutively active CD40 receptor (Eliopoulos and Rickinson, 1998). Both bind tumor necrosis factor-associated factors, resulting in the activation of NF-κB, AP-1 and STAT (Devergne et al., 1996; Izumi and Kieff, 1997; Kieser et al., 1997; Gires et al., 1999). LMP-1 appears to be more potent than CD40 in signaling activation (Brown et al., 2001), and may thus contribute to cell transformation. Germinal center B cells depend for survival on signals provided by B-cell receptor and CD40 molecules (Lam et al., 1997). Without immunoglobulin expression these cells undergo apoptosis. Since Reed–Sternberg cells do not express immunoglobulins at their surface, it is likely that LMP-1 and also LMP-2 A contribute to their survival (Jarrett, 2002). The survival mechanism of EBV-negative Reed–Sternberg cells is presently unknown.

LMP-2A increases the expression of genes engaged in cell cycle induction and prevention of apoptosis, and decreases the expression of B-cell-specific factors and genes associated with immunity (Portis et al., 2003). Thus, the function of EBV-induced membrane proteins in Reed–Sternberg cells facilitates their survival and contributes to their proliferative capacity.

Interestingly, both EBV-positive and EBV-negative Hodgkin cells reveal a constitutive strong activation of NF-κB (Bargou et al., 1996). Activation of this transcription factor appears to play a central role in HD, since the introduction of a dominant-negative mutant of IκBα, binding NF-κB irreversibly in the cytoplasm, results in apoptosis of Hodgkin and Reed–Sternberg cells (Bargou et al., 1997; Hinz et al., 2002). The constitutive activation of NF-κB results partially from mutations in the IκBα gene, from amplification of the NF-κB/REL locus, or from constitutively active CD30, CD40, Notch 1 and RANK pathways (Jundt et al., 2002; Emmerich et al., 1999; Annunziata et al., 2000; Joos et al., 2000; Martin-Subero et al., 2002). An additional group of constitutively active transcription factors in HD is represented by the STAT family (Kube et al., 2001). STAT3 and STAT6 appear to be regularly activated (Skinnider et al., 2002).

4.3.1.10.2 Immunosuppression and Hodgkin's Disease

Whereas the incidence of B-cell lymphomas dramatically increases in organ allograft recipients and AIDS patients under conditions of immunosuppression, there is a more moderate increase in risk for Hodgkin's lymphoma. In AIDS patients, the relative risk for non-Hodgkin lymphomas varies between 225 and 650 (Hessol et al., 1992; Cote et al., 1997). Solely for Burkitt's lymphomas, the risk increases 260-fold (Cote et al., 1997). For HD, the relative risk seems to be in the range of 10 to 20 (Hessol et al., 1992; Grulich et al., 1999; Dal Maso and Franceschi, 2003). The mixed cellularity type of HD is predominant in these patients, pointing to a high prevalence of EBV-associated cases (Levine, 1998).

In conclusion, several data favor a causal role of EBV in the EBV-positive cases of HD:

- Viral DNA persists within the malignant Reed–Sternberg cells and is not a contaminant of the surrounding lymphoid stroma.
- The clonality of viral DNA indicates its uptake prior to the onset of malignant growth.
- Viral antigens expressed (in particular LMP-1 and LMP-2) should promote a proliferative and transformed phenotype.
- EBV-induced infectious mononucleosis in young adults significantly increases the risk for the subsequent development of EBV-positive HD.

The major open questions at this stage concern the EBV-negative cases of HD. It has been speculated that these might result from a "hit-and-run" mechanism where, after an initial modification of the infected host cell due to genetic modifications, viral persistence may be no longer required. An alternative possibility would be the persistence of Epstein–Barr viral subgenomic fragments in those "EBV-negative" cases. There exists no evidence in either direction: ample data support the view that several of the EBV-negative HD patients had not been infected with EBV in their past

(Chapman et al., 2001; Gallagher et al., 2003). Similarly, the search for integrated EBV-fragments has been unsuccessful in EBV-negative HD materials (Staratscheck-Jox et al., 2000). Occasionally, cured Hodgkin's lymphoma patients develop EBV-induced infectious mononucleosis years after their successful treatment (H. zur Hausen, unpublished results). In addition, late first exposure and infectious mononucleosis increase the risk for EBV-positive HD cases (Alexander et al., 2003), but not for the EBV-negative form of the disease. Even the age distribution between EBV-positive and EBV-negative patients seems to differ, with EBV-negative cases commonly occurring at a greater age (Jarrett, 2002).

These considerations lead to the conclusion of a different etiology of the EBV-negative HD cases. It remains at present an open question whether a hitherto unknown infectious agent is involved, or whether merely genetic modifications suffice under certain circumstances to produce the clinical picture of HD. Thus far, the search for infectious agents has been unsuccessful. The use of consensus primers for herpes-, polyoma-, and parvoviruses did not result in the identification of an unknown agent in cell lines derived from Hodgkin biopsies or in primary biopsy material (Gallagher et al., 2002; E.-M. de Villiers and H. zur Hausen, unpublished results). Recently, TT virus-like sequences were discovered in the EBV-negative Hodgkin lymphoma line L1236 (zur Hausen and de Villiers, 2005), though the significance of this observation remains to be established.

4.3.1.11 EBV in Gastric and Esophageal Carcinomas

Gastric cancer is commonly considered as a malignancy linked to *Helicobacter pylori* infections. In 1990, Burke et al. demonstrated EBV-DNA in one lymphoepithelioma-like gastric cancer. Shortly thereafter, in 1992, Shibata and Weiss identified the presence of EBV-DNA in 16% (22 out of 138) of gastric cancers. Subsequently, a number of other groups confirmed these findings, revealing on average approximately 10% of gastric cancers as EBV-positive (Tokunaga et al., 1993; Takada, 2000). Taking into consideration the high global rate of gastric cancers of approximately 870 000 new cases every year (Parkin, 2001), an estimated number of 80 000 EBV-associated cases probably points to this cancer as the most frequent EBV-associated malignancy (zur Hausen, 2004). Major geographic differences in EBV-positivity have been reported, with the highest rates in the United States and Germany (Ott et al., 1994; Takada, 2000). It seems that EBV-positive gastric adenocarcinomas represent a distinct clinicopathological entity with a low frequency of lymph node involvement (van Beek et al., 2004).

Esophageal cancer is rarely found to be associated with EBV infection. Moreover, the scarce data available from the literature do not permit an accurate estimation of the presence of EBV genomes in these cancers. Although present in the rare undifferentiated lymphoepithelioma-like tumors of the esophagus (Mori et al., 1994), EBV was also found to be associated with esophageal squamous cell carcinomas (Jenkins et al., 1996; Yanai et al., 2003). One report describes an unusually high number of EBV DNA in squamous cell carcinomas (35%) and in adenocarcinomas

(36%), although the authors did not differentiate between EBV presence within the tumor cells and in infiltrating lymphocytes (Awerkiew et al., 2003). Thus, although rare, EBV might be etiologically involved in a small percentage of esophageal cancers.

In contrast to some other EBV-linked malignant tumors (NPC and BL), which are endemic in south-east Asia and equatorial Africa, EBV-associated gastric cancers are non-endemic throughout the world (Takada, 2000). Histomorphologically, it is difficult to differentiate them from EBV-negative gastric cancers; usually, they are characterized by a high number of infiltrating CD8 cells (Kuzushima et al., 1999). They are commonly found in the proximal part of the stomach (Takada, 2000), and occur more frequently in men than in women (Tokunaga et al., 1993). Partial gastrectomy seems to increase the risk for EBV-associated gastric cancer (Yamamoto et al., 1994).

Since the pattern of terminal repeats within the EBV genome is constant (clonal) for individual gastric cancers, the tumors clearly arose from a single EBV-infected cell (Kida et al., 1993; Imai et al., 1994; Ott et al., 1994). The expression pattern of viral antigens in EBV-positive gastric cancers is somewhat intermediate between EBV latency type I found in BLs and latency pattern II of nasopharyngeal cancer: EBNA-1, BARF-0, BARF-1, and EBER 1/2 are consistently expressed (Sugiura et al., 1996; zur Hausen et al., 2000; Luo et al., 2005), whereas the latent membrane protein LMP-2B seems to be unexpressed. In some cases LMP-1 and LMP-2A have been recorded in several cells (Kida et al., 1993; Sugiura et al., 1996).

Patients with EBV-associated gastric cancers commonly reveal high antibody titers against VCAs and viral EAs. Approximately 60% of the patients also expressed IgA antibodies against VCAs, usually at lower levels than in nasopharyngeal cancer (Imai et al., 1994,). High antibody titers seem to precede the diagnosis of EBV-linked gastric cancer (Levine et al., 1995).

Based on epidemiological studies, *H. pylori* infections have been strongly linked to gastric cancer (Parsonnet et al., 1991). It is interesting to note that there seems to be no difference in *Helicobacter* infections between EBV-positive and EBV-negative cases of gastric cancer (Yanai et al., 1999; Torlakovic et al., 2004). Based on these results, it is presently not possible to postulate an interaction between these bacterial and EBV infections of the gastric mucosa, although at this stage it is also equally impossible to rule this out.

An EBV-positive gastric cancer cell line has been established with EBNA1 and LMP-2A expression, but negative for EBNA2 and LMP-1 (Oh et al., 2004). Another EBV-positive gastric carcinoma cell line has been kept by continuous transplantation in SCID mice (Iwasaki et al., 1998). These cells also retained the same expression pattern of EBV antigens as the original tumor. Two additional lines were established from non-cancerous tissue portions of two patients with gastric cancer (Tajima et al., 1998); these lines express EBNA-2 and LMP-1 and produce infectious EBV spontaneously. This virus is able to transform primary B cells and to induce EA in Raji cells. In an EBV-negative gastric cancer line, EBV infection induced the expression of insulin-like growth factor 1 (IGF-1) (Iwakiri et al., 2003), the induction depending on the EBV-encoded EBER-RNA. The result was an accelerated growth of the infected cells. However, antibodies to IGF-1 blocked the growth stimulation, suggesting that the EBER-induced IGF-1 acts as an autocrine growth factor.

As observed in other virus-linked cancers, several modifications of host cell genes have been noted in EBV-linked gastric cancers: reduced expression and promoter methylation has been recorded in these carcinomas (Osawa et al., 2002). Promoter hypermethylation and aberrant expression was also reported for the E-cadherin promoter (Sudo et al., 2004). Methylation of the p16 as well as of the E-cadherin promoter was higher in EBV-positive than in EBV-negative cases of gastric carcinomas. Along with the p16 promoter methylation and a p16 protein loss in 90% of EBV-positive cancers, a similar percentage of tumors revealed methylation of the CDKN2A promoter, whereas EBV-negative tumors showed this methylation pattern only in 32% of cases (Vo et al., 2002). Additional observations revealed the amplification and overexpression of the c-met gene in EBV-linked gastric cancers, corresponding however to similar observations in EBV-negative gastric tumors (Kijima et al., 2002). Furthermore, up-regulation of the truncated basic hair keratin 1 (hHb1-DeltaN) has been noted in EBV-positive gastric carcinoma cells (Nishikawa et al., 2003), suggesting an interference of this unstable protein with functions of the keratin cytoskeleton and/or interference with transcriptional regulation. It may also point to an inhibition of differentiation driving the growth of NPC cells.

Distinct chromosomal aberrations were also reported in EBV-carrying gastric carcinomas. Copy number gains were recorded for chromosome 11 (Chan et al., 2001), losses of 11p and 4p were selectively found in EBV-positive tumors, while gains of 13q, 3q, and loss of 1q were solely observed in EBV-negative gastric tumors (zur Hausen et al., 2001).

Based on the published data, it is difficult to assess firmly the role of EBV in gastric cancer. Monoclonality of the infecting virus and the pattern of latent antigen expression, corresponding to other EBV-linked tumor systems, favor an etiological relationship. Several observations suggest that EBV infection occurs in the dysplastic stage and not in the normal mucosa (reviewed by Takada, 2000). According to A. zur Hausen et al. (2004), the absence of EBER 1/2 transcripts in the presumed preneoplastic gastric lesions suggests a very late infection. It is possible that EBV contributes a "malignizing" factor for pretransformed cells. This is shown in EBV-negative Akata BL cells which regain malignant growth properties after reintroduction of the EBV genome (Shimizu et al., 1994). In other EBV-positive BL lines the requirement for EBNA-1 expression for cell survival was demonstrated (Kennedy et al., 2003). The other aspect which requires further study is the possible interaction of EBV infections with pre-existing H. pylori manifestations.

4.3.1.12 EBV in NK/T-Cell Lymphomas

EBV is also found in a small percentage of T-cell and NK-cell lymphomas (Jones et al., 1988). Specifically, an extranodal angiocentric T-cell lymphoma, which is relatively common in south-east Asia, turns out to be EBV-positive (Harabuchi et al., 1990; Su et al., 1991; Zhou et al., 1994). The tumors are monoclonal and of CD4+ or

CD8+ T-cell origin. They arise after an acute primary infection or after chronic active EBV infection as a hemophagocytic syndrome, and commonly express the EBV latency pattern II (Kanegane et al., 2002; Young and Rickinson, 2004). Another EBV-linked lymphoma, again relatively common in south-east Asia, is represented by the lethal midline granuloma, which starts as an erosive lesion in the nasal cavity (Kanavaros et al., 1993; van Gorp et al., 1994). It is, however, presently included in the category of NK/T-cell lymphomas. A recent publication points to the growth promotion of T cells by EBV due to the induction of IL-9 by EBV-EBER RNA (Yang et al., 2004). Another observation by Takahara et al. (submitted for publication) that induction of LMP-1 expression in EBV-positive, but LMP-1-negative NK/T lymphoma lines, up-regulates CD25 which represents the IL-2 receptor. This may confer a growth advantage on EBV-carrying cells, as their proliferation depends on IL-2. LMP-1 induction was mediated by IL-4 and IL-10 in an EBNA-2 independent manner (Kis et al., 2006 a,b). There are at present no reports available which could hint at any specific properties of EBV strains found in these malignancies.

4.3.1.13 EBV and Other Human Cancers

Epstein–Barr virus has also been found in the rare leiomyosarcomas in AIDS patients, although detailed studies on its role in this malignancy are still not available (McClain et al., 1995; van Gelder et al., 1995; Timmons et al., 1995). Reports on a role for EBV in human breast and liver cancer (Labrecque et al., 1995; Bonnet et al., 1999; Sugawara et al., 1999) remain presently unconfirmed, and are also controversial (Herrmann and Nietobitek, 2003; Speck et al., 2003). Occasional replicating foci of EBV even in normal breast epithelium have been recently demonstrated (Huang et al., 2003), but do not lend support to a role for EBV in this malignancy.

References

Abbot, S. D., Rowe, M., Cadwallader, K, Ricksten, A., Gordon, J., Wang, F., Rymo, L., and Rickinson, A.B. Epstein–Barr virus nuclear antigen 2 induces expression of the virus-encoded latent membrane protein. *J. Virol.* 64: 2126–2134, **1990**.

Acheson, E.D. Hodgkin's disease in woodworkers. *Lancet* II: 988–989, **1967**.

Adldinger, H.K., Delius, H., Freese, U.K., Clarke, J., and Bornkamm, G.W. A putative transforming gene of the Jijoye virus differs from that of Epstein–Barr virus prototypes. *Virology* 141: 221–234, **1985**.

Akasaka, T., Akasaka, H., Ueda, C., Yonetani, N., Maesako, Y., Shimizu, A., Yamabe, H., Fukuhara, S., Uchiyama, T., and Ohno, H., Molecular and clinical features of non-Burkitt's, diffuse large-cell lymphoma of B-cell type associated with c-Myc/immunoglobulin heavy chain fusion gene. *J. Clin. Oncol.* 18: 510–518, **2000**.

Alexander, F.E., Lawrence, D.J., Freeland, J., Krajewski, A.S., Angus, B., Taylor, G.M., and Jarrett, R.F. An epidemiologic study of index and family infectious mononucleosis and adult Hodgkin's disease (HD): evidence for a specific association with EBV+ve HD in young adults. *Int. J. Cancer* 107: 298–302, **2003**.

Alfieri, C., Birkenbach, M., and Kieff, E. Early events in Epstein–Barr virus infection of human B-lymphocytes. *Virology* 181: 595–608, **1991**.

Allday, M.J., Crawford, D.H., and Thomas, J.A. Epstein–Barr virus (EBV) nuclear antigen 6 induces expression of the latent membrane protein and an activated phenotype in Raji cells. *J. Gen. Virol.* 74: 661–669, **1993**.

Allen, M.D., Young, L.S., and Dawson, C.W. The Epstein–Barr virus-encoded LMP2 A and LMP2B proteins promote epithelial cell spreading and motility. *J. Virol.* 79: 1789–1802, **2005**.

Ambinder, R.F., Shah, W.A., Rawlins, D.R., Hayward, G.S., and Hayward, S. D. Definition of the sequence requirements for binding of the EBNA-1 protein to its palindromic target sites in Epstein–Barr virus DNA. *J. Virol.* 64: 2369–2379, **1990**.

Anagnostopoulos, I., Herbst, H., Niedobitek, G., and Stein, H. Demonstration of monoclonal EBV genomes in Hodgkin's disease and in Ki-1 positive anaplastic large cell lymphoma by combined Southern blot and in situ hybridization. *Blood* 74: 810–816, **1989**.

Annunziata, C.M., Safiran, Y.J., Irving, S. G., Kasid, U.N., and Cossman, J. Hodgkin disease: pharmacologic intervention of the CD40-NF kappa B pathway by a protease inhibitor. *Blood* 96: 2841–2848, **2000**.

Awerkiew, S., Bollschweiler, E., Metzger, R., Schneider, P.M., Hölscher, A.H., and Pfister, H. Esophageal cancer in Germany is associated with Epstein–Barr virus but not with papillomaviruses. *Med. Microbiol. Immunol.* 192: 137–140, **2003**.

Babcock, G.J., Decker, L.L., Volk, M., and Thorley-Lawson, D.A. EBV persistence in memory B cells in vivo. *Immunity* 9: 395–404, **1998**.

Baer, R., Bankier, A.T., Biggin, M.D., Deininger, P.L., Farrell, P.J., Gibson, T.J., Hatfull, G., Hudson, G.S., Satchwell, S. C., Seguin, C., et al. DNA sequence and expression of the B95–8 Epstein–Barr virus genome. *Nature* 310: 207–211, **1984**.

Bargou, R.C., Leng, C., Krappmann, D., Emmerich, F., Mapara, M.Y., Bommert, K., Royer, H.D., Scheidereit, C., and Dörken, B. High-level nuclear NF-kappa B and Oct-2 is a common feature of cultured Hodgkin/Reed–Sternberg cells. *Blood* 87: 4340–4347, **1996**.

Bargou, R.C., Emmerich, F., Krappmann, D., Bommert, K., Mapara, M.Y., Arnold, W.,

Royer, H.D., Grinstein, E., Greiner, A., Scheidereit, C., and Dörken, B. Constitutive nuclear factor-kappaB-RelA activation is required for proliferation and survival of Hodgkin's disease tumor cells. *J. Clin. Invest.* 100 : 2961–2969, **1997**.

Bell, A. and Rickinson, A.B. Epstein–Barr virus, the TCL-1 oncogene and Burkitt's lymphoma. *Trends Microbiol.* 11: 495–497, **2003**.

Benschop, R.J. and Cambier, J.C. B cell development: signal transduction by antigen receptors and their surrogates. *Curr. Opin. Immunol.* 11: 143–151, **1999**.

Beral, V., Peterman, T., Berkelman, R., and Jaffe, H. AIDS-associated non-Hodgkin lymphoma. *Lancet* 337: 805–809, **1991**.

Blomme, E.A., Foy, S. H., Chappell, K.H., and La Perle, K.M. Hypereosinophilic syndrome with Hodgkin's-like lymphoma in a ferret. *J. Comp. Pathol.* 120: 211–217, **1999**.

Bonnet, M., Guinebretiere, J.M., Kremmer, E., Grunewald, V., Benhamou, E., Contesso, G., and Joab, I. Detection of Epstein–Barr virus in invasive breast cancers. *J. Natl. Cancer Inst.* 91: 1376–1381, **1999**.

Bornkamm, G.W., Hudewentz, J., Freese, U.K., and Zimber, U. Deletion of the nontransforming Epstein–Barr virus strain P3 HR-1 causes fusion of the large internal repeat to the DSL region. *J. Virol.* 43: 952–968, **1982**.

Borza, C.M., and Hutt-Fletcher, L.M. Epstein–Barr virus recombinant lacking expression of glycoprotein gp 150 infects B cells normally but is enhanced for infection of epithelial cells. *J. Virol.* 72: 7577–7582, **1998**.

Borza, C.M., Morgan, A.J., Turk, S. M., and Hutt-Fletcher, L.M. Use of gHgL for attachment of Epstein–Barr virus to epithelial cells compromises infection. *J. Virol.* 78: 5007–5014, **2004**.

Braeuninger, A., Küppers, R., Strickler, J.G., Wacker, H.H., Rajewsky, K., and Hansmann, M.L. Hodgkin and Reed–Sternberg cells in lymphocyte-predominant Hodgkin disease represent clonal populations of germinal center-derived B cells. *Proc. Natl. Acad. Sci. USA* 94: 9337–9342, **1997**.

Brielmeier, M., Mautner, J., Laux, G., and Hammerschmidt, W. The latent membrane protein 2 gene of Epstein–Barr virus is important for efficient B cell immortalization. *J. Gen. Virol.* 77: 2807–2818, **1996**.

Brown, H.J., Song, M.J., Deng, H., Wu, T.T., Cheng, G., and Sun, R. NF-κB inhibits gammaherpesvirus lytic replication. *J. Virol.* 77: 8532–8540, **2003**.

Brown, K.D., Hostager, B.S., and Bishop, G.A. Differential signaling and tumor necrosis factor receptor-associated factor (TRAF) degradation mediated by CD40 and the Epstein–Barr virus oncoprotein latent membrane protein 1 (LMP1). *J. Exp. Med.* 193: 943–954, **2001**.

Burbee, D.G., Forgacs, E., Zochbauer-Müller, S., Shivakumar, L., Fong, K., Gao, B., Randle, D., Kondo, M., Virmani, A., Bader, S., Sekido, Y., Latif, F., Milchgrub, S., Toyooka, S., Gazdar, A.F., Lerman, M.I., Zabarovsky, E.R., White, M., and Minna, J.D. Epigenetic inactivation of RASSF1 A in lung and breast cancers and malignant phenotype suppression. *J. Natl. Cancer Inst.* 93: 691–699, **2001**.

Burke, A.P., Yen, T.S., Shekitka, K.M., and Sobin, L.H. Lymphoepithelial carcinoma of the stomach with Epstein–Barr virus demonstrated by polymerase chain reaction. *Mod. Pathol.* 3: 377–380, **1990**.

Burkitt, D. A sarcoma involving the jaws of African children. *Br. J. Surg.* 46: 218–223, **1958**.

Burkitt, D. A children's cancer dependent on climatic factors. *Nature* 194: 232–234, **1962**

Capello, D., Carbone, A., Pastore, C., Gloghini, A., Saglio, G., and Gaidano, G. Point mutations of the BCL-6 gene in Burkitt's lymphoma. *Br. J. Haematol.* 99: 168–170, **1997**.

Capello, D., Vitolo, U., Pasqualucci, L., Quattrone, S., Migliaretti, G., Fassone, L., Ariatti, C., Vivenza, D., Gloghini, A" Pastore, C., Lanza, C., Nomdedeu, J., Botto, B., Freilone, R., Buonaiuto, D., Zagonel, V., Gallo, E., Palestro, G., Saglio, G., Dalla-Favera, R., Carbone, A., and Gaidano, G. Distribution and pattern of BCL-6 mutations throughout the spectrum of B-cell neoplasia. *Blood* 95: 651–659, **2000**.

Capoulade, C., Bressac-de Paillerets, B., Lefrere, I., Ronsin, M., Feunteun, J., Tursz, T., and Wiels, J. Overexpression of MDM2, due to enhanced translation, results in inactivation of wild-type p53 in Burkitt's lymphoma cells. *Oncogene* 16: 1603–1610, **1998**.

Cerimele, F., Battle, T., Lynch, R., Frank, D.A., Murad, E., Cohen, C., Macaron, N., Sixbey, J., Smith, K., Watnick, R.S., Eliopoulos, A., Shebata, B., and Arbiser, J.L. Reactive oxygen signaling and MAPK activation distinguish Epstein–Barr virus (EBV)-positive versus EBV-negative Burkitt's lymphoma. *Proc. Natl. Acad. Sci. USA* 102: 175–179, **2005**.

Cesarman, E., and Mesri, E.A. Virus associated lymphomas. *Curr. Opin. Oncol.* 11: 322–332, **1999**.

Cesarman, E., Chadburn, A., Liu, Y., Migliazza, A., Dalla-Favera, R., and Knowles, D.M. BCL-6 gene mutations in post-transplantation lymphoproliferative disorders predict response to therapy and clinical outcome. *Blood* 92: 2294–2302, **1998**.

Chan, S. H., Day, N.E., Kunaratnam, N., Chia, K.B., and Simons, M.J. HLA and nasopharyngeal carcinoma in Chinese – a further study. *Int. J. Cancer* 32: 171–176, **1983**.

Chan, W.Y. Chan, A.B., Liu, A.Y., Chow, J.H., Ng, E.K., and Chung, S. S. Chromosome 11 copy number gains and Epstein–Barr virus-associated malignancies. *Diagn. Mol. Pathol.* 10: 223–237, **2001**.

Chang, R.S. and Golden, H.D. Transformation of human leukocytes by throat washings from infectious mononucleosis patients. *Nature* 234: 359–360, **1971**.

Chang, Y., Lee, H.H., Chang, S. S., Hsu, T.Y., Wang, P.O.W., Chang, Y.S., Takada, K., and Tsai, C.H. Induction of Epstein–Barr virus latent membrane protein 1 by a lytic transactivator Rta. *J. Virol.* 78: 13 028–13 036, **2004**.

Chapman, A.L., Rickinson, A.B., Thomas, W.A., Jarrett, R.F., Crocker, J., and Lee, S. P. Epstein–Barr virus-specific cytotoxic T lymphocyte responses in the blood and tumor site of Hodgkin's disease patients: implications for a T-cell-based therapy. *Cancer Res.* 61: 6219–6226, **2001**.

Chen, H., Lee, J.M., Zong, Y., Borowitz, M., Ng, M.H., Ambinder, R.F. and Hayward, S. D. Linkage between STAT regulation and Epstein-Barr virus gene expression in tumors. *J. Virol.* 75: 2929–2937, **2001**.

Chen, H., Huang, J., Wu, F.Y., Liao, G., Hutt-Fletcher, L., and Hayward, S. D. Regulation of expression of the Epstein–Barr virus BamHI-A rightward transcripts. *J. Virol.* 79: 1724–1733, **2005**.

Cheng, Y., Chakrabarti, R., Garcia-Barcelo, M., Ha, T.J., Srivatsan, E.S., Stanbridge, E.J., and Lung, M.L. Mapping of nasopharyngeal carcinoma tumour-suppressing activity to a 1.8 megabase region of chromosome band 11q13. *Genes Chromosomes Cancer* 34: 97–103, **2002**.

Cherney, B.W., Bhatia, K.G., Sgadari, C., Gutierrez, M.I., Mostowski, H., Pike, S. E., Gupta, G., Magrath, I.T., and Tosato, G. Role of the p53 tumor suppressor gene in the tumorigenicity of Burkitt's lymphoma cells. *Cancer Res.* 57: 2 508–2515, **1997**.

Cheung, A. and Kieff, E. Long internal direct repeat in Epstein–Barr virus DNA. *J. Virol.* 44: 286–294, **1982**.

Cho, E.Y., Hildesheim, A., Chen, C.J., Hsu, M.M., Chen, I.H., Mittl, B.F., Levine, P.H., Liu, M.Y., Chen, J.Y., Brinton, L.A., Cheng, Y.J., and Yang, C.S. Nasopharyngeal carcinoma and genetic polymorphisms of DNA repair enzymes XRCC1 and hOGG1. *Cancer Epidemiol. Biomarkers Prev.* 12: 1100–1104, **2003**.

Cinti, C., Leoncini, L., Nyongo, A., Ferrari, F., Lazzi, S., Bellan, C., Vatti, R., Zamparelli, A., Cevenini, G., Tosi, G. M., Claudio, P.P., Maraldi, N. M., Tosi, P., and Giordano, A. Genetic alterations of the retinoblastoma-related gene RB2/p130 identify different pathogenetic mechanisms in and among Burkitt's lymphoma subtypes. *Am. J. Pathol.* 156: 751–760, **2000a**.

Cinti, C., Claudio, P.P., Howard, C.M., Neri, L.M., Fu, Y., Leoncini, L., Tosi, G.M., Maraldi, N.M., and Giordano, A. Genetic alterations disrupting the nuclear localization of the retinoblastoma-related gene RB2/p130 in human tumor cell lines and primary tumors. *Cancer Res.* 60: 383–389, **2000b**.

Coffey, A.J., Brooksbank, R.A., Brandau, O., Oohashi, T., Howell, G.R., Bye, J.M., Cahn, A.P., Durham, J., Heath, P., Wray, P., Pavitt, R., Wilkinson, J. et al. Host response to EBV infection in X-linked lymphoproliferative disease results from mutations in an SH2 domain encoding gene. *Nat. Genet.* 20: 129–135, **1998**.

Cohen, J., Wang, F., Mannick, J., and Kieff, E. Epstein–Barr virus nuclear protein 2 is a key determinant of lymphocyte transformation. *Proc. Natl. Acad. Sci. USA* 86: 9558–9562, **1989**.

Cohen, O., Inbal, B., Kissil, J.L., Raveh, T., Berissi, H., Spivak-Kroizaman, T., Feinstein, E., and Kimchi, A. DAP-kinase participates in TNF-alpha- and Fas-induced apoptosis and its function requires the death domain. *J. Cell Biol.* 146: 141–148, **1999**.

Contreras-Brodin, B.A., Anvret, M., Imreh, S., Altiok, E., Klein, G., and Masucci, M. B cell phenotype dependent expression of the Epstein–Barr virus nuclear antigens EBNA-2 to EBNA-6: studies with somatic cell hybrids. *J. Gen. Virol.* 72: 3025–3033, **1991**.

Cordier, M., Calender, A., Billaud, M., Zimber, U., Rousselet, G., Pavlish, O., Banchereau, J., Tursz, T., Bornkamm, G., and Lenoir, G.M. Stable transformation of Epstein–Barr virus (EBV) nuclear antigen 2 in lymphoma cells containing the EBV P3 HR-1 genome induces expression of B cell activation molecules CD21 and CD23. *J. Virol.* 64: 1002–1113, **1990**.

Corn, P.G., Kuerbitz, S. J., van Noesel, M.M., Esteller, M., Compitello, N., Baylin, S. B., and Herman, J.G. Transcriptional silencing of the p73 gene in acute lymphoblastic leukemia and Burkitt's lymphoma is associated with 5' CpG island methylation. *Cancer Res.* 59: 3352–3356, **1999**.

Correa, P. and O'Conor, G.T. Epidemiologic patterns of Hodgkin's disease. *Int. J. Cancer* 8: 192–201, **1971**.

Cote, T.R., Biggar, R.F., Rosenberg, P.S., Devesa, S. S., Percy, C., Yellin, F.J., Lemp, G., Hardy, C., Goedert, J.J., and Blattner, W.A. Non-Hodgkin's lymphoma among people with AIDS: incidence, presentation and public health burden. AIDS/Cancer Study Group. *Int. J. Cancer* 73: 645–650, **1997**.

Counter, C.M., Botelho, F.M., Wang, P., Harley, C.B., and Bacchetti, S. Stabilization of short telomeres and telomerase activity accompany immortalization of Epstein–Barr virus – transformed human B lymphocytes. *J. Virol.* 68: 3410–3414, **1994**.

Dalla-Favera, R., Bregni, M., Erikson, J., Patterson, D., Gallo, R.C., and Croce, C.M. Human c-myc onc gene is located on the region of chromosome 8 that is translocated in Burkitt lymphoma cells. *Proc. Natl. Acad. Sci. USA* 79: 7824–7827, **1982**.

Dal Maso, L., and Franceschi, S. Epidemiology of non-Hodgkin lymphomas and other haemolymphopoietic neoplasms in people with AIDS. *Lancet Oncol.* 4: 110–119, **2003**.

Dambaugh, T., Hennessy, K., Chamnankit, L., and Kieff, E. U2 region of Epstein–Barr virus DNA may encode Epstein–Barr virus nuclear antigen 2. *Proc. Natl. Acad. Sci. USA* 81: 7632–7636, **1984**.

Dammann, R., Li, C., Yoon, J.H., Chin, P.L., Bates, S., and Pfeifer, G.P. Epigenetic inactivation of a RAS association domain family protein from the lung tumour suppressor locus 3 p21.3. *Nat. Genet.* 25: 315–319, **2000**.

Dawson, C.W., Tramountanis, G., Eliopoulos, A.G., and Young, L.S. Epstein–Barr virus latent membrane protein 1 (LMP1) activates the phosphatidylinositol 3-kinase/Akt pathway to promote cell survival and induce actin filament remodeling. *J. Biol. Chem.* 278: 3694–3704, **2003**.

Decaussin, G., Sbih-Lammali, F., de Turenne-Tessier, M., Bouguermouh, A., and Ooka, T. Expression of BARF1 gene encoded by Epstein–Barr virus in nasopharyngeal carcinoma biopsies. *Cancer Res.* 60: 5584–5588, **2000**.

Delecluse, H.-J., Bartnizke, S., Hammerschmidt, W., Bullerdiek, J., and Bornkamm, G.W. Episomal and integrated copies of Epstein–Barr virus coexist in Burkitt lymphoma cell lines. *J. Virol.* 67: 1292–1299, **1993**.

de Schryver, A., Friberg, S., Jr., Klein, G., Henle, W., Henle, G., de Thé, G., Clifford, P., and Ho, H.C. Epstein–Barr virus-associated antibody patterns in carcinoma of the post-nasal space. *Clin. Exp. Immunol.* 5: 443–459, **1969** .

Devergne, O., Hatzivassiliou, E., Izumi, K.M., Kaye, K.M., Kleijnen, M.F., Kieff, E., and Mosialos, G. Association of TRAF1, TRAF2, and TRAF3 with an Epstein–Barr virus LPM1 domain important for B cell transformation: role in NK-kappaB activation. *Mol. Cell. Biol.* 16: 7096–7108, **1996**.

Devergne, O., Cahir McFarland, E.D., Mosialos, G., Izumi, K.M., Ware, C.F., and Kieff, E. Role of the TRAF binding site and NF-κB activation in Epstein–Barr virus latent membrane protein 1-induced cell gene expression. *J. Virol.* 72: 7900–7908, **1998**.

Dörken, H.M. Hodgkin: Eine epidemiologische Studie über 140 Kinder; Stadt/Land Relation, Berufe der Eltern, Kontakte mit Haustieren. *Arch. Geschwulstforsch.* 45: 283–298, **1975**.

Dotti, G., Fiocchi, R., Motta, T., Gamba, A., Gotti, E., Gridelli, B., Borleri, G., Manzoni, C., Viero, P., Remuzzi, G., Barbui, T., and Rambaldi, A. Epstein–Barr virus-negative lymphoproliferative disorders in long-term survivors after heart, kidney, and liver transplant. *Transplantation* 69: 827–833, **2000**.

Dreijerink, K., Braga, E., Kuzmin, I., Geil, L., Duh, F.M., Angeloni, D., Zbar, B., Lerman, M.I., Stanbridge, E.J., Minna, J.D., Protopopov, A., Li, J., Kashuba, V., Klein, G., and Zabarovsky, E.R. The candidate tumor suppressor gene, RASSF1 A, from human chromosome 3 p21.3 is involved in kidney tumorigenesis. *Proc. Natl. Acad. Sci. USA* 98: 7504–7509, **2001**.

Drotar, M.E., Silva, S., Barone, E., Campbell, D., Tsimbouri, P., Jurvansu, J., Bhatia, P., Klein, G., and Wilson, J.B. Epstein–Barr virus nuclear antigen-1 and Myc cooperate in lymphomagenesis. *Int. J. Cancer* 106: 388–395, **2003** .

D'Souza, B.N., Edelstein, L.C., Pegman, P.M., Smith, S. M., Loughran, S. T., Clarke, A., Mehl, A., Rowe, M., Gelinas, C., and Walls, D. Nuclear factor κB-dependent activation of the antiapoptotic bfl-1 gene by the Epstein–Barr virus latent membrane protein 1 and activated CD40 receptor. *J. Virol.* 78: 1800–1816, **2004**.

Dykstra, M.L., Longnecker, R., and Pierce, S. K. Epstein–Barr virus coopts lipid rafts to block the signaling and antigen transport functions of the BCR. *Immunity* 14: 57–67, **2001**.

Ehlers, B., Ochs, A., Leendertz, F., Goltz, M., Boesch, C., and Mätz-Rensing, K. Novel simian homologues of Epstein–Barr virus. *J. Virol.* 77: 10 695–10 699, **2003**.

Eliopoulos, A.G. and Rickinson, A.B. Epstein–Barr virus: LMP1 masquerades as an active receptor. *Curr. Biol.* 8: R196 –R198, **1998**.

Eliopoulos, A.G., Stack, M., Dawson, C.W., Kaye, K.M., Hodgkin, L., Sihota, S., Rowe, M., and Young, L.S. Epstein–Barr virus-encoded LMP1 and CD40 mediate IL-6 production in epithelial cells via an NF-κB pathway involving TNF receptor-associated factors. *Oncogene* 14: 2899–2916, **1997**.

Eliopoulos, A.G., Gallagher, N.J., Blake, S. M., Dawson, C.W., and Young, L.S. Activation of the p38 mitogen-activated protein kinase pathway by Epstein–Barr virus-encoded latent membrane protein 1 coregulates interleukin-6 and interleukin-8 production. *J. Biol. Chem.* 274: 16085–16096, **1999**.

Eliopoulos, A.G., Caamano, J.H., Flavell, J., Reynolds, G.M., Murray, P.G., Poyet, J.L., and Young, L.S. Epstein–Barr virus-encoded latent infection membrane protein 1 regulates the processing of p100 NF-κB2 to p52 via an IKKγ/NEMO-independent signalling pathway. *Oncogene* 22: 7557–7569, **2003**.

Emmerich, F., Meiser, M., Hummel, M., Demel, G., Foss, H.D., Jundt, F., Mathas, S., Krappmann, D., Scheidereit, C., Stein, H., and Dörken, B. Overexpression of I kappa B alpha without inhibition of NF-kappaB activity and mutations in the I kappa B alpha gene in Reed–Sternberg cells. *Blood* 94: 3129–3134, **1999**.

Engel, P., Eck, M.J., and Terhorst, C. The SAP and SLAM families in immune responses and X-linked lymphoprolifera-tive disease. *Nat. Rev. Immunol.* 3: 813–821, **2003**.

Epstein, M.A., Achong, B.G., and Barr, Y.M. Virus particles in cultured lymphoblasts from Burkitt's lymphoma. *Lancet* 1: 702–703, **1964**.

Epstein, M.A., Hunt, R.D., and Rabin, H. Pilot experiments with EB virus in owl monkeys (*Aotus trivirgatus*) I. Reticulo-proliferative disease in an inoculated animal. *Int. J. Cancer* 12: 309–318, **1973**.

Everly, D.N., Jr., Mainou, B.A., and Raab-Traub, N. Induction of Id1 and Id3 by latent membrane protein 1 of Epstein–Barr virus and regulation of p27/Kip and cyclin-dependent kinase 2 in rodent fibroblast transformation. *J. Virol.* 78: 13 470–13 478, **2004**.

Fahraeus, R., Fu, H.L., Ernberg, I., Finke, J., Rowe, M., Klein, G., Falk, K., Nilsson, E., Yadav, M., Busson, P., et al. Expression of Epstein–Barr virus-encoded proteins in nasopharyngeal carcinoma. *Int. J. Cancer* 42: 329–338, **1988** .

Fahraeus, R., Jansson, A., Ricksten, A., Sjo-blom, A., and Rymo, L. Epstein–Barr virus-encoded nuclear antigen 2 activates the viral latent membrane protein promoter by modulating the activity of a negative regulatory element. *Proc. Natl. Acad. Sci. USA* 87: 7390–7394, **1990**.

Feichtinger, H., Li, S. -L., Kaaya, E., Putkonen, P., Grünewald, K., Weyrer, K., Böttiger, D., Ernberg, I., Linde, A., Biber-feld, G., and Biberfeld, P. A monkey model for Epstein–Barr virus-associated lym-phomagenesis in human acquired immunodeficiency syndrome. *J. Exp. Med.* 176: 281–286, **1992**.

Feldhahn, N., Schwering, I., Lee, S., War-tenberg, M., Klein, F., Wang, H., Zhou, G., Wang, S. M., Rowley, J.D., Hescheler, J., Krönke, M., Rajewsky, K., and Muschen, M. Silencing of B cell receptor signals in human naïve B cells. *J. Exp. Med.* 196: 1291–1305, **2002**.

Filipovich, A.H., Mathur, A., Kamat, D., and Shapiro, R.S. Primary immunodeficien-cies: genetic risk factors for lymphoma. *Cancer Res.* (Suppl.) 52: 5465 S– 5467 S, **1992**.

Frappier, L., Goldsmith, K., and Bendell, L. Stabilization of the EBNA-1 protein on the Epstein–Barr virus latent origin of DNA replication by a DNA looping mechanism. *J. Biol. Chem.* 269: 1057–1062, **1994**.

Fraumeni, J.F., Jr. and Li, F.P. Hodgkin's dis-ease in childhood: an epidemiologic study. *J. Natl. Cancer Inst.* 42: 681–691, **1969**.

Frech, B., Zimber-Strobl, U., Yip, T.T., Lau, W.H., Müller-Lantzsch, N. Characteriza-tion of the antibody response to the latent infection terminal proteins of Epstein–Barr virus in patients with nasopharyngeal car-cinoma. *J. Gen. Virol.* 74: 811–818, **1993**.

Gahn, T. and Schildkraut, C. The Epstein–Barr virus origin of plasmid replication, oriP, contains both the initiation and ter-mination sites of DNA replication. *Cell* 58: 527–535, **1989**.

Gaidano, G., Ballerini, P., Gong, J.Z., Inghirami, G., Neri, A., Newcomb, E.W., Magrath, I.T., Knowles, D.M., and Dalla-Favera, R. p53 mutations in human lym-phoid malignancies: association with Burkitt lymphoma and chronic lympho-cytic leukemia. *Proc. Natl. Acad. Sci. USA* 88: 5413–5417, **1991**.

Gallagher, A., Perry, J., Shield, L., Freeland, J., MacKenzie, J., and Jarrett, R.F. Viruses and Hodgkin disease: no evidence of novel her-pesviruses in non-EBV-associated lesions. *Int. J. Cancer* 101: 259–264, **2002**.

Gallagher, A., Perry, J., Freeland, J., Alexander, F.E., Carman, W.F., Shield, L., Cartwright, R. and Jarrett, R.F. Hodgkin lymphoma and Epstein–Barr virus (EBV): no evidence to support hit-and-run mechanism in cases classified as non-EBV-associated. *Int. J. Cancer* 104: 624–630, **2003**.

Gerber, P., Lucas, S., Nonoyama, M., Perlin, E., and Goldstein, L.I. Oral excretion of Epstein–Barr virus by healthy subjects and patients with infectious mononucleosis. *Lancet* 2: 988–989, **1972**.

Gerbitz, A., Mautner, J., Geltinger, C., Hortnagel, K., Christoph, B., Asenbauer, H., Klobeck, G., Polack, A., and Bornkamm, G.W. Deregulation of the proto-oncogene c-myc through t(8;22) translocation in Burkitt's lymphoma. *Oncogene* 18: 1745–1753, **1999**.

Gilligan, K., Rajadurai, P., Resnick, L., and Raab-Traub, N. Epstein–Barr virus small nuclear RNAs are not expressed in permissively infected cells in AIDS-associated leukoplakia. *Proc. Natl. Acad. Sci. USA* 87: 8790–8794, **1990 a**.

Gilligan, K., Sato, H., Rajadurai, P., Busson, P., Young, L., Rickinson, A.B., Tursz, T., and Raab-Traub, N. Novel transcription from the Epstein–Barr virus terminal EcoRI fragment, DIJhet, in a nasopharyngeal carcinoma. *J. Virol.* 64: 4948–4956, **1990 b**.

Gires, O., Kohlhuber, F., Kilger, E., Baumann, M., Kieser, A., Kaiser, C., Zeidler, R., Scheffer, B., Ueffing, M., and Hammerschmidt, W. Latent membrane protein 1 of Epstein–Barr virus interacts with JAK3 and activates STAT proteins. *EMBO J.* 18: 3064–3073, **1999**.

Glaser, S. L. and Jarrett, R.F. The epidemiology of Hodgkin's disease. In: Diehl, V. (Ed.), *Hodgkin's disease*, Ninth edition. London, Baillieres Clin. Haematol. pp. 401–416, **1996**.

Gong, M., Ooka, T., Matsua, T., and Kieff, E. Epstein–Barr virus glycoprotein homologous to herpes simplex virus gB. *J. Virol.* 61: 499–508, **1987**.

Gordadze, A.V., Peng, R., Tan, J., Liu, G., Sutton, R., Kempkes, B., Bornkamm, G.W., and Ling, P.D. Notch 1 Ic partially replaces EBNA-2 function in B cells immortalized by Epstein–Barr virus. *J. Virol.* 75: 5899–5912, **2001** .

Grossman, S. R., Johannsen, E., Tong, X., Yalamanchili, R., and Kieff, E. The Epstein–Barr virus nuclear antigen 2 transactivator is directed to response elements by the Jκ recombination signal binding protein. *Proc. Natl. Acad. Sci. USA* 91: 7568–7572, **1994**.

Grulich, A.E., Wan, X., Law, M.G., Coates, M., and Kaldor, J.M. Risk of cancer in people with AIDS. *AIDS* 13: 839–843, **1999**.

Gutierrez, M.I., Bhatia, K., Barriga, F., Diez, B., Muriel, F.S., de Andreas, M.L., Epelman, S., Risueno, C, and Magrath, I.T. Molecular epidemiology of Burkitt's lymphoma from South America: Differences in breakpoint location and Epstein–Barr virus association from tumors in other world regions. *Blood* 79: 3261–3266, **1992**.

Gutensohn, N.M. and Cole, P. Epidemiology of Hodgkin's disease. *Semin. Oncol.* 7: 92–102, **1980**.

Hammerschmidt, W. and Sugden, B. Genetic analysis of immortalizing functions of Epstein–Barr virus in human B lymphocytes. *Nature* 340: 393–397, **1989**.

Harabuchi, Y., Yamanaka, N., Kataura, A., Imai, S., Kinoshita, T., Mizuno, F., and Osato, T. Epstein–Barr virus in nasal T-cell lymphomas in patients with lethal midline granuloma. *Lancet* 335: 128–130, **1990**.

Harris, N.L., Jaffe, E.S., Stein, H., Banks, P.M., Chan, J.K., Cleary, M.L., Delsol, G., De Wolf-Peeters, C., Falini, B., Gatter, K.C. et al. A revised European–American classification of lymphoid neoplasms: A proposal from the International Lymphoma Study Group. *Blood* 84: 1361–1392, **1994**.

Hayes, D.P., Brink, A.A.T.P., Vervoort, M.B.H.J., Middeldorp, J.M., Meijer, C.J., and van den Brule, A.J. Expression of Epstein–Barr virus (EBV) transcripts encoding homologues to important human proteins in diverse EBV associated diseases. *Mol. Pathol.* 52: 97–103, **1999**.

Hecht, J.L. and Aster, J.C. Molecular Biology of Burkitt's lymphoma. *J. Clin. Oncol.* 18: 3707–3721, **2000**.

Hemann, M.T., Bric, A., Teruya-Feldstein, J., Herbst, A., Nilsson, J.A., Cordon-Cardo, C., Cleveland, J.L., Tansey, W.P., and Lowe, S. W. Evasion of the p53 tumour surveillance network by tumour-derived MYC mutants. *Nature* 436: 807–811, **2005**.

Henderson, B.E., Dworsky, R., Menck, H., Alena, B., Henle, W., Henle, G., Terasaki, P., Newell, G.R., Rawlings, W., and Kinnear, B.K. Case-control study of Hodgkin's disease. II. Herpesvirus group antibody titers and HL-A type. *J. Natl. Cancer Inst.* 51: 1443–1447, **1973**.

Henderson, S., Huen, D., Rowe, M., Dawson, C., Johnson, G., and Rickinson, A.B. Epstein–Barr virus encoded BHRF1 protein, a viral homologue of bcl-2, protects human B cells from programmed cell death. *Proc. Natl. Acad. Sci. USA* 90: 8479–8483, **1993**.

Henkel, T., Ling, P.D., Hayward, S. D., and Peterson, M.G. Mediation of Epstein–Barr virus EBNA2 transactivation by recombination signal-binding protein J kappa. *Science* 265: 92–95, **1994**.

Henle, G. and Henle, W. Immunofluorescence in cells derived from Burkitt's lymphoma. *J. Bacteriol.* 91: 1248–1256, **1966**.

Henle, G. and Henle, W. Epstein–Barr virus-specific IgA serum antibodies as an outstanding feature of nasopharyngeal carcinoma. *Int. J. Cancer* 17: 1–7, **1976**.

Henle, G., Henle, W., and Diehl, V. Relation of Burkitt's tumour associated herpes-type virus to infectious mononucleosis. *Proc. Natl. Acad. Sci. USA* 59: 94–101, **1968**.

Henle, G., Henle, W., Clifford, P., Diehl, V., Kafuko, G.W., Kirya, B.G., Klein, G., Morrow, R.H., Munube, G.M.R., Pike, P., Tukei, P.M., and Ziegler, J.L. Antibodies to Epstein–Barr virus in Burkitt's lymphoma and control groups. *J. Natl. Cancer Inst.* 43: 1147–1157, **1969**.

Henle, G., Henle, W., and Klein, G. Demonstration of two distinct components in the early antigen complex of Epstein–Barr virus-infected cells. *Int. J. Cancer* 8: 272–282, **1971**.

Henle, W. and Henle, G. The relation between the Epstein–Barr virus and infectious mononucleosis, Burkitt's lymphoma and cancer of the postnasal space. *East Afr. Med. J.* 46: 402–406, **1969**.

Henle, W. and Henle, G. Epstein–Barr virus-related serology in Hodgkin's disease. *Nat. Cancer Inst. Monograph* 36: 79–84, **1973**.

Henle, W. and Henle, G. Seroepidemiology of the virus. In: Epstein, M.A. and Achong, B.G. (Eds.), *The Epstein–Barr virus.* Berlin, Springer-Verlag, pp. 61–78, **1979**.

Henle, W., Diehl, V., Kohn, G., zur Hausen, H., and Henle, G. Herpes-type virus and chromosome marker in normal leukocytes after growth with irradiated Burkitt cells. *Science* 157, 1064–1065, **1967**.

Henle, W., Henle, G., Zajac, B.A., Pearson, G., Waubke, R., and Scriba, M. Differential reactivity of human serums with early antigens induced by Epstein–Barr virus. *Science* 169: 188–190, **1970**.

Hennessy, K., Heller, M., van Santen, V., and Kieff, E. Simple repeat array in Epstein–Barr virus DNA encodes part of the Epstein–Barr virus nuclear antigen. *Science* 220: 1396–1398, **1983**.

Hennessy, K., Wang, F., Woodland Bushman, E., and Kieff, E. Definitive identification of a member of the Epstein–Barr nuclear protein 3 family. *Proc. Natl. Acad. Sci. USA* 83: 5693–5697, **1986**.

Herbst, H., Dallenbach, F., Hummel, M., Niedobitek, G., Pileri, S., Müller-Lantzsch. N., and Stein, H. Epstein–Barr virus latent membrane antigen expression in Hodgkin and Reed–Sternberg cells. *Proc. Natl. Acad. Sci. USA* 88: 4766–4770, **1991**.

Herrmann, K. and Niedobitek, G. Lack of evidence for an association of Epstein–Barr virus infection with breast carcinoma. *Breast Cancer Res.* 5: R13–R17, **2003**.

Hesse, J., Andersen, E., Levine, P.H., Ebbesen, P., Halberg, P., Reisher, J.I. Antibodies to Epstein–Barr virus and cellular immunity in Hodgkin's disease and chronic lymphatic leukaemia. *Int. J. Cancer* 11: 237–243, **1973**.

Hessol, N.A., Katz, M.H., Liu, J.Y., Buchbinder, S. P., Rubino, C.J., and Holmberg, S. D., Increased incidence of Hodgkin's disease in homosexual men with HIV infection. *Ann. Intern. Med.* 117: 309–311, **1992**.

Hildesheim, A., Anderson, L.M., Chen, C.J., Cheng, Y.J., Brinton, L.A., Daly, A.K., Reed, C.D., Chen, I.H., Caporaso, N.E., Hsu, M.M., Chen, J.Y., Idle, J.R., Hoover, R.N., Yang, C.S., and Chhabra, S. K. CYP2E1 genetic polymorphisms and risk of nasopharyngeal carcinoma in Taiwan. *J. Natl. Cancer Inst.* 89: 1207–1212, **1997**.

Hildesheim, A., Apple, R.J., Chen, C.J., Wang, S. S., Cheng, Y.J., Klitz, W., Mack, S. J., Chen, I.H., Hsu, M.M., Yang, C.S., Brinton, L.A., Levine, P.H., and Erlich,

H.A. Association of HLA class I and II alleles and extended haplotypes with nasopharyngeal carcinoma in Taiwan. *J. Natl. Cancer Inst.* 94: 1780–1789, **2002**.

Hinz, M., Lemke, P., Anagnostopoulos, I., Hacker, C., Krappmann, D., Mathas, S., Dörken, B., Zenke, M., Stein, H., and Scheidereit, C. Nuclear factor kappaB-dependent gene expression profiling of Hodgkin's disease tumor cells, pathogenetic significance, and link to constitutive signal transducer and activator of transcription 5 a activity. *J. Exp. Med.* 196: 605–617, **2002**.

Ho, J.H. Nasopharyngeal carcinoma. *Adv. Cancer Res.* 15: 57–92, **1972**.

Hoagland, R.J. The transmission of infectious mononucleosis. *Am. J. Med. Sci.* 229: 262–272, **1955**.

Hochberg, D., Middeldorp, J.M., Catalina, M., Sullivan, J.L., Luzuriaga, K., and Thorley-Lawson, D.A. Demonstration of the Burkitt's lymphoma Epstein–Barr virus phenotype in dividing latently infected memory cells in vivo. *Proc. Natl. Acad. Sci. USA* 101: 239–244, **2004**.

Hoover, R.N. Lymphoma risks in populations with altered immunity – a search for a mechanism. *Cancer Res.* 52 (Suppl.): 5477S–5478S, **1992**.

Hsieh, J.J. and Hayward, S. D. Masking of the CBF1/RFPJκ transcriptional repression domain by Epstein–Barr virus EBNA2. *Science* 268: 560–563, **1995**.

Hu, L.F., Zabarovsky, E.R., Chen, F., Cao, S. L., Ernberg, I., Klein, G., and Winberg, G. Isolation and sequencing of the Epstein–Barr virus BNLF-1 gene (LMP1) from a Chinese nasopharyngeal carcinoma. *J. Gen. Virol.* 72: 2399–2409, **1991**.

Huang, J., Chen, H., Hutt-Fletcher, L., Ambinder, R.F., and Hayward, S. D. Lytic viral replication as a contributor to the detection of Epstein–Barr virus in breast cancer. *J. Virol.* 77: 13 267–13 274, **2003**.

Humme, S., Reisbach, G., Feederle, R., Delecluse, H.J., Bousset, K., Hammerschmidt, W., and Schepers, A. The EBV nuclear antigen 1 (EBNA1) enhances B cell immortalization several thousandfold. *Proc. Natl. Acad. Sci. USA* 100: 10 989–10 994, **2003**.

Ichikawa, A., Hotta, T., and Saito, H. Mutations of the p53 gene in B-cell lymphoma. *Leuk. Lymphoma* 11: 21–25, **1993**.

Imai, S., Koizumi, S., Sugiura, M., Tokunaga, M., Uemura, Y., Yamamoto, N., Tanaka, S., Sato, E., and Osato, T. Gastric carcinoma: monoclonal epithelial malignant cells expressing Epstein–Barr virus latent infection protein. *Proc. Natl. Acad. Sci. USA* 91: 9131–9135, **1994**.

Ito, Y., Tokuda, H., Ohigashi, H., and Koshimizu, K. Distribution and characterization of environmental promoter substances as assayed by synergistic Epstein–Barr virus-activating system. *Princess Takamatsu Symp.* 14: 125–137, **1983 a**.

Ito, Y., Yanase, S., Tokuda, H., Kishishita, M., Ohigashi, H., Hirota, M., and Koshimizu, K. Epstein–Barr virus activation by tung oil, extracts of *Aleurite fordii* and its diterpene ester 12-O-hexadecanoyl-16-hydroxyphorbol-13-acetate. *Cancer Lett.* 18: 87–95, **1983 b**.

Ito, Y., Ohigahshi, H., Koshimizu, K., and Yi, Z. Epstein–Barr virus-activating principle in the ether extracts of soils collected under plants which contain active diterpene esters. *Cancer Lett.* 19: 113–117, **1983 c**.

Iwakiri, D., Eizuru, Y., Tokunaga, M., Takada, K. Autocrine growth of Epstein–Barr virus-positive gastric carcinoma cells mediated by an Epstein–Barr virus-encoded small RNA. *Cancer Res.* 63: 7062–7067, **2003**.

Iwakiri, D., Sheen, T.S., Chen, J.Y., Huang, D.P., and Takada, K. Epstein–Barr virus-encoded small RNA induces insulin-like growth factor 1 and supports growth of nasopharyngeal carcinoma –derived cell lines. *Oncogene* 24: 1767–1773, **2005**.

Iwasaki, Y., Chong, J., Hayashi, Y., Ikeno, R., Arai, K., Kitamura, M., Koike, M., Hirai, K., and Fukayama, M. Establishment and characterization of a human Epstein–Barr virus-associated gastric carcinoma in SCID mice. *J. Virol.* 72: 8321–8326, **1998**.

Izumi, K.M., and Kieff, E.D. The Epstein–Barr virus oncogene product latent membrane protein 1 engages the tumor necrosis factor receptor-associated death domain protein to mediate B lymphocyte transformation and activate NF-κB. *Proc. Natl. Acad. Sci. USA* 94, 12 592–12 597, **1997**.

Jalbout, M., Bouaouina, N., Gargouri, J., Corbex, M., Ben Ahmed, S., and Chouchane, L. Polymorphism of the stress protein HSP70–2 gene is associated with the susceptibility to the nasopharyngeal carcinoma. *Cancer Lett.* 193: 75–81, **2003**.

Jarrett, R.F. Viruses and Hodgkin's lymphoma. *Ann. Oncol.* (Suppl.) 13: 23–29. **2002**.

Jenkins, T.D., Nakagawa, H., and Rustgi, A.K. The association of Epstein–Barr virus DNA with esophageal squamous cell carcinoma. *Oncogene* 13: 1809–1813, **1996**.

Ji, L., Arcinas, M., Boxer, L.M. NF-κB sites function as positive regulators of expression of the translocated c-myc allele in Burkitt's lymphoma. *Mol. Cell Biol.* 14: 7967–7974, **1994**.

Johansson, B., Klein, G., Henle, W., and Henle, G. Epstein–Barr virus (EBV)-associated antibody patterns in malignant lymphoma and leukemia. *Int. J. Cancer* 6: 450–462, **1970**.

Johnson, R.J., Stack, M., Hazlewood, S. A., Jones, M., Blackmore, C.G., Hu, L.F., and Rowe, M. The 30-base-pair deletion in Chinese variants of the Epstein–Barr virus LMP1 gene is not the major effector of functional differences between variant LMP1 genes in human lymphocytes. *J. Virol.* 72: 4038–4048, **1998**.

Jones, C., Hayward, S. D., and Rawlins, D.R. Interaction of the lymphocyte-derived Epstein–Barr virus nuclear antigen EBNA-1 with its DNA-binding sites. *J. Virol.* 63: 101–110, **1989**.

Jones J.F., Shurin, S., Abramowsky, C., Tubbs, R.R., Sciotto, C.G., Wahl, R., Sands, J., Gottman, D., Katz, B.Z., and Sklar, J. T-cell lymphomas containing Epstein–Barr viral DNA in patients with chronic Epstein–Barr virus infections. *N. Engl. J. Med.* 318: 733–741, **1988**.

Joos, S., Falk, M.H., Lichter, P., Haluska, F.G., Henglein, B., Lenoir, G.M., and Bornkamm, G.W. Variable breakpoints in Burkitt lymphoma cells with chromosomal t(8;14) translocation separate c-myc and the IgH locus up to several hundred kb. *Hum. Mol. Genet.* 1: 625–632, **1992**.

Joos, S., Küpper, M., Ohl, S., von Bonin, F., Mechtersheimer, G., Bentz, M., Marynen, P., Möller, P., Pfreundschuh, M., Trümper, L., and Lichter, P. Genomic imbalances including amplification of the tyrosine kinase gene JAK2 in CD30+ Hodgkin cells. *Cancer Res.* 60: 549–552, **2000**.

Joseph, A.M., Babcock, G.J., and Thorley-Lawson, D.A. EBV persistence involves strict selection of latently infected B cells. *J. Immunol.* 165: 2975–2981, **2000**.

Jox, A., Zander, T., Küppers, R., Irsch, J. Kanzler, H., Kornacker, M., Bohlen, H., Diehl, V., and Wolf, J. Somatic mutations within the untranslated regions of rearranged Ig genes in a case of classical Hodgkin's disease as a potential cause for the absence of Ig in the lymphoma cells. *Blood* 93: 3964–3972, **1999**.

Jundt, F., Anagnostopoulos, I., Forster, R., Mathas, S., Stein, H., and Dörken, B. Activated Notch1 signaling promotes tumor cell proliferation and survival in Hodgkin and anaplastic large cell lymphomas. *Blood* 99: 3398–3403, **2002** .

Kallin, B., Dillner, J., Ernberg, I, Ehlin-Henriksson, B., Rosen, A., Henle, W., Henle, G., and Klein, G. Four virally determined nuclear antigens are expressed in Epstein–Barr virus transformed cells. *Proc. Natl. Acad. Sci. USA* 83: 1499–1503, **1986**.

Kanavaros, P., Lescs, M.C., Briere, J., Divine, M., Galateau, F., Joab, I., Bosq, J., Farcet, J.P., Reyes, F., and Gaulard, P. Nasal T-cell lymphoma: a clinicopathologic entity with peculiar phenotype and with Epstein–Barr virus. *Blood* 81: 2688–2695, **1993**.

Kanda, K., Hu, H.M., Zhang, L., Grandchamps, J., and Boxer, L.M. NF-κB activity is required for the deregulation of c-myc expression by the immunoglobulin heavy chain enhancer. *J. Biol. Chem.* 275: 32 338–32 346, **2000**.

Kanegane, H., Nomura, K., Miyawaki, T., and Tosato, G. Biological aspects of Epstein–Barr virus (EBV)-infected lymphocytes in chronic active EBV infection and associated malignancies. *Crit. Rev. Oncol. Haematol.* 44: 239–249, **2002** .

Kang, M.S., Lu, H., Yasui, T., Sharpe, A., Warren, H., Cahir-MacFarland, E., Bronson, R., Hung, S. C., and Kieff, E. Epstein–Barr virus nuclear antigen 1 does not induce lymphomas in transgenic FVB mice. *Proc. Natl. Acad. Sci. USA* 102: 820–825, **2005**.

Kanzler, H., Küppers, R., Hansmann, M.L., and Rajewsky, K. Hodgkin and Reed–Sternberg cells in Hodgkin's disease represent the outgrowth of a dominant tumor clone derived from (crippled) germinal center B cells. *J. Exp. Med.* 184: 1495–1505, **1996**.

Kaplan, H.S. *Hodgkin's disease*. Harvard University Press, Cambridge, Massachusetts, **1980**.

Karran, L., Gao, Y., Smith, P.R., and Griffin, B.E. Expression of a family of complementary-strand transcripts in Epstein–Barr virus-infected cells. *Proc. Natl. Acad. Sci. USA* 89: 8058–8062, **1992**.

Kashuba, E., Yurchenko, M., Szirak, K., Stahl, J., Klein, G., and Szekely, L. Epstein–Barr virus – encoded EBNA-5 binds to Epstein–Barr virus-induced Fte/S3a protein. *Exp. Cell Res.* 303: 47–55, **2005**.

Katzenellenbogen, R.A., Baylin, S. B., Herman, J.G. Hypermethylation of the DAP-kinase CpG island is a common alteration in B-cell malignancies. *Blood* 93: 4347–4353, **1999**.

Kennedy, G., Komano, J., and Sugden, B. Epstein–Barr virus provides a survival factor to Burkitt's lymphomas. *Proc. Natl. Acad. Sci. USA* 100: 14 269–14 274, **2003**.

Kerr, B.M., Lear, A.L., Rowe, M., Croom-Carter, D., Young, L.S., Rookes, S. M., Gallimore, P.H., and Rickinson, A.B. Three transcriptionally distinct forms of Epstein–Barr virus latency in somatic cell hybrids: cell phenotype dependence of virus promoter usage. *Virology* 187: 189–201, **1992**.

Kida, Y., Miyauchi, K., and Takano, Y. Gastric adenocarcinoma with differentiation to sarcomatous components associated with monoclonal Epstein–Barr virus infection and LMP1 expression. *Virchows Arch. A Pathol. Anat. Histopathol.* 423: 383–387, **1993**.

Kieff, E. In: Fields, B.N., Knipe, P.M. and Howley, P.M. (Eds.), *Fields Virology*, Third Edition, Lippincott-Raven Publishers, Philadelphia, vol. 2: 2343–2396, **1996**.

Kieser, A., Kilger, E., Gires, O., Ueffing, M., Kolch, W., and Hammerschmidt, W. Epstein–Barr virus latent membrane protein-1 triggers AP-1 activity via the c-Jun N-terminal kinase cascade. *EMBO J.* 16: 6478–6485, **1997**.

Kijima, Y., Hokita, S., Yoshinaka, H., Itoh, T., Koriyama, C., Eizuru, Y., Akiba, S., and Aikou, T. Amplification and overexpression of c-met gene in Epstein–Barr virus-associated gastric carcinomas. *Oncology* 62: 60–65, **2002**.

Kim, L.H., Eow, G.I., Peh, S. C., and Poppema, S. The role of CD30, CD40 and CD95 in the regulation of proliferation and apoptosis in classical Hodgkin's lymphoma. *Pathology* 35: 428–435, **2003**.

Kim, O.J. and Yates, J.L. Mutants of Epstein–Barr virus with a selective marker disrupting the TP gene transform B cells and replicate normally in culture. *J. Virol.* 67: 7634–7640, **1993**.

King, W., Dambaugh, T., Heller, M., Dowling, J., and Kieff, E. Epstein–Barr virus DNA XII. A variable region of the Epstein–Barr virus genome is included in the P3HR-1 deletion. *J. Virol.* 43: 979–986, **1982**.

Kiss, C., Nishikawa, J., Takada, K., Trivedi, P., Klein, G., and Szekely, L. T cell leukemia I oncogene expression depends on the presence of Epstein–Barr virus in the virus-carrying Burkitt lymphoma lines. *Proc. Natl. Acad. Sci. USA* 100: 4813–4818, **2003**.

Kis, L.L., Takahara, M., Nagy, N., Klein, G., and Klein, E. Cytokine mediated induction of the major Epstein–Barr virus (EBV)-encoded transforming protein, LMP-1. *Immunol. Lett.* 104: 83–88, **2006 a**.

Kis, L.L., Takahara, M., Nagy, N., Klein, G., and Klein, E. IL-10 can induce the expression of EBV-encoded latent membrane protein-1 (LMP-1) in the absence of EBNA-2 in B-lymphocytes, in Burkitt lymphoma-, and in NK-lymphoma derived cell lines. *Blood* 107: 2928–2935, **2006 b**.

Klein, G. Lymphoma development in mice and humans: diversity at initiation is followed by convergent cytogenetic evolution. *Proc. Natl. Acad. Sci. USA* 76: 2442–2446, **1979**.

Klein, G., Giovanella, B.C., Lindahl, T., Fialkow, P.J., Singh, S., and Stehlin, J.S. Direct evidence for the presence of Epstein–Barr virus DNA and nuclear antigen in malignant epithelial cells from patients with poorly differentiated carcinoma of the nasopharynx. *Proc. Natl. Acad. Sci. USA* 71: 4737–4741, **1974**.

Knowles, D.M. The molecular genetics of post-transplantation lymphoproliferative disorders. *Springer Semin. Immunopathol.* 20: 357–373, **1998**.

Knutson, J.C. The level of c-fgr RNA is increased by EBNA-2, an Epstein–Barr virus gene required for B-cell immortalization. *J. Virol.* 64: 2530–2536, **1990**.

Komano, J., Sugiura, M., and Takada, K. Epstein–Barr virus contributes to the malignant phenotype and to apoptosis resistance in Burkitt's lymphoma cell line Akata. *J. Virol.* 72: 9150–9156, **1998**.

Kube, D., Holtick, U., Vockerodt, M., Ahmadi, T., Haier, B., Behrmann, I., Heinrich, P.C., Diehl, V., and Tesch, H. STAT3 is constitutively activated in Hodgkin cell lines. *Blood* 98: 762–770, **2001**.

Kripalani-Joshi, S. and Law, H.Y. Identification of integrated Epstein–Barr virus in nasopharyngeal carcinoma using pulse field gel electrophoresis. *Int. J. Cancer* 56: 187–192, **1994**.

Kuppers, D.A., Lan, K., Knight, J.S., and Robertson, E.S. Regulation of matrix metalloproteinase 9 expression by Epstein–Barr virus nuclear antigen 3C and the suppressor of metastasis Nm23-H1. *J. Virol.* 79: 9714–9724, **2005** .

Küppers, R., Rajewsky, K., Zhao, M., Simons, G., Laumann, R., Fischer, R., Hansmann, M.LK. Hodgkin disease: Hodgkin and Reed–Sternberg cells picked from histological sections show clonal immunoglobulin gene rearrangements and appear to be derived from B cells at various stages of development. *Proc. Natl. Acad. Sci. USA* 91: 10962–10966, **1994**.

Kurosaki, T. Genetic analysis of B cell antigen receptor signaling. *Annu. Rev. Immunol.* 17: 555–592, **1999**.

Kusano, S. and Raab-Traub, N. An Epstein–Barr virus protein interacts with Notch in epithelial cells. *J. Virol.* 75: 384–395, **2001**.

Kuzushima, K., Nakamura, S., Nakamura, T., Yamamura, Y., Yokoyama, N., Fujita, M., Kiyono, T., and Tsurumi, T. Increased frequency of antigen-specific CD8(+) cytotoxic T lymphocytes infiltrating an Epstein–Barr virus-associated gastric carcinoma. *J. Clin. Invest.* 104: 163–171, **1999**.

Labrecque, L.G., Barnes, D.M., Fentiman, I.S., and Griffin, B.E. Epstein–Barr virus in epithelial cell tumors: a breast cancer study. *Cancer Res.* 55: 39–45, **1995**.

Laherty, C.D., Hu, H.M., Opipari, A.W., Wang, F., and Dixit, V.M. The Epstein–Barr virus LMP1 gene product induces A20 zinc finger protein expression by activating nuclear factor κB. *J. Biol. Chem.* 267: 24157–24160, **1992**.

Laichalk, L.L. and Thorley-Lawson, D.A. Terminal differentiation into plasma cells initiates the replicative cycle of Epstein–Barr virus in vivo. *J. Virol.* 79: 1296–1307, **2005**.

Lam, K.P., Kuhn, R., and Rajewsky, K. In vivo ablation of surface immunoglobulin on mature B cells by inducible gene targeting results in rapid cell death. *Cell* 90: 1073–1083, **1997**.

Lang, D.J., Garruto, R.M., and Gajdusek, D.C. Early acquisition of cytomegalovirus and Epstein-Barr virus antibody in several isolated Melanesian populations. *Am. J. Epidemiol.* 105: 480–487, **1977**.

Latour, S. and Veillette, A. Molecular and immunological basis of X-linked lymphoproliferative disease. *Immunol. Rev.* 192: 212–224, **2003**.

Latour, S., Gish, G., Helgason, C.D., Humphries, R.K., Pawson, T., and Veilette, A. Regulation of SLAM-mediated signal transduction by SAP, the X-linked lymphoproliferative gene product. *Nat. Immunol.* 2: 681–690, **2001**.

Lawrence, J.B., Villnave, C.A., and Singer, R.H. Sensitive, high resolution chromatin and chromosome mapping in situ: presence and orientation of two closely integrated copies of EBV in a lymphoma line. *Cell* 52: 51–61, **1988**.

Lee, S. P., Brooks, J.M., Al-Jarrah, H., Thomas, W.A., Haigh, T.A., Taylor, G.S., Humme, S., Schepers, A., Hammerschmidt, W., Yates, J.L., Rickinson, A.B., and Blake, N.W. CD8T cell recognition of endogenously expressed Epstein–Barr virus nuclear antigen 1. *J. Exp. Med.* 199: 1409–1420, **2004**.

Levine, A.M. Hodgkin's disease in the setting of human immunodeficiency virus infection. *J. Natl. Cancer Inst. Monogr.* 23: 37–42, **1998**.

Levine, P.H., Ablashi, D.V., Berard, C.W., Carbone, P.P., Waggoner, D.E., and Malan, L. Elevated antibody titers to Epstein–Barr virus in Hodgkin's disease. *Cancer* 27: 416–421, **1971**.

Levine, P.H., Stemmermann, G., Lennette, E.T., Hildesheim, A., Shibata, D., and Nomura, A. Elevated antibody titers to Epstein–Barr virus prior to the diagnosis of Epstein–Barr virus-associated gastric adenocarcinoma. *Int. J. Cancer* 60: 642–644, **1995**.

Levitskaya, J., Coram, M., Levitsky, V., Imreh, S., Steigerwald-Mullen, P.M., Klein, G.,

Kurilla, M.G., and Masucci, M.G. Inhibition of antigen processing by the internal repeat region of the Epstein–Barr virus nuclear antigen-1. *Nature*375: 685–688, **1995**.

Levy-Strumpf, N. and Kimchi, A. Death-associated proteins (DAPs): From gene identification to the analysis of their apoptotic and tumor suppressive functions. *Oncogene* 17: 3331–3340, **1998**.

Li, C., Iosef, C., Jia, C.Y., Han, V.K., and Li, S. S. Dual functional roles for the X-linked lymphoproliferative syndrome gene product SAP/SH2D1A in signaling through the signaling activating lymphocyte molecule (SLAM) family of immune receptors. *J. Biol. Chem*. 278: 3852–3859, **2003**.

Limpens, J., Stad, R., Vos, C., de Vlaam, C., de Jong, D., van Ommen, G.C., Schuuring, E., and Kluin, P.M. Lymphoma-associated translocation t(14;18) in blood B cells of normal individuals. *Blood* 85: 2528–2536, **1995**.

Lin, J., Johannsen, E., Robertson, E., and Kieff, E. Epstein–Barr virus nuclear antigen 3C putative repression domain mediates coactivation of the LMP1 promoter with EBNA-2. *J. Virol*. 76: 232–242, **2002**.

Lindstrom, M.S., Klangby, U., and Wiman, K.G. p14ARF homozygous deletion or MDM2 overexpression in Burkitt lymphoma lines carrying wild type p53. *Oncogene* 20: 2171–2177, **2001**.

Linet, M.S., Ries, L.A., Smith, M.A., Tarone, R.E., and Devesa, S. S. Cancer surveillance series: recent trends in childhood cancer incidence and mortality in the United States. *J. Natl. Cancer Inst*. 91: 1051–1058, **1999**.

Lo, K.-W., Huang, D.P., and Lau, K.M. p16 gene alterations in nasopharyngeal carcinoma. *Cancer Res*. 55: 2039–2043, **1995**.

Lo, K.-W., Kwong, J., Hui, A.B., Chan, S. Y., To, K.F., Chan, A.S., Chow, L.S., Teo, P.M., Johnson, P.J., and Huang, D.P. High frequency of promoter hypermethylation of RASSF1A in nasopharyngeal carcinoma. *Cancer Res*. 61: 3877–3881, **2001**.

Lo, K.-W. and Huang, D.P. Genetic and epigenetic changes in nasopharyngeal carcinoma. *Semin. Cancer Biol*. 12: 451–462, **2002**.

Lombardi, L., Newcomb, E.W., Dalla-Favera, R. Pathogenesis of Burkitt lymphoma: expression of an activated c-myc oncogene causes the tumorigenic conversion of EBV-infected human B lymphoblasts. *Cell* 49: 161–170, **1987**.

Longnecker, R., Miller, C., Miao, X.Q., Tomkinson, B., and Kieff, E. The last seven transmembrane and carboxy-terminal cytoplasmic domains of Epstein–Barr virus latent membrane protein 2 (LMP2) are dispensable for lymphocyte infection and growth transformation in vitro. *J. Virol*. 67: 2006–2013, **1993**.

Lu, S. -J., Day, N.E., Degos, L., Lepage, V., Wang, P.C., Chan, S. H., Simons, M., McKnight, B., Easton, D., Zeng, Y., et al. Linkage of nasopharyngeal carcinoma susceptibility locus to the HLA region. *Nature* 346: 470–471, **1990**.

Lukes, R.J., Craver, L.F., Hall, T.C., Rapaport, H., and Rubin, P. Report on the nomenclature committee. *Cancer Res*. 26: 1311, **1966**.

Luo, B., Wang, Y., Wang, X.F., Liang, H., Yan, L.P., Huang, B.H., and Zhao, P. Expression of Epstein–Barr virus genes in EBV-associated gastric carcinomas. *World J. Gastroenterol*. 11: 629–633, **2005**.

Macfarlane, G.J., Evstifeeva, T., Boyle, P., and Grufferman, S. International patterns in the occurrence of Hodgkin's disease in children and young adult males. *Int. J. Cancer* 61: 165–169, **1995**.

Maeda, H., Ozaki, K., Honaga, S., and Narama, I. Hodgkin's-like lymphoma in a dog. *Zentralbl. Veterinärmed. A*. 40: 200–204, **1993**.

Magrath, I. The pathogenesis of Burkitt's lymphoma. *Adv. Cancer Res*. 55: 133–270, **1990**.

Magrath, I., Adde, M., Shad, A., Venzon, D., Seibel, N., Gootenberg, J., Neely, J., Arndt, C., Nieder, M., Jaffe, E., Wittes, R.A., and Horak, I.D. Adults and children with small non-cleaved-cell lymphoma have a similar excellent outcome when treated with the same chemotherapy regimen. *J. Clin. Oncol*. 14: 925–934, **1996**.

Mannick, J.B, Cohen, J.I., Birkenbach, M., Marchini, A., and Kieff, E. The Epstein–Barr virus nuclear protein encoded by the leader of the EBNA RNAs (EBNA-LP) is important in B lymphocyte transformation. *J. Virol*. 65: 6826–6837, **1991**.

Manolov, G. and Manolova, Y. Marker band in one chromosome 14 from Burkitt lymphomas. *Nature* 237: 33–34, **1972**.

Marafioti, T., Hummel, M., Anagnostopoulos, I., Foss, H.D., Falini, B., Delsol, G., Isaacson, P.G., Pileri, S., and Stein, H. Origin of nodular lymphocyte-predominant Hodgkin's disease from a clonal expansion of highly mutated germinal-center B cells. *N. Engl. J. Med.* 337: 453–458, **1997**.

Marafioti, T., Hummel, M., Foss, H.D., Laumen, H., Korbjuhn, P., Anagnostopoulos, I., Lammert, H., Demel, G., Theil, J., Wirth, T., and Stein, H. Hodgkin and Reed–Sternberg cells represent an expansion of a single clone originating from a germinal center B-cell with functional immunoglobulin gene rearrangements but defective immunoglobulin transcription. *Blood* 95: 1443–1450, **2000**.

Martin-Subero, J.I., Gesk, S., Harder. L., Sonoki, T., Tucker, P.W., Schlegelberger, B., Grote, W., Novo, F.J., Calasanz, M.J., Hansmann, M.L., Dyer, M.J., and Siebert, R. Recurrent involvement of the REL and BCL11A loci in classical Hodgkin lymphoma. *Blood* 99: 1474–1477, **2002**.

McClain, K.L., Leach, C.T., Jenson, H.B., Joshi, V.V., Pollock, B.H., Parmley, R.T., DiCarlo, F.J., Chadwick, E.G., and Murphy, S. B. Association of Epstein–Barr virus with leiomyosarcomas in children with AIDS. *N. Engl. J. Med.* 332: 12–18, **1995**.

McCunney, R.J. Hodgkin's disease, work, and the environment. A review. *J. Occup. Environ. Med.* 41: 36–46, **1999**.

Middleton, T. and Sugden, B. Retention of plasmid DNA in mammalian cells is enhanced by binding of the Epstein–Barr virus replication protein EBNA1. *J. Virol.* 68: 4067–4071, **1994**.

Milham, S., Jr. and Hesser, J.E. Hodgkin's disease in woodworkers. *Lancet* 2: 136–137, **1967**.

Miller, C.L., Lee, J.H., Kieff, E., and Longnecker, R. An integral membrane protein (LMP2) blocks reactivation of Epstein–Barr virus from latency following surface immunoglobulin crosslinking. *Proc. Natl. Acad. Sci. USA* 91: 772–776, **1994**.

Miller, G., Shope, T., Lisco, H., Stitt, D., and Lipman, M. Epstein–Barr virus: transformation, cytopathic changes, and viral antigens in squirrel monkey and marmoset leukocytes. *Proc. Natl. Acad. Sci. USA* 69: 383–387, **1972**.

Miller, W.E., Edwards, R.H., Walling, D.M., and Raab-Traub, N. Sequence variation in the Epstein–Barr virus latent membrane protein 1. *J. Gen. Virol.* 75: 2729–2740, **1994**.

Miller, W.E., Cheshire, J.L., Baldwin, AS., Jr., and Raab-Traub, N. The NPC-derived C15 LMP1 protein confers enhanced activation of NF-kappa B and induction of the EGFR in epithelial cells. *Oncogene* 16: 1869–1877, **1998**.

Mitelman, F., Andersson-Anvret, M., Brandt, L., Catovsky, D., Klein, G., Manolov, G., Manolova, Y., Mark-Vendel, E., and Nilsson, P.G. Reciprocal 8:14 translocation in EBV-negative B-cell acute lymphocytic leukemia with Burkitt-type cells. *Int. J. Cancer* 24: 27–33, **1979**.

Miyazaki, I., Cheung, R.K., and Dosch, H.M. Viral interleukin-10 is critical for the induction of B cell growth transformation by Epstein–Barr virus. *J. Exp. Med.* 178: 439–447, **1993**.

Morgan D.G., Niederman, J.C., Miller, G., Smith, H.W., and Dowaliby, J.M. Site of Epstein–Barr virus replication in the oropharynx. *Lancet* 2: 1154–1157, **1979**.

Mori, M., Watanabe, M., Tanaka, S., Mimori, K., Kuwano, H., and Sugimachi, K. Epstein–Barr virus-associated carcinomas of the esophagus and stomach. *Arch. Pathol. Lab. Med.* 118: 998–1001, **1994**.

Morra, M., Howie, D., Grande, M.S., Sayos, J., Wang, N., Wu, C., Engel, P., and Terhorst, C. X-linked lymphoproliferative disease: a progressive immunodeficiency. *Annu. Rev. Immunol.* 19: 657–682, **2001 a**.

Morra, M., Lu, J., Poy, F., Martin, M., Sayos, J., Calpe, S., Gullo, C., Howie, D., Rietdijk, S., Thompson, A., Coyle, A.J., Denny, C., Yaffe, M.B., Engel, P., Eck, M.J., and Terhorst, C. Structural basis for the interaction of the free SH2 domain EAT-2 with SLAM receptors in hematopoietic cells. *EMBO J.* 20: 5840–5852, **2001 b**.

Mosier, D.E., Gulizia, R.J., Baird, S. M., and Wilson, D.B. Transfer of a functional human immune system to mice with severe combined immunodeficiency. *Nature* 335: 256–259, **1988**.

Munoz, N., Davidson, R.J.L., Withoff, B., Ericsson, J.E., and de Thé, G. Infectious mononucleosis and Hodgkin's disease. *Int. J. Cancer* 22: 10–13, **1978**.

Murakami, M., Lan, K., Subramanian, C., and Robertson, E.S. Epstein–Barr virus nuclear antigen 1 interacts with Nm23-H1 in lymphoblastoid cell lines and inhibits its ability to suppress cell migration. *J. Virol.* 79: 1559–1568, **2005** .

Murono, S., Inoue, H., Tanabe, T., Joab, I., Yoshizaki, T., Furukawa, M., Pagano, J.S. Induction of cyclooxygenase-2 by Epstein–Barr virus latent membrane protein 1 is involved in vascular endothelial growth factor production in nasopharyngeal carcinoma cells. *Proc. Natl. Acad. Sci. USA* 98: 6905–6910, **2001**.

Müschen, M., Rajewsky, K., Bräuninger, A., Baur, A.S., Oudejans, J.J., Roers, A., Hansmann, M.L., and Küppers, R. Rare occurrence of classical Hodgkin's disease as a T cell lymphoma. *J. Exp. Med.* 191: 387–394, **2000**.

Nanbo, A., Inoue, K., Adachi-Takasawa, K., and Takada, K. Epstein–Barr virus RNA confers resistance to interferon-α-induced apoptosis in Burkitt's lymphoma. *EMBO J.* 21: 954–965, **2002**.

Nanbo, A., Yoshiyama, H., and Takada, K. Epstein–Barr virus-encoded poly(A)⁻ RNA confers resistance to apoptosis mediated through Fas by blocking the PKR pathway in human epithelial intestine 407 cells. *J. Virol.* 79: 12 280–12 285, **2005**.

Narducci, M.G., Pescarmona, E., Lazzeri, C., Signoretti, S., Lavinia, A.M., Remotti, D., Scala, E., Baroni, C.D., Stoppacciaro, A., Croce, C.M., and Russo, G. Regulation of TCL-1 expression in B- and T-cell lymphomas and reactive lymphoid tissues. *Cancer Res.* 60: 2095–2100, **2000**.

Nelson, B.P., Nalesnik, M.A., Bahler, D.W., Locker, J., Fung, J.J., and Swerdlow, S. H. Epstein–Barr virus-negative post-transplant lymphoproliferative disorders: a distinct entity? *Am. J. Surg. Pathol.* 24: 375–385, **2000**.

Neri, A., Barriga, F., Knowles, D.M., Magrath, I., and Dalla-Favera, R. Different regions of the immunoglobulin heavy-chain locus are involved in chromosomal translocations in distinct pathogenetic forms of Burkitt lymphoma. *Proc. Natl. Acad. Sci. USA* 85: 2748–2752, **1988**.

Neri, A., Barriga, F., Ighirami, G., Knowles, D.M., Neequaye, J., Magrath, I.T., and Dalla-Favera, R. Epstein–Barr virus infection precedes clonal expansion in Burkitt's and acquired immunodeficiency syndrome-associated lymphoma. *Blood* 77: 1092–1095, **1991**.

Neuhierl, B., Feederle, R., Hammerschmidt, W., and Delecluse, H.J. Glycoprotein gp110 of Epstein–Barr virus determines viral tropism and efficiency of infection. *Proc. Natl. Acad. Sci. USA* 99: 15 036–15 041, **2002**.

Nichols, K.E., Harkin, D.P., Levitz, S., Krainer, M., Kolquist, K.A., Genovese, C., Bernard, A., Ferguson, M., Zuo, L., Snyder, E., Buckler, A.J., Wise, C., Ashley, J., Lovett, M., Valentine, M.B., Look, A.T., Gerald, W., Housman, D.E., and Haber, D.A. Inactivating mutations in an SH2 domain-encoding gene in X-linked lymphoproliferative syndrome. *Proc. Natl. Acad. Sci. USA* 95: 13 765–13 770, **1998**.

Niedobitek, G., Hansmann, M.L., Herbst, H., Young, L.S., Dienemann, D., Hartmann, C.A., Finn, T., Pitteroff, S., Welt, A., Anagnostopoulos, I., et al. Epstein–Barr virus and carcinomas: undifferentiated carcinomas but not squamous cell carcinomas of the nasopharynx are regularly associated with EBV. *J. Pathol.* 165: 17–24, **1991**.

Niedobitek, G., Young, L.S., Sam, C.K., Brooks, L., Prasad, U., and Rickinson, A.B. Expression of Epstein–Barr virus genes and of lymphocyte activation molecules in undifferentiated nasopharyngeal carcinomas. *Am. J. Pathol.* 140: 879–887, **1992**.

Niedobitek, G., Agathanggelou, A., Finerty, S., Tierney, R., Watkins, P., Jones, E.L., Morgan, A., Young, L.S., and Rooney, N. Latent Epstein–Barr virus infection in cottontop tamarins. A possible model for Epstein–Barr virus infection in humans. *Am. J. Pathol.* 145: 969–978, **1994**.

Nishikawa, J., Kiss, C., Imai, S., Takada, K., Okita, K., Klein, G., and Szekely, L. Upregulation of the truncated basic hair keratin 1 (hHb1-DeltaN) in carcinoma cells by Epstein–Barr virus (EBV). *Int. J. Cancer* 107: 597–602, **2003** .

Nonoyama, M. and Pagano, J.S. Homology between Epstein-Barr virus DNA and viral DNA from Burkitt's lymphoma and nasopharyngeal carcinoma determined by DNA-DNA reassociation kinetics. *Nature* 242: 44–47, **1973**.

Nonoyama, M., Huang, C.H., Pagano, J.S., Klein, G., and Singh, S. DNA of Epstein–Barr virus detected in tissue of Burkitt's lymphoma and nasopharyngeal carcinoma. *Proc. Natl. Acad. Sci. USA* 70: 3265–3268, **1973**.

Nonoyama, M., Kawai, Y., Huang, C.H, Pagano. J.S., Hirshaut, Y., and Levine, P.H. Epstein–Barr virus DNA in Hodgkin's disease, American Burkitt's lymphoma, and other human tumors. *Cancer Res.* 34: 1228–1231, **1974**.

Oh, S. T., Seo, J.S., Moon, U.Y., Kang, K.H., Shin, D.J., Yoon, S. K., Kim, W.H., Park, J.G., and Lee, S. K. A naturally derived gastric cancer cell line shows latency I Epstein–Barr virus infection closely resembling EBV-associated gastric cancer. *Virology* 320: 330–336, **2004**.

Old, L.J., Boyse, E.A., Oettgen, H.F., De Harven, E., Geering, G., Williamson, B., and Clifford, P. Precipitating antibody in human serum to an antigen present in cultured Burkitt's lymphoma cells. *Proc. Natl. Acad. Sci. USA* 56: 1699–1704, **1966**.

O'Reilly, R.J., Small, T.N., Papadopoulos, E., Lucas, K., Lacerda, J., and Koulova, L. Adoptive immunotherapy for Epstein–Barr virus-associated lymphoproliferative disorders complicating marrow allografts. *Springer Semin. Immunopathol.* 20: 455–491, **1998**.

Osawa, T., Chong, J.M., Sudo, M., Sakuma, K., Uozaki, H., Shiabahara, J., Nagai, H., Funata, N., and Fukayama, M. Reduced expression and promoter methylation of p16 gene in Epstein–Barr virus-associated gastric carcinoma. *Jpn. J. Cancer Res.* 93: 1195–1200, **2002**.

Ott, G., Kirchner, T., and Müller-Hermelink, H.K. Monoclonal Epstein–Barr virus genomes but lack of EBV-related protein expression in different types of gastric carcinoma. *Histopathology* 25: 323–329, **1994**.

Pallesen, G., Hamilton-Dutoit, S. J., Rowe, M., and Young, L.S. Expression of Epstein–Barr virus latent gene products in tumour cells of Hodgkin's disease. *Lancet* 337: 320–322, **1991**.

Pallesen, G., Hamilton-Dutoit, S. J., and Zhou, X. The association of Epstein–Barr virus (EBV) with T lymphoproliferations and Hodgkin's disease: two new developments in the EBV field. *Adv. Cancer Res.* 62: 179–239, **1993**.

Parker, G.A., Crook, T., Bain, M., Sara, E.A., Farrell, P.J., and Allday, M.J. Epstein–Barr virus nuclear antigen (EBNA)3C is an immortalizing oncoprotein with similar properties to adenovirus E1A and papillomavirus E7. *Oncogene* 13: 2541–2549, **1996**.

Parkin, D.M. Global cancer statistics in the year 2000. *Lancet Oncol.* 2: 533–543, **2001**.

Parkin, D.M., Whelan, S. L., Ferlay, J., Teppo, L., and Thomas, D.B. *Cancer Incidence in Five Continents*, Vol. VIII, IARC Sci. Publ. 155, **2002**.

Parsa, N.Z., Gaidano, G., Mukherjee, A.B., Hauptschein, R.S., Lenoir, G., Dalla-Favera, R., and Chaganti, R.S. Cytogenetic and molecular analysis of 6q deletions in Burkitt's lymphoma cell lines. *Genes Chromosomes Cancer* 9: 13–18, **1994**.

Parsonnet, J., Friedman, G.D., Vandersteen, D.P., Chang, Y., Vogelman, J.H., Orentreich, N., and Sibley, R.K. *Helicobacter pylori* infection and the risk of gastric carcinoma. *N. Engl. J. Med.* 325: 1127–1131, **1991**.

Pellicci, P.G., Knowles, D.M., Magrath, I., Dalla-Favera, R. Chromosomal breakpoints and structural alterations of the c-myc locus differ in endemic and sporadic forms of Burkitt lymphoma. *Proc. Natl. Acad. Sci. USA* 83: 2984–2988, **1986**.

Pegtel, D.M., Subramanian, A., Sheen, T.-S., Tsai, C.-H., Golub, T.R., and Thorley-Lawson, D.A. Epstein–Barr virus encoded LMP2A induces primary epithelial cell migration and invasion: possible role in nasopharyngeal carcinoma metastasis. *J. Virol.* 15 430–15 442, **2005**.

Petti, L. and Kieff, E. A sixth Epstein–Barr virus nuclear protein (EBNA3B) is expressed in latently infected growth transformed lymphocytes. *J. Virol.* 62: 2173–2178, **1988**.

Petti, L., Sample, C., and Kieff, E. Subnuclear localization and phosphorylation of Epstein–Barr virus latent infection nuclear proteins. *Virology* 176: 563–574, **1990**.

Pfeffer, S., Zavolan, M., Grässer, F.A., Chien, M., Russo, J.J., Ju, J., John, B., Enright, A.J., Marks, D., Sander, C., and Tuschl, T. Identification of virus-encoded microRNAs. *Science* 304: 734–736, **2004**.

Polack, A., Hortnagel, K., Pajic, A., Christoph, B., Baier, B., Falk, M., Mautner, J., Grettinger, C., Bornkamm, G.W., and

Kempkes, B. c-myc activation renders proliferation of Epstein–Barr virus (EBV)-transformed cells independent of EBV nuclear antigen 2 and latent protein 1. *Proc. Natl. Acad. Sci. USA* 93: 10411–10416, **1996**.

Pope, J.H., Horne, M.K., and Scott, W. Transformation of foetal human leukocytes in vitro by filtrates of a human leukaemic cell line containing herpes-like virus. *Int. J. Cancer* 3: 857–866, **1968**.

Pope, J.H., Horne, M.K., and Wetters, E.J. Significance of a complement-fixing antigen associated with herpes-like virus and detected in the Raji cell line. *Nature* 222: 186–187, **1969**.

Portis, T., Dyck, P., and Longnecker, R. Epstein–Barr virus (EBV) LMP2A induces alterations in gene transcription similar to those observed in Reed–Sternberg cells of Hodgkin lymphoma. *Blood* 102: 4166–4178, **2003**.

Purtilo, D.T., Cassel, C.K., Yang, J.P., and Harper, R. X-linked recessive progressive combined variable immunodeficiency (Duncan's disease). *Lancet* 1: 935–940, **1975**.

Raab-Traub, N. and Flynn, K. The structure of the termini of the Epstein–Barr virus as a marker of clonal cellular proliferation. *Cell* 47: 883–889, **1986**.

Raab-Traub, N., Hood, R., Yang, C.S., Henry, B.D., and Pagano, J.S. Epstein–Barr virus transcription in nasopharyngeal carcinomas. *J. Virol.* 48: 580–590, **1983**.

Raab-Traub, N., Flynn, K., Pearson, G., Huang, A., Levine, P., Lanier, A., and Pagano, J.S. The differentiated form of nasopharyngeal carcinoma contains Epstein–Barr virus DNA. *Int. J. Cancer* 39: 25–29, **1987**.

Rabson, M., Gradoville, L., Heston, L., and Miller, G. Non-immortalizing P3J-HR-1 Epstein–Barr virus: a deletion mutant of its transforming parent, Jijoye. *J. Virol.* 44: 834–844, **1982**.

Ramiro, A.R., Jankovic, M., Eisenreich, T., Difilippantonio, S., Chen-Kiang, S., Muramatsu, M., Honjo, T., Nussenzweig, A., and Nussenzweig, M.C. AID is required for c-myc/IgH chromosome translocations in vivo. *Cell* 118: 431–438, **2004** .

Rawlins, D.R., Milman, G., Hayward, S. D., and Hayward, G.S. Sequence-specific DNA binding of the Epstein–Barr virus nuclear antigen (EBNA-1) to clustered sites in the plasmid maintenance region. *Cell* 42: 859–868, **1985**.

Re, D., Muschen, M., Ahmadi, T., Wickenhauser, C., Staratschek-Jox, A., Holtick, U., Diehl, V., and Wolf, J. Oct-2 and Bob-1 deficiency in Hodgkin and Reed–Sternberg cells. *Cancer Res.* 61: 2080–2084, **2001**.

Reedman, B.M. and Klein, G. Cellular localisation of an Epstein–Barr virus (EBV)-associated complement-fixing antigen in producer and non-producer lymphoblastoid cell lines. *Int. J. Cancer* 11: 499–520, **1973**.

Reisman, D., Yates, J., and Sugden, B. A putative origin of replication of plasmids derived from Epstein–Barr virus is composed of two *cis*-acting components. *Mol. Cell. Biol.* 5: 1822–1832, **1985**.

Rickinson, A.B., Young, L.S., and Rowe, M. Influence of the Epstein–Barr virus nuclear antigen EBNA 2 on the growth phenotype of virus-transformed B cells. *J. Virol.* 61: 1310–1317, **1987**.

Rickinson, A.B. and Kieff, E. In: Fields, B.N., Knipe, P.M. and Howley, P.M. (Eds.), *Fields Virology*, Third Edition, Lippincott-Raven Publishers, Philadelphia, vol. 2: 2397–2446, **1996**.

Robertson, E.S., Lin, J., and Kieff, E. The amino-terminal domains of Epstein–Barr virus nuclear proteins 3A, 3B, and 3C interact with RBPJ(κ). *J. Virol.* 70: 3068–3074, **1996**.

Rooney, C.M., Gregory, C.D., Rowe, M., Finerty, S., Edwards, C., Rupani, H., and Rickinson, A.B. Endemic Burkitt's lymphoma: phenotypic analysis of tumor biopsy cells and of derived tumor cell lines. *J. Natl. Cancer Inst.* 77: 681–687, **1986**.

Rosa, M.D., Gottlieb, E., Lerner, M.R., and Steitz, J.A. Striking similarities are exhibited by two small Epstein–Barr virus-encoded ribonucleic acids and the adenovirus-associated ribonucleic acids VAI and VAII. *Mol. Cell. Biol.* 1: 785–796, **1981**.

Rosdahl, N., Larsen, S. O., and Clemmesen, J. Hodgkin's disease in patients with previous infectious mononucleosis: 30 years' experience. *Br. Med. J.* 2: 253–256, **1974**.

Rosendorff, A., Illanes, D., David, D., Lin, J., Kieff, E., and Johannsen, E. EBNA3C coactivation with EBNA2 requires a SUMO homology domain. *J. Virol.* 78: 367–377, **2004**.

Rowe, D.T., Rowe, M., Evan, G.I., Wallace, L.E., Farrell, P.J., and Rickinson, A.B. Restricted expression of EBV latent genes and T-lymphocyte-detected membrane antigen in Burkitt's lymphoma cells. *EMBO J.* 5: 2599–2607, **1986**.

Rowe, M., Rowe, D.T., Gregory, C.D., Young, L.S., Farrell, P.J., Rupani, H., and Rickinson, A.B. Differences in B cell growth phenotype reflect novel patterns of Epstein–Barr virus latent gene expression in Burkitt's lymphoma cells. *EMBO J.* 6: 2743–2751, **1987**.

Sadler, R.H. and Raab-Traub, N. The Epstein–Barr virus 3.5 kilobase latent membrane protein 1mRNA initiates from a TATA-Less promoter within the first terminal repeat. *J. Virol.* 69: 4577–4581, **1995**.

Sakai T, Taniguchi, Y., Tamura, K., Minoguchi, S., Fukuhara, T., Strobl, L.J., Zimber-Strobl, U., Bornkamm, G.W., and Honjo, T. Functional replacement of the intracellular region of the Notch1 receptor by Epstein–Barr virus nuclear antigen 2. *J. Virol.* 72: 6034–6039, **1998**.

Sample, J., Young, L., Martin, B., Chatman, T., Kieff, E., and Rickinson, A.B. Epstein–Barr virus types 1 and 2 differ in their EBNA 3A, EBNA-3B, and EBNA-3C genes. *J. Virol.* 64: 4084–4092, **1990**.

Sample, J., Brooks, L., Sample, C., Young, L.S., Rowe, M., Gregory, C., Rickinson, A.B., and Kieff, E. Restricted Epstein–Barr virus protein expression in Burkitt lymphoma is due to a different Epstein–Barr nuclear antigen 1 transcriptional initiation site. *Proc. Natl. Acad. Sci. USA* 88: 6343–6347, **1991**.

Sawyer, J.R., Waldron, J.A., Jagannath, S., Barlogie B. Cytogenetic findings in 200 patients with multiple myeloma. *Cancer Genet. Cytogenet.* 82: 41–49, **1995**.

Sayos, J., Wu, C., Morra, M., Wang, N., Zhang, X., Allen, D., van Schaik, S., Notarangelo, L., Geha, R., Roncarolo, M.G., Oettgen, H., De Vries, J.E., Aversa, G., and Terhorst, C. The X-linked lymphoproliferative-disease gene product SAP regulates signals induced through the co-receptor SLAM. *Nature* 395: 462–469, **1998**.

Schaefer, B.C., Woisetschlaeger, M., Strominger, J.L., and Speck, S. H. Exclusive expression of Epstein–Barr virus nuclear antigen 1 in Burkitt lymphoma arises from a third promoter, distinct from the promoters used in latently infected lymphocytes. *Proc. Natl. Acad. Sci. USA* 88: 6550–6554, **1991**.

Schatzl, H., Tschikobava, M., Rose, D., Voevodin, A., Nitschko, H., Sieger, E., Busch, U., von der Helm, K., and Lapin, B. The Sukhumi primate monkey model for viral lymphomogenesis: high incidence of lymphomas with presence of STLV-1 and EBV-like virus. *Leukemia* 7 (Suppl. 2): S86–S92, **1993**.

Schoch, C., Rieder, H., Stollmann-Gibbels, B., Freund, M., Tischler, H.J., Silling-Engelhardt, G., and Fonatsch, C. 17p anomalies in lymphoid malignancies: diagnostic and prognostic implications. *Leuk. Lymphoma* 17: 271–279, **1995**.

Seemayer, T.A., Gross, T.G., Egeler, R.M., Pirruccello, S. J., Davis, J.R., Kelly, C.M., Okano, M., Lanyi, A., and Sumegi, J. X-linked lymphoproliferative disease: Twenty-five years after the discovery. *Pediatr. Res.* 38: 471–478, **1995** .

Seitz, V., Hummel, M., Marafioti, T., Anagnostopoulos, I., Assaf, C., and Stein, H. Detection of clonal T-cell receptor gamma-chain gene rearrangements in Reed–Sternberg cells of classic Hodgkin disease. *Blood* 95: 3020–3024, **2000** .

Shanmugaratnam, K. Histological typing of nasopharyngeal carcinoma. *IARC Sci. Publ.* 20: 3–12, **1978**.

Sharma, S. K., Chattopadhyay, R., Chakrabarti, K., Pati, S. S., Srivastava, V.K., Tyagi, P.K., Mahanty, S., Misra, S. K., Adak, T., Das, B.S., and Chitnis, C.E. Epidemiology of malaria transmission and development of natural immunity in a malaria-endemic village, San Dulakudar, in Orissa state, India. *Am. J. Trop. Med. Hyg.* 71: 457–465, **2004**.

Sheng, W., Decaussin, G., Sumner, S., and Ooka, T. N-terminal domain of BARF-1 gene encoded by Epstein–Barr virus is essential for malignant transformation of rodent fibroblasts and activation of BCL-2. *Oncogene* 20: 1176–1185, **2001** .

Sheng, W., Decaussin, G., Ligout, A., Takada, K., and Ooka, T. Malignant transformation of Epstein–Barr virus-negative Akata cells by introduction of the BARF1 gene carried by Epstein–Barr virus. *J. Virol.* 77: 3859–3865, **2003**.

Shibata, D. and Weiss, L.M. Epstein–Barr virus-associated gastric adenocarcinoma. *Am. J. Pathol.* 140: 769–774, **1992**.

Shimizu, N., Tanabe-Tochikura, A., Kuroiwa, Y., and Takada, K. Isolation of Epstein–Barr virus (EBV)-negative cell clones from the EBV-positive Burkitt's lymphoma (BL) line Akata: malignant phenotypes of BL cells are dependent on EBV. *J. Virol.* 68: 6069–6073, **1994**.

Shiramizu, B., Barriga, F., Neequaye, J., Jafri, A., Dalla-Favera, L., Neri, A., Gutierrez, M., Levine, P., and Magrath, I. Patterns of chromosomal breakpoint locations in Burkitt's lymphoma: relevance to geography and Epstein–Barr virus association. *Blood* 77: 1516–1526, **1991**.

Shope, T., Dechairo, D., and Miller, G. Malignant lymphoma in cottontop marmosets after inoculation with Epstein–Barr virus. *Proc. Natl. Acad. Sci. USA* 70: 2487–2491, **1973**.

Shou, Y., Martelli, M.L., Gabrea, A., Qi, Y., Brents, L.A., Roschke, A., Dewald, G., Kirsch, I.R., Bergsagel, P.L., and Kuehl, W.M. Diverse karyotypic abnormalities of the c-myc locus associate with c-myc dysregulation and tumor progression in multiple myeloma. *Proc. Natl. Acad. Sci. USA* 97: 228–233, **2000**.

Shu, C.H., Chang, Y.S., Liang, C.L., Liu, S. T., Lin, C.Z., and Chang, P. Distribution of type A and type B EBV in normal individuals and patients with head and neck carcinomas in Taiwan. *J. Virol. Methods* 38: 123–130, **1992**.

Sigaux, F., Berger, R., Bernheim, A., Valensi, F., Daniel, M.T., and Flandrin, G. Malignant lymphomas with band 8q24 chromosome abnormality: A morphologic continuum extending from Burkitt's to immunoblastic lymphoma. *Br. J. Haematol.* 57: 393–405, **1984**.

Sixbey, J.W., Nedrud, J.G., Raab-Traub, N., Hanes, R.A., and Pagano, J.S. Epstein–Barr virus replication in oropharyngeal epithelial cells. *N. Engl. J. Med.* 310: 1225–1230, **1984**.

Skinnider, B.F., Elia, A.J., Gascoyne, R.D., Patterson, B., Trümper, L., Kapp, U., and Mak, T.W. Signal transducer and activator of transcription 6 is frequently activated in Hodgkin and Reed–Sternberg cells of Hodgkin lymphoma. *Blood*, 99: 618–626, **2002**.

Slavutsky, I., Andreoli, G., Gutierrez, M., Narbaitz, M., Lucero, G., and Eppinger, M. Variant (8;22) translocation in lymphoblastic lymphoma. *Leuk. Lymphoma* 21: 169–172, **1996**.

Smith, P.R. and Griffin, B.E. Transcription of the Epstein–Barr virus gene EBNA-1 from different promoters in nasopharyngeal carcinoma and B-lymphoblastoid cells. *J. Virol.* 66: 706–714, **1992**.

Smith, P.R., de Jesus, O., Turner, D., Hollyoake, M., Karstegl, C.E., Griffin, B.E., Karran, L., Wang, Y., Hayward, S. D., and Farrell, P.J. Structure and coding content of CST (BART) family RNAs of Epstein–Barr virus. *J. Virol.* 74: 3082–3092, **2000**.

Speck, P., Callen, D.F., and Longnecker, R. Absence of the Epstein–Barr virus genome in breast cancer-derived cell lines. *J. Natl. Cancer Inst.* 95: 1253–1254, **2003**.

Staege, M.S., Lee, S. P., Frisan, T., Mautner, J., Scholz, S., Pajic, A., Rickinson, A.B., Masucci, M.G., Polack, A., and Bornkamm, G.W. Myc overexpression imposes a nonimmunogenic phenotype on Epstein–Barr virus-infected B cells. *Proc. Natl. Acad. Sci. USA* 99: 4550–4555, **2002**.

Staratschek-Jox, A., Kotkowski, S., Belge, G., Rüdiger, T., Bullerdiek, J., Diehl, V., and Wolf, J. Detection of Epstein–Barr virus in Hodgkin–Reed–Sternberg cells: no evidence for the persistence of integrated viral fragments in latent membrane protein-1 (LMP-1)-negative classical Hodgkin's disease. *Am. J. Pathol.* 156: 209–216, **2000**.

Stein, H., Marafioti, T., Foss, H.D., Laumen, H., Hummel, M., Anagnostopoulos, I., Wirth, T., Demel, G., and Falini, B. Downregulation of BOB.1/OBF.1 and Oct2 in classical Hodgkin disease but not in lymphocyte-predominant Hodgkin disease correlates with immunoglobulin transcription. *Blood* 97: 496–501, **2001**.

Stewart, S., Dawson, C.W., Takada, K., Curnow, J., Moody, C.A., Sixbey, J.W., and Young, L.S. Epstein–Barr virus-encoded LMP2A regulates viral and cellular gene expression by modulation of the NF-κB transcription factor pathway. *Proc. Natl. Acad. Sci. USA* 101: 15730–15735, **2004**.

Strockbine, L.D., Cohen, J.I., Farrah, T., Lyman, S. D., Wagener, F., DuBose, R.F., Armitage, R.J., and Spriggs, M.K. The Epstein–Barr virus BARF1 gene encodes a novel, soluble colony-stimulating factor-1 receptor. *J. Virol.* 72: 4015–4021, **1998**.

Su, I.J., Hsieh, H.C., Lin, K.H., Uen, W.C., Kao, C.L., Chen, C.J., Cheng, A.L., Kadin, M.E., and Chen, J.Y. Aggressive peripheral T-cell lymphomas containing Epstein–Barr viral DNA: A clinicopathological and molecular analysis. *Blood* 77: 799–808, **1991**.

Subar, M., Neri, A., Inghirami, G., Knowles, D.M., and Dalla-Favera, R. Frequent c-myc oncogene activation and infrequent presence of Epstein–Barr virus genome in AIDS-associated lymphoma. *Blood* 72: 667–671, **1988**.

Sudo, M., Chong, J.M., Sakuma, K., Ushiku, T., Uozaki, H., Nagai, H., Funata, N., Matsumoto, Y., and Fukayama, M. Promoter hypermethylation of E-cadherin and its abnormal expression in Epstein-Barr virus-associated gastric carcinoma. *Int. J. Cancer* 109: 194–199, **2004**.

Sugawara, Y., Mizugaki, Y., Uchida, T., Torii, T., Imai, S., Makuuchi, M., and Takada, K. Detection of Epstein–Barr virus (EBV) in hepatocellular carcinoma tissue: a novel EBV latency characterized by the absence of EBV-encoded small RNA expression. *Virology* 256: 196–202, **1999**.

Sugimoto, M., Ide, T., Goto, M., and Furuichi, Y. Reconsideration of senescence, immortalization and telomere maintenance of Epstein–Barr virus-transformed human B lymphoblastoid cell lines. *Mech. Ageing Dev.* 107: 51–60, **1999**.

Sugimoto, M., Tahara, H., Ide, T., and Furuichi, Y. Steps involved in immortalization and tumorigenesis in human B-lymphoblastoid cell lines transformed by Epstein–Barr virus. *Cancer Res.* 64: 3361–3364, **2004**.

Sugiura, M., Imai, S., Tokunaga, M., Koizumi, S., Uchizawa, M., Okamoto, K., and Osato, T. Transcriptional analysis of Epstein–Barr virus gene expression in EBV-positive gastric carcinoma: unique viral latency in the tumour cells. *Br. J. Cancer* 74: 625–631, **1996**.

Sumegi, J., Huang, D., Lanyi, A., Davis, J.D., Seemayer, T.A., Maeda, A., Klein, G., Seri, M., Wakiguchi, H., Purtilo, D.T., and Gross, T.G. Correlation of mutations of the SH2D1A gene and Epstein–Barr virus infection with clinical phenotype and out-

come in X-linked lymphoproliferative disease. *Blood* 96: 3118–3125, **2000**.

Sung, N.S., Edwards, R.H., Seillier-Moiseiwitsch, F., Perkins, A.G., Zeng, Y., and Raab-Traub, N. Epstein–Barr virus strain variation in nasopharyngeal carcinoma from the endemic and non-endemic regions of China. *Int. J. Cancer* 76: 207–215, **1998**.

Sutkowski, N., Conrad, B., Thorley-Lawson, D.A., and Huber, B.T. Epstein–Barr virus transactivates the human endogenous retrovirus HERV-K18 that encodes a superantigen. *Immunity* 15: 579–589, **2001**.

Szekely, L., Selivanova, G., Magnusson, K.P., Klein, G., and Wiman, K.G. EBNA-5, an Epstein–Barr virus-encoded nuclear antigen, binds to the retinoblastoma and p53 proteins. *Proc. Natl. Acad. Sci. USA* 90:5455–5459, **1993** .

Tajima, M., Komuro, M., and Okinaga, K. Establishment of Epstein–Barr virus-positive human gastric epithelial cell lines. *Jpn. J. Cancer Res.* 89: 262–268, **1998**.

Takada, K. Epstein–Barr virus and gastric carcinoma. *Mol. Pathol.* 53: 255–261, **2000**.

Takada, K. and Nanbo, A. The role of EBERs in oncogenesis. *Semin. Cancer Biol.* 11: 461–467, **2001**.

Takahara, M., Kis, L.L., Nagy, N., Liu, A., Klien, G., and Klein, E. Cytokine-induced increase of the EBV encoded latent membrane protein 1 (LMP1) leads to elevated expression of CD25 (IL-2R alpha) on NK lymphoma cells and thereby potentiates their proliferative response to IL-2. Submitted for publication.

Takakuwa, T., Luo, W.J., Ham, M.F., Sakane-Ishikawa, F., Wada, N., and Aozasa, K. Integration of the Epstein–Barr virus into chromosome 6q15 of Burkitt lymphoma cell line (Raji) induces loss of BACH2 expression. *Am. J. Pathol.* 164: 967–974, **2004**.

Tannenbaum, S. R., Bishop, W., Yu, M.C., and Henderson, B.E. Attempts to isolate N-nitroso compounds from Chinese-style salted fish. *Natl. Cancer Inst. Monogr.* 69: 209–211, **1985**.

Taub, R., Kirsch, I., Morton, C., Lenoir, G., Swan, D., Tronick, S., Aaronson, S., and Leder, P. Translocation of the c-myc gene into the immunoglobulin heavy chain locus in human Burkitt lymphoma and murine plasmocytoma cells. *Proc. Natl. Acad. Sci. USA* 79: 7837–7841, **1982**.

Teitell, M., Damore, M.A., Sulur, G.G., Turner, D.E., Stern, M.H., Said, J.W., Denny, C.T., and Wall. R. TCL1 oncogene expression in AIDS-related lymphomas and lymphoid tissues. *Proc. Natl. Acad. Sci. USA* 96: 9809–9814, **1999**.

Thangevelu, M., Olopade, O., Beckman, E., Vardiman, J.W., Larson, R.A., McKeithan, T.W., Le Beau, M.M., and Rowley, J.D. Clinical, morphologic, and cytogenetic characteristics of patients with lymphoid malignancies characterized by both t(14;18)(q32;q21) and t(8;14)(q24;q32) or t(8;22)(q24;q11). *Genes Chromosomes Cancer* 2: 147–158, **1990**.

Theil, J., Laumen, H., Marafioti, T., Hummel, M., Lenz, G., Wirth, T., and Stein, H. Defective octamer-dependent transcription is responsible for silenced immuno-globulin transcription in Reed–Sternberg cells. *Blood* 97: 3191–3196, **2001** .

Thomas, R.K., Re, D., Wolf, J., and Diehl, V. Part I: Hodgkin's lymphoma – molecular biology of Hodgkin and Reed–Sternberg cells. *Lancet Oncol.* 5: 11–18, **2004**.

Thornburg, N.J., Pathmanathan, R., Raab-Traub, N. Activation of nuclear factor-κB p50 homodimer/Bcl-3 complexes in nasopharyngeal carcinoma. *Cancer Res.* 63: 8293–8301, **2003**.

Thornburg, N.J., Kusano, S., and Raab-Traub, N. Identification of Epstein–Barr virus RK-BARF0-interacting proteins and characterization of expression pattern. *J. Virol.* 78: 12848–12856, **2004**.

Timmons, C.F., Dawson, D.B., Richards, C.S., Andrews, W.S., and Katz, J.A. Epstein–Barr virus-associated leiomyosarcomas in liver transplantation recipients. Origin from either donor or recipient tissue. *Cancer* 76: 1481–1489, **1995** .

Tierney, R.J., Steven, N., Young, L.S., and Rickinson, A.B. Epstein–Barr virus latency in blood mononuclear cells: analysis of viral gene transcription during primary infection and in the carrier state. *J. Virol.* 68: 7374–7385, **1994** .

Tokunaga, M., Land, C.E., Uemura, Y., Tokudome, T., Tanaka, S., and Sato, E. Epstein–Barr virus in gastric carcinoma. *Am. J. Pathol.* 143: 1250–1254, **1993**.

Tomkinson, B., Robertson, E., and Kieff, E. Epstein–Barr virus nuclear proteins EBNA-3A and EBNA-3C are essential for B-lymphocyte growth transformation. *J. Virol.* 67: 2014–2025, **1993**.

Torlakovic, E., Tierens, A., Dang, H.D., and Delabie, J. The transcription factor PU.1, necessary for B-cell development is expressed in lymphocyte predominance, but not in classical Hodgkin's disease. *Am. J. Pathol.* 159: 1807–1814, **2001**.

Torlakovic, G., Snover, D.C., and Torlakovic, E. Simultaneous EBV-positive lymphoepithelioma-like carcinoma and EBV-negative intestinal-type adenocarcinoma in a patient with *Helicobacter pylori*-associated chronic gastritis. *Am. J. Clin. Pathol.* 121: 237–243, **2004**.

Tsimbouri, P., Drotar, M.E., Coy, J.L., and Wilson, J.B. Bcl-xL and RAG genes are induced and the response to IL-2 enhanced in EmuEBNA-1 transgenic mouse lymphocytes. *Oncogene* 21: 5182–8187, **2002**.

Uchihara, J.N., Krensky, A.M., Matsuda, T., Kawakami, H., Okudaira, T., Masuda, M., Ohta, T., Takasu, N., and Mori, N. Transactivation of the CCL4/RANTES gene by Epstein–Barr virus latent membrane protein 1. *Int. J. Cancer*, 114: 747–755, **2005**.

Unniraman, S., Zhou, S., and Schatz, D.G. Identification of an AID-independent pathway for chromosomal translocations between the Igh switch region and Myc. *Nat. Immunol.* 5: 1117–1123, **2004**.

van Beek, J., zur Hausen, A., Klein Kranenbarg, E., van de Velde, C.J., Middeldorp, J.M., van den Brule, A.J., Meijer, C.J.M., and Bloemena, E. EBV-positive gastric adenocarcinomas: a distinct clinicopathological entity with a low frequency of lymph node involvement. *J. Clin. Oncol.* 22: 664–670, **2004**.

van Gelder, T., Vuzevski, V.D., and Weimar, W. Epstein–Barr virus in smooth-muscle tumors. *N. Engl. J. Med.* 332: 1719, **1995**.

van Gorp, J., Doornewaard, H., Verdonck, L.F., Klopping, C., Vos, P.F., and van den Tweel, J.G.. Posttransplant T-cell lymphoma. Report of three cases and a review of the literature. *Cancer* 73: 3064–3072, **1994**.

Vieira, P., de Waal-Malefyt, R., Dang, M.N., Johnson, K.E., Kastelein, R., Fiorentino, D.F., de Vries, J.E., Roncarolo, M.G.,

Mosmann, T.R., and Moore, K.W. Isolation and expression of human cytokine synthesis inhibitory factor cDNA clones: homology to Epstein–Barr virus open reading frame BCRF1. *Proc. Natl. Acad. Sci. USA* 88: 1172–1176, **1991**.

Vo, Q.N., Geradts, J., Gulley, M.L., Boudreau, D.A., Bravo, J.C., and Schneider, B.G. Epstein–Barr virus in gastric adenocarcinomas: association with ethnicity and CDKN2A promoter methylation. *J. Clin. Pathol.* 55: 669–675, **2002** .

Vockerodt, M., Pinkert, D., Smola-Hess, S., Michels, A., Ransohoff, R.M., Tesch, H., and Kube, D. The Epstein–Barr virus oncoprotein latent membrane protein 1 induces expression of the chemokine IP-10: importance for mRNA half-life regulation. *Int. J. Cancer* 114: 598–605, **2005**.

von Knebel Doeberitz, M., Bornkamm, G.W., and zur Hausen, H. Establishment of spontaneously outgrowing lymphoblastoid cell lines with Cyclosporin A. *Med. Microbiol. Immunol. (Berl.)* 172: 87–99, **1983**.

Vose, J.M., Chiu, B.C., Cheson, B.D., Dancey, J., and Wright, J. Update on epidemiology and therapeutics for non-Hodgkin's lymphoma. *Hematology (Am. Soc. Hematol. Educ. Program)* 241–262, **2002**.

Walton, R.M. and Hendrick, M.J. Feline Hodgkin's-like lymphoma: 20 cases. *Vet. Pathol.* 38: 504–511, **2001**.

Waltzer, L., Perricaudet, M., Sergeant, A., and Manet, E. Epstein–Barr virus EBNA3A and EBNA3C proteins both repress RBP-Jκ-EBNA2-activated transcription by inhibiting the binding of RBP-Jκ to DNA. *J. Virol.* 70: 5909–5915, **1996**.

Wang, F., Gregory, C.D., Rowe, M., Rickinson, A.B., Wang, D., Birkenbach, M., Kikutani, H., Kishimoto, T., and Kieff, E. Epstein–Barr virus nuclear antigen 2 specifically induces expression of the B-cell activation antigen CD23. *Proc. Natl. Acad. Sci. USA* 83: 3452–3457, **1987a**.

Wang, F., Petti, L., Braun, D., Seung, S., and Kieff, E. A bicistronic Epstein–Barr virus mRNA encodes two nuclear proteins in latently infected, growth transformed lymphocytes. *J. Virol.* 61: 945–954, **1987b**.

Wang, F., Gregory, C., Sample, C., Rowe, M., Liebowitz, D., Murray, R., Rickinson, A.B., and Kieff, E. Epstein–Barr virus latent membrane protein (LMP1) and nuclear proteins 2 and 3C are effectors of phenotypic changes in B lymphocytes, EBNA-2 and LMP1 cooperatively induce CD23. *J. Virol.* 64: 2309–2318, **1990**.

Wedderburn, N., Edwards, J.M., Desgranges, C., Fontaine, C., Cohen, B., and de Thé, G. Infectious mononucleosis-like response in common marmosets infected with Epstein–Barr virus. *J. Infect. Dis.* 150: 878–882, **1984**.

Weiss, L.M., Strickler, J.G., Warnke, R.A., Purtilo, D.T., and Sklar, J. Epstein–Barr viral DNA in tissues of Hodgkin's disease. *Am. J. Pathol.* 129: 86–91, **1987**.

Weiss, L.M., Movahed, L.A., Warnke, R.A., and Sklar, J. Detection of Epstein–Barr viral genomes in Reed–Sternberg cells of Hodgkin's disease. *N. Engl. J. Med.* 320: 502–506, **1989**.

Wilson, J.B., Bell, J.L., and Levine, A.J. Expression of Epstein–Barr virus nuclear antigen-1 induces B cell neoplasia in transgenic mice. *EMBO J.* 15: 3117–3126, **1996**.

Wolf, H., zur Hausen, H., and Becker, V. EB viral genomes in epithelial nasopharyngeal carcinoma cells. *Nat. New Biol.* 244: 245–247, **1973**.

Wolf, H., Haus, M., and Wilmes, E. Persistence of Epstein–Barr virus in the parotid gland. *J. Virol.* 51: 795–798, **1984**.

Wu, T.C., Mann, R.B., Epstein, J.I., MacMahon, E., Lee, W.A., Charache, P., Hayward, S. D., Kurman, R.J., Hayward, G.S., and Ambinder, R.F. Abundant expression of EBER1 small nuclear RNA in nasopharyngeal carcinoma. A morphologically distinctive target for detection of Epstein–Barr virus in formalin-fixed paraffin-embedded carcinoma specimens. *Am. J. Pathol.* 138: 1461–1469, **1991**.

Wysokenski, D.A. and Yates, J.L. Multiple EBNA1-binding sites are required to form an EBNA1-dependent enhancer and to activate a minimal replicative origin within oriP of Epstein-Barr virus. *J. Virol.* 63: 2657–2666, **1989**.

Yamamoto, N., Tokunaga, M., Uemura, Y., Tanaka, S., Shirahama, H., Nakamura, T., Land, C.E., and Sato, E. Epstein–Barr virus and gastric remnant cancer. *Cancer* 74: 805–809, **1994**.

Yanai, H., Murakami, T., Yoshiyama, H., Takeuchi, H., Nishikawa, J., Nakamura, H., Okita, K., Miura, O., Shimuzu, N., and

Takada, K. Epstein–Barr virus-associated gastric carcinoma and atrophic gastritis. *J. Clin. Gastroenterol.* 29: 39–43, **1999**.

Yanai, H., Hirano, A., Matsusaki, K., Kawano, T., Miura, O., Yoshida, T., Okita, K., and Shimizu, N. Epstein–Barr virus association is rare in esophageal squamous cell carcinoma. *Int. J. Gastrointest. Cancer* 33: 165–170, **2003**.

Yanase, S. and Ito, Y. Heat durability of Epstein–Barr virus-activating substances of plant origin: 12-O-tetradecanoylphorbol-13-acetate, 12-O-hexadecanoyl-16hydrophorbol-13-acetate, croton oil, tung oil, and *Croton megalocarpus*extract. *Cancer Lett.* 22: 183–186, **1984**.

Yang, L., Aozasa, K., Oshimi, K., and Takada, K. Epstein–Barr virus (EBV)-encoded RNA promotes growth of EBV-infected T cells through interleukin-9 induction. *Cancer Res.* 64: 5332–5337, **2004**.

Yano, T., Sander, C.A., Clark, H.M., Dolezal, M.V., Jaffe, E.S., and Raffeld, M. Clustered mutations in the second exon of the myc gene in sporadic Burkitt's lymphoma. *Oncogene* 8: 2741–2748, **1993**.

Yeung, W.M., Zong, Y.S., Chiu, C.T., Chan, K.H., Sham, J.S., Choy, D.T., and Ng, M.H. Epstein–Barr virus carriage by nasopharyngeal carcinoma in situ. *Int. J. Cancer* 53: 746–750, **1993**.

Young, L.S. Infection control: the immunocompromised host. *Infect. Control Hosp. Epidemiol.* 10: 274–275, **1989**.

Young, L.S. and Murray, P.G. Epstein–Barr virus and oncogenesis: from latent genes to tumours. *Oncogene* 22: 5108–5121, **2003**.

Young, L.S. and Rickinson, A.B. Epstein–Barr virus: 40 years on. *Nat. Rev. Cancer* 4: 757–768, **2004**.

Young, L.S., Dawson, C.W., Clark, D., Rupani, H., Busson, P., Tursz, T., Johnson, A., and Rickinson, A.B. Epstein–Barr virus gene expression in nasopharyngeal carcinoma. *J. Gen. Virol.* 69: 1051–1065, **1988**.

Young, L.S., Finerty, S., Brooks, L., Scullion, F., Rickinson, A.B., and Morgan, A.J. Epstein–Barr virus gene expression in malignant lymphomas induced by experimental virus infection of cottontop tamarins. *J. Virol.* 63: 1967–1974, **1989**.

Yu, M.C. and Henderson, B.E. Intake of Cantonese-style salted fish as a cause of nasopharyngeal carcinoma. *IARC Sci. Publ.* 84; 547–549, **1987**.

Yu, M.C., Ho, J.H.C., Lai, S. H., and Henderson, B.E. Cantonese-style salted fish as a cause of nasopharyngeal carcinoma: report of a case-control study in Hong Kong. *Cancer Res.* 46: 956–961, **1986**.

Yu, M.C., Huang, T.B., and Henderson, B.E. Diet and nasopharyngeal carcinoma: a case-control study in Guangzhou, China. *Int. J. Cancer* 43: 1077–1082, **1989**.

Zeng, M.-S., Li, D.-J., Liu, Q.-L., Song, L.-B., Li, M.-Z., Zhang, R.-H., Yu, X.-J., Wang, H.-M., Ernberg, I., and Zeng, Y.-X. Genomic sequence analysis of Epstein–Barr virus strain GD1 from a nasopharyngeal carcinoma patient. *J. Virol.*79: 15 323–15 330, **2005**.

Zhang, C.X., Lowrey, P., Finerty, S., and Morgan, A.J. Analysis of Epstein–Barr virus gene transcription in lymphoma induced by the virus in the cottontop tamarin by construction of a cDNA library with RNA extracted from a tumour biopsy. *J. Gen. Virol.* 74: 509–514, **1993**.

Zhou, X.G., Hamilton-Dutoit, S. J., Yan, Q.H., and Pallesen, G. High frequency of Epstein–Barr virus in Chinese peripheral T cell lymphoma. *Histopathology* 24: 115–122, **1994**.

Zimber-Strobl, U., Suentzenich, K., Falk, M., Laux, G., Cordier, M., Calender, A., Billaud, M., Lenoir, G.M., and Bornkamm, G.W. Epstein–Barr virus terminal protein gene transcription is dependent on EBNA2 expression and provides evidence for viral integration into the host genome. *Curr. Top. Microbiol. Immunol.* 166: 359–366, **1990**.

Zimber-Strobl, U., Strobl, U.J., Meitinger, C., Hinrichs, R., Sakai, T., Furukawa, T., Honjo, T., and Bornkamm, G.W. Epstein–Barr virus nuclear antigen 2 exerts its transactivating function through interaction with recombination signal binding protein RBP-J kappa, the homologue of Drosophila Suppressor of Hairless. *EMBO J.* 13: 4973–4982, **1994**.

zur Hausen, A. Epstein–Barr virus-carrying gastric carcinomas: pathogenesis and clinical aspects. Academisch Proefschrift, Vrije Universiteit, Amsterdam, **2004**.

zur Hausen, A., Brink, A.A.T.P., Craanen, M.E., Middeldorp, J.M., Meijer, C.J.L.M., and van den Brule, A.J.C. Unique transcription pattern of Epstein–Barr virus

---

(EBV) in EBV-carrying gastric adenocarcinomas: expression of the transforming BARF 1 gene. *Cancer Res.* 60: 2745–2748, **2000**.

zur Hausen, A., van Grieken, N.C.T., Meijer, G.A., Hermsen, M.A.J.A., Bloemena, E., Meuwissen, S. G.M., Braak, J.P.A., Meijer, C.J.L.M., Kuipers, E.J., van den Brule, A.J.C. Distinct chromosomal aberrations in Epstein–Barr virus-carrying gastric carcinomas tested by comparative genomic hybridization. *Gastroenterology* 121: 612–618, **2001**.

zur Hausen, A., van Rees, B.P., van Beek, J., Craanen, M.E., Bloemena, E., Offerhaus, G.J.A., Meijer, C.J.L.M., van den Brule, A.J.C. Epstein–Barr virus in gastric carcinomas and gastric stump carcinomas: a late event in gastric carcinogenesis. *J. Clin. Pathol.* 57: 487–491, **2004**.

zur Hausen, H. and de Villiers, E.-M. A virus target cell conditioning model to explain some epidemiological characteristics of childhood leukemias and lymphomas. *Int. J. Cancer* 115: 1–5, **2005**.

zur Hausen, H. and Schulte-Holthausen, H. Presence of EB virus nucleic acid homology in a "virus-free" line of Burkitt tumour cells. *Nature* 227: 245–247, **1970**.

zur Hausen, H., Henle, W., Hummeler, K., Diehl, V., and Henle, G. Comparative study of cultured Burkitt tumor cells by immunofluorescence, autoradiography and electron microscopy. *J. Virol.* 1: 830–837, **1967**.

zur Hausen, H., Schulte-Holthausen H., Klein, G., Henle, W., Henle, G., Clifford, P., and Santesson, L. EBV DNA in biopsies of Burkitt tumors and anaplastic carcinomas of the nasopharynx. *Nature* 228: 1056–1058, **1970**.

zur Hausen, H., Bornkamm, G.W., Schmidt, R., and Hecker, E. Tumor initiators and promoters in the induction of Epstein–Barr virus. *Proc. Natl. Acad. Sci. USA* 76: 782–785, **1979**.

4.4
Rhadinoviruses

4.4.1
Human Herpesvirus Type 8 (HHV-8, Kaposi's sarcoma-associated herpesvirus)

4.4.1.1 Historical Background

In 1872, a Hungarian dermatologist, Moriz Kaposi, working at that time in Vienna, described a new tumor type of the skin that he characterized as an "idiopathic multiple pigmented sarcoma of the skin". He observed these rare tumors on the legs and arms of elderly men, particularly among inhabitants of the Mediterranean region, of Eastern Europe, and in males of Jewish descent. Subsequently this tumor, which was designated as Kaposi's sarcoma (KS), remained rare in Europe for more than 100 years. Besides this sporadic and "classic" form of KS, an endemic form of the tumor was detected in equatorial Africa (reviewed in Hutt, 1983). In addition, in the years between 1969 and 1973 it was noted that organ transplant recipients were at increased risk of developing this tumor (Siegel et al., 1969; Penn and Starzl, 1970; Fahey, 1971; Haim et al., 1972; Birkeland and Kemp, 1973) (Fig. 4.12).

In 1981, highly aggressive forms of KS were identified in homosexual men who had previously acquired the newly identified AIDS infection (Borkovic and Schwartz, 1981; Gottlieb et al., 1981; Hymes et al., 1981). Subsequently, it was shown that close to 30% of HIV-1-positive homosexual men developed AIDS-associated KS (Beral, 1991). This and another study suggested that KS should have an infectious

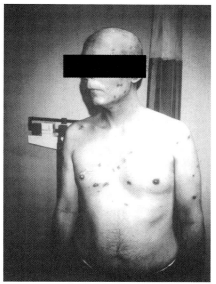

Fig. 4.12 Kaposi's sarcoma. (Source: Centers of Disease Control and Prevention (CDC), Atlanta, and courtesy of D.P. Drotman and H. Haverkos.)

etiology activated under immunosuppression (Weiss and Biggar, 1986). A DNA fragment of the putative responsible agent was identified in 1994 by Chang and Moore and their colleagues, and this resulted in the identification of a new human herpesvirus, human herpesvirus type 8 (HHV-8) or Kaposi sarcoma-associated human herpesvirus (KSHV) (Russo et al., 1996; Neipel et al., 1997). The availability of viral DNA sequences permitted the detection of HHV-8 in two additional lympho-proliferative conditions, primary effusion lymphoma (PEL) (Cesarman et al., 1995, 1996), and in a variable percentage in multicentric Castleman disease (MCD) (Soulier et al., 1995; Corbellino et al., 1996). During the past 10 years the epidemiology and the molecular biology of this interesting virus infection have been intensively studied.

4.4.1.2 Epidemiology and Mode of Transmission

The epidemiology of KS has been described in detail in a recent review (Dourmishev et al., 2003), wherein differentiation was made between the classic or sporadic form, the African endemic, the AIDS-epidemic, and the iatrogenic (immunosuppression of allograft recipients) forms of the lesion. Although all of these forms seem to differ in their histology, aggressiveness, morbidity and mortality, they are all linked with HHV-8 infections. This infection emerges as a prerequisite for the development of KS.

The classic form has been more often observed in elderly men in Mediterranean regions in Italy, Greece, Turkey, and Israel (Schwartz, 1996; Iscovich et al., 2000). In Italy, the seroprevalence of antibodies against HHV-8 differs substantially from the north to the south. In northern Italy, 7.3% of blood donors are HHV-8-positive, in central Italy 9.5%, and in the south 24.6% (Whitby et al., 1998). Kaposi's sarcoma develops in the Mediterranean in only 0.03% of HHV-8-infected men above the age of 50 years (Vitale et al., 2001), and this suggests the involvement of additional cofactors in tumor development. It has been proposed that a combination of mild immunosuppression (lower lymphocyte and CD4 cell numbers) and of immune activation (increased serum neopterin and β_2-microglobulin levels) may account for the sporadic KS cases (Touloumi et al., 1999).

Since family members and heterosexual partners of sporadic KS patients reveal increased HHV-8 seroprevalence (Angeloni et al., 1998; Brambilla et al., 2000; Plancoulaine et al., 2004), transmission of the virus probably occurs by sexual as well as by nonsexual contacts. Tonsillar swabs from KS patients are frequently HHV-8-positive, suggesting that saliva contact, similar to EBV transmission (Cattani et al., 1999), and possibly also breast milk (Dedicoat et al., 2004), are the most important routes for HHV-8 transmission in sporadic KS cases. In endemic populations from Central Africa, the most likely route of HHV-8 transmission occurs from mother to child and between siblings (Plancoulaine et al., 2004). Thus far, no evidence has been reported for vertical transmission of HHV-8 during pregnancy (Sarmati et al., 2004), although vertical transmission has been suggested for African HHV-8 infections (Dupin and Calvez, 2000).

Today, the African endemic form of KS is difficult to study in view of the high prevalence of HIV infections in virtually all of those countries in which KS was previously endemic. These were mainly the north-eastern regions of the Congo (Zaire), western Uganda and Tanzania, although KS covered a broad band of equatorial Africa (Dourmishev et al., 2003). In the pre-AIDS period from 1954 to 1960, KS amounted to 6.2–6.6% of male cancer patients in Uganda without female cases; about 30 years later, the prevalence in males rose to 48.6%, and in females to 17.9% (Wabinga et al., 1993). Today, two age groups are mainly affected by KS: adults at an average age of 35 years, and children with an average age of 3 years. In Cameroon, approximately 4% of all childhood cancers are due to KS (Kasolo et al., 1997). Besides oral and sexual modes of virus transmission, in certain African regions ritual skin piercing and tattooing may also contribute to transmission of the virus (Enbom et al., 2002).

HHV-8 infects a number of target cells (B cells, macrophages, endothelial cells and keratinocytes) *in vivo* via cell surface heparan sulfate, and uses $\alpha_3\beta_1$ integrin as one of its entry receptors (Akula et al., 2002; Naranatt et al., 2003). The infection of endothelial cells results in a semipermissive response: the cells are converted into spindle shape, part of them produce virus, resulting in cell death, while surviving cells enter the stage of viral latency (Gao et al., 2003). In addition, HHV-8, similar to other members of the herpesvirus group, induces chromosomal instability in primary human endothelial cells (Pan et al., 2004), and is also able to transform these cells (Flore et al., 1998). Early in the course of infection HHV-8 induces acetylation of microtubules and the activation of *RhoA* and *Rac* GTPases (Naranatt et al., 2005). The activation of Rho GTPases significantly enhances the nuclear delivery of viral DNA.

AIDS-associated KS is strikingly linked to the epidemiology of HIV infections. Dual infections by HHV-8 and HIV-1 are high in the AIDS epicenters, such as California and New York (Dourmishev et al., 2003). During the early 1980s, the incidence of AIDS-associated KS in homosexual men in San Francisco was about 40% (Beral et al., 1990), but by the mid-1900 – due to the introduction of effective anti-AIDS therapy – it had declined to 15–25% (Whitby et al., 1995; Moore et al., 1996a; Gao et al., 1996; Kedes et al., 1996). In Thailand, where there is a low incidence of KS but a high rate of HIV infections, only 2–12% of homosexual men were reported HHV-8-positive in 2002 (Ayuthaya et al., 2002). It is interesting to note that the introduction of highly active antiretroviral therapy (HAART) resulted, in the United States, to an 8.8% annual decline in KS incidence (Jones et al., 2000). Clearly, the immune restoration occurring due to this therapy plays the most important role in this respect; typically, a long period of treatment (> 24 months) results in undetectable HHV-8 viremia (Bourboulia et al., 2004). Since HIV-specific protease inhibitors (e.g., indinavir and sequenivir) are also anti-angiogenic (Sgadari et al., 2002), this may, in addition, contribute to the effect of HAART therapy in preventing KS.

Sexual transmission is clearly the most prominent route of HHV-8 infection in HIV-infected populations (Martin et al., 1998). The risk for KS development is calculated to be more than 10 000-fold higher in HIV-infected homosexuals than in the general population (Goedert, 2000). Correspondingly, hemophiliacs and injection drug addicts have a markedly reduced HHV-8 infection rate and a low KS risk (Beral et al., 1990; Atkinson et al., 2004). Orogenital sex seems to represent a particularly high-risk factor (Dukers et al., 2000).

Immunosuppressive therapy in organ allograft recipients in HHV-8-positive patients may lead to the iatrogenic form of KS. This occurs in about 0.4% of transplant patients in the United States and Western Europe (Farge et al., 1993; Penn, 1997), in contrast to 4.0–5.3% of renal transplant patients in Saudi-Arabia (Qunibi et al., 1988; Penn, 1993). The type of immunosuppressive therapy plays an important role, in particular cyclosporine treatment results more frequently in KS development (Penn, 1993), possibly due to the reactivation of latent HHV-8 (Hudnall et al., 1999). Although the vast majority of these patients is HHV-8-seropositive before organ transplantation, seronegative patients may also become infected from the donated organ (Parravicini et al., 1997; Barozzi et al., 2003).

4.4.1.3 Pathogenesis: Other Diseases Associated with HHV-8 Infections

Besides Kaposi's sarcoma, primary effusion lymphoma (PEL) is a rare HHV-8-associated cancer. This lesion constitutes only 0.13% of all AIDS-associated lymphomas, but AIDS patients who previously acquired KS are at increased risk for this lymphoma (Mbulaiteye et al., 2002).

Another partially HHV-8 associated rare angiolymphoproliferative disorder is that of multicentric Castleman disease (MCD) (Soulier et al., 1995; Corbellino et al., 1996). Among AIDS patients with MCD, more than 90% are positive for HHV-8, whereas among HIV-seronegative MCD patients only 40% are HHV-8-infected

(Grandadam et al., 1997). Lytic infection is more frequently detectable in MCD lesions, which suggests that the viral gene expression program differs here from that of KS and PEL (Teruya-Feldstein et al., 1998; Katano et al., 2000; Oksenhendler et al., 2000; Parravicini et al., 2000). A viral involvement in the HHV-8-negative MCD proliferations has not yet been identified.

Several other diseases were suspected of being linked to HHV-8 infection (for a review, see Dourmishev et al., 2003), but as yet no reproducible results have been recorded.

4.4.1.4 Viral Genes Expressed in Viral Latency

Detailed reports of viral genes and genome functions have been provided in three excellent recent reviews by Dormishev et al. (2003), Moore and Chang (2003), and Verma and Robertson (2003). Consequently, this chapter will only detail those genes and their functions that are engaged in viral latency and tumorigenesis, and which permit escape of the virus from host cell immune functions.

One gene that is highly expressed in all HHV-8-associated malignancies and all infected cells is the latency-associated nuclear protein *LANA* (Kedes et al., 1997; Dupin et al., 1999). This gene is located in ORF 73 and is expressed as a polycistronic mRNA jointly with viral cyclin, originating from ORF 72, and viral Fas-associated death domain IL-1B converting enzyme inhibitory protein encoded by ORF 71 (Sarid et al., 1999). LANA represents a 222 to 232-kDa nuclear protein, and is important for viral episome maintenance during latent infection. It tethers the viral episomes to host cell chromosomes, and is also bound to the terminal repeat elements of the viral genome (Ballestas et al., 1999; Cotter and Robertson, 1999). The binding site at the terminal repeat region covers the carboxy-terminal 200 amino acids of LANA (Ballestas and Kaye, 2001; Cotter et al., 2001), whereas the N-terminus of this protein plays an important role in binding to chromatin (Barbera et al., 2004; Wong et al., 2004). Binding to this region as oligomer (Komatsu et al., 2004) is sufficient to permit replication of terminal-repeat-containing plasmids (Fejer et al., 2003; Grundhoff and Ganem, 2003). Disruption of LANA leads to abortive episome persistence (Ye et al., 2004; Barbera et al., 2004). LANA also binds to histone H1 (Cotter and Robertson, 1999) and to the SUV39H1 histone methyltransferase (Sakakibara et al., 2004).

A large number of functions have recently been ascribed to LANA. This protein has a transcriptionally regulatory role and affects gene expression both positively and negatively. LANA regulates its own promoter positively via its C-terminal domain, and binds to a defined site within the core promoter (Jeong et al., 2004). LANA interacts with p53 and down-regulates p53-mediated activation of p53-responsive promoters, thus protecting against apoptosis (Friborg et al., 1999). The 223 amino acids of the LANA C-terminus are sufficient to inhibit p53-mediated activation of the human BAX promoter (Wong et al., 2004). LANA also associates with hypophosphorylated ("active") pRB *in vitro* and under conditions of transient transfections, thus transactivating E2F-responsive promoters. In combination with *H-ras* it transforms primary rat cells and renders them tumorigenic in the nude mouse system (Radkov et al., 2000). It also prolongs the life span of human primary umbilical vein endothelial cells (Watanabe et al., 2003). A further interesting feature of LANA is the activation of the activator protein 1 (AP-1) response element and the induction of the binding of a *c-Jun-Fos* heterodimer, which in turn results in IL-6 expression (An et al., 2004). In another system, cervical cancer, *c-Jun-Fos* heterodimer formation seems to be one of the characteristics of the malignant phenotype (Soto et al., 2000). LANA also induces the inhibitor of the basic helix-loop-helix transcription factor Id-1 (Tang et al., 2003). The multifunctional activities of LANA are further underlined by the activation of the human telomerase transcriptase promoter (Knight et al., 2001) by directly interacting with the transcription factor SP1 (Verma et al., 2004). LANA interferes with the Wnt signaling pathway by interacting with the glycogen synthase kinase 3 (GSK-3). This overcomes the GSK-3 mediated inhibition of β-catenin and results in increased levels of β-catenin (Fujimuro and Hayward, 2003). Another cellular transcriptional repressor, KLIP1, repressing herpes simplex thymidine kinase promoter activity, interacts with LANA which alleviates its activity (Pan et al., 2003). It seems that LANA also plays a critical role in maintaining viral latency, as it suppresses the replication and transcription activator (*Rta*) of HHV-8, thus, controlling the switch between viral latency and lytic replication (Lan et al., 2004).

The multiple functions of LANA are summarized in Table 4.5. It is somewhat surprising that this protein combines various functions of other viral oncogenes, including the EBNAs, papilloma-, polyoma- and adenovirus oncogenes.

A second important gene product in latently infected cells is the *viral cyclin D* protein, coded for by ORF 72, revealing a 32 % identity and 54 % similarity to cellular cyclin D2 (Chang et al., 1996; Godden-Kent et al., 1997; Li et al., 1997 a; Swanton et al., 1997). This protein forms functional complexes with the cellular cdk-6, phosphory-

Table 4.5 Interaction of the LANA protein with cellular proteins, and resulting consequences

Interacting gene product	Activation/repression	Consequence
p53	Inactivation	Inactivation fo p53-responsive promoters (e.g., BAX)
pRB	Inactivation	Activation of E2F and cdk2
AP-1	Co-activation	Formation of c-jun/Fos heterodimers
Id-1 (helix-loop-helix transcription factor)	Activation	
SP-1	Activation	Activation of telomerase reverse transcriptase
Glycogen kinase 3 GSK-3	Inactivation and altered distribution	β-catenin overexpression
HHV-8 replication and transcription activator Rta	Inactivation	Latency maintenance

lates RB1 and histone H1, and stimulates the G_1 to S transition. The complex v-cyclin/cdk-6 is resistant to the inhibitory functions of the cyclin-dependent kinase inhibitors p16, p21, and p27 and phosphorylates and down-regulates p27 (Swanton et al., 1997; Ellis et al., 1999; Mann et al., 1999; Card et al., 2000). Phosphorylation of Bcl-2 by this complex may lead to apoptosis. In latent infection this is probably counteracted by the inactivation of p53 by interaction with LANA (see above). Similar to LANA, v-cyclin is invariably expressed in biopsies from Kaposi's sarcomas and primary effusion lymphomas (Dittmer, 2003; Jarviluoma et al., 2004). v-Cyclin overrides growth-suppressive signals of the signal transducer and activator 3 (STAT3) by suppressing its activity. This prevents the growth-suppressive effect by the IL-6 type cytokine, oncostatin M (Lundquist et al., 2003). The targeted expression of v-cyclin to B- and T-lymphocyte compartments results in lymphoma development by nine months of age (Verschuren et al., 2004), and all lymphomas had lost p53 expression. This suggests a role for p53 in interacting with v-cyclin.

A third protein originating from ORF 74 clearly represents a viral oncoprotein and possesses homology to the cellular G-protein-coupled receptor (GPCR) (Swanton et al., 1997). It is relatively closely related to the IL-8 receptors CXCR1 and CXCR2, and activates the phosphoinositide pathway. Although the protein appears to be difficult to detect in latently infected tumor cells, the respective RNA is constitutively expressed. Upon transfection, vGPCR transforms rat fibroblasts (Arvanitakis et al., 1997) and NIH 3 T3 cells (Bais et al., 1998). It also has been shown to immortalize human endothelial cells by activating the VEGF receptor-2/KDR (Bais et al., 2003) and to induce angioproliferative tumors in transgenic mice that strikingly resemble human KS (Montaner et al., 2003). These data point to a central role for vGPCR as one of the major pathogenic determinants of KS. cGPCR has been considered as a gene expressed in lytic infection, yet, it has been proposed that its dysregulated expression by HIV-1 Tat, inflammation, or aborted cell cycle progression may trigger its expression and the up-regulation of oncogenic signaling pathways (Sodhi et al., 2004). The demonstration of lytic replication-defective HHV-8 genomes in Kaposi's tumors and PEL cell lines may lend some support for this speculation (Deng et al., 2004). The mode by which vGPCR may contribute to the neoplastic growth was analyzed by Pati et al. (2003) and Montaner et al. (2004). According to these and other authors, vGPCR up-regulates the expression and secretion of several cytokines by stimulating NF-κB, AP-1, and nuclear factor of activated T cells (NF-AT) by the activation of the small G protein Rac1 and its effector, the p21-activated kinase 1 (Pak1) (Dadke et al., 2003). Inhibition of the latter blocked vGPCR-induced transcription and the secretion of cytokines, including IL-6 and IL-8 and the growth-regulated oncogene α (GROα). The constitutive activation of NK-κB and the induction of pro-inflammatory and angiogenetic factors are consistent with the inflammatory hyperproliferative nature of Kaposi lesions (Pati et al., 2003). NF-AT activation depended on signaling through the phosphatidylinositol 3-kinase-Akt-glycogen synthetase kinase 3 (P13-K/Akt/GSK-3) pathway. Interestingly, NF-AT and NF-κB activation by vGPCR was greatly increased by the HIV-1 Tat protein, whereas Tat alone had little effect. Thus, there seems to exist a collaborative stimulation by vGPCR and Tat.

There exists another latency-expressed protein originating from an adjacent genomic region, ORF 71 (also labeled K13), the v-FLICE-inhibitory protein, v-FLIP. This possesses two death effector domains, and functions as a dominant-negative inhibitor of Fas-receptor-mediated apoptosis by binding to Fas-associated death domain protein and caspase 8 (FLICE) (Belanger et al., 2001). v-FLIP is constitutively expressed. Upon transduction it enhances tumorigenicity of mouse B lymphoma cells in immunocompetent mice (Djerbi et al., 1999) and transforms Rat-1 and Balb/3 T3 fibroblast cells to soft agar growth and tumor formation in nude mice (Sun et al., 2003). v-FLIP activates NF-κB by activating the IκB kinase γ (Chaudhary et al., 1999; Kataoka et al., 2000; Liu et al., 2002; Field et al., 2003). Specifically, the up-regulation of p100/NF-κB2 expression and its subsequent procession into the p52 subunit are effected by v-Flip (Matta and Chaudhary, 2004). Silencing of ORF 71 expression by siRNA inhibits the processing of p100 and blocks cell proliferation. v-FLIP is largely responsible for NF-κB activation in latently infected PEL cells, and its elimination results in decreased NF-κB activity, induction of apoptosis, and increased sensitivity to external apoptotic stimuli (Guasparri et al., 2004). It has also been documented that v-FLIP activates the JNK/AP-1 pathway in a TRAF-dependent fashion (An et al., 2003). This results in cellular IL-6 expression, the promoter of which becomes active after NF-κB and AP-1 activation.

Kaposin (K12) represents a small hydrophobic protein of 60 amino acids. It has also been reported to represent a transforming protein after transfection of its gene into Rat-3 tissue culture cells, which then form tumors after inoculation into nude mice (Kliche et al., 2001; Muralidhar et al., 1998, 2000). The K12 locus is complex, it encodes many potential ORFs, the relative importance of which is unclear (Li et al., 2002). Its complex transcripts are abundantly present in KS cells and in PEL cell lines (Zhong et al., 1996; Staskus et al., 1997; Sturzl et al., 1997). Kaposin reorganizes cellular actin (Kliche et al., 2001) and associates with cytohesin-1, a guanine nucleotide exchange factor, regulating integrin activity. Three different Kaposins – A, B, and C – have been identified in PEL cell lines. Induction of the lytic cycle by phorbol ester TPA treatment of HHV-8-positive cells increases the transcription substantially (Li et al., 2002).

The HHV-8 genome contains four tandemly arranged genes coding for viral interferon regulatory factors (vIRF1–4). During the lytic cycle vIRFs 1, 2, and 4 are induced, whereas vIRF-3 is not inducible and constitutively present at low abundancy in PEL cells (Fakhari and Dittmer, 2002; Cunningham et al., 2003; Dittmer, 2003). The protein is also designated as LANA-2. It inhibits p53-mediated transactivation and PKR-triggered apoptosis, and abrogates activation of caspase 3 (Esteban et al., 2003). It seems to be latently expressed exclusively in B cells (Rivas et al., 2001). vIRF3 stimulates the transcriptional activity of cellular IRF-3 and -7 by directly interacting with IRF-3 and -7 through its C-terminal region (Lubyova et al., 2004). It also binds to the transcriptional co-activator CBP/p300. It is recruited to the interferon α-promoters by IRF-3 and -7 and activates genes controlled by these proteins.

Besides vIRF-3, which is not inducible after TPA treatment, the inducible vIRF-1 is transcribed at a low rate during viral latency (Cunningham et al., 2003). The function of vIRF-1 differs from that of vIRF-3, as it blocks the interaction between IRF-3 and p300 and inhibits histone acetylation (Lubyova et al., 2004). Similar to the other two vIRFs (vIRF-2 and -4), there is at this stage no recognizable direct role of vIRF-1 for the viral state of latency, or for events linked to cell transformation.

The last latency-associated protein which apparently plays an important role in cell transformation originates from a family of alternatively sliced transcripts of approximately 7.5 kb, translated with hypervariable protein epitopes (Stebbing et al., 2003). The coding gene (K1) is located between ORF 75 and the terminal repeats at the right end of the HHV-8 genome (Glenn et al., 1999). The gene product represents a latent membrane protein (LAMP). The K1 gene consists of eight alternatively spliced exons and is supposed to encode a 45-kDa transmembrane protein with 12 predicted transmembrane regions (Brinkmann et al., 2003). The C-terminal cytoplasmic domain contains binding sites for SH2 and SH3 domains, and binds in addition tumor necrosis factor receptor-associated proteins. In its organization it shows a remarkable similarity to EBV LMP-1 and LMP-1A. It activates the Ras/mitogen-activated protein kinase (MAPK) and NF-κB pathways. This requires phosphorylation of tyrosine residue 481 within one of the SH2-binding sites which is mediated by tyrosine kinases *Src, Lck, Yes, Hck,* and *Fyn* (Brinkmann et al., 2003). Additional experimental data point to a central role of K1-mediated constitutive *Lyn kinase* activation for the production of VEGF and NK-κB activation (Prakash et al., 2005). Smaller K1 isoforms of the K1 protein activate these pathways to a much lesser degree.

The transforming potential of the K1 gene was first reported by Lee et al. (1998). The expression of K1 in rodent fibroblasts resulted in morphologic changes and focus formation. In case of replacement of a gene encoding the herpesvirus saimiri-transforming protein (which shows no structural relationship to K1) by K1, this recombinant herpesvirus immortalizes primary T lymphocytes to IL-2-independent growth and induces lymphoma in cottontop marmosets. In B lymphocytes, K1 targets the phosphatidylinositol kinase pathway, activates the *Akt* kinase, and inhibits the phosphatase PTEN (Tomlinson and Damania, 2004). Activation of *Akt* results in phosphorylation and inhibition of members of the forkhead transcription factor family which regulate cell cycle progression and apoptosis. Thus, K1 promotes cell survival pathways and prevents cells from undergoing premature apoptosis. K1 probably represents the most important transforming protein of HHV type 8, although the pathogenic spectrum of HHV-8-induced tumors in all likelihood originates from the cooperation of various viral oncogenes.

Our current knowledge of genes expressed under conditions of viral latency is summarized in Table 4.6.

4.4.1.5 Cellular Genes Regulating Viral Latency

Activation of the replication and transcription factor (RTA) of γ-herpesviruses initiates the lytic cycle of HHV-8. This transactivator is preserved among all known γ-2-herpesviruses (Damiana et al., 2004). Its transcriptional activation is suppressed by cellular poly(ADP-ribose) polymerase 1 (PARP-1) and the Ste20-like kinase hKFC

Table 4.6 Transforming genes of HHV-8 an genes expressed in
latent infection

Gene	Function	Transformation of
LANA	Episome maintenance, transcript. regulator	Transforms primary rat cells jointly with H-ras
v-cyclin D	Binds to cdk-6, phosphorylates Rb1 and histone H1	Lymphomas in transgenic mice after loss of p53 expression
v-FLIP (K13)	Blocks Fas-mediated apoptosis and caspase 8, activates NF-κB	Promotes tumor establishment due to evasion form NK cell killing
LAMP (K15)	Membrane protein, resembles EBV LMP1 and LMP 2 A. Activates Ras and NF-κB pathways	Transforms rodent fibroblasts; immortalizes T-lymphocytes; induces lymphomas in cotton-top marmosets
Kaposin (K12)	Reorganizes cellular actin, regulates integrin activity	Malignant transformation of rat-3 cells
v-IRF-3 (K10.5, LANA-2)	Inhibition of p53-mediated transactiv. stimulates activity of cell. IRF-3 + IRF-7	Constitutively expressed only in hematopoietic cells
G-protein-coupled receptor (GPCR)	Activates VEGF-R, NF-êB, AP-1, and NF-AT	Transforms rat fibroblasts and NIH-3 T3 cells

which interact with the serine/threonine region of γ-herpesvirus RTA (Gwack et al., 2003). The genetic ablation of PARP-1 and hKFC substantially enhances the replication of these viruses. Suppression of the RTA-promoter is also mediated in *in-vitro*-infected endothelial cells by the joint action of interferon-γ, tumor necrosis factor-α, IL-1β, and IL-6 (Milligan et al., 2004), whereas interferon-γ alone effectively induces HHV-8 in PEL cells (Blackbourn et al., 2000; Chang et al., 2000; Mercader et al., 2000).

The expression of the cellular protein *Raf* significantly enhances HHV-8 infection of target cells (Akula et al., 2004). The Raf-induced vascular endothelial growth factor (VEGF) is apparently responsible for this effect since the treatment of cells with a VEGF receptor inhibitor significantly reduced the infection (Ford et al., 2004). Thus, *Raf* seems to modulate the pathogenesis of Kaposi's sarcoma.

4.4.1.6 Interaction Between HIV and HHV-8

The frequency of HHV-8-associated KS development in patients infected by human immunodeficiency viruses (HIV) could suggest that, besides the induction of immunosuppression, HIV infection may specifically activate latent HHV-8 genomes. Indeed, several observations point in this direction. Conditioned media from HIV-1-infected T cells induce the lytic reactivation of HHV-8 in PEL cells (Mercader et al., 2000). Replication of HIV in PEL cells has the same effect (Varthakavi et al., 1999).

Specific HIV proteins (*Tat* and *Vpr*) can induce HHV-8 gene expression; conversely, the *Rta* protein of HHV-8 synergizes with *Tat* in activating the HIV long terminal repeat (Huang et al., 2001). Overexpression of Tat in transgenic mice induces KS-like lesions (Vogel et al., 1988); extracellular Tat is also able to support the growth and survival of KS cells (Ensoli et al., 1990; Barillari et al., 1993; Albini et al., 1995). Tat mediates an anti-apoptotic gene expression program, in part by direct interactions with VEGF receptor 2 and IGF receptor I (Deregibus et al., 2002). In addition, Tat enhances the infectivity of HHV-8. The full-length HIV Tat and a 13-amino acid peptide corresponding to the basic region of Tat enhance the entry of HHV-8 into endothelial and other cells (Aoki and Tosato, 2004). Correspondingly, the median HHV-8 viral load is substantially higher in Kaposi's sarcomas of HIV-1-positive patients than in HIV-negative KS patients (Chandra et al., 2003).

All of these data underline the existence of a remarkable synergism between two virus infections, belonging to two very different virus families.

4.4.1.7 Viral Homologues to Host Cell Genes and Evasion from the Host's Immune Mechanisms

HHV-8 is particularly effective in immune evasion strategies (Moore and Chang, 2003). These strategies involve the MIR proteins, v-FLIP, and viral chemokines. Established strategies and related proteins from other viruses are listed in Table 4.7.

Table 4.7 Genes of HHV-8 with immune modulatory functions.
(Reproduced from Moore, 1996b. With permission)

KSHV protein	KSHV gene	Features and functions	Related proteins from other viruses
vKCP	ORF4	Homologue of cellular complement control regulators; inhibits C3 deposition on cell surface	HVS-ORF4, HSV1-gC, Vaccinia-vCP/C21 L, Cowpox-IMP, Vaccinia-SPICE
KIS	ORF K1	Constitutively active membrane protein containing ITAM motif; interacts with mu chains of B-cell receptor complex to block surface transport; transforms rodent fibroblasts and primary T cells; activates Syk signaling pathway; variable ectodomain used for KSHV strain analysis	HVS-STP
MIR1/MIR2	ORF K3/K5	Enhanced endocytosis of surface MHCI via ubiquitination; MIR2 also ubiquitinates and down-regulates ICAM-1 and B7.2	MHV 68-K3, CMV-US2
vCCL-2 (vMIP-II)	ORF K4	Binds to CCR3 and induces angiogenesis *in ovo*; induces eosinophil and Th2 chemotaxis; CCR8 and vGPCR antagonist	Molluscum-MC148

Table 4.7 (Continued)

KSHV protein	KSHV gene	Features and functions	Related proteins from other viruses
vCCL-3 (vMIP-III)	*ORF K4.1*	Agonist for CCR4 and induces Th2 chemotaxis; induces angiogenesis *in ovo*; protein expressed in KS lesions (by Western blot)	
vCCL-1 (vMIP-I)	*ORF K6*	Bids CCR5 and induces angiogenesis *in ovo*; CCR8 agonist; induces Th2 chemotaxis	Molluscum-MC148
vIRF-1	*ORF K9*	Inhibits IFN signaling; binds CBP/p300; transforms rodent fibroblasts; protein expressed in MCD and PEL cell lines, not detectable in KS or PEL	EBV-EBNA2, Adeno-E1 A, EBV-EBNA2, Adeno-E1 A, SV40-LT, HTLV-Tax
vFLIP	*ORF K13*	Homologue of cellular apoptosis inhibitor (FLIP); transcribed on major latency transcripts (LT)1 and LT2; post-transcriptionals regulation of protein expression *in vivo*	HSV-ORF71
ORF45	*ORF45*	Binds to and inhibits IRF7 nuclear translocation	Vaccinia-E3 L

The two transmembrane proteins MIR1 and MIR2 efficiently inhibit MHC 1 surface expression (Ishido et al., 2000; Stevenson et al., 2000). MHC I is removed from the plasma membrane by endocytosis, lysosomal targeting, and subsequent degradation of the MHC molecules (Coscoy and Ganem, 2000). In addition to MHC I, MIR2 also ubiquitates and down-regulates the accessory immune receptors ICAM-1 and B7.2 (Ishido et al., 2000; Coscoy and Ganem, 2001). MHC I-depleted HHV-8-infected cells escape from the resulting risk of being attacked by NK killer cells (Natarajan et al., 2002) by presenting virus-encoded MHC-like molecules at the cell surface (Tortorella et al., 2000). This is mediated by the expression of v-FLICE-inhibitory protein (v-FLIP) (Thome et al., 1997), which possesses two death effector domains and acts as a dominant-negative inhibitor of *Fas*-induced apoptosis and of caspase 8 (FLICE) (Belanger et al., 2001). Under these conditions, caspase 8 can no longer be recruited into the death-signaling process (Krueger et al., 2001). v-FLIP constitutively activates the NF-κB pathway by directly interacting with the IκB kinase (Liu et al., 2002).

HHV-8 effectively inhibits cell-mediated immune responses through the secretion of virus-encoded chemoattractant proteins (chemokines). The virus codes for three secreted chemokines, v-CCL1 (ORF K6), v-CCL2 (ORF K4), and v-CCL3 (ORF K4.1). All of these differ in their receptor specificities and possess broad antagonistic activities for chemokine receptors and block the chemotaxis for Th1 and NK lymphocytes (Boshoff et al., 1997; Chen et al., 1998; Dairaghi et al., 1999; Endres et al., 1999). v-CCL1 and v-CCL2 are only expressed in lytic infections, while v-CCL3 is also found in KS, stimulates angiogenesis, and may thus play a role in the pathogenesis

(Stine et al., 2000). v-CCL2 signals play a pivotal role in directing antiviral effector cells toward virus-infected organs, and potently inhibit type 1 T-cell-mediated inflammation (Lindow et al., 2003).

A number of additional HHV-8 proteins permit the evasion from innate immunity: the mechanisms involve complement binding, down-regulation of the B-cell receptor, and inhibition of interferon initiation and signaling (Moore and Chang, 2003). A complement control protein (KCP) has homology to human complement regulators (Russo et al., 1996). This blocks human complement-mediated lysis of erythrocytes and serves as a cofactor for factor I-mediated inactivation of complement proteins C3 b and C4 b (Mullick et al., 2003). This protein originates from ORF4 and occurs in three isoforms (Spiller et al., 2003).

The B-cell receptor (BCR) interacts with the complement-binding proteins CD19 and CD21 and regulates the development and functions of B cells. ORF K1 of HHV-8 encodes a small transmembrane glycoprotein, *KIS* (K ITAM-signaling), which possesses immunoglobulin-like properties. Its overexpression causes the transformation of rat fibroblasts, in the context of KIS substitution for the STP oncogene in recombinant herpesvirus saimiri it immortalizes T lymphocytes and induces lymphomas in marmosets (Lee et al., 1998). By interacting with the µ-chain, KIS blocks the intracellular transport of BCR complexes to the cell surface (Lee et al., 2000).

A number of viral proteins act as antagonists of cellular interferons. The secretion of v-interleukin 6 (v-IL-6) results in the activation of STAT1 and STAT3 phosphorylation, the MAP kinase and other serine/threonine kinases (Osborne et al., 1999). N-linked glycosylation at N78 and N89 is required for optimal function of v-IL-6, but not for cellular IL-6 (Dela Cruz et al., 2004). Similar to human IL-6, v-IL-6 maintains the B-cell proliferation in IL-6-dependent murine and human cell lines (Moore et al., 1996 b; Burger et al., 1998). The growth of lymphoma cells, carrying HHV-8 DNA, depends on the autocrine stimulation by v-IL-6 (Chatterjee et al., 2002). v-IL-6 is directly activated by interferon-α, but blocks intracellular interferon signaling. Whereas interferon-α down-regulates the IL-6 receptor, gp 80, v-IL-6 bypasses gp80 and binds directly to the gp130 transducer molecule. v-IL-6 has developed a unique molecular strategy to interact with gp130 with an almost entirely divergent structure of its receptor binding sites (Boulanger et al., 2004). Thus, v-IL-6 prevents the induction of an antiviral state by interferon and sustains the proliferation of HHV-8-positive B-lymphoma cells.

Another HHV-8-encoded protein, v-interferon-responsive factor 1 (v-IRF1), prevents the recruitment of p300 and the CREB-binding protein (CBP) histone acetyltransferase coactivators into the interferon transcriptional complex by cellular IRF3 (Weaver et al., 1998; Li et al., 2000). v-IRF1 acts as transactivator for v-IL-6, but its effect on histone acetylation represses a number of other genes (Li et al., 1997 b; Roan et al., 1999; Li et al., 2000). Expression of v-IRF1 in NIH 3T3 cells causes full transformation of these cells (Gao et al., 1997).

Besides the inhibition of p53-mediated apoptosis by LANA-1 and LANA-2 (v-IRF-3), v-IRF1 also blocks this p53 effect (Nakamura et al., 2001; Seo et al., 2001). HHV-8 has developed an additional mechanism to interfere with cellular apoptotic signals: it codes for a viral BCL-2-like protein, v-BCL2, which escapes the normally operating caspase-mediated conversion of its cellular homologue BCL-2 to pro-apoptotic proteins (Bellows et al., 2000). It blocks apoptosis which would be effected by the overexpression of latent v-cyclin/CDK6 complexes. The latter complex inactivates cellular BCL-2 by phosphorylation (Ojala et al., 2000). A further anti-apoptotic factor which acts at the mitochondrial membrane is v-IAP; this is structurally similar to cellular survivin (Feng et al., 2002; Wang et al., 2002). v-IAP stabilizes mitochondrial Ca^{2+} flux under conditions of cellular stress, and blocks apoptosis induced by a variety of different agents (Feng et al., 2002).

HHV-8 emerges as an extremely well-adapted virus in the human host. A larger number of HHV-8-encoded proteins reveal a remarkable molecular mimicry with host cell proteins, commonly interfering with the function of the latter. This permits an efficient evasion from host immune surveillance, as well as from intracellular control mechanisms.

4.4.1.8 HHV-8-Related Herpesviruses in Nonhuman Primates

Rhadinoviruses are found in Old and New World monkeys. A new rhadinovirus was reported in 1997 in Old World rhesus monkeys (Desrosiers et al., 1997). Cynomolgus and pig-tailed macaques contain closely related, but species-specific viral sequences (Strand et al., 2000). In addition, two distinct γ-2 herpesviruses were found in African green monkeys (Greensill et al., 2000). B lymphocytes emerge as the major site of viral persistence (Bergquam et al., 1999). In simian immunodeficiency virus (SIV)-infected monkeys only specific strains of rhesus rhadinovirus seem to induce multicentric lymphoproliferative disorders (Wong et al., 1999), whereas others apparently do not contribute to lymphoma development (Ruff et al., 2003).

A novel HHV-8 homologue (PapRV2) was reported in captive baboon species (*Papio anubis* and others) (Whitby et al., 2003). The viral DNA has substantial sequence identity to two HHV-8 genes, viral polymerase, and thymidilate synthase. A colony of almost 200 animals revealed cross-reacting antibodies recognizing HHV-8 or macaque rhadinovirus antigens.

Replication of HHV-8 after infection of rhesus macaques has been reported (Renne et al., 2004), though even rhesus monkeys positive for SIV failed to develop Kaposi-like sarcomas or lymphoproliferative disease.

Among New World monkeys two members of the rhadinovirus family – herpesvirus saimiri and herpesvirus ateles – rapidly produce leukemias and lymphomas in some non-natural hosts (Melendez et al., 1972). Leukemias arise in cotton-top marmosets almost like an acute infection upon inoculation of one of these two virus types. Although an initial report claimed propagation of herpesvirus saimiri in human cells (Ablashi et al., 1971), subsequent studies indicated that in spite of synthesis of early genes most of these infections are abortive (Daniel et al., 1975; Dahlberg et al., 1988). Herpesvirus saimiri may, however, persist in various human hematopoietic and epithelial cell lines (Grassmann and Fleckenstein, 1989; Simmer et al., 1991), and strains of the herpesvirus saimiri subgroup C are even able to stably transform human T lymphocytes (Biesinger et al., 1992). The same strains also immortalize Old World monkey T lymphocytes (Akari et al., 1996).

4.4.2
Marek's Disease of Chickens

Marek's disease was first described by Marek (1907) as a polyneuritis of chicken. Subsequently, it was characterized as a neurolymphomatosis and fowl paralysis, but the causative agent, a herpesvirus, was not discovered until 1967 (Churchill and Biggs, 1967). Viral DNA codes for the RNA subunit of telomerase (Fragnet et al., 2003). The occupational infection of humans with this agent has been suspected to occur, based on the presence of antibodies to Marek's virus in human sera (Choudat et al., 1996; Laurent et al., 2001); however, Marek's disease DNA has been detected only in chicken, and not in human plasma (Hennig et al., 2003). It remains to be seen whether the reported serological reactivity may originate from a related, presently unknown herpesvirus infection. Marek's virus, like several other herpesviruses, has also been reported to transactivate the terminal repeat promoter of the Rous sarcoma retrovirus (Tieber et al., 1990)

References

Ablashi, D.V., Armstrong, G.R., Heine, U., and Manaker, R.A. Propagation of Herpesvirus saimiri in human cells. *J. Natl. Cancer Inst.* 47: 241–244, **1971**.

Akari, H., Mori, K., Terao, K., Otani, I., Fukasawa, M., Mukai, R., and Yoshikawa, Y. In vitro immortalization of Old World monkey T lymphocytes with Herpesvirus saimiri: its susceptibility to infection with simian immunodeficiency viruses. *Virology* 218: 382–388, **1996**.

Akula, S. M., Pramod, M.P., Wang, F.Z., and Chandran, B. Integrin alpha3 beta1 (CD49 c/29) is a cellular receptor for Kaposi's sarcoma-associated herpesvirus (KSHV/HHV-8) entry into its target cells. *Cell* 108: 407–419, **2002**.

Akula, S. M., Ford, P.W., Whitman, A.G., Hamden, K.E., Shelton, J.G., and McCubrey, J.A. Raf promotes human herpesvirus-8 (HHV-8/KSHV) infection. *Oncogene* 23: 5227–5241, **2004**.

Albini, A., Barillari, G., Benelli, R., Gallo, R.C., and Ensoli, B. Angiogenic properties of human immunodeficiency virus type 1 Tat protein. *Proc. Natl. Acad. Sci. USA* 92: 4838–4842, **1995**.

An, J., Sun, Y., Sun, R., and Rettig, M.B. Kaposi's sarcoma associated herpesvirus encoded vFLIP induces cellular IL-6 expression: the role of the NF-κB and JNK/AP1 pathways. *Oncogene* 22: 3371–3385, **2003**.

An, J., Sun, Y., Rettig, M.B. Transcriptional coactivation of c-Jun by the KSHV-encoded LANA. *Blood* 103: 222–228, **2004**.

Angeloni, A., Heston, L., Uccini, S., Sirianni, M.C., Cottoni, F., Masala, M.K., Cerimele, D., Lin, S. -F., Sun, R., Rigsby, M., Faggioni, A., and Miller, G. High prevalence of antibodies to human herpesvirus 8 in relatives of patients with classic Kaposi's sarcoma from Sardinia. *J. Infect. Dis.* 177: 1715–1718, **1998**.

Aoki, Y. and Tosato, G. HIV-1 Tat enhances Kaposi sarcoma-associated herpesvirus (KSHV) infectivity. *Blood* 104: 810–814, **2004**.

Arvanitakis, L., Geras-Raaka, E., Varma, A., Gershengorn, M.C., and Cesarman, E. Human herpesvirus KSHV encodes a constitutively active G-protein-coupled receptor linked to cell proliferation. *Nature* 385: 347–350, **1997**.

Atkinson, J.O., Biggar, R.J., Goedert, J.J., and Engels, E.A. The incidence of Kaposi sarcoma among injection drug users with AIDS in the United States. *J. Acquir. Immune Defic. Syndr.* 37: 1282–1287, **2004**.

Ayuthaya, P.I., Katano, H., Inagi, R., Auwanit, W., Sata, T., Kurata, T., and Yamanishi, K. The seroprevalence of human herpesvirus 8 infection in the Thai population. *Southeast Asian J. Trop. Med. Public Health* 33: 297–305, **2002** .

Bais, C., Santomasso, B., Coso, O., Arvanitakis, L., Raaka, E.G., Gutkind, J.S., Asch, A.S., Cesarman, E., Gershengorn, M.C., and Mesri, E.A. G-protein-coupled receptor of Kaposi's sarcoma-associated herpesvirus is a viral oncogene and angiogenesis activator. *Nature* 391: 86–89, **1998**.

Bais, C., van Geelen, A., Eroles, P., Mutlu, A., Chiozzini, C., Dias, S., Silverstein, R.L., Rafii, S., and Mesri, E.A. Kaposi's sarcoma associated herpesvirus G protein-coupled receptor immortalizes human endothelial cells by activation of the VEGF receptor-2/KDR. *Cancer Cell* 3: 131–143, **2003**.

Ballestas, M.E. and Kaye, K.M. Kaposi's sarcoma-associated herpesvirus latency-associated nuclear antigen 1 mediates episome persistence through cis-acting terminal repeat (TR) sequence and specifically binds TR DNA. *J. Virol.* 75: 3250–3258, **2001**.

Ballestas, M.E., Chatis, P.A., and Kaye, K.M. Efficient persistence of extrachromosomal KSHV DNA mediated by latency-associated nuclear antigen. *Science* 284: 641–644, **1999**.

Barbera, A.J., Ballestas, M.E., and Kaye, K.M. The Kaposi's sarcoma-associated herpesvirus latency-associated nuclear antigen 1N terminus is essential for chromosome association, DNA replication, and episome persistence. *J. Virol.* 78: 294–301, **2004**.

Barillari, G., Gendelman, R., Gallo, R.C., and Ensoli, B. The Tat protein of human immunodeficiency virus type 1, a growth factor for AIDS Kaposi sarcoma and cytokine-activated vascular cells, induces adhesion of the same cell types by using integrin receptors recognizing the RDG amino acid sequence. *Proc. Natl. Acad. Sci. USA* 90: 7941–7945, **1993**.

Barozzi, P., Luppi, M., Facchetti, F., Mecucci, C., Alu, M., Sarid, R., Rasini, V., Ravazzini, L., Rossi, E., Festa, S., Crescenzi, B., Wolf, D.G., Schulz, T.F., and Torelli, G. Post-transplant Kaposi sarcoma originates from the seeding of donor-derived progenitors. *Nature Med.* 9: 554–561, **2003**.

Belanger, C., Gravel, A., Tomoiu, A., Janelle, M.E., Gosselin, J., Tremblay, M.J., and Flamand, L. Human herpesvirus 8 viral FLICE-inhibitory protein inhibits Fas-mediated apoptosis through binding and prevention of procaspase-8 maturation. *J. Hum. Virol.* 4: 62–73, **2001**.

Bellows, D.S., Chau, B.N., Lee, P., Lazebnik, Y., Burns, W.H., and Hardwick, J.M. Anti-apoptotic herpesvirus bcl-2 homologs escape caspase-mediated conversion to proapoptotic proteins. *J. Virol.* 74: 5024–5031, **2000**.

Beral, V. Epidemiology of Kaposi's sarcoma. *Cancer Surv.* 10: 5–22, **1991**.

Beral, V., Peterman, T., Berkelman, R., and Jaffe, H.W. Kaposi's sarcoma among persons with AIDS: a sexually transmitted infection? *Lancet* 335: 123–127, **1990**.

Bergquam, E.P., Avery, N., Shiigi, S. M., Axthelm, M.K., and Wong, S. W. Rhesus rhadinovirus establishes a latent infection in B lymphocytes in vivo. *J. Virol.* 73: 7874–7876, **1999**.

Biesinger, B., Muller-Fleckenstein, I., Simmer, B., Lang, G., Wittmann, S., Platzer, E., Desrosiers, R.C., and Fleckenstein, B. Stable growth transformation of human T lymphocytes by herpesvirus saimiri. *Proc. Natl. Acad. Sci. USA* 89: 3116–3119, **1992**.

Birkeland, S. A. and Kemp, E. Malignant tumours following immunosuppression in renal transplantation. *Proc. Eur. Dial. Transplant. Assoc.* 10: 429–433, **1973**.

Blackbourn, D.J., Fujimura, S., Kutzkey, T., and Levy, J.A. Induction of human herpesvirus-8 gene expression by recombinant interferon-gamma. *AIDS* 14: 98–99, **2000**.

Borkovic, S. P. and Schwartz, R.A. Kaposi's sarcoma presenting in the homosexual man – a new and striking phenomenon. *Ariz. Med.* 38: 902–904, **1981**.

Boshoff, C., Endo, Y., Collins, P.D., Takeuchi, Y., Reeves, J.D., Schweickart, V.L., Siani, M.A., Sasaki, T., Williams, T.J., Gray, P.W., Moore, P.S., Chang, Y., and Weiss, R.A. Angiogenic and HIV inhibitory functions of KSHV-encoded chemokines. *Science* 278, 290–294, **1997**.

Bourboulia, D., Aldam, D., Lagos, D., Allen, E., Williams, I., Cornforth, D., Copas, A., and Boshoff, C. Short- and long-term effects of highly active antiretroviral therapy on Kaposi sarcoma-associated herpesvirus immune responses and viraemia. *AIDS* 18: 485–493, **2004**.

Boulanger, M.J., Chow, D.C., Brevnova, E., Martick, M., Sandford, G., Nicholas, J., and Garcia, K.C. Molecular mechanism for viral mimicry of a human cytokine: activation of gp130 by HHV-8 interleukin-6. *J. Mol. Biol.* 335: 641–654, **2004**.

Brambilla, L., Boneschi, V., Ferrucci, S., Taglioni, M., and Berti, E. Human herpesvirus infection among heterosexual partners of patients with classical Kaposi's sarcoma. *Br. J. Dermatol.* 143: 1021–1025, **2000**.

Brinkmann, M.M., Glenn, M., Rainbow, L., Kieser, A., Henke-Gendo, C., and Schulz, T.F. Activation of mitogen-activated protein kinase and NF-κB pathways by a Kaposi's sarcoma-associated herpesvirus K15 membrane protein. *J. Virol.* 77: 9346–9358, **2003**.

Burger, R., Neipel, F., Fleckenstein, B., Savino, R., Ciliberto, G., Kalden, J.R., and Gramatzki, M. Human herpesvirus type 8 interleukin-6 homologue is functionally active in human myeloma cells. *Blood* 91: 1858–1863, **1998** .

Card, G.L., Knowles, P., Laman, H., Jones, N., and McDonald, N.Q. Crystal structure of a gamma-herpesvirus cyclin-cdk complex. *EMBO J.* 19: 2877–2888, **2000**.

Cattani, P., Capuano, M., Cerimele, F., La Parola, I.L., Santangelo, R., Masini, C., Cerimele, D., and Fadda, G. Human herpesvirus 8 seroprevalence and evaluation o nonsexual transmission routes by detection of DNA in clinical specimens from human immunodeficiency virus-seronegative patients from central and southern Italy, with and without Kaposi's sarcoma. *J. Clin. Microbiol.* 37: 1150–1153, **1999**.

Cesarman, E., Moore, P.S., Rao, P.H., Inghirami, G., Knowles, D.M., and Chang, Y. In vitro establishment and characterization of two acquired immunodeficiency syndrome-related lymphoma cell lines (BC-1 and BC-2) containing Kaposi's sarcoma-associated herpesvirus-like (KSHV) DNA sequences. *Blood* 86: 2708–2714, **1995**.

Cesarman, E., Nador, R.G., Aozasa, K., Delsol, G., Said, J.W., and Knowles, D.M. Kaposi's sarcoma-associated herpesvirus in non-AIDS related lymphomas occurring in body cavities. *Am. J. Pathol.* 149: 53–57, **1996**.

Chandra, A., Demirhan, I., Massambu, C., Pyakurel, P., Kaaya, E., Enbom, M., Urassa, W., Linde, A., Heiden, T., Biberfeld, P., Doerr, H.W., Cinatl, J., Loewer, J., and Chandra, P. Cross-talk between human herpesvirus 8 and the transactivator protein in the pathogenesis of Kaposi's sarcoma in HIV-infected patients. *Anticancer Res.* 23: 723–728, **2003**.

Chang, J., Renne, R., Dittmer, D., and Ganem, D. Inflammatory cytokines and the reactivation of Kaposi's sarcoma-associated herpesvirus lytic replication. *Virology* 266: 17–25, **2000**.

Chang, Y., Cesarman, E., Pessin, M.S., Lee, F., Culpepper, J., Knowless, D.M., and Moore, P.S. Identification of herpesvirus-like DNA sequences in AIDS-associated Kaposi's sarcoma. *Science* 266: 1865–1869, **1994**.

Chang, Y., Moore, P.S., Talbot, S. J., Boshoff, C.H., Zarkowska, T., Godden, K., Paterson, H., Weiss, R.A., and Mittnacht, S. Cyclin encoded by KS herpesvirus. *Nature* 382: 410, **1996**.

Chatterjee, M., Osborne, J., Bestetti, G., Chang, Y., and Moore, P.S. Viral IL-6-induced cell proliferation and immune evasion of interferon activity. *Science* 298: 1432–1435, **2002**.

Chaudhary, P.M., Jasmin, A., Eby, M.T., and Hood, L. Modulation of the NF-κB pathway by virally encoded death effector domains-containing proteins. *Oncogene* 18: 5738–5746, **1999**.

Chen, S., Bacon, K.B., Li, L., Garcia, G.E., Xia, Y., Lo, D., Thompson, D.A., Siani, M.A., Yamamoto, T., Harrison, J.K., and Feng, L. In vivo inhibition of CC and CX3C chemokine-induced leukocyte infiltration and attenuation of glomerulonephritis in Wistar-Kyoto (WKY) rats by vMIP-II. *J. Exp. Med.* 188: 193–198, **1998**.

Choudat, D., Dambrine, G., Delemotte, B., and Coudert, F. Occupational exposure to poultry and prevalence of antibodies against Marek's disease virus and avian retroviruses. *Occup. Environ. Med.* 53: 403–410, **1996**.

Churchill, A.E. and Biggs, P.M. Agent of Marek's disease in tissue culture. *Nature* 215: 528–530, **1967**.

Corbellino, M., Poirel, L., Aubin, J.T., Paulli, M., Magrini, U., Bestetti, G., Galli, M., and

Parravicini, C. The role of human herpesvirus 8 and Epstein–Barr virus in the pathogenesis of giant lymph node hyperplasia (Castleman's disease). *Clin. Infect. Dis.* 22: 1120–1121, **1996**.

Coscoy, L. and Ganem, D. Kaposi's sarcoma-associated herpesvirus encodes two proteins that block cell surface display of MHC class I chains by enhancing their endocytosis. *Proc. Natl. Acad. Sci. USA* 97: 8051–8056, **2000**.

Coscoy, L. and Ganem, D. A viral protein that selectively downregulates ICAM-1 and B7–2 and modulates T cell costimulation. *J. Clin. Invest.* 107: 1599–1606, **2001**.

Coscoy, L., Sanchez, D.J., and Ganem, D. A novel class of herpesvirus-encoded membrane-bound E3 ubiquitin ligases regulates endocytosis of proteins involved in immune recognition. *J. Cell Biol.* 155: 1265–1273, **2001**.

Cotter, M.A., II, and Robertson, E.S. The latency-associated nuclear antigen tethers the Kaposi's sarcoma-associated herpesvirus genome to host chromosomes in body cavity-based lymphoma cells. *Virology* 264: 254–264, **1999**.

Cotter, M.A., II, Subramanian, C., and Robertson, E.S. The Kaposi's sarcoma-associated herpesvirus latency-associated nuclear antigen binds to specific sequences at the left end of the viral genome through its carboxy-terminus. *Virology* 291: 241–259, **2001**.

Cunningham, C., Barnard, S., Blackbourn, D.J., and Davison, A.J. Transcription mapping of human herpesvirus 8 genes encoding viral interferon regulatory factors. *J. Gen. Virol.* 84: 1471–1483, **2003**.

Dadke, D., Fryer, B.H., Golemis, E.A., and Field, J. Activation of p21-activated kinase 1-nuclear factor κB signaling by Kaposi's sarcoma-associated herpes virus G protein-coupled receptor during cellular transformation. *Cancer Res.* 63: 8837–8847, **2003**.

Dahlberg, J.E., Ablashi, D.V., Rhim, J.S., Fladger, A., and Salahuddin, S. Z. Replication of Herpesvirus saimiri is semipermissive in human cells because of a block in the synthesis of certain late proteins. *Intervirology* 29: 277–234, **1988**.

Dairaghi, D.J., Fan, R.A., McMaster, B.E., Hanley, M.R., and Schall, T.J. HHV8-encoded vMIP-I selectively engages chemokine receptor CCR8. Agonist and antagonist profiles of viral chemokines. *J. Biol. Chem.* 274, 21 569–21 574, **1999**.

Damania, B., Jeong, J.H., Bowser, B.S., DeWire, S. M., Staudt, M.R., and Dittmer, D.P. Comparison of the Rta/Orf50 transactivator proteins of gamma-2-herpesviruses. *J. Virol.* 78: 5491–5499, **2004**.

Daniel, M.D., Silva, D., Jackman, D., Sehgal, P., Baggs, R.B., Hunt, R.D., King, N.W., and Melendez, L.V. Reactivation of squirrel monkey heart isolate (Herpesvirus saimiri strain) from latently infected human cell cultures and induction of malignant lymphoma in marmoset monkeys. *Bibl. Haematol.* 43: 392–395, **1975**.

Dedicoat, M., Newton, R., Alkharsah, K.R., Sheldon, J., Szabados, I., Ndlovu, B., Page, T., Casabonne, D., Gilks, C.F., Cassol, S. A., Whitby, D., and Schulz, T.F. Mother-to-child transmission of human herpesvirus-8 in South Africa. *J. Infect. Dis.* 190: 1068–1075, **2004**.

Dela Cruz, C.S., Lee, Y., Viswanathan, S. R., El-Guindy, A.S., Gerlach, J., Nikiforow, S., Shedd, D., Gradoville, L., and Miller, G. N-linked glycosylation is required for optimal function of Kaposi's sarcoma herpesvirus-encoded, but not cellular, interleukin 6. *J. Exp. Med.* 199: 503–514, **2004**.

Deng, J.H., Zhang, Y.J., Wang, X.P., and Gao, S. J. Lytic replication-defective Kaposi's sarcoma associated herpesvirus: potential role in infection and malignant transformation. *J. Virol.* 78: 11 108–11 120, **2004**.

Deregibus, M.C., Cantaluppi, V., Doublier, S., Brizzi, M.F., Deambrosis, I., Albini, A., and Camussi, G. HIV-1-Tat protein activates phosphatidylinositol 3-kinase/AKT-dependent survival pathways in Kaposi's sarcoma cells. *J. Biol. Chem.* 277: 25 195–25 202, **2002**.

Desrosiers, R.C., Sasseville, V.G., Czajak, S. C., Zhang, X., Mansfield, K.G., Kaur, A., Johnson, R.P., Lackner, A.A., and Jung, J.U. A herpesvirus of rhesus monkeys related to the human Kaposi's sarcoma-associated herpesvirus. *J. Virol.* 71: 9764–9769, **1997**.

Dittmer, D.P. Transcription profile of Kaposi's sarcoma-associated herpesvirus in primary Kaposi's sarcoma lesions as determined by real-time PCR arrays. *Cancer Res.* 63: 2010–2015, **2003**.

Djerbi, M., Screpanti, V., Catrina, A.I., Bogen, B., Biberfeld, P., and Grandien, A. The inhibitor of death receptor signaling, FLICE-inhibitory protein defines a new class of tumor progression factors. *J. Exp. Med.* 190: 1025–1032, **1999**.

Dourmishev, L.A., Dourmishev, A.L., Palmeri, D., Schwartz, R.A., and Lukac, D.M. Molecular genetics of Kaposi's sarcoma-associated herpesvirus (human herpesvirus 8) epidemiology and pathogenesis. *Microbiol. Molec. Biol. Rev.* 67: 175–212, **2003**.

Dukers, N.H., Renwick, N., Prins, M., Geskus, R.B., Schulz, T.F., Weverling, G.J., Coutinho, R.A., and Goudsmit, J. Risk factors for human herpesvirus 8 seropositivity and seroconversion in a cohort of homosexual men. *Am. J. Epidemiol.* 151: 213–224, **2000**.

Dupin, N. and Calvez, V. Virus HHV8/KSHV.1. Aspects épidémiologiques et moléculaires. *Ann. Dermatol. Venereol.* 127: 528–531, **2000**.

Dupin, N., Fisher, C., Kellam, P., Ariad, S., Tulliez, M., Franck, N., van Marck, E., Salmon, D., Gorin, I., Escande, J.-P., Weiss, R.A., Alitalo, K., and Boshoff, C. Distribution of human herpesvirus-8 latently infected cells in Kaposi's sarcoma, multicentric Castleman's disease, and primary effusion lymphoma. *Proc. Natl. Acad. Sci. USA* 96: 4546–4551, **1999**.

Ellis, M., Chew, Y.P., Fallis, L., Freddersdorf, S., Boshoff, C., Weiss, R.A., Lu, X., and Mittnacht, S. Degradation of p27(Kip) cdk inhibitor triggered by Kaposi's sarcoma virus cyclin.cdk6 complex. *EMBO J.* 18: 644–653, **1999**.

Enbom, M., Urassa, W., Massambu, C., Thorstensson, R., Mhalu, F., and Linde, A. Detection of human herpesvirus 8 DNA in serum from blood donors with HHV-8 antibodies indicates possible bloodborne transmission. *J. Med. Virol.* 68: 264–267, **2002**.

Endres, M.J., Garlisi, C.G., Xiao, H., Shan, L., and Hedrick, J.A. The Kaposi's sarcoma-related herpesvirus (KSHV)-encoded chemokine vMIP-I is a specific agonist for the CC chemokine receptor (CCR)8. *J. Exp. Med.* 189: 1993–1998, **1999** .

Ensoli, B., Barillari, G., Salahuddin, S. Z., Gallo, R.C., and Wong-Staal, F. Tat protein of HIV-1 stimulates growth of cells derived from Kaposi's sarcoma lesions of AIDS patients. *Nature* 345: 84–86, **1990**.

Esteban, M., Garcia, M.A., Domingo-Gil, E., Arroyo, J., Nombela, C., and Rivas, C. The latency protein LANA2 from Kaposi's sarcoma-associated herpesvirus inhibits apoptosis induced by dsRNA-activated protein kinase but not RNase L activation. *J. Gen. Virol.* 84: 1463–1470, **2003**.

Fahey, J.L. Cancer in the immunosuppressed patient. *Ann. Intern. Med.* 75: 310–312, **1971**.

Fakhari, F.D. and Dittmer, D.P. Charting latency transcripts in Kaposi's sarcoma-associated herpesvirus by whole genome real-time quantitative PCR. *J. Virol.* 76: 6213–6223, **2002**.

Farge, D., and the Collaborative Transplantation Research Group of Ile de France. Kaposi's sarcoma in organ transplant recipients. *Eur. J. Med.* 2: 339–343, **1993**.

Fejer, G., Medveczky, M.M., Horvath, E., Lane, B., Chang, Y., and Medveczky, P.G. The latency-associated nuclear antigen of Kaposi's sarcoma-associated herpesvirus interacts preferentially with the terminal repeats of the genome in vivo and this complex is sufficient for episomal DNA replication. *J. Gen. Virol.* 84: 1451–1462, **2003**.

Feng, P., Park, J., Lee, B.S., Lee, S. H., Bram, R.J., and Jung, J.U. Kaposi's sarcoma-associated herpesvirus mitochondrial K7 protein targets a cellular calcium-modulating cyclophilin ligand to modulate intracellular calcium concentration and to inhibit apoptosis. *J. Virol.* 76: 11491–11504, **2002**.

Field, N., Low, W., Daniels, M., Howell, S., Daviet, L., Boshoff, C., and Collins, M. KSHV vFLIP binds to IKK-γ to activate IKK. *J. Cell Sci.* 116: 3721–3728, **2003**.

Flore, O., Rafii, S., Ely, S., O'Leary, J.J., Hyjeck, E.M., and Cesarman, E. Transformation of primary human endothelial cells by Kaposi's sarcoma – associated herpesvirus. *Nature* 394: 588–592, **1998**.

Ford, P.W., Hamden, K.E., Whitman, A.G., McCubrey, J.A., and Akula, S. M. Vascular endothelial growth factor augments human herpesvirus-8 (HHV-8/KSHV) infection. *Cancer Biol. Ther.* 3: 876–881, **2004**.

Fragnet, L., Blasco, M.A., Klapper, W., and Rasschaert, D. The RNA subunit of telomerase is encoded by Marek's disease virus. *J. Virol.* 77: 5985–5996, **2003**.

Friborg, J., Jr., Kong, W., Hottiger, M.O., and Nabel, G.J. p53 inhibition by the LANA protein of KSHV protects against cell death. *Nature* 402: 889–894, **1999**.

Fujimuro, M. and Hayward, S. D. The latency-associated nuclear antigen of Kaposi's sarcoma-associated herpesvirus manipulates the activity of glycogen synthase kinase 3-β. *J. Virol.* 77: 8019–8030, **2003**.

Gao, S. J., Kingsley, L., Hoover, D.R., Spira, T.J., Rinaldo, C.R., Saah, A., Phair, J., Detels, R., Parry, P., Chang, Y. and Moore, P.S. Seroconversion to antibodies against Kaposi's sarcoma-associated herpesvirus-related latent nuclear antigens before the development of Kaposi's sarcoma. *N. Engl. J. Med.* 335: 233–241, **1996**.

Gao, S. J., Boshoff, C., Jayachandra, S., Weiss, R.A., Chang, Y., and Moore, P.S. KSHV ORF K9 (vIRF) is an oncogene which inhibits the interferon signaling pathway. *Oncogene* 15: 1979–1986, **1997**.

Gao, S. J., Deng, J.H., and Zhou, F.C. Productive lytic replication of a recombinant Kaposi's sarcoma-associated herpesvirus in efficient primary infection of primary human endothelial cells. *J. Virol.* 77: 9738–9749, **2003**.

Glenn, M., Rainbow, L., Aurade, F., Davison, A., and Schulz, T.F. Identification of a spliced gene from Kaposi's sarcoma-associated herpesvirus encoding a protein with similarities to latent membrane proteins 1 and 2A of Epstein–Barr virus *J. Virol.* 73: 6953–6963, **1999**.

Godden-Kent, D., Talbot, S. J., Boshoff, H.C., Chang, Y., Moore, P.S., Weiss, R.A., and Mittnacht, S. The cyclin encoded by Kaposi's sarcoma-associated herpesvirus stimulates cdk6 to phosphorylate the retinoblastoma protein and histone H1. *J. Virol.* 71: 4193–4198, **1997**.

Goedert, J.J. The epidemiology of acquired immunodeficiency syndrome malignancies. *Semin. Oncol.* 27: 390–401, **2000**.

Gottlieb, G.J., Ragaz, A., Vogel, J.V., Friedman-Kien, A., Rywlin, A.M., Weiner, E.A., and Ackerman, A.B. A preliminary communication on extensively disseminated Kaposi's sarcoma in young homosexual men. *Am. J. Dermatopathol.* 3: 111–114, **1981**.

Grandadam, M., Dupin, N., Calvez, V., Gorin, I., Blum, L., Kernbaum, S., Sicard, D., Buisson, Y., Agut, H., Escande, J.P., and Huraux, J.M. Exacerbations of clinical symptoms in human immunodeficiency virus type 1-infected patients with multicentric Castleman's disease are associated with a high increase in Kaposi's sarcoma herpesvirus DNA load in peripheral blood mononuclear cells. *J. Infect. Dis.* 175: 1198–1201, **1997**.

Grassmann, R. and Fleckenstein, B. Selectable recombinant herpesvirus saimiri is capable of persisting in a human T-cell line. *J. Virol.* 63: 1818–1821, **1989**.

Greensill, J., Sheldon, J.A., Renwick, N.M., Beer, B.E., Norley, S., Goudsmit, J., and Schultz, T.F. Two distinct gamma-2 herpesviruses in African green monkeys: a second gamma-2 herpesvirus lineage among old world primates? *J. Virol.* 74: 1572–1577, **2000**.

Grundhoff, A. and Ganem, D. The latency-associated nuclear antigen of Kaposi's sarcoma-associated herpesvirus permits replication of terminal repeat-containing plasmids. *J. Virol.* 77: 2779–2783, **2003**.

Guasparri, I., Keller, S. A., and Cesarman, E. KSHV vFLIP is essential for the survival of infected lymphoma cells. *J. Exp. Med.* 199: 993–1003, **2004**.

Gwack, Y., Nakamura, H., Lee, S. H., Souvlis, J., Yustein, J.T., Gygi, S., Kung, H.J., and Jung, J.U. Poly(ADP-ribose) polymerase 1 and Ste20-like kinase hKFC act as transcriptional repressors for γ-herpesvirus lytic replication. *Mol. Cell. Biol* . 23: 8282–8294, **2003**.

Haim, S., Shafrir, A., Better, O.S., Robinson, E., Chaimowitz, C., and Erlik, D. Kaposi's sarcoma in association with immunosuppressive therapy. Report of two cases. *Isr. J. Med. Sci.* 8: 1993–1997, **1972**.

Hennig, H., Osterrieder, N., Müller-Steinhardt, M., Teichert, H.M., Kirchner, H., and Wandinger, K.P. Detection of Marek's disease virus DNA in chicken but not in human plasma. *J. Clin. Microbiol.* 41: 2428–2432, **2003**.

Huang, L.M., Chao, M.F., Chen, M.Y., Shih, H.M., Chiang, Y.P., Chuang, C.Y., and Lee,

C.Y. Reciprocal regulatory interaction between human herpesvirus 8 and human immunodeficiency virus type 1. *J. Biol. Chem.* 276: 13 427–13 432, **2001**.

Hudnall, S. D., Rady, P.L., Tyring, S. K., and Fish, J.C. Hydrocortisone activation of human herpesvirus 8 viral DNA replication and gene expression in vitro. *Transplantation* 67: 648–652, **1999**.

Hutt, M.S. Classical and endemic form of Kaposi's sarcoma. A review. *Antibiot. Chemother.* 32: 12–17, **1983**.

Hymes, K.B., Cheung, T., Greene, J.B., Prose, N.S., Marcus, A., Ballard, H., William, D.C., and Laubenstein, L.J. Kaposi's sarcoma in homosexual men – a report of eight cases. *Lancet* II: 598–600, **1981**.

Iscovich, J., Boffetta, P., Franceschi, S., Azizi, E., and Sarid, R. Classic Kaposi sarcoma: epidemiology and risk factors. *Cancer* 88: 500–517, **2000**.

Ishido, S., Wang, C., Lee, B.S., Cohen, G.B., and Jung, J.U., Downregulation of major histocompatibility complex class I molecules by Kaposi's sarcoma-associated herpesvirus K3 and K5 proteins. *J. Virol.* 74: 5300–5309, **2000**.

Jarviluoma, A., Koopal, S., Rasanen, S., Makela, T.P., and Ojala, P.M. KSHV viral cyclin binds to p27KIP1 in primary effusion lymphomas. *Blood* 104: 3349–3354, **2004**.

Jeong, J.H., Orvis, J., Kim, J.W., McMurtrey, C.P., Renne, R., and Dittmer, D.P. Regulation and autoregulation of the promoter for the latency-associated nuclear antigen of Kaposi's sarcoma-associated herpesvirus. *J. Biol. Chem.* 279: 16 822–16 831, **2004**.

Jones, J.L., Hanson, D.L., Dworkin, M.S., and Jaffe, H.W. Incidence and trends in Kaposi's sarcoma in the era of effective antiretroviral therapy. *J. Acquir. Immune Defic. Syndr.* 24: 270–274, **2000**.

Kaposi, M. Idiopathisches multiples Pigmentsarkom der Haut. *Arch. Dermatol. Syphilis* 4: 265–273, **1872**.

Kasolo, F.C., Mpabalwani, E., and Gompels, U.A. Infection with AIDS-related herpesviruses in human immunodeficiency virus-negative infants and endemic childhood sarcoma Kaposi's sarcoma in Africa. *J. Gen. Virol.* 78: 847–855, **1997** .

Katano, H., Sato, Y., Kurata, T., Mori, S., and Sata, T. Expression and localization of human herpesvirus 8-encoded proteins in primary effusion lymphoma, Kaposi's sarcoma, and multicentric Castleman's disease. *Virology* 269: 335–344, **2000**.

Kataoka, T., Budd, R.C., Holler, N., Thome, M., Martinon, F., Irmler, M., Burns, K., Hahne, M., Kennedy, N., Kovacsovics, M., and Tschopp, J. The caspase-8 inhibitor FLIP promotes activation of NF-κB and Erk signaling pathways. *Curr. Biol* . 10: 640–648, **2000**.

Kedes, D.H., Operskalski, E., Busch, M., Kohn, R., Flood, J., and Ganem, D. The seroepidemiology of human herpesvirus 8 (Kaposi's sarcoma-associated herpesvirus): distribution of infection in KS risk groups and evidence for sexual transmission. *Nat. Med.* 2: 918–924, **1996**.

Kedes, D.H., Lagunoff, M., Renne, R., and Ganem, D. Identification of the gene encoding the major latency-associated nuclear antigen of the Kaposi's sarcoma-associated herpesvirus. *J. Clin. Invest.* 100: 2606–2610, **1997**.

Kliche, S., Nagel, W., Kremmer, E., Atzler, C., Ege, A., Knorr, T., Koszinowski, U., Kolanus, W., and Haas, J. Signaling by human herpesvirus 8 kaposin A through direct membrane recruitment of cytohesin-1. *Mol. Cell* 7: 833–843, **2001** .

Knight, J.S., Cotter, M.A., II, and Robertson, E.S. The latency-associated nuclear antigen of Kaposi's sarcoma-associated herpesvirus transactivates the telomerase reverse transcriptase promoter. *J. Biol. Chem.* 276: 22 971–22 978, **2001**.

Komatsu, T., Ballestas, M.E., Barbera, A.J., Kelley-Clarke, B., and Kaye, K.M. KSHV LANA 1 binds DNA as an oligomer and residues N-terminal to the oligomerization domain are essential for DNA binding, replication, and episome persistence. *Virology* 319: 225–236, **2004**.

Krueger, A., Baumann, S., Krammer, P.H., and Kirchhoff, S. FLICE-inhibitory proteins: regulators of death-receptor-mediated apoptosis. *Mol. Cell. Biol.* 21: 8247–8254, **2001**.

Lan, K., Kuppers, D.A., Verma, S. C., and Robertson, E.S. Kaposi's sarcoma-associated herpesvirus-encoded latency-associated nuclear antigen inhibits lytic replication by targeting Rta: a potential mechanism for virus-mediated control of latency. *J. Virol.* 78: 6585–6594, **2004**.

Laurent, S., Esnault, E., Dambrine, G., Goudeau, A., Choudat, D., and Rasschaert, D. Detection of avian oncogenic Marek's disease herpesvirus DNA in human sera. *J. Gen. Virol.* 82: 233–240, **2001**.

Lee, B.S., Alvarez, X., Ishido, S., Lackner, A.A., and Jung, J.U. Inhibition of intra-cellular transport of B cell antigen receptor complexes by Kaposi's sarcoma-associated herpesvirus K1. *J. Exp. Med.* 192: 11–21, **2000**.

Lee, H., Veazey, R., Williams, K., Li, M., Guo, J., Neipel, F., Fleckenstein, B., Lackner, A., Desrosiers, R.C., and Jung, J.U. Deregulation of cell growth by the K1 gene of Kaposi's sarcoma-associated herpesvirus. *Nat. Med.* 4: 435–440, **1998**.

Li, H., Komatsu, T., Dezube, D.J., and Kaye, K.M. The Kaposi's sarcoma-associated herpesvirus K12 transcript from primary effusion lymphoma contains complex repeat elements, is spliced, and initiates from a novel promoter. *J. Virol.* 76: 11 880–11 888, **2002**.

Li, M., Lee, H., Yoon, D.W., Albrecht, J.C., Fleckenstein, B., Neipel, F., and Jung, J.U. Kaposi's sarcoma-associated herpesvirus encodes a functional cyclin. *J. Virol.* 71: 1984–1991, **1997 a**.

Li, M., Lee, H., Guo, J., Neipel, F., Fleckenstein, B., Ozato, K., and Jung, J.U. Kaposi's sarcoma-associated herpesvirus viral interferon regulatory factor. *J. Virol.* 72: 5433–5440, **1997 b**.

Li, M., Damania, B., Alvarez, X., Ogryzko, V., Ozato, K., and Jung, J.U. Inhibition of p300 histone acetyltransferase by viral interferon regulatory factor. *Mol. Cell. Biol.* 20: 8254–8263, **2000**.

Lindow, M., Nansen, A., Bartholdy, C., Stryhn, A., Hansen, N.J., Boesen, T.P., Wells, T.N., Schwartz, T.W., and Thomsen, A.R. The virus-encoded chemokine vMIP-II inhibits virus-induced Tc1-driven inflammation. *J. Virol.* 77: 7393–7400, **2003**.

Liu, L., Eby, M.T., Rathore, N., Sinha, S. K., Kumar, A., and Chaudhary, M. The human herpes virus 8-encoded viral FLICE inhibitory protein physically associates with and persistently activates IκB kinase complex.

*J. Biol. Chem.*277: 13 745–13 751, **2002**.

Lubyova, B., Kellum, M.J., Frisancho, A.J., and Pitha, P.M. Kaposi's sarcoma-associated herpesvirus-encoded vIRF-3 stimulates the transcriptional activity of cellular IRF-3 and IRF-7. *J. Biol. Chem.* 279: 7643–7654, **2004**.

Lundquist, A., Barre, B., Bienvenu, F., Hermann, J., Avril, S., and Coqueret, O. Kaposi sarcoma-associated viral cyclin K overrides cell growth inhibition mediated by oncostatin M through STAT3 inhibition. *Blood* 101: 4070–4077, **2003** .

Mann, D.J., Child, E.S., Swanton, C., Laman, H., and Jones, N. Modulation of p27 (Kip1) levels by the cyclin encoded by Kaposi's sarcoma-associated herpesvirus. *EMBO J.* 18: 654–663, **1999**.

Marek, J. Multiple Nervenentzündung (Polyneuritis) bei Hühnern. *Dtsch. Tierärztl. Wschr.* 15: 417–421, **1907**.

Martin, J.N., Ganem, D.E., Osmond, D.H., Page-Shafer, K.A., Macrae, D., and Kedes, D.H. Sexual transmission and the natural history of human herpesvirus 8 infection. *N. Engl. J. Med.* 338: 948–954, **1998**.

Matta, H. and Chaudhary, P.M. Activation of alternative NF-κB pathway by human herpesvirus 8-encoded Fas-associated death domain-like IL-1β-converting enzyme inhibitory protein (vFLIP). *Proc. Natl. Acad. Sci. USA* 101: 9399–9404, **2004**.

Mbulaiteye, S. M., Biggar, R.J., Goedert, J.J., and Engels, E.A: Pleural and peritoneal lymphoma among people with AIDS in the United States. *J. Acquir. Immune Defic. Syndr.* 29: 418–421, **2002**.

Melendez, L.V., Hunt, R.D., Daniel, M.D., Fraser, C.E.O., Barahona, H.H., King, N.W., and Garcia, F.G. Herpesvirus saimiri and ateles – their role in malignant lymphomas of monkeys. *Fed. Proc.* 31: 1643–1650, **1972**.

Mercader, M., Taddeo, B., Panella, J.R., Chandran, B., Nickoloff, B.J., and Foreman, K.E. Induction of HHV-8 lytic cycle replication by inflammatory cytokines produced by HIV-infected T cells. *Am. J. Pathol.* 156: 1961–1971, **2000** .

Milligan, S., Robinson, M., O'Donnell, E., and Blackbourn, D.J. Inflammatory cytokines inhibit Kaposi sarcoma-associated herpesvirus lytic gene transcription in in vitro-infected endothelial cells. *J. Virol.* 78: 2591–2596, **2004**.

Montaner, S., Sodhi, A., Molinolo, A., Bugge, T.H., Sawai, E.T., He, Y., Li, Y., Ray, P.E., and Gutkind, J.S. Endothelial infection with KSHV genes in vivo reveals that vGPCR initiates Kaposi's sarcomagenesis and can promote the tumorigenic potential of viral latent genes. *Cancer Cell* 3: 23–36, **2003**.

Montaner, S., Sodhi, A., Servitja, J.M., Ramsdell, A.K., Barac, A., Sawai, E.T., and Gutkind, J.S. The small GTPase Rac1 links the Kaposi sarcoma-associated herpesvirus vGPCR to cytokine secretion and paracrine neoplasia. *Blood* 104: 2903–2911, **2004**.

Moore, P.S. and Chang, Y. Kaposi sarcoma-associated herpesvirus immunoevasion and tumorigenesis: two sides of the same coin? *Annu. Rev. Microbiol.* 57: 609–639, **2003**.

Moore, P.S., Kingsley, L.A., Holmberg, S. D., Spira, T., Gupta, P., Hoover, D.R., Parry, J.P., Conley, L.J., Jaffe, H.W., and Chang, Y. Kaposi's sarcoma-associated herpesvirus infection prior to onset of Kaposi's sarcoma. *AIDS* 10: 175–180, **1996 a**.

Moore, P.S., Boshoff, C., Weiss, R.A., and Chang, Y. Molecular mimicry of human cytokine and cytokine response pathway genes by KSHV. *Science* 274: 1739–1744, **1996 b**.

Mullick, J., Bernet, J., Singh, A.K., Lambris, J.D., and Sahu, A. Kaposi's sarcoma-associated herpesvirus (human herpesvirus 8) open reading frame 4 protein (kaposica) is a functional homolog of complement control proteins. *J. Virol.* 77: 3878–3881, **2003**.

Muralidhar, S., Pumfery, A.M., Hassani, M., Sadaie, M.R., Kishishita, M., Brady, J., Doniger, J., Medveczky, P., and Rosenthal, L. Identification of kaposin (open reading frame K12) as a human herpesvirus 8 (Kaposi's sarcoma-associated herpesvirus) transforming gene. *J. Virol.* 72: 4980–4988, **1998**.

Muralidhar, S., Veytsmann, G., Chandran, B., Ablashi, D., Doniger, J., and Rosenthal, L.J. Characterization of the human herpesvirus 8 (Kaposi's sarcoma-associated herpesvirus) oncogene, kaposin (ORF K12). *J. Clin. Virol.* 16: 203–213, **2000**.

Nador, R.G., Cesarman, E., Chadburn, A., Dawson, D.B., Ansari, M.Q., Said, J., and Knowles, D.M. Primary effusion lymphoma: a distinct clinicopathologic entity associated with the Kaposi's sarcoma-associated herpes virus. *Blood* 88: 645–656, **1996**.

Nakamura, H., Li, M., Zarycki, J. and Jung, J.U. Inhibition of p53 tumor suppressor by viral interferon regulatory factor. *J. Virol.* 75: 7572–7582, **2001**.

Naranatt, P.P., Akula, S. M., Zien, C.H., Krishnan, H.H., and Chandran, B. Kaposi's sarcoma-associated herpesvirus induces the phosphatidylinositol 3-kinase-PCK-zeta-MEK-ERK signaling pathway in target cells early during infection: implications for infectivity. *J. Virol.* 77: 1524–1539, **2003**.

Naranatt, P.P., Krishnan, H.H., Smith, M.S., and Chandran, B. Kaposi's sarcoma-associated herpesvirus modulates microtubule dynamics via RhoA-GTP-diaphanous 2 signaling and utilizes the dynein motors to deliver its DNA to the nucleus. *J. Virol.* 79: 1191–1206, **2005**.

Natarajan, K., Dimasi, N., Wang, J., Mariuzza, R.A., and Margulies, D.H. Structure and function of natural killer cell receptors: multiple molecular solutions to self, non-self discrimination. *Annu. Rev. Immunol.* 20: 853–885, **2002** .

Neipel, F., Albrecht, J.C., and Fleckenstein, B. Cell-homologous genes in the Kaposi's sarcoma-associated rhadinovirus human herpesvirus 8: determinants of its pathogenicity? *J. Virol.* 71: 4187–4192, **1997**.

Ojala, P.M., Yamamoto, K., Castanos-Velez, E., Biberfeld, P., Korsmeyer, S. J., and Makela, T.P. The apoptotic v-cyclin-CDK6 complex phosphorylates and inactivates Bcl-2. *Nat. Cell Biol.* 2: 819–825, **2000**.

Oksenhendler, E., Carcelain, G., Aoki, Y., Boulanger, E., Maillard, A., Clauvel, J.P., and Agbalika, F. High levels of human herpesvirus 8 viral load, human interleukin-6, interleukin-10, and C-reactive protein correlate with exacerbation of multicentric Castleman disease in HIV-infected patients. *Blood* 96: 2069–2073, **2000**.

Osborne, J., Moore, P.S., and Chang, Y. KSHV-encoded viral IL-6 activates multiple human IL-6 signaling pathways. *Hum. Immunol.* 60: 921–927, **1999**.

Pan, H.Y., Zhang, Y.J., Wang, X.P., Deng, J.H., Zhou, F.C., and Gao, S. J. Identification of a novel cellular transcriptional repressor interacting with the latent nuclear antigen of Kaposi's sarcoma-associated herpesvirus. *J. Virol.* 77: 9758–9768, **2003**.

Pan, H., Zhou, F., and Gao, S. -J. Kaposi's sarcoma-associated herpesvirus induction of chromosome instability in primary human endothelial cells. *Cancer Res.* 64: 4064–4068, **2004**.

Parravicini, C., Olsen, S. J., Capra, M., Poli, F., Sirchia, G., Gao, S. J., Berti, E., Nocera, A., Rossi, E., Bestetti, G., Pizzuto, M., Galli, M., Moroni, M., Moore, P.S., and Corbellino, M. Risk of Kaposi's sarcoma-associated herpesvirus transmission from donor allografts among Italian posttransplant Kaposi's sarcoma patients. *Blood* 90: 2826–2829, **1997**.

Parravicini, C., Chandran, B., Corbellino, M., Berti, E., Paulli, M., Moore, P.S., and Chang, Y. Differential viral protein expression in Kaposi's sarcoma-associated herpesvirus-infected diseases: Kaposi's sarcoma, primary effusion lymphoma, and multicentric Castleman's disease. *Am. J. Pathol.* 156: 743–749, **2000**.

Pati, S., Foulke, J.S., Jr., Barabitskaya, O., Kim, J., Nair, B.C., Hone, D., Smart, J., Feldman, R.A., and Reitz. M. Human herpesvirus 8-encoded vGPCR activates nuclear factor of activated T cells and collaborates with human immunodeficiency virus type 1 Tat. *J. Virol.* 77: 5759–5773, **2003**.

Penn, I. Tumors after renal and cardiac transplantation. Review. *Hematol. Oncol. Clin. North Am.* 7: 431–445, **1993**.

Penn, I. Kaposi's sarcoma in transplant recipients. *Transplantation* 64: 669–673, **1997**.

Penn, I. and Starzl, T.E. Malignant lymphomas in transplantation patients: a review of the world experience. *Int. Z. Klin. Pharmakol. Toxikol.* 3: 49–54, **1970**.

Plancoulaine, S., Abel, L., Tregouet, D., Duprez, R., van Beveren, M., Tortevoye, P., Froment, A., and Gessain, A. Respective roles of serological status and blood specific antihuman herpesvirus 8 antibody levels in human herpesvirus 8 intrafamilial transmission in a highly endemic area. *Cancer Res.* 64: 8782–8787, **2004**.

Prakash, O., Swamy, O.R., Peng, X., Tang, Z.Y., Li, L., Larson, J.E., Cohen, J.C., Gill, J., Farr, G., Wang, S., and Samaniego, F. Activation of Src kinase Lyn by the Kaposi sarcoma-associated herpesvirus K1 protein: implications for lymphomagenesis. *Blood* 105: 3987–3994, **2005**.

Qunibi, W., Akhtar, M., Sheth, K., Ginn, H.E., Al-Furayh, O., DeVol, E.B., and Taher, S. Kaposi sarcoma: the most common tumor after renal transplantation in Saudi-Arabia. *Am. J. Med.* 84: 225–232, **1988**.

Radkov, S. A., Kellam, P., and Boshoff, C. The latent nuclear antigen of Kaposi's sarcoma-associated herpesvirus targets the retino-blastoma-E2F pathway and with the oncogene H-ras transforms primary rat cells. *Nat. Med.* 6: 1121–1127, **2000**.

Renne, R., Dittmer, D., Kedes, D., Schmidt, K., Desrosiers, R.C., Luciw, P.A., and Ganem, D. Experimental transmission of Kaposi's sarcoma-associated herpesvirus (KSHV/HHV-8) to SIV-positive and SIV-negative rhesus macaques. *J. Med. Primatol*. 33: 1–9, **2004**.

Rivas, C., Thlick, H.E., Parravicini, C., Moore, P.S., and Chang, Y. Kaposi's sarcoma-associated herpesvirus LANA2 is a B-cell-specific latent viral protein that inhibits p53. *J. Virol.* 75: 429–438, **2001**.

Roan, F., Zimring, J.C., Goodbourn, S., Offermann, M.K. Transcriptional activation by the human herpesvirus-8-encoded interferon regulatory factor. *J. Gen. Virol.* 80: 2205–2209, **1999**.

Ruff, K., Baskin, G.B., Simpson, L., Murphey-Corb, M., and Levy L.S. Rhesus rhadinovirus infection in healthy and SIV-infected macaques at Tulane National Primate Research Center. *J. Med. Primatol.* 32: 1–6, **2003**.

Russo, J.J., Bohenzky, R.A., Chien, M.C., Chen, J., Yan, M., Maddalena, D., Parry, J.P., Peruzzi, D., Edelman, I.S., Chang, Y., and Moore, P.S. Nucleotide sequence of the Kaposi sarcoma-associated herpesvirus (HHV8). *Proc. Natl. Acad. Sci. USA* 93: 14 862–14 867, **1996**.

Sakakibara, S., Ueda, K., Nishimura, K., Do, E., Ohsaki, E., Okuno, T., and Yamanishi, K. Accumulation of heterochromatin components on the terminal repeat sequence of Kaposi's sarcoma-associated herpesvirus mediated by the latency-associated nuclear antigen. *J. Virol.* 78: 7299–7310, **2004**.

Sarid, R., Wiezorek, J.S., Moore, P.S., and
Chang, Y. Characterization and cell cycle
regulation of the major Kaposi's sarcoma-
associated herpesvirus (human herpesvirus 8) latent genes and their promoter. *J. Virol.* 73: 1438–1446, **1999**.

Sarmati, L., Carlo, T., Rossella, S., Montano,
M., Adalgisa, P., Rezza, G., and Andreoni,
M. Human herpesvirus-8 infection in pregnancy and labor: lack of evidence of vertical
transmission. *J. Med. Virol.* 72: 462–466,
2004.

Schwartz, R.A. Kaposi's sarcoma: advances
and perspectives. *J. Am. Acad. Dermatol.*
34: 804–814, **1996**.

Seo, T., Park, J., Lee, D., Hwang, S. G., and
Choe, J. Viral interferon regulatory factor 1
of Kaposi's sarcoma-associated herpesvirus
binds to p53 and represses p53-dependent
transcription and apoptosis. *J. Virol.* 75:
6193–6198, **2001** .

Sgadari, C., Barillari, G., Toschi, E., Carlei,
D., Bacigalupo, I., Baccarini, S., Palladino,
C., Leone, P., Bugarini, R., Malavasi, L.,
Cafaro, A., Falchi, M., Valdembri, D.,
Rezza, G., Bussolino, F., Monini, P., and
Ensoli, B. HIV protease inhibitors are
potent anti-angiogenic molecules and pro-
mote regression of Kaposi sarcoma. *Nat.
Med.* 8: 225–232, **2002**.

Siegel, J.H., Janis, R., Alper, J.C., Schutte, H.,
Robbins, L., and Blaufox, M.D. Disseminated visceral Kaposi's sarcoma. Appearance after human renal homograft opera-
tion. *JAMA* 207: 1493–1496, **1969**.

Simmer, B., Alt, M., Buckreus, I., Berthold,
S., Fleckenstein, B., Platzer, E., and
Grassmann, R. Persistence of selectable
herpesvirus saimiri in various human hae-
matopoietic and epithelial cell lines. *J. Gen.
Virol.* 72: 1953–1958, **1991**.

Sodhi, A., Montaner, S., and Gutkind, J.S.
Does dysregulated expression of a deregulated viral GPCR trigger Kaposi's sarcomagenesis? *FASEB J.* 18: 422–427, **2004**.

Soto, U., Denk, C., Lengert, M., Finzer, P.,
Hutter, K.-J., zur Hausen, H., and Rösl, F.
Genetic complementation to non-
tumorigenicity in cervical carcinoma cells
correlates with alterations in AP-1 composition. *Int. J. Cancer,* 86: 811–817, **2000**.

Soulier, J., Grollet, L., Oksenhendler, E.,
Cacoub, B., Cazals-Hatem, D., Babinet, P.,
d'Agay, M.F., Clauvel, J.P., Raphael, M.,

Degos, L., et al. Kaposi's sarcoma-
associated herpesvirus-like DNA
sequences in multicentric Castleman's disease. *Blood* 86: 1276–1280, **1995**.

Spiller, O.B., Robinson, M., O'Donell, E., Milligan, S., Morgan, B.P., Davison, A.J., and
Blackbourn, D.J. Complement regulation
by Kaposi's sarcoma-associated herpesvirus
ORF4 protein. *J. Virol.* 77: 592–599, **2003**.

Staskus, K.A., Zhong, W., Gebhard, K.,
Herndier, B., Wang, H., Renne, R.,
Beneke, J., Pudney, J., Anderson, D.J.,
Ganem, D., and Haase, A.T. Kaposi's sar-
coma-associated herpesvirus gene expres-
sion in endothelial (spindle tumor) cells. *J.
Virol.* 71: 715–719, **1997**.

Stebbing, J., Bourboulia, D., Johnson, M.,
Henderson, S., Williams, I., Wilder, N.,
Tyrer, M., Youle, M., Imami, N., Kobu, T.,
Kuon, W., Sieper, J., Gotch, F., and Boshoff, C. Kaposi's sarcoma-associated herpesvirus cytotoxic T lymphocytes recognize
and target Darwinian positively selected
autologous K1 epitopes. *J. Virol.* 77: 4306–
4314, **2003**.

Stevenson, P.G., Efstathiou, S., Doherty, P.C.,
and Lehner, P.J. Inhibition of MHC class I-
restricted antigen presentation by gamma-
2-herpesviruses. *Proc. Natl. Acad. Sci. USA*
97: 8455–8460, **2000**.

Stine, J.T., Wood, C., Hill, M., Epp, A.,
Raport, C.J., Schweickart, V.L., Endo, Y.,
Sasaki, T., Simmons, G., Boshoff, C.,
Clapham, P., Chang, Y., Moore, P., Gray,
P.W., and Chantry, D. KSHV-encoded CC
chemokine vMIP-III is a CCR4 agonist,
stimulates angiogenesis, and selectively
chemoattracts TH2 cells. *Blood* 95: 1151–
1157, **2000**.

Strand, K., Harper, E., Thormahlen, S., Thou-
less, M.E., Tsai, C., Rose, T., and Bosch,
M.L. Two distinct lineages of macaque
gamma herpesviruses related to the
Kaposi's sarcoma-associated herpesvirus. *J.
Clin. Virol.* 16: 253–269, **2000** .

Sturzl, M., Blasig, C., Schreier, A., Neipel, F.,
Hohenadl, C., Cornali, E., Ascherl, G.,
Esser, S., Brockmeyer, N.H., Ekman, M.,
Kaaya, E.E., Tschachler, E., and Biberfeld,
P. Expression of HHV-8 latency-associated
T0.7 RNA in spindle cells and endothelial
cells of AIDS-associated classical and Afri-
can Kaposi's sarcoma. *Int. J. Cancer* 72:
68–71, **1997**.

Sun, Q., Zachariah, S., and Chaudhary, P.M. The human herpes virus 8-encoded viral FLICl inhibitory protein induces cellular transformation via NF-κB activation. *J. Biol. Chem.* 278: 52 437–52 445, **2003**.

Swanton, C., Mann, D.J., Fleckenstein, B., Neipel, F., Peters, G., and Jones, N. Herpes viral cyclin/Cdk6 complexes evade inhibition by CDK inhibitor proteins. *Nature* 390: 184–187, **1997**.

Tang, J., Gordon, G.M., Muller, M.G., Dahiya, M., and Foreman, K.E. Kaposi's sarcoma-associated herpesvirus latency-associated nuclear antigen induces expression of the helix-loop-helix protein Id-1 in human endothelial cells. *J. Virol.* 77: 5975–5984, **2003**.

Teruya-Feldstein, J., Zauber, P., Setsuda, J.E., Berman, E.L., Sorbara, L., Raffeld, M., Tosato, G., and Jaffe, E.S. Expression of human herpesvirus-8 oncogene and cytokine homologues in an HIV-seronegative patient with multicentric Castleman's disease and primary effusion lymphoma. *Lab. Investig.* 78: 1637–1642, **1998**.

Thome, M., Schneider, P., Hofmann, K., Fickenscher, H., Meinl, E., Neipel, F., Mattmann, C., Burns, K., Bodmer, J.L., Schroter, M., Scaffidi, C., Krammer, P.H., Peter, M.E., and Tschopp, J. Viral FLICE-inhibitory proteins (FLIPs) prevent apoptosis induced by death receptors. *Nature* 386: 517–521, **1997**.

Tieber, V.L., Zalinskis, L.L., Silva, R.F., Finkelstein, A., and Coussens, P.M. Transactivation of the Rous sarcoma virus long terminal repeat promoter by Marek's disease virus. *Virology* 179: 719–727, **1990**.

Tomlinson, C.C. and Damania, B. The K1 protein of Kaposi's sarcoma-associated herpesvirus activates the Akt signaling pathway. *J. Virol.* 78: 1918–1927, **2004**.

Tortorella, D., Gewurz, B.E., Furman, M.H., Schust, D.J., and Ploegh, H.L. Viral subversion of the immune system. *Annu. Rev. Immunol.* 18: 861–926, **2000**.

Touloumi, G., Hatzakis, A., Potouridou, I., Milona, I., Strarigos, J., Katsambas, A., Giraldo, G., Beth-Giraldo, E., Biggar, R.J., Mueller, N., and Trichopoulos, D. The role of immunosuppression and immune-activation in classic Kaposi's sarcoma. *Int. J. Cancer* 82: 817–821, **1999**.

Varthakavi, V., Browning, P.J., and Spearman, P. Human immunodeficiency virus replication in primary effusion lymphoma cell line stimulates lytic-phase replication of Kaposi's sarcoma-associated herpesvirus. *J. Virol.* 73: 10 329–10 338, **1999**.

Verma, S. C. and Robertson, E.S. Molecular biology and pathogenesis of Kaposi sarcoma-associated herpesvirus. *FEMS Microbiol. Lett.* 222: 155–163, **2003**.

Verma, S. C., Borah, S., and Robertson, E.S. Latency-associated nuclear antigen of Kaposi's sarcoma-associated herpesvirus up-regulates transcription of human telomerase reverse transcriptase promoter through interaction with transcription factor Sp1. *J. Virol.* 78: 10 348–10 359, **2004**.

Verschuren, E.W., Hodgson, J.G., Gray, J.W., Kogan, S., Jones, N., and Evan, G.I. The role of p53 in suppression of KSHV cyclin-induced lymphomagenesis. *Cancer Res.* 64: 581–589, **2004**.

Vitale, F., Briffa, D.V., Whitby, D., Maida, I., Grochowska, A., Levin, A., Romano, N., and Goedert, J.J. Kaposi's sarcoma herpes virus and Kaposi's sarcoma in the elderly populations of 3 Mediterranean islands. *Int. J. Cancer* 91: 588–591, **2001**.

Vogel, J., Hinrichs, S., Reynolds, R., Luciw, P., and Jay, G. The HIV tat gene induces dermal lesions resembling Kaposi's sarcoma in transgenic mice. *Nature* 335: 606–611, **1988**.

Wabinga, H.R., Parkin, D.M., Wabwire-Mangen, F., and Mugerwa, J.W. Cancer in Kampala, Uganda, in 1989–1991: changes in incidence in the era of AIDS. *Int. J. Cancer* 54: 26–36, **1993**.

Wang, H.W., Sharp, T.V., Koumi, A., Koentges, G., and Boshoff, C. Characterization of an anti-apoptotic glycoprotein encoded by Kaposi's sarcoma-associated herpesvirus which resembles a spliced variant of human survivin. *EMBO J.* 21: 2602–2615, **2002**.

Watanabe, T., Sugaya, M., Atkins, A.M., Aquilino, E.A., Yang, A., Borris, D.L., Brady, J., and Blauvelt, A. Kaposi's sarcoma-associated herpesvirus latency-associated nuclear antigen prolongs the life span of primary human umbilical vein endothelial cells. *J. Virol.* 77: 6188–6196, **2003**.

Weaver, B.K., Kumar, K.P., and Reich, N.C. Interferon regulatory factor 3 and CREB-binding protein/p300 are subunits of double-stranded RNA-activated transcription factor DRAF1. *Mol. Cell. Biol.* 18: 1359–1368, **1998**.

Weiss, S. and Biggar, R. The epidemiology of human retrovirus-associated illness. *Mt. Sinai J. Med.* 53: 579–591, **1986**.

Whitby, D., Howard, M.R., Tenant-Flowers, M., Brink, N.S., Copas, A., Boshoff, C., Hatzioannou, T., Suggett, F.E., Aldam, D.M., Denton, A.S. et al. Detection of Kaposi sarcoma associated herpesvirus in peripheral blood of HIV-infected individuals and progression to Kaposi's sarcoma. *Lancet* 346: 799–802, **1995**.

Whitby, D., Luppi, M., Barzozi, P., Boshoff, C., Weiss, R.A., and Torelli, G. Human herpesvirus 8 seroprevalence in blood donors and lymphoma patients from different regions of Italy. *J. Natl. Cancer Inst.* 90: 395–397, **1998**.

Whitby, D., Stossel, A., Gamache, C., Papin, J., Bosch, M., Smith, A., Kedes, D.H., White, G., Kennedy, R., and Dittmer, D.P. Novel Kaposi's sarcoma-associated herpesvirus homolog in baboons. *J. Virol.* 77: 8159–8165, **2003**.

Wong, L.Y., Matchett, G.A., and Wilson, A.C. Transcriptional activation by the Kaposi's sarcoma-associated herpesvirus latency-associated nuclear antigen is facilitated by an N-terminal chromatin-binding motif. *J. Virol.* 78: 10074–10 085, **2004**.

Wong, S. W., Bergquam, E.P., Swanson, R.M., Lee, F.W., Shiihi, S. M., Avery, N.A" Fanton, J.W., and Axthelm, M.K. Induction of B cell hyperplasia in simian immunodeficiency virus-infected rhesus macaques with the simian homologue of Kaposi sarcoma-associated herpesvirus. *J. Exp. Med.* 190: 827–840, **1999**.

Ye, F.C., Zhou, F.C., Yoo, S. M., Xie, J.P., Browning, P.J., and Gao, S. J. Disruption of Kaposi's sarcoma-associated herpesvirus latent nuclear antigen leads to abortive episome persistence. *J. Virol.* 78: 11 121–11 129, **2004**.

Zhong, W., Wang, H., Herndier, B., and Ganem, D. Restricted expression of Kaposi sarcoma-associated herpesvirus (human herpesvirus 8) genes. *Proc. Natl. Acad. Sci. USA* 93: 6641–6646, **1996**.

5

Papillomavirus Infections: A Major Cause of Human Cancers

5.1
Introduction

This was the heading of a review which appeared during the mid-1990s (zur Hausen, 1996) and, indeed, papillomaviruses have emerged today as one of the most important group of infectious carcinogens.

As outlined in Chapter 1, the infectious nature of warts became evident around the turn of the twentieth century. The first link of papillomavirus infection to cancer originated from studies on cancer induction by the cottontail rabbit papillomavirus in domestic rabbits and the subsequent elegant studies performed by Peyton Rous and his associates on synergistic effects between these infectious carcinogens and chemical factors (Rous and Beard, 1934; Rous and Kidd, 1938; Rous and Friedewald, 1944). The molecular analysis of papillomaviruses had a slow start. The viruses were first visualized electronmicroscopically in 1949 (Strauss et al.), and their circular double-stranded DNA genome was demonstrated in 1963 (Crawford and Crawford, 1963). Yet, the unavailability of a tissue culture system for viral replication hampered the progress for several additional years.

First evidence for biological functions of a member of this virus group originated from studies with bovine papillomaviruses (BPV). This virus was able to induce urinary bladder tumors in cattle (Olson et al., 1959), was found to be tumorigenic after inoculation into newborn hamsters (Friedmann et al., 1963; Boiron et al., 1964), and transformed calf and murine cells in tissue culture (Black et al., 1963; Thomas et al., 1963). In humans, a detailed analysis of potentially oncogenic papillomaviruses began during the early 1970s, with a publication by Stefania Jablonska in Warsaw (Jablonska et al., 1972), who considered a rare hereditary papillomatosis, *epidermodysplasia verruciformis*, "...as model in studies of papillomaviruses in oncogenesis".

Shortly thereafter it was postulated that papillomaviruses may play a major role in the induction of carcinomas of the cervix (zur Hausen et al., 1974 a,b, 1975; zur Hausen, 1975, 1976, 1977). At about the same time, the heterogeneity of human papillomaviruses (HPV) became evident (Gissmann and zur Hausen, 1976; Gissmann et al., 1977; Orth et al., 1977), and a specific HPV type was frequently discovered in skin cancers of epidermodysplasia patients (Orth et al., 1978, 1979). The isolation and identification of specific HPV types in genital warts and laryngeal

Infections Causing Human Cancer. Harald zur Hausen
Copyright © 2006 WILEY-VCH Verlag GmbH & Co. KGaA, Weinheim
ISBN: 3-527-31056-8

papillomas (Gissmann and zur Hausen, 1980; de Villiers et al., 1981; Gissmann et al., 1982) and directly from cervical cancer (HPV 16 and HPV 18) (Dürst et al., 1983; Boshart et al., 1984) and from premalignant genital lesions (Ikenberg et al., 1983) resulted subsequently in an explosion of studies on the role of HPV in anogenital cancers.

Although a number of subsequent experimental studies supported a causal role of "high risk" HPV infections (zur Hausen, 1986 a) in cervical cancer, it took almost a decade, before epidemiologic studies came to the same conclusion (Muñoz et al., 1992; Schiffman et al., 1993; Bosch et al., 1995; Matsukura and Sugase, 1995).

Today, mechanistic aspects of HPV-induced carcinogenesis have been partially unraveled and specific types of HPV have emerged as the most common "human carcinoma viruses" (zur Hausen, 1989 a). There exist remarkable differences in HPV-caused cancers between females and males (Fig. 5.1).

The practical application of our present knowledge in diagnosing patients at risk, in the treatment of early and late lesions, and in particular in preventing these infections by vaccination dominate the research issues in this field.

5.1.1
Structure of the Viral Particle, Transcriptional Regulation, and Taxonomy

Papillomavirus particles have a diameter of approximately 55 nm and contain a double-stranded circular DNA genome. The viral DNA is associated with histone-like proteins (Favre et al., 1977; Pfister and zur Hausen, 1978) and encapsidated by 72 capsomeres (Klug and Finch, 1965). The major capsid protein is encoded by the L1 open reading frame (ORF) which contains type-specific antigenic domains. The L2 ORF codes for a minor L2-component of the viral capsid. This protein possesses group-specific antigenic domains. Virus-like particles can be obtained by expressing either L1 only or L1 and L2 proteins in recombinant systems (Zhou et al., 1991, 1992; Kirnbauer et al., 1992). The L1 protein is highly conserved among different papillomavirus types, whereas the L2 protein is less conserved. The structure of the papillomavirus particle without a lipid-containing envelope renders these viruses relatively resistant to heating and organic solvents (Bonnez et al., 1994).

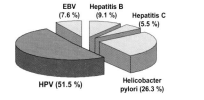
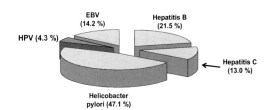

Fig. 5.1 Global percentage of human papillomavirus (HPV)-linked cancers in females and males in relation to other cancers linked to infections.

Papillomavirus genomes contain between 7200 and 8000 base pairs (bp), with up to 10 ORFs. Only one strand of the viral genome is transcriptionally active, transcription occurs only in one direction, and the ORFs of different HPV types reveal a high degree of topic correspondence (Chen et al., 1982; Danos et al., 1982). A long-control region (LCR) or upstream regulatory region (URR) covers about 12% of the genome. As its main functions, the URR regulates the epithelial-specific transcription, the differential expression of viral genes during the course of cell differentiation, receives feed-back signals to control viral gene expression, and responds to host factors on viral gene expression.

The regulation of viral gene expression is complex and controlled by viral and cellular transcription factors. Most of these regulations occur within the URR region, which varies substantially in nucleotide composition between individual HPV types. Additional regulatory mechanisms involve the use of different promoters, differential splicing, particularly affecting the E1 gene, differential transcription termination signals, and variations in the stability of different viral mRNAs. The URRs of anogenital HPVs range in size between 88 and 900 bp, but in other HPV genera – particularly in those found in genus β – they are somewhat shorter. Within the URR, cis-active elements regulate transcription of the E6 and E7 genes, which represent the most important transforming genes for immortalization and the maintenance of the malignant phenotype of HPV-positive cervical cancer cells (Schwarz et al., 1985; Yee et al., 1985; Münger et al., 1989; Hawley-Nelson et al., 1989; von Knebel Doeberitz et al., 1992).

Analysis of the URR regions of different papillomavirus genotypes resulted in the identification of several binding sites shared among most HPV types, as well as a few unique ones. The common sequences include TFIID binding to TATA boxes located approximately 30 bp upstream from early start sites (Longworth and Laimins, 2004a). Sp-1 and AP-1 binding sites, upstream of these sequences, have been identified in all HPV types studied (del Mar Pena and Laimins, 2001). Many different HPV types share binding sites for additional factors, including those for NF-1, TEF-1, TEF-2, Oct-1, AP-2, KRF-1, and YY-1 (Mack and Laimins, 1991; Bauknecht et al., 1992; Ishiji et al., 1992; Butz and Hoppe-Seyler, 1993; O'Connor and Bernard, 1995). The keratinocyte-specific enhancers seem to regulate the tropism of papillomaviruses for epithelial cells. Glucocorticoid-responsive elements emerge as particularly important for anogenital papillomavirus types (Gloss et al., 1987).

In genital HPV types the transcription of late genes is activated in differentiated cells from start sites within the E7 ORF. This seems to be due to a rearrangement of chromatin around the late promoter region during the course of epithelial differentiation (del Mar Pena and Laimins, 2001).

At present, 106 human and 22 animal papillomavirus genotypes have been fully described, yet it is very likely that the total number of human – and certainly also of animal genotypes – will be much higher (de Villiers et al., 2004a; E.-M. de Villiers, personal communication). All known human papillomavirus types, isolation sites and appropriate references are listed in Table 5.1.

The heterogeneity of the HPV family is not restricted to the human members, and the large number of human prototypes reflects the intensity of investigations in our

Table 5.1 All presently known human papillomavirus (HPV) types and sites of their isolation (courtesy of E.-M. de Villiers).

HPV-type	Original isolation from
1	plantar warts
2	common warts
3	flat warts
4	common warts
5	benign and malignant epidermodysplasia verruciformis (EV) lesions
6	genital warts, laryngeal papillomatosis
7	"butcher's warts", oral papillomas of HIV patients
8	benign and malignant EV lesions
9	EV lesions
10	flat warts
11	laryngeal papillomas, genital warts
12	EV lesions
13	oral focal epithelial hyperplasia
14	EV lesions
15	EV lesions
16	CIN III and anogenital and oral cancers
17	EV lesions
18	CIN III and anogenital cancers
19	EV lesions
20	EV lesions and cutaneous squamous cell carcinomas
21	EV lesions
22	EV lesions
23	EV lesions
24	EV lesions
25	EV lesions
26	common warts under immunosuppression
27	common warts
28	flat warts
29	common warts
30	anogenital and oral intraepithelial lesions
31	CIN III and anogenital cancers
32	oral focal epithelial hyperplasia, oral florid papillomatosis
33	CIN III and anogenital and oral cancers
34	low-grade CINs
35	usually low-grade CIN
36	actinic keratoses, EV lesions
37	keratoacanthoma
38	papillomas under immunosuppression and skin cancers
39	CIN lesions and anogenital cancers
40	anogenital intraepithelial neoplasias
41	cutaneous squamous cell carcinomas
42	low-grade CIN
43	low-grade CIN
44	low-grade CIN, condylomata acuminata
45	anogenital intraepithelial neoplasias
46	now designated as HPV 20b
47	EV lesions
48	cutaneous lesions

Table 5.1 (Continued)

HPV-type	Original isolation from
49	flat warts under immunosuppression
50	EV lesion
51	CIN and anogenital cancers
52	CIN III and anogenital cancers
53	anogenital intraepithelial neoplasias
54	anogenital intraepithelial neoplasias
55	anogenital intraepithelial neoplasias
56	anogenital intraepithelial neoplasias and cancers
57	oral and inverted maxillary sinus papillomas
58	CIN III and anogenital cancers
59	anogenital intraepithelial neoplasias
60	epidemoid cysts
61	anogenital intraepithelial neoplasias
62	anogenital intraepithelial neoplasias
63	myrmecia warts
64	anogenital intraepithelial neoplasias
65	pigmented warts
66	CIN and anogenital cancer
67	anogenital intraepithelial neoplasia
68	anogenital intraepithelial neoplasia
69	CIN and anogenital cancers
70	vulvar papillomas
71	anogenital intraepithelial neoplasias
72	oral papillomas in HIV patients
73	oral papillomas in HIV patients
74	anogenital intraepithelial neoplasia
75	common warts in organ allograft recipients
76	common warts in organ allograft recipients
77	common warts in organ allograft recipients
78	skin wart
79	erroneous designation, no longer existing
80	normal skin and ear canal
81	vaginal intraepithelial neoplasia I
82	CIN II and CIN III
83	anal condyloma
84	normal cervical smear
85	cervical scraping and wart
86	CIN I
87	koilocytotic atypia
88	skin wart
89	normal cervical smear
90	normal cervical smear
91	normal cervical smear
92	basal cell carcinoma
93	actinic keratosis
94	squamous cell carcinoma skin
95	skin wart
96	perilesional skin of squamous cell carcinoma
97	genital isolate

Table 5.1 (Continued)

HPV-type	Original isolation from
98	normal skin
99	normal skin
100	premalignant lesion and squamous cell carcinoma skin
101	normal skin
102	genital isolate
103	genital isolate
104	skin wart
105	premalignant skin lesion
106	genital isolate

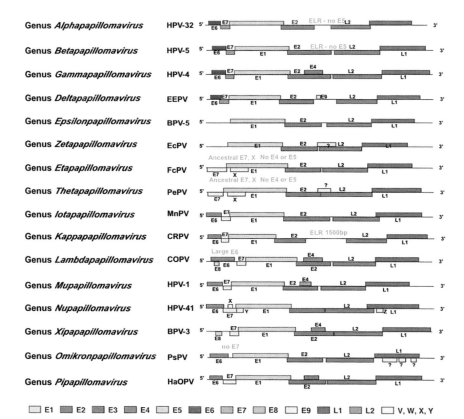

Fig. 5.2 Open reading frames of various HPV types. (Reprinted from VIRUS TAXONOMY, Eighth Report of the International Committee on Taxonomy of Viruses, Vol 1, Fauquet, C.M., Mayo, M.A., Maniloff, J., Desselberger, U. and Ball, L.A. (Eds.), Part II – The Double Stranded DNA Viruses, Papillomaviridae, 241. Copyright 2005, with permission from Elsevier.)

species. The 22 animal papillomavirus types that have been fully characterized originate mainly from nonhuman primates and from cattle. The genomic organization of the various papillomavirus genera is depicted in Figure 5.2.

It warrants attention that a number of animal papillomavirus types are more closely related to individual members of the human subgroups than are the latter among each other. A papillomavirus, isolated from a penile carcinoma of a rhesus monkey, is very closely related to HPV 52 (Ostrow et al., 1991). Likewise, a pygmy chimpanzee papillomavirus is most closely related to HPV 13 (van Ranst et al., 1992), while the cottontail rabbit papillomavirus and the canine oral papillomavirus, a finch papillomavirus and a porcupine papillomavirus reveal some relatedness to genus µ, containing HPV types 1 and 63 (Giri et al., 1985; Delius et al., 1994; Rector et al., 2005). These observations stress the assumption that, in developmental terms, the papillomavirus genera split off in prehistoric times, probably even before the development of nonhuman primates.

Although originally combined with Polyomaviruses into the family of Papovaviridae, the differences in genetic organization and functional properties resulted in their recognition as a new family of Papillomaviridae. The family is subdivided into 16 genera, labeled by letters of the Greek alphabet form α (alpha) to π (pi). The relative relatedness of individual types is indicated in the phylogenetic tree (Fig. 5.3).

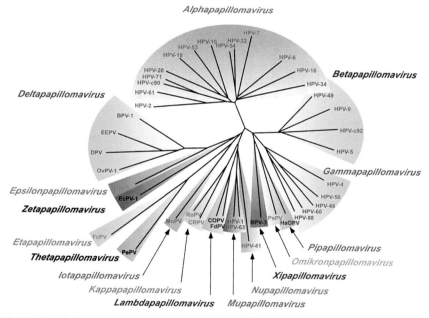

Fig. 5.3 The phylogenetic tree and nomenclature of papillomaviruses. (Reprinted from VIRUS TAXONOMY, Eighth Report of the International Committee on Taxonomy of Viruses, Vol 1, Fauquet, C.M., Mayo, M.A., Maniloff, J., Desselberger, U. and Ball, L.A. (Eds.), Part II – The Double Stranded DNA Viruses, Papillomaviridae, 252. Copyright 2005, with permission from Elsevier.)

Genotypes are defined by a difference of more than 10% within the most conserved region (L1 ORF), while differences of less than 10% characterize subtypes (de Villiers, 2001). It is interesting to note that this arbitrary separation also seems to define HPV serotypes.

There exist some structural differences between individual genera, as exemplified by the absence of an E5 ORF in genera β, γ, ε, φ and ι. The E4 ORF is missing in genera ε and φ, no typical E6 is present in genera ε and φ, and some genera contain an additional ORF (E8) within the E6 region (genera κ and ζ).

5.1.2
Transmission and Natural History of Papillomavirus Infections

The transmission of HPVs is facilitated by microlesions in the skin and mucosa, and/or by abraded or macerated epithelial surfaces (Oriel, 1971). Anogenital HPV infections are mainly transmitted by sexual contacts, but are rarely detected in sexually inexperienced young women (Fairley et al., 1992; Andersson-Ellström et al., 1994; Gutman et al., 1994; Rylander et al., 1994). It was noted at an early stage that there exists a correlation between the number of sexual partners and the prevalence of HPV infection (Rosenfeld et al., 1989; Moscicki et al., 1990; Bauer et al., 1993; Critchlow and Koutsky, 1995). Occasionally, anogenital HPV infections are also transmitted digitally from one epithelial site to the other (Moy et al., 1989; Euvrard et al., 1993). In addition, they may be transmitted by fomites, by medical instruments, and also by laser plumes (Garden et al., 1988; Ferenczy et al., 1990).

Oral–genital contact may lead to infections at oral sites by anogenital papillomaviruses (Kashima et al., 1992a). Salivary transmission probably accounts for additional infections in the oral region.

Skin infections by papillomaviruses originate from close skin contact, from contaminated materials, by walking barefoot on abrasive surfaces (Rasmussen et al., 1958; Koutsky et al., 1988), or from accidental wounding with contaminated equipment (Melchers et al., 1993).

The life cycle of HPVs is tightly linked to the differentiation program of human keratinocytes. The production of viral particles occurs exclusively in suprabasal differentiated layers. Recently, however, a replication- and differentiation-independent system for the production of infectious HPV particles has been developed (Pyeon et al., 2005). Infection seems to require the availability of a cell which is still in the proliferation program (for a review, see zur Hausen, 1996). This most commonly appears to occur in microlesions, where basal layer cells are exposed to the surface. It may also happen at the periphery of junctions between different types of epithelial cells. At the distal periphery of the cervical transformation zone, particularly in very young women, proliferating cells touch the surface. This is the most vulnerable region for high-risk anogenital HPV infections.

5.1.3
Functions of Viral Proteins

5.1.3.1 **E6**

The following sections will mainly deal with functions of high-risk HPV proteins (e.g., HPV 16, 18, and 31); the differing properties of corresponding proteins in low-risk viruses will be detailed separately.

The E6 protein of HPV 16 contains 151 nucleic acids and reveals four Cys-X-X-Cys motifs that mediate zinc binding and which should result in the formation of two zinc finger structures (Barbosa et al., 1989; Grossman and Laimins, 1989; Kanda et al., 1991). E6 proteins are found in the nucleus as well as in the cytoplasm, and bind a larger number of cellular proteins. Expression of the *E6* gene alone results in immortalization of various types of human cells, though at low efficiency and commonly accompanied by the loss of p16^{INK4} expression (Band et al., 1990; Wazer et al., 1995; Reznikoff et al., 1996; Kiyono et al., 1997; Liu et al., 1999). E6, in addition, cooperates with the *ras* oncogene in the immortalization of primary rodent cells (Storey and Banks, 1993). E6 cooperates with the E7 protein in the efficient immortalization of human cells (Münger et al., 1989). It induces anchorage-independent growth of NIH 3 T3 cells and transactivates the adenovirus E2 promoter (Sedman et al., 1991).

The binding and degradation of p53 represents one of the most intensively studied functions of the E6 protein (Werness et al., 1990; Scheffner et al., 1990). p53 has been characterized as a tumor suppressor gene, regulating the expression of genes involved in cell cycle control. Among these, the cyclin-dependent kinase inhibitor p21 plays an important role. DNA damage results in activation of p53 and in the induction of high levels of p21, leading to cell cycle arrest and apoptosis (Ko and Prives, 1996). The activation of apoptotic pathways represents a cellular defense mechanism against the spread of virus infections, as well as a protective function against an undesired accumulation of mutational modifications. A number of viruses – in particular members of the herpesvirus group (see Chapter 4) – have developed mechanisms to interfere with apoptotic pathways. E6 binds to p53 in a ternary complex with E6-AP (Huibregtse et al., 1991). The formation of this complex results in ubiquitination of p53 and subsequent degradation of the latter by the 26 S proteasome (Hubbert et al., 1992; Huibregtse et al., 1993, 1995). E6 also binds to p300/CBP, which is a coactivator of p53 (Lechner and Laimins, 1994; Patel et al., 1999; Zimmermann et al., 1999), and thus interferes also indirectly with p53. High-risk HPV E6 binds and functionally inactivates the cyclin-dependent kinase inhibitors p21 (Funk et al., 1997; Jones et al., 1997), a transcriptional target of p53 (el-Deiry et al., 1993; Harper et al., 1993; Xiong et al., 1993), and p27 (Zerfass-Thome et al., 1996).

p53 also acts as a transcriptional activator by binding to specific DNA sequences (Kern et al., 1991). It is required for growth arrest following cellular DNA damage (Kuerbitz et al., 1992; Lin et al., 1992). Failure of this function results in continued DNA replication after DNA damage and in chromosomal instability (Livingstone et al., 1992; Yin et al., 1992). The transcriptional activation function of p53 is also inhibited by high-risk HPV E6 (Gu et al., 1994). Interference with the p53/PUMA/Bax cascade was recently shown to be responsible for the anti-apoptotic function of the E6 protein in cervical cancer cells (Vogt et al., 2006).

Binding of E6 to E6-AP mediates also a self-ubiquitination of the E6-AP protein (Kao et al., 2000). Therefore, it is likely that the reduction of E6-AP concentrations in E6-positive cells will negatively affect the proteolysis of other E6-AP-binding cellular proteins, among them members of the *src*-family of tyrosine kinases (Oda et al., 1999; Frame, 2002). It becomes increasingly apparent that binding of E6 to E6-AP or to other ubiquitin ligases is one of the central events in E6 functions, and influences all other E6-mediated effects described below (Kelley et al., 2005).

Another functionally important interaction results from the carboxy-terminal PDZ (PSD-95, Dlg, and ZO-1 proteins) domain protein-binding motive X-(S/T)-X-(V/I/L)-COOH which can bind a number of cellular PDZ domain-containing proteins. Clearly important here are *hDlg* (human homologue of *Drosophila melanogaster* tumor suppressor protein discs large), *MUPP1* (multi-PDZ domain protein), *hScrib* (human homologue of *Drosophila melanogaster* tumor suppressor *scribble*) (Kiyono et al., 1997; Lee et al., 1997, 2000; Nakagawa and Huibregtse, 2000), and *MAGI-1* (Glaunsinger et al., 2000). The PDZ domains seem to act as molecular scaffold to mediate signal transduction (Gomperts, 1996; Craven and Bredt, 1998). Binding of E6 to these proteins results in their degradation. This binding and degradation process is clearly of substantial importance for cell immortalization by E6, since E6 transgenic mice devoid of PDZ protein expression but expressing a functional p53 do not develop epidermal hyperplasias, regularly observed in wild-type transgenics (Nguyen et al., 2003). Yet, even deletion of the hDlg binding motif of HPV16 E6 permitted the bypass of senescence of human mammary epithelial cells (Kiyono et al., 1998). In this system the activation of telomerase appears to be the major determinant of cellular immortalization. At least in the cervical carcinoma cell line HeLa, containing multiple copies of HPV18 DNA, continued expression of telomerase is not sufficient for the maintenance of the malignant phenotype. Repression of the *E6* gene in these cells, stably expressing an exogenous *hTERT* gene which encodes the catalytic subunit of telomerase, elevated telomerase activity and elongated telomeres did not prevent senescence and apoptosis (Horner et al., 2004). On the other hand, overexpression of the catalytic subunit of telomerase, murine TERT, in basal keratinocytes of transgenic mice results in increased epidermal tumors (Gonzáles-Suárez et al., 2001). This may underline the existing differences in transformability of human and murine cells. Human keratinocytes expressing *hTERT* are able to bypass p16[INK4]-mediated senescence and become immortal, yet they retain normal growth and differentiation characteristics (Dickson et al., 2000).

One report describes that hDlg and MAGIs are degraded by E6 complexing in an E6-AP-independent pathway (Grm and Banks, 2004). It is likely that other E6-associated ubiquitin ligases than E6-AP are important for the degradation of certain E6 targets. One PDZ protein which is degraded by E6/E6-AP is TIP-2/GIPC (Favre-Bonvin et al., 2005); this protein has been found to be involved in transforming growth factor-β (TGF-β) signaling and enhances the expression of TGF-β type III receptor at the cell membrane. Its degradation diminishes the antiproliferative effect of TGF-β in high-risk HPV E6-expressing cells.

The degradation of PDZ domain-carrying proteins by E6 or E6/E6-AP complexes may also affect the *Notch* signaling pathway. DELTA1 and DELTA4, both Notch ligands, interact with Dlg1 (Six et al., 2004) which is directly affected by the E6/E6-AP complex. JAGGED1, a cell-bound ligand for Notch receptors, contains a PDZ domain, although mutation of the PDZ ligand did not affect the ability of JAGGED1 to initiate Notch signaling (Ascano et al., 2003). Another PDZ domain-containing member of the E3 ubiquitin ligase family, *LNX*, can enhance Notch signaling (Nie et al., 2002). It has been reported that JAGGED1 and Notch ligand are up-regulated in high-grade cervical lesions and in invasive cervical cancer, whereas a negative regulator of JAGGED1-Notch signaling, *Manic Fringe*, is down-regulated (Veeraraghavalu et al., 2004).

E6 has been shown to induce suprabasal DNA synthesis and is alone sufficient to induce carcinomas in transgenic animals (Song et al., 1999). This activity is p53-independent, and correlates with the ability of E6 to bind PDZ domain proteins (Nguyen et al., 2003).

The activation of the catalytic subunit hTERT by E6 emerges as an important factor in cell immortalization (Klingelhutz et al., 1996; Meyerson et al., 1997; Nakamura et al., 1997). Clues of the mechanism leading to hTERT activation by high-risk HPVs originated from experiments conducted by Veldman et al. (2003). A complex of E6/*Myc/Max* binds to the hTERT promoter and results in its activation. This effect is specific for high-risk HPV E6. Gewin et al. (2004) proposed that complexes of E6/E6-AP, forming an E3 ubiquitin ligase, target an hTERT repressor, NFX1–91, which becomes highly ubiquitinated and destabilized. E6-independent knock-down of NFX1–91 also results in derepression of the endogenous hTERT promoter and elevated levels of telomerase activity. E6 mutants that fail to bind E6-AP are also defective for increasing telomerase activity and transactivating the hTERT promoter (Liu, X., et al., 2005). E6 functions in solely E6-expressing p16^{INK4}-positive or -negative cells are summarized in Figures 5.4 and 5.5.

The induction of chromosomal instability by *E6* oncogene expression is probably one of the very important aspects in the long-term progression of latently high-risk HPV-infected cells. One major reason is the degradation of p53 and the resulting loss of G_1/S checkpoint control and the disruption of p53-dependent G_1 arrest after DNA damage. Kessis and colleagues (1996) showed that either E6 or E7 proteins of high-risk, but not of low-risk HPV, increase the frequency of foreign DNA integration into the host genome. This could be related to the observed HPV DNA integration at late stages of tumor progression – for example, in cervical intraepithelial neoplasia (CIN) III lesions (Klaes et al., 1999) which commonly reveal a similarly high level of viral oncoprotein expression as cervical cancer cells (Dürst et al., 1991; Stoler et al., 1992).

Suppression of both, caspase 3 and 8, by E6 results in the suppression of apoptosis induced by TNF-α via the Fas pathway (Filippova et al., 2004). This seems to be mediated by binding of E6 to cellular FADD and subsequent degradation of the latter. Repression of the E6 gene on the other hand initiates p53-dependent, telomerase-inde-

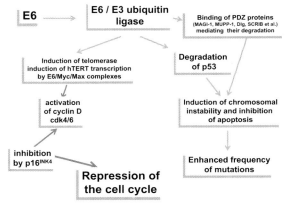

Fig. 5.4 Consequences of E6 expression in p16[INK4]-expressing cells. The activation of the cell cycle is counteracted by p16[INK4] which interferes by blocking cyclin D/cdk4/6 complexes.

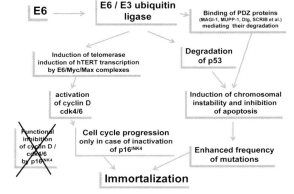

Fig. 5.5 In cells where p16[INK4] is inactivated (either due to DNA methylation, mutation or deletion), pE6 expression may lead directly to immortalization.

pendent senescence and apoptosis in HeLa cervical carcinoma cells (Horner et al., 2004). The E6 protein also interacts with other pre-apoptotic proteins, most notably with Bak (Thomas and Banks, 1999; Jackson et al., 2000). Restoration of p53 expression sensitizes HPV 16-immortalized human keratinocytes to CD95-mediated apoptosis (Aguilar-Lemarroy et al., 2002).

Several other protein interactions have been reported for E6: among others, with the adhesion and cellular polarity determining factor paxillin, the interferon regulatory factor IRF-3, and the calcium-binding protein E6-BP (Ronco et al., 1998; Tong and Howley, 1997; Chen et al., 1998; Elston et al., 1998). By binding to tuberin, a negative regulator for insulin-induced phosphorylation of S6 kinase and eIF4 E-binding protein 1, E6 also interferes with the insulin signaling pathway (Lu et al., 2004). In addition, E6 seems to be able to promote phosphorylation of the retinoblastoma protein (Malanchi et al., 2004). A compendium of E6 interacting factors has been published by Mantovani and Banks (2001). At present, the significance of the data in this section in terms of cell immortalization and transformation is difficult to assess.

5.1.3.2 E6*

A series of polypeptides expressed by high-risk HPV types through alternative splic-ing of E6 and labeled as E6* may point to a viral pathway regulating E6 activity (Schneider-Gädicke et al., 1988). One of these, E6*I, interacts with full-length E6 as well as with E6-AP and blocks the degradation of p53 (Pim et al., 1997). Mantovani and Banks (2001) argue that a possible E6* function could ensure the presence of a limited amount of p53 at viral replication sites. This seems to be supported by the observation that HPV recruits DNA polymerase α for its DNA replication and that p53 may enhance the replicative fidelity of this enzyme (Albrechtsen et al., 1999). It is interesting to note that p53 is also found in replication centers of herpes simplex, cytomegalovirus, and adenoviruses (Wilcock and Lane, 1991; Fortunato and Spector, 1998; König et al., 1999). In addition, an interaction between the HPV ori-complex binding and p53 has been noted (Massimi et al., 1999). A recent study suggests that E6* expression may result in a higher resistance to UV B radiation, and that this is related to a high glutathione peroxidase activity (Mouret et al., 2005). In general, functions of E6* polypeptides have as yet been poorly studied.

5.1.3.3 E7

The HPV16 E7 protein represents a zinc finger-binding phosphoprotein with two Cys-X-X-Cys domains composed of 98 amino acids. The zinc finger-binding domain and the two Cys-X-X-Cys motifs show similarity to the E6 protein, suggesting an evo-lutionary relationship between the two proteins. The amino-terminal part of the E7 protein contains two domains corresponding partially to the conserved region 1 (CR-1) and completely to the conserved region 2 (CR-2) of adenovirus E1 A proteins and to an analogous region in SV40 large T antigen (Phelps et al., 1989). Both of the E1 A regions are involved in cell transformation (Moran and Mathews, 1987). Both corresponding domains in E7 (cd-1 and cd-2) contribute to the immortalizing poten-tial of E7 (Phelps et al., 1992). The E7 protein is able to undergo pH-dependent con-formational transitions, exposing hydrophobic surfaces to the solvent (Alonso et al., 2004). Under these conditions it self-assembles into defined spherical oligomeres.

The phosphorylation of E7 is mediated by casein kinase II (CKII). Two S100 family calcium-binding proteins, macrophage inhibitor-related factor 8 (MRP-8) and MRP-14, form a protein complex that inactivates CKII (Tugizov et al., 2005). This complex consequently also inhibits CKII-mediated phosphorylation of E7. Treatment of HPV-immortalized cells with exogenous MRP-8/14 resulted in E7 hy-pophosphorylation and growth inhibition.

Expression of E7 is able to transform immortalized NIH 3T3 cells and, at very low frequency, also human keratinocytes (Münger et al., 1989; Wazer et al., 1995; Zerfass et al., 1995). This frequency is enhanced by overexpression of hTERT to induce telomerase (Kiyono et al., 1998).

One of the key features of E7 function is its complex formation with the retino-blastoma protein pRb and the related pocket proteins p107 and p130 (Dyson et al.,

1989; Berezutskaya et al., 1997; Classon and Dyson, 2001). The three proteins are differently expressed throughout the cell cycle: Whereas Rb is constitutively expressed, p107 is predominantly expressed during S-phase and p130 prevails in G_0 (Classon and Dyson, 2001; Longworth and Laimins, 2004 a). While the unphosphorylated forms of pocket proteins form complexes with E2F/DP1 transcription factors, upon progression from G_1 into S-phase, Rb becomes phosphorylated by cyclin-kinase complexes, releasing E2 F transcription factors. Binding of E7 has the same effect, resulting in the constitutive activation of E2F proteins that activate promoters of genes involved in S-phase progression and apoptosis (Edmonds and Vousden, 1989; Weintraub et al., 1995). This involves genes that are required for DNA synthesis, such as DNA polymerase α and thymidine kinase (La Thangue, 1994; Slansky and Farnham, 1996). There exists a good correlation between the inactivation of pocket proteins by E7 and its transforming potential (Heck et al., 1992; Phelps et al., 1992; Kiyono et al., 1998). Complex formation between E7 and Rb is not restricted to high-risk viruses; indeed, HPV 6 and 11 E7 also bind Rb, though at lower affinity (Piboonniyom et al., 2003). HPV 1 E7 binds Rb with high affinity, yet it is unable to activate E2F-inducible genes or to degrade Rb (Ciccolini et al., 1994; Schmitt et al., 1994). Recently, an association of E7 with the 600-kDa retinoblastoma protein-associated factor, p600, has been reported (Huh et al., 2005). This association is independent of the pocket proteins and is mediated through the N-terminal domain which contributes to cellular transformation independently of pRb binding.

E7 also mediates degradation of the pocket proteins through the ubiquitin proteasome pathway (Edmonds and Vousden, 1989; Jewers et al., 1992; Berezutskaya et al., 1997; Wang et al., 2001). Since Rb also regulates cell cycle exit during differentiation, the abrogation of its function by E7 also permits suprabasal cells to enter DNA replication (Chellappan et al., 1992). Binding of E7 to Rb seems also to be important for maintenance of the episomal state of HPV DNA, though the mechanism is poorly understood (Longworth and Laimins, 2004 b). Rb-bound E7 of high-risk HPV types also trans-activates the promoter of p73 (Brooks et al., 2002). In normal cervical epithelium, p73 expression is confined to the basal and suprabasal layers. In neoplastic lesions, however, expression is detected throughout the epithelium and increases with the grade of neoplasia. In addition, a deregulation of expression of the N-terminal splice variant p73Δ2 was observed in a significant proportion of cancers, but not in normal epithelium.

B-myb, a growth-promoting gene regulated by the release of E2 F, is also transcriptionally activated by HPV 16 E7 (Lam et al., 1994). It is inappropriately transcribed during G_1 and constitutively overexpressed in cycling cells containing E7. Regulation of the *B-myb* promoter is apparently mediated by p107-containing complexes binding to the E2 F binding site.

Several other interactions of high-risk HPV E7 with cellular proteins appear to be of substantial importance for its growth-promoting properties: the oncoprotein inhibits the function of the cyclin-dependent inhibitors p21 and p27 (Zerfass-Thome et al., 1996; Funk et al., 1997; Jones et al., 1997). High-risk E7 proteins bind directly to cyclin A/cdk-2 complexes and, through p107, indirectly to cyclin E/cdk-2 complexes by retaining their cdk2-associated kinase activity (Dyson et al., 1992; Arroyo et al., 1993; Tommasino et al., 1993; McIntyre et al., 1996). In contrast to low-risk E7 proteins, they even increase the levels of cyclin A and E proteins (Martin et al., 1998). The blocking of the cdk inhibitors p21 and p27 by E7 may contribute to the latter effect.

The promyelocytic leukemia (PML) protein induces senescence when overexpressed in primary human fibroblasts. E7 circumvents PML-induced senescence (Bischof et al., 2005). In this case, Rb-related and Rb-independent mechanisms of E7 are necessary to overcome the PML-induced senescence. A senescence inhibitor, DEK, represents an up-regulated target for high-risk HPV E7, but not for low-risk HPVs (Wise-Draper et al., 2005). This up-regulation emerges as a common event in high-risk HPV-driven carcinogenesis.

Another important group of cellular proteins bound to high-risk HPV E7 are the histone deacetylases (HDACs). They also repress E2 F-inducible promoters by binding to Rb proteins (Weintraub et al., 1995; Brehm et al., 1998). Binding of E7 to HDACs occurs independently of E7/Rb interactions (Longworth and Laimins, 2004 b). HDACs remove acetyl groups from the lysine-rich amino-terminal tails of histone proteins and functionally inactivate directly E2F proteins by deacetylation (Marks et al., 2001). Mutation in the HDAC binding domain of E7 results in an inability to stably maintain viral episomes and to extend the lifespan of transfected cells (Longworth and Laimins, 2004 a). Thus, similar to Rb-binding, the association of E7 with HDACs has profound consequences for the E7-expressing cell. The E7 transactivation of the cdc25A tyrosine phosphatase promoter depends on the binding of Rb and HDACs (Nguyen et al., 2002). E7, via HDAC recruitment, also silences the interferon regulatory factor 1 (IRF-1) gene that is important for interferon signaling and immune surveillance of persisting HPV infections (Park et al., 2000). This seems to affect in particular interferon α-inducible genes, but has no effect on interferon γ-inducible genes (Barnard and McMillan, 1999). On the other hand, E7-transfected mouse lymphoma cells were greatly sensitized to interferon α-induced apoptosis (Thyrell et al., 2005).

Besides interactions with the histone deacetylases, one report also describes binding of E7 with the acetyltransferase domain of pCAF which is supposed to function as a co-activator for a variety of transcription factors including p53 (Avvakumov et al., 2003). This interaction reduces the acetyltransferase activity *in vitro*.

Several additional cellular proteins are affected by E7 interactions: these include the S4 subunit of the 26S proteasome (Berezutskaya and Bagchi, 1997), Mi2β, as a component of the NURD histone deacetylase complex (Brehm et al., 1998), the transcription factor AP-1 (Antinore et al., 1996), the fork-head domain transcription factor MPP2 (Lüscher-Firzlaff et al., 1999), insulin-like growth factor (IGF) binding protein 3 (Mannhardt et al., 2000), the TATA box binding protein TBP (Massimi et al., 1996, 1997; Phillips and Vousden, 1997), and a human DnaJ protein, hTid-1 (Schilling et al., 1998).

By blocking Rb and p21, high-risk HPV E7 effectively overcomes cell cycle arrest (Helt et al., 2002) (Fig. 5.6). This seems to represent one reason for the genetic instability of E7-transfected cells, also evidenced by the increased integration of foreign DNA in such cells (Kessis et al., 1996).

Although E6 and E7 can both independently induce chromosomal instability (White et al., 1994), they cooperate in generating mitotic defects and aneuploidy (Münger et al., 2004). The latter appears to be primarily the result of centrosome abnormalities. E6 and E7 become apparent during episomal HPV 16 persistence (Duensing et al., 2001), and levels increase in cells containing integrated HPV DNA (Pett et al., 2004). HPV 16 E7 expression induces primary centrosome and centriole duplication errors in normal diploid cells (Duensing et al., 2001). The mechanism appears to be independent of Rb interactions, since expression of E7 in mouse embryo fibroblasts that lack pRb, p107 and p130 expression also results in increased centrosome abnormalities (Duensing and Münger, 2003). Further data indicate that disruption of the p16^{INK4a}/pRb checkpoint of epithelial cell immortalization does not necessarily lead to centrosome-associated genomic instability (Piboonniyom et al., 2003).

In addition to centrosome abnormalities, anaphase bridges and lagging chromosomes, indicating errors in mitotic spindle attachment, and double-stranded DNA breaks are commonly observed in these cells (Duensing and Münger, 2002). Dysregulation of mitotic pathways in cervical cancer and high-risk HPV-expressing cells lines have also been observed by genomic analyses (Patel et al., 2004; Thierry et al., 2004)

Some of the pathways influenced by E7 expression are shown in Figure 5.6.

A newly arising (and doubtless important) aspect of the regulation of E7 expression originates from observations pointing to the importance of the ARF locus (p19^{ARF} for mouse and p14^{ARF} for human) for E7 regulation. The *ARF* gene codes for a tumor suppressor protein with potent cell cycle inhibitory function (Quelle et al., 1995). It acts upstream of p21 by stabilizing and activating p53 (reviewed by Sherr, 1998). This activation occurs by binding of ARF to MDM2, which is an inhibitor of p53. In addition, however, p14^{ARF} seems to act via a p53-independent mechanism in the regulation of cell cycle arrest and apoptosis, which may depend entirely on p21 (Hemmati et al., 2005). ARF also associates with certain members of the E2F family and induces their degradation through the ubiquitin-proteasome pathway (Martelli et al., 2001; Eymin et al., 2002).

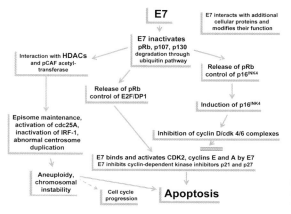

Fig. 5.6 Schematic outline of some of the important pathways influenced by high-risk HPV E7 oncoproteins. The regular consequence of the sole expression of E7 is apoptosis, presumably mediated by the release of E2 F following pRb inactivation.

In 2003, Pan and colleagues demonstrated an effective inhibition of E7 functions by exogenously expressed murine p19[ARF]. ARF caused relocalization of E7 from the nucleoplasm to the nucleolus, and blocked the proteolysis of Rb induced by E7. Although this finding requires confirmation, it could suggest that human p14[ARF] may provide a natural protective mechanism against E7 expression. It is interesting to note that immunohistochemical data, at the first glance, appear to contradict this expectation: Sano et al. (2002) and Wang, J.L., et al. (2004) reported an increased expression of p16[INK4] and p14[ARF] in cervical premalignant and malignant lesions. This was supported by polymerase chain reaction (PCR) analysis revealing an increased transcription of p14[ARF] (Kanao et al., 2004). On the other hand, this situation is somewhat reminiscent of p16[INK4] which is commonly inactivated in solely E6-immortalized cells (Reznikoff et al., 1996), but overexpressed in E6/E7-transformed lesions and cell lines. There, the overexpression is due to the inactivation of Rb by E7 and the resulting transcriptional activation of p16 by E2F. Since p16[INK4] blocks cyclin D/cdk 4/6 complexes, its growth-inhibitory effect is circumvented by E7 by directly stimulating cyclins E and A. The overexpression of p14[ARF] in advanced cervical lesions may point to a similar effect, where its blocking function on E7, however – for as yet unknown reasons – is no longer functioning. In spite of a high p14[ARF] expression in cervical cancer cells, this protein does not seem to interfere with the E7 function. Under conditions of hyperproliferation, p14[ARF] stabilizes p53 by binding HDM2 and inhibiting its HDM2-mediated ubiquitination and degradation (reviewed in Bothner et al., 2001). Upon binding, the conformation of p14[ARF] and HDM2 changes substantially to extended structures comprised of β-strands. It might be suspected that the preferential binding of E6 to p53 could result in p14[ARF]/HDM2 complexes (Tao and Levine, 1999) which may block the p14[ARF] inhibitory function for E7 and, at the same time, the functions of HDM2. It has been shown previously that HDM2 negatively regulates the hTERT promoter (Zhao et al., 2005). In HPV-positive cancer cells, however, the HDM2 pathway is completely inactive (Hengstermann et al., 2001), which suggests therefore that binding of p53 by E6 of high-risk HPV may inactivate HDM2 by forming complexes with p14[ARF] activity. For these reasons, an analysis of p14[ARF] expression in solely E7-immortalized cells should be of particular interest.

The suspected regulatory networks triggered by E7 and E6 are shown schematically in Figures 5.7 and 5.8.

Effects of E6 and E7 in non-transformed cells

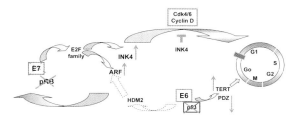

Fig. 5.7 E6 and E7 functions in nontransformed epithelial cells. The initial expression of E7 results in the release of pRb-mediated suppression of E2 F, which activates p16[INK4] and p14[ARF]. P16[INK4] expression blocks cell cycle progression at the G_0/G_1 boundary, and p14[ARF] in turn down-regulates E7.

Effects of E6 and E7 in cervical cancer cells

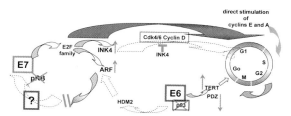

Fig. 5.8 E6 and E7 functions in cervical carcinoma cells. The high expression of E7 results in the release of pRb-mediated suppression of E2 F, which activates p16^{INK4} and p14^{ARF}. The inhibition of cell cycle progression by p16 ^{INK4} expression is circumvented by the direct E7 activation of cyclins E and A. It is presently not clear whether a possible modification of p14^{ARF} is the reason for its failing inhibition of E7, in spite of high levels of p14^{ARF}.

Figures 5.7 and 5.8 depict the individual as well as joint functions of E6 and E7 proteins, and speculate on an important role for p14^{ARF}. In particular, the direct activation of cyclins E and A by E7 circumvents the block exerted by p16 ^{INK4} on cyclinD/ cdk4/6 complexes. The inactivation of p53 by E6, on the other hand, blocks the E2F-mediated apoptosis as the common consequence of sole E7 expression, and is likely to result in an inhibition of p14^{ARF}.

5.1.3.4 E5

The E5 protein is the major transforming protein in BPVs (Schiller et al., 1986; Di-Maio et al., 1986; Rabson et al., 1986). In HPV infections tested thus far, E5 has only weak transforming activity (Leptak et al., 1991; Leechanachai et al., 1992; Pim et al., 1992). The high-risk HPV *E5* genes code for a protein of approximately 80 amino acids which is highly hydrophobic and mainly localized in the membranes of endosomes, the Golgi apparatus and, to a lesser extent, in the cytoplasmic membranes (Bubb et al., 1988; Halbert and Galloway, 1988; Conrad et al., 1993). In contrast to BPV 1, HPV 16 E5 forms complexes with EGF receptors (Hwang et al., 1995), but does not activate growth factor receptors (Suprynowicz et al., 2005). The E5 proteins associate with the membrane-bound protease-ATPase which is part of the gap-junction complex (Conrad et al., 1993; Finbow and Pitts, 1993). These proteins have the ability to inhibit endosomal acidification, yet they do not uniformly alkalinize intracellular compartments (Disbrow et al., 2005).

High- and low-risk E5 proteins modulate EGF-mediated ERK1/2 MAP kinase activation and down-regulate MHC class I molecules (Cartin and Alonso, 2003; Ashrafi et al., 2005). Expression of HPV 16 E5 also perturbs MHC class II antigen maturation (Zhang et al., 2003). Thus, the interference with cell-mediated immune functions seems to represent an important step in early interactions between virus-infected cells and the host. The inhibition of apoptosis in human foreskin keratino-cytes and of TRAIL and FasL-mediated apoptosis in human keratinocyte raft cul-tures also seem to represent an important contribution to early virus – host cell in-teractions (Zhang et al., 2002; Kabsch et al., 2004).

The *E5* gene of not only high-risk, but also of some low-risk HPV (HPV 6), cooper-ates with the *E7* gene to stimulate proliferation of primary cells and of murine 3T3 cells (Bouvard et al., 1994b; Valle and Banks, 1995). This cooperation may lead to transformation of the murine cells. HPV 16 E5 enhances the immortalization of pri-mary human keratinocytes after transfection with E6/E7 genes (Stoppler et al., 1996). Transformation of rodent fibroblast cell lines by HPV 11 and 16 has been re-ported (Straight et al., 1993; Suprynowicz et al., 2005). Thus, high-risk HPV *E5* genes seem to play an important role in early events following infection. The frequent loss of this gene in cervical cancers does not support its role in later events of virus-induced oncogenesis.

5.1.3.5 **E1**

E1 shares several properties with SV40 large T antigen (Sun et al., 1990; Seo et al., 1993). The ORF is transcribed into a polycistronic RNA. The protein fulfills an im-portant function in HPV DNA replication, and possesses site-specific DNA-binding functions (Ustav et al., 1991; Ustav and Stenlund, 1991), in that it binds and hydro-lyzes ATP and has ATP-dependent helicase activity (Yang et al., 1993). E1 interacts with cellular DNA polymerase α (Bonne-Andrea et al., 1995). The E1 protein binds to the proximal region of the LCR, where the binding site also represents the origin of viral replication (Holt et al., 1994). Bidirectional unwinding of this region repre-sents a prerequisite for viral DNA replication (Li et al., 1993). E1 as a nonstructural protein and the major structural protein L1 are the two most highly conserved re-gions among different HPV genotypes.

E1 acts as a helicase and is required for efficient viral DNA replication. In HPV 11, a plasmid with the E1 coding region alone supports transient replication of an ori-carrying plasmid, whereas a plasmid containing both the E1 and E2 regions and the viral origin of replication resulted in a self-contained replicon (Deng et al., 2003). Sumoylation of the papillomavirus origin-binding E1 protein emerges as a critical factor for its function (Malcles et al., 2002; Rosas-Acosta et al., 2005). This seems to be mediated by the SUMO E3 ligases of the PIAS protein family, as determined for BPV and HPV 11 E1. HPV replication also requires E1 phosphorylation by cyclin/cdk, which also regulates its nucleocytoplasmic localization (Deng et al., 2004). Another important factor seems to be the recruitment of the major human single-stranded DNA-binding protein, replication protein A (RPA) (Loo and Melendy, 2004).

The crystal structure of E1 has been analyzed (Enemark et al., 2000, 2002; Auster and Joshua-Tor, 2004), the studies having shown that the E1 DNA-binding domain orchestrates assembly of the hexameric helicase on the ori. The results also suggest a mechanism for the transition between double- and single-stranded DNA-binding required for a functional helicase. The DNA-binding domain of HPV 18 does not share the same nucleotide and amino acid requirements for specific DNA recognition as BPV 1 and HPV 11 E1s. Rather, as discussed in the following section, E1 and E2 form a complex which regulates the efficient replication of papillomavirus DNA.

5.1.3.6 **E2**

The properties of papillomavirus E2 proteins have been reviewed extensively (Hegde, 2002). The *E2* gene codes for at least two proteins which act as transcription factors and regulators of viral DNA replication (Androphy et al., 1987; Ustav and Stenlund, 1991; Chiang et al., 1992; Bouvard et al., 1994a; Demeret et al., 1997). They represent major intragenomic regulators of viral gene expression. The E2 protein is composed of a C-terminal DNA-binding domain and an N-terminal *trans*-activation domain, and forms dimers at specific binding sites (Dostatni et al., 1988; Doorbar et al., 1990). In human cervical keratinocytes the HPV 16 and 18 E2 proteins function as transcriptional activators (Cripe et al., 1987; Phelps and Howley, 1987; Bouvard et al., 1994a). Four positions for E2 binding are highly conserved in the LCR of high-risk HPVs. Three of these emerge as essential for the viral life cycle; their specific arrangement within the URR appears to be of importance (Stubenrauch et al., 1998). If E2 binds to the promoter-proximal binding site 1, it interferes with the recognition of the neighboring TATA box by TATA-box-binding protein (Dostatni et al., 1991). Conversely, human TATA binding protein inhibits HPV 11 DNA replication by antagonizing E1/E2 complex formation on the viral origin of replication (Hartley and Alexander, 2002). This suggests a role for this transcription factor in regulating also viral DNA replication. In addition, binding of E2 to binding sites 2 and 3 may contribute to promoter repression. This is probably due to competition with cellular transcription factors such as Sp1 (Demeret et al., 1997). The HPV 18 E2 protein binds with greatest affinity to binding site 4, and with reduced affinities to binding sites 1 and 2 (Sanders and Maitland, 1994; Demeret et al., 1997). This results in an activation of the E6/E7 promoter at low concentrations of E2, and in repression at higher concentrations, when E2 occupies the binding sites 1 and 2. The recognition of sequences by E2 in the DNA appears to effect sequence-specific conformational changes, depending on the sites occupied by E2 (Bedrosian and Bastia, 1990). The nucleic acid composition of the preferred binding site is 5′AACCGN(4)CGGTT3′, where the E2 proteins bind preferentially to sites containing an A:T-rich central spacer (Dell et al., 2003). The fidelity of HPV16 E1/E2-mediated DNA replication seems to depend mainly on the cellular environment; for example, cells which are deficient in XP30RO (deficient in the bypass polymerase ε) reveal a high rate of mutations which can be restored by expressing the enzyme again (Taylor et al., 2003). A cellular protein TopBP1 (topoisomerase II β-binding protein) has been described as a transcriptional co-activator of E2, enhancing the E2 ability to activate transcription and replication (Boner et al., 2002). Chaperone proteins Hsp70 and Hsp 40 abrogate an inhibition of the E1 replicative helicase by the E2 protein (Lin et al., 2002).

Overexpression of E2 acts anti-proliferatively, and results in cell cycle arrest and apoptosis. The latter effect is induced through the extrinsic pathway, involving caspase 8. E2 itself is cleaved by caspases, whereby the cleaved E2 protein exhibits an enhanced apoptotic activity (Blachon and Demeret, 2003).

The crystal structure of the E2 DNA-binding domain has been analyzed for BPV type 1 (Hegde et al., 1992), for high-risk HPV types (Bussiere et al., 1998; Harris and Botchan, 1999), and for the low-risk HPV 11 (Wang, Y., et al., 2004). In addition, the X-ray structure of the papillomavirus E1 helicase in complex with E2 has been un-raveled (Abbate et al., 2004). The E2 binding domains are structurally similar among the different papillomavirus types.

Deletion of the E2 ORF occurs relatively frequently in cervical cancer cells as a consequence of viral DNA integration into the host cell genome (Schwarz et al., 1985). This commonly seems to lead to a deregulated expression of viral *E6* and *E7* genes, facilitating further progression to more advanced stages of carcinogenesis. Mutations in the E2 ORF, and specifically also in the E2 DNA binding sites within the viral URR, result in enhanced immortalizing properties of HPV 16 DNA (Romanczuk and Howley, 1992). In cervical carcinogenesis, disruption of the E2 ORF due to integration of the viral DNA is commonly a late event, usually not occurring before the development of CIN III lesions (Matsukura et al., 1989; Dürst et al., 1992; Daniel et al., 1995; Klaes et al., 1999). E2 interacts with E1 in stimulating viral DNA replication (Chiang et al., 1992; Sverdrup and Khan, 1994; Chow and Broker, 1994), and also seems to facilitate the binding of E1 to the origin of replication (Seo et al., 1993).

5.1.3.7 E4

E4 originates from a viral transcript formed by a single splice between the beginning of the E1 ORF and the E4 ORF. Its mRNA is the major transcript in HPV-induced lesions (Chow et al., 1987 a,b). E4 is not required for transformation or episomal persistence of viral DNA (Neary et al., 1987); rather, the protein is exclusively localized within the differentiating layer of the epithelium (Doorbar et al., 1986; Breitburd et al., 1987). It probably has been incorrectly assigned as an early gene product, as it seems to play a role in productive infection, apparently by disrupting normal differentiation and by establishing favorable conditions for viral maturation.

The association of E4 proteins with the keratin cytoskeleton has been demonstrated by Doorbar et al. (1991) and by Roberts et al. (1993). E4 tonofilament-like structures which cause a collapse of the cytokeratin network can be visualized electron- microscopically. In HPV 16-infected cells, collapse of the cytokeratin intermediate filament structures is directly mediated by E4, and results from a strong interaction with cytokeratin 18 (Wang, Q., et al., 2004). In addition, E4 sequesters Cdk1/cyclin B1 onto the cytokeratin network (Davy et al., 2005). This prevents an accumulation of active Cdk1/cyclin B1 complexes in the nucleus, and explains the previously observed G_2 arrest of cells expressing E4 (Nakahara et al., 2002; Raj et al., 2004). The G_2 arrest of the infected cells seems to play a significant role in the promotion of HPV genome amplification and S-phase genome maintenance during differentiation (Knight et al., 2004; Davy et al., 2005; Wilson et al., 2005). HPV 16 E4 also associates with a member of the DEAD box protein family of RNA helicases (Doorbar et al., 2000), and binds to mitochondria (Raj et al., 2004). Due to the progressive cleaving of N-terminal sequences, a series of E4 polypeptides is produced which cooperates to negatively influence keratinocyte proliferation (Knight et al., 2004).

Thus, E4 emerges as an important HPV protein, creating optimal conditions for viral DNA replication in suprabasal keratinocytes and the concomitant production of late viral proteins.

5.2
The Concept of Cellular Interfering Cascades: Immunological, Intracellular and Paracrine Host Factors Influencing Viral Oncogene Expression or Function

A cellular interfering factor (CIF) was initially postulated to explain the restriction of tumorvirus gene expression in proliferating cells, and the long latency period between primary infection and the eventual emergence of invasive cancer (zur Hausen, 1986 b, see chapter 3.3.1). Originally, it was proposed that an intracellular function suppresses either transcription of viral oncogenes or functions of viral oncoproteins. When applied to high-risk HPV infections, the suppression of viral transcription in proliferating basal layer cells of low-grade CIN lesions (Dürst et al., 1991, 1992; Stoler et al., 1992) seemed to point initially to a regulatory interference at the level of transcription. The interruption of this cellular function by mutational events or by epigenetic modifications, affecting both coding alleles of the respective gene, was thought to be necessary prior to malignant conversion.

During the following years it became apparent that cellular interference is much more complex: It is based in part not only on innate immunity and cell-mediated immune functions, on intracellular functional inhibition of viral oncoproteins, but also on the paracrine suppression of viral transcription. These findings led in turn to a modification of the original concept which foresees gene silencing in at least three cellular signaling cascades, as shown schematically in Figure 5.9.

The pathogenesis of high-risk HPV-induced cancers, which commonly span a period of more than 20 years, can also be visualized, as outlined in Figure 5.10. The stepwise progression from persistent infection to early lesions, high-grade dysplasias and invasive cancer, which usually covers two to three decades, is interpreted as the consequence of increasing mutations or epigenetic modifications within these three signaling cascades, affecting an allelic set of genes within each of the cascades, respectively. Thus, the number of cellular genes which could be modified in this process should roughly correspond to the number of genes required for the function of these signaling cascades and is, in all likelihood, substantial.

Evidence for the existence of these gene cascades is briefly summarized in the following sections.

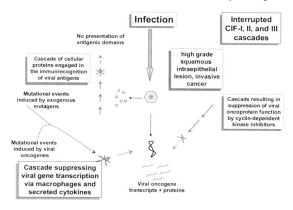

Fig. 5.9 Interruption of at least three signaling cascades by silencing of cellular genes engaged in the control of persistent HPV infection, permitting malignant conversion of the infected cell.

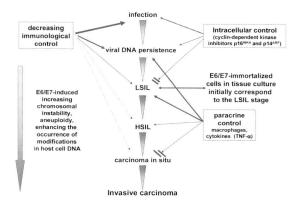

Fig. 5.10 Individual steps required in the progression of a high-risk HPV infection to invasive carcinoma. The time period elapsing between primary infection and invasive growth is commonly in the order of 20 to 25 years.

5.2.1
Immunological Control

The immune response of infected humans to papillomavirus antigens commonly occurs only late after infection, and usually leads only to a low reactivity. Some infected persons remain seronegative, this being most likely due to localization of the virus infection at the surfaces of skin or mucosa, and hence to a low concentration of viral antigens reaching the immunoreactive cells (Ho et al., 2004). Seropositivity is not necessarily protective against reinfections by the same virus type (Viscidi et al., 2004). The immune control of anogenital HPV infections has been recently reviewed (Stern, 2005). It has been suggested that an innate immune response by dendritic cells and Langerhans cells in the skin continuously senses the environment and coordinates with innate immune effectors (macrophages, polymorphic leucocytes and natural killer [NK] cells). As a result, immunemodulatory molecules are synthesized including various interferons, transforming growth factor-β (TGF-β), tumor necrosis factor α (TNF-α) and several interleukins. The Langerhans cells present a combination of MHC peptides, co-stimulatory molecules (CD80, CD86, and CD40), and interleukins

(IL-12 or IL-10) and activate naïve T cells (Niedergang et al., 2004). The subsequent T-cell response shapes the T-cell immunity into a T helper (Th) type 1 or type 2 response (Kalinski et al., 1999; Wang, J.L., et al., 2004). Whereas a Th1 response favors the production of cytotoxic T-cell effectors, Th2 facilitates the stimulation of B cells and their isotype switching to provide neutralizing antibodies.

5.2.2
CIF-I: Recognition System and its Disturbance

The development of immunity and T-cell recognition of HPV target antigens emerge as the prime mechanisms to clear a persisting HPV infection by destruction of the virus-positive cells. E7-specific activity at low systemic levels can be detected in patients with HPV-linked lesions and cancers. This has been revealed by the demonstration of Th cells (Kadish et al., 1997; De Gruijl et al., 1998), cytotoxic T lymphocytes (Bontkes et al., 2000), γ-interferon production (van der Burg et al., 2001), and HLA tetramer assays (Youde et al., 2000).

Clearly, escape from immunological surveillance emerges as one of the prime factors for persistent infection and the subsequent development of lesions. In anogenital neoplasias, a high frequency of HLA class I down-regulation has been noted (Keating et al., 1995), and was found to represent an early change, linked to progressing lesions (Bontkes et al., 1998; Abdel-Hady et al., 2001). Multiple genetic changes may cause the HLA dysregulation (Brady et al., 2000) which is found in 90% of cervical cancers (Koopman et al., 2000). Such changes could involve the transportation activating pathway, the interferon-γ responsiveness of HLA expression, or auxiliary functions required for HLA interactions. The reported hereditary susceptibility and increased risk for cervical cancer of specific HLA haplotypes fits into this consideration (Little and Stern, 1999; Hildesheim and Wang, 2002).

The important role of the immune system in the control of HPV infections is further underlined by the increased incidence of HPV infections of the anogenital tract (Tindle and Frazer, 1994) and the skin (Shamanin et al., 1994a, 1996; Stark et al., 1994; Bouwes Bavinck and Berkhout, 1997) under conditions of immunosuppression. Since 1995, an increasing number of reports have been made analyzing the role of HIV infections on anogenital HPV-linked lesions (Sun et al., 1995; Palefsky et al., 1999; Moscicki et al., 2000; Strickler et al., 2005). Interestingly, the cited studies – and most of many others – identified an increased risk for squamous intraepithelial lesions in HIV-infected women, but failed to demonstrate any significant increase in cervical cancer rates. This may be due to the long latency periods required for malignant conversion of premalignant clones and the high mortality rate of HIV-infected individuals.

Although E5 proteins of high- and low-risk HPVs down-regulate MHC class I molecules (Ashrafi et al., 2005), and the expression of HPV 16 E5 also perturbs MHC class II antigen maturation (Zhang et al., 2003), this seems to facilitate a delayed early recognition by immune functions, though it is clearly not sufficient for prolonged viral DNA persistence. Thus, the interference with cell-mediated immune functions seems to represent an important step in early interactions between virus-infected cells and the host. The breakdown of immunological control of latently HPV-infected host cells emerges as a critical factor for viral long-term latency, and favors further progression of the affected cells towards invasive growth. It also has negative consequences for attempts to attack later stages of HPV-modified cells by immunotherapeutic approaches. The modifications of cellular genes involved in the presentation of viral antigens may affect different cellular pathways, but merge in one consequence: the inability of the immune system to present or recognize specific antigenic domains of viral oncoproteins. This seems to justify the conclusion of including the control of one major interference factor (the immune system and its failure in tumor progression) as one important regulatory principle. It is here considered as cellular interference factor (CIF) cascade I.

5.2.3
CIF-II: Intracellular Control of Viral Oncoprotein Functions

Transforming properties of sole transfection with the *E6* oncogene of HPV 16 or 18 were initially reported by Band et al. (1990, 1991) for human mammary epithelial cells. Later, Reznikoff et al. (1996) provided indirect evidence for the existence of intracellular mechanisms suppressing E6 viral oncoprotein functions. These authors observed inactivation of the $p16^{INK4}$ gene in all cells immortalized by E6. Four of five clones showed hemizygous deletion of the 9p21 region. In a subsequent study, Foster et al. (1998) showed that the reduction in p16 expression is mainly due to methylation of CpG islands in the p16 promoter. A number of subsequent reports described the absence of $p16^{INK4}$ expression in solely E6 immortalized cells (Kiyono et al., 1998; Jarrard et al., 1999; Tsutsui et al., 2002; Yamamoto et al., 2003). $p16^{INK4}$ causes disruption of the cyclin D/cdk4/6 complexes and replaces them by cdk4/6-$p16^{INK4}$ complexes (Xiong et al., 1996). This disrupts progression of the cell cycle, as shown schematically in Figure 5.11. This disruption, however, is circumvented by the direct activation of cyclins E and A by the high-risk HPV oncoprotein E7, stressing again the cooperative effect of both viral oncoproteins.

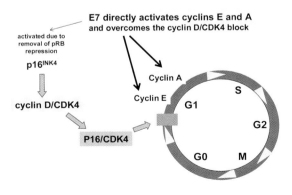

E7 effects on the cell cycle

Fig. 5.11 Inactivation of $p16^{INK4}$ permits the unimpaired stimulation of the cell cycle by high-risk HPV E6.

These observations demonstrate the existence of an intracellular control for high-risk HPV E6 proteins at the functional level exerted by p16^{INK4}. Clearly, this functional control does not affect cells immortalized or transformed by E6 and E7, since under those conditions p16^{INK4} is overexpressed.

It is therefore a clear question of whether a similar control may exist for E7 protein. This control should become inactivated in solely E7-immortalized cells. A clue to the existence of such a control seems to originate from data published by Pan et al. (2003). These authors demonstrate that the expression of p19^{ARF} (the murine homologue of human p14^{ARF}) causes relocalization of E7 from the nucleoplasm to the nucleolus. Two distinct regions in p19^{ARF} overlapping with MDM2 binding sites are necessary for this relocalization of E7. Under these conditions, proteolysis of Rb induced by E7 is blocked. Although these results still need to be confirmed, they do suggest that p19^{ARF} is an effective inhibitor of E7.

Similar to p16^{INK4}, p14^{ARF} is overexpressed in HPV-positive cervical cancers (Sano et al., 2002; Kanao et al., 2004). For p16^{INK4}, this overexpression apparently finds its explanation in the release of its pRb control by E7-mediated pRb degradation. The direct stimulation of cyclins E and A by Hr-HPV E7 circumvents the potential block of cyclin D/cdk4 complexes by this abundant cyclin-dependent kinase inhibitor. For p14^{ARF}, the dysregulation is less well understood, but it seems that *E6* gene expression overcomes a potential E7 inhibition of p14^{ARF} (Stott et al., 1998). In mouse embryo fibroblasts lacking p19^{ARF}, E7 stabilizes p53 (Seavey et al., 1999). This effect is probably due to the binding of E7 to MDM2, an inhibitor of p53 in an autoregulatory loop. The cells do not accumulate p53, apparently due to the inactivation of MDM2 functions by E7 binding (Alunni-Fabbroni et al., 2000). As outlined previously, the preferential binding of E6 to p53 may result in p14^{ARF}/HDM2 complexes (Tao and Levine, 1999) which may block the p14^{ARF} inhibitory function for E7 and, at the same time, the functions of HDM2. It has been shown previously that HDM2 negatively regulates the hTERT promoter (Zhao et al., 2005). In HPV-positive cancer cells, however, the HDM2 pathway is completely inactive (Hengstermann et al., 2001), which suggests that the binding of p53 by E6 of high-risk HPV may inactivate HDM2 by forming complexes with p14 ^{ARF} activity.

Clearly, the specific inhibition of E7 by p14^{ARF} requires further investigation. One would predict suppression of p14^{ARF} expression or of its function in solely E7-immortalized cells, but such studies are not presently available. It is tempting to speculate that the presence of E6 is the reason for a functionally inactive overexpression of p14^{ARF} in cervical cancer cells.

To summarize the points of this section, evidence exists for an intracellular control of *E6* and *E7* oncogene functions, and the disruption of this control probably plays a role in the progression of preneoplastic lesions to invasive cancer. Yet, it is difficult to exclude at this stage that the disruption of another signaling cascade (paracrine regulation, see below) may result in the transcriptional activation of both oncogenes which paralyze the described functional control in a joint and coordinated function.

5.2.4
CIF-III: Paracrine Control

The important role of paracrine factors in controlling the potentially deleterious effects of high-risk HPV infections can be easily deduced from studies on the hetero-implantation of HPV-immortalized or malignantly transformed lines into immuno-suppressed mice. Immortalized cells are quickly growth-inhibited and do not form tumors, whereas cervical carcinoma-derived cell lines are commonly tumorigenic. The first evidence that a paracrine control acts at the level of HPV transcription originated from studies analyzing the HPV transcription in heterotransplanted non-malignant HeLa cell – human fibroblast hybrids in comparison to parental HeLa cells (Bosch et al., 1990). In these studies, HPV transcription in the nonmalignant hybrid cells was rapidly suppressed, whereas in the tumorigenic parental cells a high rate of HPV transcription continued. Similar observations were recorded for heterografted HPV-immortalized keratinocytes, when compared to a malignant line derived from these cells (Dürst et al., 1991). These results corresponded to later studies demonstrating suppression of HPV transcription in basal and suprabasal cells of early HPV 16 containing clinical lesions (CIN I/II) in comparison to late stages (CIN III) and invasive cervical cancer which regularly revealed intensive transcription of *E6/E7* genes (Dürst et al., 1992; Stoler et al., 1992).

Preceding experiments had demonstrated a cytostatic and/or cytolytic activity of activated murine macrophages against HPV 16-transformed, but not against HPV 18-transformed, murine NIH 3T3 and A31 3T3 cells (Denis et al., 1989). Since these cells, as well as their nontransformed counterparts, were resistant to recombinant TNF-α, these authors claimed that the cell killing was independent of TNF-α. Rösl and colleagues (1994) revealed a selective down-regulation of HPV 18 transcription in nonmalignant HeLa – fibroblast hybrids by activated macrophages, and showed that this effect could be reproduced by the addition of low concentrations of TNF-α. Under these conditions the monocyte chemoattractant protein MCP-1 was highly up-regulated. HPV 16 E6 expression in human or murine cells sensitized these to lysis by macrophages, but not by NK cells (Routes et al., 2005), the lysis being shown to depend on the production of TNF-α or nitric oxide.

A number of additional studies confirmed the selective growth inhibition of nonmalignant HPV-immortalized cells or of low-grade cervical intraepithelial lesions, but not of malignant cells, by TNF-α (Malejczyk et al., 1992; Villa et al., 1992; Kyo et al., 1994; Delvenne et al., 1995; Vieira et al., 1996; Soto et al., 1999). Some of these studies indicate that HPV 18-immortalized cells are less sensitive to TNF-α than those immortalized by HPV 16 (Boccardo et al., 2004), although HPV 18-positive nonmalignant HeLa – fibroblast hybrids proved to be highly sensitive. In contrast to these reports, one group reported stimulation of growth of HPV-immortalized cervical keratinocytes and cervical carcinoma-derived cell lines by TNF-α in epidermal growth factor- and serum-depleted media (Woodworth et al., 1995; Gaiotti et al., 2000).

The mechanism of transcriptional regulation of nonmalignant high-risk HPV-immortalized cells was analyzed in a number of additional studies. Induction of the

MCP-1 gene in nonmalignant HPV-containing cells and low-grade cervical intraepithelial neoplasias (Rösl et al., 1994; Kleine et al., 1995; Kleine-Lowinski et al., 1999), but not in high-grade lesions and invasive carcinomas, by TNF-α emerges as a defense mechanism attracting more macrophages to the respective lesion. On the other hand, *MCP-1* expression is suppressed by a higher level of either *E6* or *E7* expression (Kleine-Lowinski et al., 2003). This suppression seems to be selective, since other chemokines were not affected.

Clues for the molecular basis of TNF-α-mediated transcriptional effects originated from studies analyzing the composition of the transcription factor AP-1, which seems to control the proliferation of HPV-positive cells in clinical lesions (Soto et al., 1999, 2000). AP-1 consists of jun family members (c-jun/junD/junB) either homodimerized or frequently heterodimerized with Fra-1, a member of the c-fos family. In nonmalignant HPV-containing cells, the AP-1 binding site contains to some extent c-jun/Fra-1 heterodimers, and the Fra-1 involvement is substantially increased after TNF-α treatment. Cervical carcinoma cell lines either express low amounts of Fra-1 or are negative for Fra-1 expression, but commonly express high quantities of c-fos. Ectopic expression of c-fos under a heterologous promoter in nonmalignant HeLa – fibroblast hybrids induces tumorigenicity and a change in the jun/Fra-1 ratio towards jun/c-fos heterodimers (Soto et al., 1999; Prusty and Das, 2005). These data suggest that the composition of AP-1 in the HPV promoter plays a crucial role in determining the growth properties of the respective cells, and that this composition is steered by paracrine regulatory factors, prominent among them TNF-α. In most cervical carcinoma cells the TNF-α-mediated pathway is interrupted and functionally inactive. This is further supported by observations showing that the endogenous TNF-α-induced interferon-β synthesis does not function in cervical carcinoma cell lines, in contrast to nonmalignant cells (Bachmann et al., 2002). Apparently, TNF-α-mediated activation of IRF-1 and p48 as key regulatory molecules in the differential interferon-β response fails to function in these malignant cells.

The constitutively increased c-fos transcription in cervical cancer cells seems to be based on a disturbance in c-fos regulation. In malignant cells, c-fos is constitutively expressed even after serum starvation (van Riggelen et al., 2005). c-fos expression is mainly controlled by the serum response element (SRE) motif in the c-fos promoter. Constitutive c-fos activity results from the inefficient expression of the ternary complex factor Net, which negatively regulates endogenous c-fos synthesis. Stable ectopic expression of Net results in a disappearance of c-fos protein from the AP-1 transcription complex. These data seem to place loss of Net and constitutive c-fos expression at the center of the transformation process of cervical carcinoma cells, although the induction of Net by TNF-α requires further study.

One target for the disturbance of TNF-α-mediated signaling could originate from polymorphisms in the TNF-α promoter. Indeed, a number of reports describe such polymorphisms as a risk factor for cervical cancer. In one study, CIN patients had a significantly higher frequency of TNF-α-308 low secretor genotypes compared to controls (Kirkpatrick et al., 2004). New significant associations between several TNF-α single-nucleotide polymorphisms and susceptibility to cervical cancer were reported very recently (Deshpande et al., 2005). In combination with the HLA DQ6

(DQA1*0102-DBQ 1*0602) haplotype, the TNF-α-11 haplotype increased the risk for cervical cancer significantly (Ghaderi et al., 2000, 2001). These data, which revealed a specific modification in the TNF-α promoter, may explain the higher risk for cervical cancer in specific populations, and underline studies demonstrating a hereditary factor in the development of cervical cancer (Magnusson and Gyllensten, 2000). However, they do not provide a reasonable explanation for those cervical cancers in which signaling pathways are blocked after exogenous addition of TNF-α. Possible polymorphisms of the TNF-α receptor which could explain this failure are described as a putative factor in autoimmune and inflammatory pathomechanisms (Csarzar and Abel, 2001); however, for cervical cancers they remain presently unexplored. Alterations in other genes which regulate the TNF-α-mediated signaling cascade may also contribute to the observed disturbances in cervical cancers.

These observations seem to underline a central role of TNF-α in the paracrine regulation of HPV transcriptional activity. They do not exclude, however, the possibility of an involvement of other cytokines or chemokines as regulatory factors. Indeed, TGF-β, IL-1, IL-6, IL-10, amphiregulin and others have been implicated in other studies (Braun et al., 1990; Woodworth et al., 1990, 1995; Gaiotti et al., 2000; Azar et al., 2004). Thus, nonresponsiveness to paracrine signals emerges as one hallmark of cervical cancer. Modifications to this signaling cascade emerge as one *conditio sine qua non* for malignant transformation of human cells containing HPV.

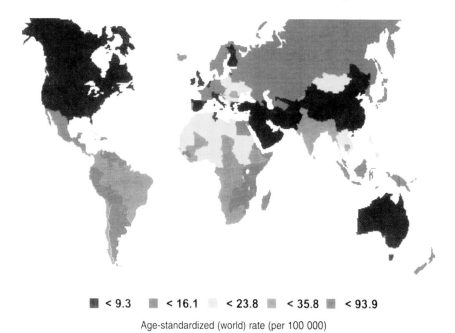

■ < 9.3　　■ < 16.1　　< 23.8　　■ < 35.8　　■ < 93.9

Age-standardized (world) rate (per 100 000)

Fig. 5.12 The global age-standardized rate of cancer of the cervix. (Globocan 2002, Cancer Incidence, Mortality and Prevalence Worldwide, IARC CancerBase No. 5, Ferlay, J., Bray, F., Pisani, P., Parkin, D.M. (editors), version 2.0, IARCPress, Lyon, 2004.)

5.3
Cancers Linked to HPV Infections

5.3.1
Cancer of the Cervix

The global distribution of cancer of the cervix differs substantially between the developed and developing regions of the world (Fig. 5.12).

Today, cancer of the cervix probably represents the best-documented case of a human cancer caused by specific viral infections. The evidence has been documented in previous reviews (zur Hausen, 1996; IARC, 2006), and will not be repeated here in all details. The earliest data originated from the demonstration of HPV 16 and 18 DNA in the majority of cervical cancer biopsies (Dürst et al., 1983; Boshart et al., 1984), and the subsequent demonstration of the specific DNA integration pattern and the selective transcription of *E6/E7* genes (Schwarz et al., 1985; Yee et al., 1985). The identification of the same high-risk HPV types in precursor lesions of anogenital cancers lent further support for their role in this malignancy (Ikenberg et al., 1983; Crum et al., 1984). Subsequently, it was shown that the DNA of these viruses possesses transforming properties for murine cells (Watts et al., 1984; Yasumoto et al., 1986) and immortalizes human epithelial cells (Dürst et al., 1987; Pirisi et al., 1987, Kaur and McDougall, 1988). The *E6/E7* genes were sufficient for these transforming and immortalizing events (Bedell et al., 1987; Schlegel et al., 1988; Münger et al., 1989). Mice transgenic for the high-risk HPV oncoproteins developed carcinomas at sites determined by the selected promoters (Tinsley et al., 1992; Arbeit et al., 1993, 1996; Lambert et al., 1993; Greenhalgh et al., 1994; Sasagawa et al., 1994).

During the following years, the malignant phenotype of cervical cancer cells was shown to depend on continued expression of the two viral oncogenes (von Knebel Doeberitz et al., 1992, 1994; Lappalainen et al., 1994; Rorke, 1997, Alvarez-Salas et al., 1999). Even sole suppression of the E6 oncoprotein by specific peptide aptamers (Butz et al., 2000) or by selective expression and inhibition of HPV 16 E6 in HeLa cells by bovine papillomavirus type 1 E2 protein (Horner et al., 2004), resulted in apoptosis or senescence. Based on these experimental data, it was evident that the HPV infection must play an essential role in cervical cancer development and in the maintenance of malignant growth.

Support for a role of high-risk HPV in cervical cancer was obtained at a relatively late stage, from epidemiologic studies. Although the wide variation in methodological approaches during the late 1980s prohibited useful comparison of the available data (zur Hausen, 1989b), such comparisons were made and resulted in the statement that "...the available data, although suggestive, do not allow further inferences on causality." (Bosch and Muñoz, 1989). A few years later, large case-control and prospective studies provided full support of the experimental data (Muñoz et al., 1992; Bosch et al., 1992, 1995). Today, numerous additional epidemiologic studies have confirmed these results (for a review, see IARC, 2006), leaving no doubt that cervical cancer is caused by high-risk HPVs. Recently, the definition of papil-

IARC Evaluation on Carcinogenicity of Human Papillomaviruses

Anogenital tract:

Sufficient evidence for carcinogenicity for types

16, 18, 31, 33, 35, 39, 45, 51, 52, 56, 58, 59, 66

Some studies also point to
a possible role of HPVs 6, 11, 26, 30, 68, 73, and 82,
which are rarely found in human cancers.

Fig. 5.13 Evidence for a role of specific papillomavirus types in causing human cancers. (Modified from IARC, Volume 90.)

lomavirus types linked to cervical cancer was attempted by an expert group at the IARC (IARC, 2006). Current knowledge on the carcinogenicity of HPV is summarized in Figure 5.13.

As shown in Figure 5.13, there exist a number of HPV types which have been rarely found in malignant tumors, and thus their carcinogenic potential remains to be proven.

The data on high-risk HPV infections in carcinomas of the anogenital tract, as well as of non-anogenital cancers, are summarized in Table 5.2.

The data in Table 5.2 reveal the high prevalence of HPV 16 infections in all of these cancers. Besides HPV 18, all other papillomavirus infections are relatively rare in anogenital and oral cancers; their relative distribution in cervical cancer is shown graphically in Figure 5.14. These data underline the dominating role of HPV 16 and, to a lesser degree, of HPV 18.

The typical precursor lesions of cancer of the cervix are CIN III. Most of these lesions again contain HPV 16 and, to a limited degree, other high-risk viruses. Low-grade CINs frequently contain also other HPV types, such as 6, 11, 34, 35, 40, 42,43, 44, 53, 54, 55, 61, 62, 70, 71, and 74.

One of the early hallmarks of high-risk HPV infection is the development of aneuploidy, most likely due to the uneven amplification of centrosomes (Duensing and Münger, 2003). This event precedes integration of viral DNA in high-grade lesions (Melsheimer et al., 2004). A number of chromosomal aberrations have been noted during the course of progression of the lesions. These involve various chromosomal sites, gains in chromosomes 3 q and deletions in 2 q33-q37 (Rao et al., 2004), loss of heterozygosity in 3p and 6 q (Acevedo et al., 2002), but also 9pter-p13 (Manolaraki et al., 2002), and deletions in 3p (Wistuba et al., 1997). It seems that one of the most consistent changes affects the fragile histidine triad (FHIT) locus on the short arm

Table 5.2 HPV-positivity in anogenital and non-anogenital human cancer

Type of cancer	Papillomavirus types involved	Percent HPV-positive
Cervical cancer	16, 18, 31, 33, 35, 39, 45, 51, 52, 56, 58, 59, 66 (26, 68, 73, 82)	> 95%
Vulva carcinoma		
basaloid	16, 18	> 50%
"warty"	16, 18	> 50%
keratinizing	16	< 10%
Penile carcinoma		
basaloid	16, 18	> 50%
"warty"	16, 18	> 50%
keratinizing	16	< 10%
Vaginal carcinoma	16, 18	> 50%
Anal cancer	16, 18	> 70%
Oral cavity and tonsils	16, 18, 33	~25%
Nail bed	16	~70%

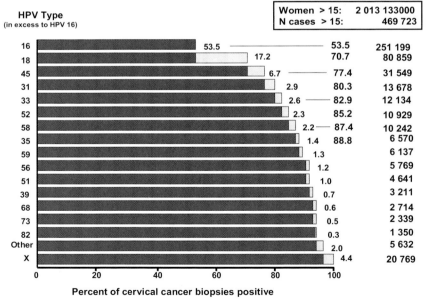

Fig. 5.14 Relative percentages of HPV types found in cervical cancer.

of chromosome 3 (Greenspan et al., 1997; Krivak et al., 2001). In addition to these changes, methylation of the HPV long control region and the flanking L1 gene were noted, low in dysplasia but increasing substantially in carcinomas (Kalantari et al., 2004). Interestingly, microcell-mediated transfer of chromosome 4 into HeLa cells suppresses telomerase activity and results in cellular senescence (Baksch et al., 2001). A mortality gene has been identified in this cell line, mapping to a 130 kb region of human chromosome 4q22-q23 (Bryce et al., 2002). At present, it is unclear as to what extent these chromosomal modifications affect the signaling cascades engaged in the control of HPV infections.

5.3.2
Penile Cancer

The relative positivity of penile cancers for persistent high-risk papillomavirus DNA is indicated in Table 5.2 (for a review, see IARC, 2006). Penile cancer represents a relatively rare malignancy in most parts of the world, although there exist interesting geographical correlations between incidences of cervical and penile cancer (Nandakumar et al., 2005). The histology of this tumor has been extensively reviewed; for relatively recent reviews, see Cubilla et al. (2000) and Bezerra et al. (2001).

A number of clinical observations have documented the malignant transition of genital warts (condylomata acuminata) into penile carcinomas. Some of the older observations were summarized in zur Hausen (1977). Although the majority of virus-positive penile cancers contain HPV 16 DNA, several tumors appeared to be only positive for HPV 6 or 11 DNA (Noel et al., 1992; Pilotti et al., 1993; Dianzani et al., 1998). This correlates with the observation that the invasively growing Buschke–Löwenstein tumors regularly contain DNA of these low-risk viruses (Boshart and zur Hausen, 1986).

5.3.3
Vulvar Cancer

In vulvar cancer the situation is very reminiscent of penile cancers. Typical squamous cell carcinomas of basaloid or warty histology occurring at younger age are commonly HPV-positive, whereas those occurring preferentially at higher age with lichen sclerosus-like lesions are mainly devoid of detectable HPV DNA (Neill et al., 1990; Hørding et al., 1991). To date, the relative rarity of these tumors has prevented a large-scale analysis of the latter for the possible persistence of cutaneous HPV types.

The detection of p16^{INK4} expression seems to represent a useful marker to differentiate even premalignant vulvar and penile lesions for infection with high-risk HPV (Riethdorf et al., 2004; Ruhul Quddus et al., 2005; Rufforny et al., 2005).

The development of a specific T-cell response to HPV E7 antigenic epitopes occasionally results in the clearance of vulvar intraepithelial neoplasias III (Bourgault Villada et al., 2004); however, in the majority of cases it remains ineffective at this stage of progression (Todd et al., 2004). Measurable antibody titers in premalignant lesions against HPV 16 VLPs were noted in 43 to 82% of cases, even in lichen sclerosus hyperplasia (Heim et al., 2005).

Comparative genomic hybridization of vulvar carcinomas revealed a pattern which corresponded to similar changes in cervical cancer (Huang et al., 2005). Gains were frequently found in 1q, 3q, 5p, and 8q. A high level of amplification was found in some of these tumors. Losses in 2q, 3p, 4p, and 11p were less consistent. Occasionally, integration of viral DNA is seen already in VIN II and III lesions (for a review, see Wentzensen et al., 2004).

5.3.4
Vaginal Cancer

Vaginal cancer accounts for approximately 2% of all female genital malignancies, and has a worse prognosis than cervical cancer (Goodman, 1998). Early tests of vaginal cancer revealed a high degree of HPV positivity (Kiyabu et al., 1989; Ikenberg et al., 1990). Approximately 30% of all cases had been treated for prior occurrence of other anogenital tumors, most often of the cervix (Daling et al., 2002). A prospective seroepidemiological study revealed that seropositivity for HPV 16 was associated with an increased risk of developing vulvar or vaginal cancers (Bjorge et al., 1997). Patients undergoing radiotherapy for advanced cervical or endometrial cancer bear a considerable risk of developing vaginal preneoplastic lesions. High-grade lesions are then commonly positive for HPV 16 DNA (Barzon et al., 2002).

In most other characteristics, vaginal HPV-associated cancers correspond to those described for vulvar cancer (see Section 5.3.3).

5.3.5
Perianal and Anal Cancer

Perianal and anal cancers represent about 4% of all anogenital tumors (Clark et al., 2004), and are highly linked to anogenital high-risk HPV infections, particularly to HPV 16. The rate of positive biopsies usually exceeds 70% (Palefsky et al., 1991; Zaki et al., 1992). The incidence of these cancers, as well as the incidence of the precursor lesions, is high in men who have sex with men (Chin-Hong et al., 2004), and is higher in HIV-positive patients (Haga et al., 2001). Increasing with the histological grade, genetic changes accumulate and a copy gain was mapped to chromosome 3q, a modification also frequently observed in cervical and vulvar cancer (Huang et al., 2005).

Besides cervical and about 25% of oropharyngeal cancers, perianal and anal cancers represent the third most important malignancy consistently linked to high-risk HPV infections.

5.3.6
Cancer of the Head and Neck

The role of papillomavirus infections in head and neck cancer was recently reviewed by Gillison (2004). Early suggestions for a role of HPV in oral squamous cell carcinomas were based on cytological features (presence of koilocytotic atypia) in precursor lesions and tumors (Syrjänen et al., 1983). The first demonstration of HPV 16 DNA in carcinomas and their precursor lesions was reported in 1985 (Löning et al., 1985). A number of additional publications subsequently confirmed the presence of HPV DNA in a subset of oral cancers, in particular in tumors arising in the Waldeyer's ring (Niedobitek et al., 1990; Snijders et al., 1992; Franceschi et al., 1996; Schwartz et al., 1998). Cancer of the oropharynx is causing substantial morbidity and mortality on a global scale, with an annual incidence rate of approximately 275 000 cases (Parkin et al., 2005). Tonsillar carcinomas reveal a particularly high rate of HPV positivity (Niedobitek et al., 1990; Snijders et al., 1992). The prevalence of these tumors increased between 1973 and 1995, from 1.9 % to 2.7 % per year in Caucasian and African-American males, whereas the prevalence of cancers at other oral sites, except for carcinomas of the tongue, remained unchanged (Frisch et al., 2000 a; Gillison, 2004; Shiboski et al., 2005). HPV infections appear to be more common in carcinomas of the base of tongue than in mobile parts of the tongue (Dahlgren et al., 2004).

High rates of HPV positivity were reported from India (31–71 %), where betel nut chewing emerges as a major contributing factor (Balaram et al., 1995; D'Costa et al., 1998; Nagpal et al., 2002; Koppikar et al., 2005). Figures from 20 publications of data mainly obtained from Northern America and Europe provide an average rate of HPV positivity of 23.5 % (reviewed in Gillison, 2004). By analyzing 60 studies, Kreimer et al. (2005) reported HPV prevalence in 5046 head and neck cancers of 25.9 %, with a higher rate in oropharyngeal cancers (35.6 % of 969) than oral squamous cell carcinomas (23.5 % of 2646) and a surprisingly high rate of HPV-positive laryngeal squamous cell carcinomas (24 % of 1.435). Based on these reviews and a large set of individual publications, a positivity rate of ~25 % for oropharyngeal cancers appears to be a realistic assumption.

The majority of oropharyngeal cancers, positive for papillomavirus DNA, contain HPV 16 (~90 %); in addition, HPV 18, 33 and 31 have also been detected. HPV 6 has been detected in rare cases (Kahn et al., 1994). Transcription of viral *E6* and *E7* genes has been consistently demonstrated within the positive cancers (Snijders et al., 1992; Wilczynski et al., 1998; Ke et al., 1999; Wiest et al., 2002; Balz et al., 2003), and the integration of viral DNA and overexpression of p16^{INK4} revealed a similar pattern as in cervical carcinomas (Steenbergen et al., 1995; Hafkamp et al., 2003). Loss of the viral E2 region has also been reported (Mellin et al., 2002; Koskinen et al., 2003). These observations underline a similar role of HPV 16 infection in oropharyngeal cancers as established for cervical cancers.

The HPV-positive cancers of the oropharyngeal region reveal molecular, pathohistological and prognostic differences when compared to HPV-negative carcinomas at these sites. In the positive tumors, p53 is targeted by E6 (Balz et al., 2003), although some tumors revealed the coexistence of HPV DNA and mutated p53 (Snijders et al., 1994; Sisk et al., 2002). Similarly, due to the targeting of pRb by E7, the expression of the former is decreased in HPV-positive oral tumors (Wilczynski et al., 1998; Mork et al., 2001; Wiest et al., 2002).

HPV-positive oropharyngeal cancers arise preferentially from the lingual and palatine tonsils, and reveal distinct basaloid pathology (Brandsma and Abramson, 1989; Fouret et al., 1997; Paz et al., 1997; Gillison et al., 2000). Some of the tumors are also poorly differentiated (van Houten et al., 2001; Klussmann et al., 2003; El-Mofty et al., 2003; Poetsch et al., 2003). The prognosis of HPV-positive cancers is significantly better than that of negative tumors. After adjustment for possible confounding factors, the risk of dying with the former cancer is 59% (Gillison et al., 2000) to 83% (Schwartz et al., 2001) lower than that for HPV-negative cancers of this region. Some studies also report a more favorable response to radiotherapy (Mellin et al., 2000; Lindel et al., 2001; Strome et al., 2002).

An elevated risk for acquiring HPV-positive oropharyngeal cancers is associated with increasing numbers of sexual partners, with a history of practicing oral sex, and also with a history of condylomata acuminata (Schwartz et al., 1998; Herrero et al., 2003; Rajkumar et al., 2003; Smith, E.M., et al., 2004). Seroepidemiologic case-control and prospective studies also revealed an increased risk of exposure to HPV 16 and the development of oral or oropharyngeal cancers (Schwartz et al., 1998; Mork et al., 2001; Herrero et al., 2003), even after adjustment for tobacco and alcohol use (Smith et al., 1998). A history of HPV-linked malignancy represents a risk factor for tonsillar cancer. Women older than 50 years with a history of cervical cancer, and husbands of women with in-situ or invasive cervical cancer also increase the risk for this malignancy (Hemminki et al., 2001). Fanconi's anemia represents a specific risk factor; the risk for head and neck cancers in this population is approximately 500-fold higher than in the general population (Kutler et al., 2003 a) with a high rate of HPV positivity (Kutler et al., 2003 b).

In-vitro immortalization of oral keratinocytes with HPV 16 has been achieved (Kang and Park, 2001). Although nonmalignant for immunocompromised mice, exposure of these cells to tobacco carcinogens enhanced expression of E6 and E7 and resulted in tumor formation in nude mice (Li et al., 1992; Kim et al., 1993). Yet, the relationship of HPV 16 infections to premalignant oropharyngeal lesions is presently less clear. Dysplasias adjacent to HPV-containing cancers in Fanconi lesions have been reported to be devoid of HPV DNA (Kutler et al., 2003 b). There exists a wide variation in HPV positivity of leukoplakias and oral dysplastic lesions in the literature (reviewed in Gillison, 2004). The situation may be analogous to that described for Epstein–Barr virus (EBV) in gastric and nasopharyneal cancers (see chapters 4.3.1.9 and 4.3.1.11), where virus infection seems to occur in dysplastic cells and apparently contributes to late steps in malignant conversion. Clearly, this point requires further investigation.

5.3.7
Other Cancers

Cancers of several additional sites have been described as containing papillomavirus DNA. These involve cancers of the breast, prostate, lung, colon and rectum, ovary, bladder, nasal, sinonasal and conjunctival cancers, larynx, and esophagus. The relevant evidence is discussed briefly in the following sections.

5.3.7.1 Breast Cancer

Several reports have documented negative findings for HPVs 6, 11, 16, 18, 31, 33, and 35 (Ostrow et al., 1987; Wrede et al., 1992; Bratthauer et al., 1992; Czerwenka et al., 1996) in breast cancer. In contrast, a number of laboratories have claimed to find HPV 16 (Di Leonardo et al., 1992), HPV 33 (Yu et al., 2000), HPV 11, 16 and 18 (Liu et al., 2001), and HPV 16 and 18 (Damin et al., 2004), in several of the investigated breast cancer biopsies. Recently, de Villiers et al. (2005) cloned several HPV types from ductal breast carcinomas and from corresponding samples of the mamilla of the same patients. The most prevalent types were HPV 11 and 6. At present, the significance of these findings is presently difficult to assess, but further studies should clarify the existing situation.

5.3.7.2 Prostate Cancer

Similar to cancer of the breast, the data on HPV presence in prostate cancer are conflicting. A few case reports have claimed HPV DNA in these tumors (Serth et al., 1999; Carozzi et al., 2004) or elevated odds ratios for an association between HPV 16 antibodies and prostate cancer (Hisada et al., 2000; Dillner et al., 1998), whereas this was not confirmed in other studies (Dennis and Dawson, 2002; Rosenblatt et al., 2003). It is interesting, however, to note that prostate cancer and sexually transmitted diseases reveal a clear-cut positive association, although responsible factors have not yet been identified (Key, 1985; Hayes at al., 2000; Strickler and Goedert, 2001; Rosenblatt et al., 2001; Taylor et al., 2005; Fernández et al., 2005).

Based on the available data, a relationship between HPV infection and prostate cancer is unlikely. The positive serologic findings may result from a generally increased risk for prostate cancer in individuals exposed to sexually transmitted diseases.

5.3.7.3 Lung Cancer

Although an early study revealed HPV 16 DNA in an anaplastic carcinoma of the lung (Stremlau et al., 1985), it seems that high-risk HPVs are only rarely found in lung cancers (Stoler et al., 1991; Shamanin et al., 1994 b; Szabo et al., 1994; Brouchet et al., 2005). Yet, occasionally HPV 16- and HPV 18-positive tumors are found. An exceptionally high rate of HPV 16- and 18-positive lung cancers has been reported among non-smoking women from Taiwan (Cheng et al., 2001).

In rare lung cancers developing in patients with recurrent laryngeal and bronchial papillomatosis, however, several reports describe the presence of mainly HPV 11, but also of HPV 6 DNA, in part integrated and transcribed in the malignant lesions (Byrne et al., 1987; Bejui-Thivolet et al., 1990; Guillou et al., 1991; DiLorenzo et al., 1992; Rady et al., 1998; Cook et al., 2000; Lele et al., 2002; Xu et al., 2004). Thus, for this type of cancer there exists good evidence for a role of the low-risk anogenital types 11 and 6. HPV 11 represents the prevailing type in laryngeal papillomatosis.

5.3.7.4 Colon and Rectum Cancers

In contrast to anal and perianal cancers, for cancers of the rectum and colon there exists no convincing evidence for an involvement of papillomavirus infections. Except for three reports finding HPV 16, 18 or 45 DNA in a substantial percentage of colon cancers at low copy numbers and in none of 10 control tissues (Sayhan et al., 2001; Buyru et al., 2003; Bodaghi et al., 2005), a number of other publications reported negative results (reviewed in IARC, 2006). Thus, the evidence for HPV involvement in these tumors is far from conclusive.

5.3.7.5 Ovarian Cancer

The majority of attempts to demonstrate HPV DNA in primary ovarian cancers have been unsuccessful (reviewed in IARC, 2006). It is of interest, however, that occasionally HPV 16-positive CIN III lesions may spread to the endometrium, fallopian tubes and ovaries (Mai et al., 1996; Pins et al., 1997; Manolitsas et al., 1998), while HPV 6 and 11 may even colonize regions of squamous metaplasia of the endometrium and cause adenoacanthomas (Sherwood et al., 1997; O'Leary et al., 1998).

5.3.7.6 Bladder Cancer

There exists no clear-cut evidence for a role of papillomavirus infections in transitional cell carcinomas of the bladder. Most studies analyzing these tumors produced negative results (reviewed in IARC, 2006). In several other PCR-based studies the rate of positivity was about 3%.

Squamous cell carcinomas of the bladder, mainly occurring in *Schistosoma*-endemic countries, were more frequently reported to be HPV-positive. Up to 8% were reported to be positive for HPV 6, 11 or 16 (Kerley et al., 1991; Anwar et al., 1992; Wilczynski et al., 1993; Maloney et al., 1994; Westenend et al., 2001).

In carcinomas of the urethra, HPV 6 and HPV 16 DNA has been discovered repeatedly (Grussendorf-Conen et al., 1987; Mevorach et al., 1990; Wiener et al., 1992; Wiener and Walther, 1994).

5.3.7.7 Nasal, Sinonasal and Conjunctival Cancers

The rare inverted papillomas of the nasal cavity and paranasal sinuses frequently start to grow invasively and convert into malignant tumors in up to 13 % of cases (Bernauer et al., 1997). Several of these tumors contain HPV 11 or 6 (Syrjänen et al., 1987; Respler et al., 1987; Kashima et al., 1992 b; Harris et al., 1998) or HPV 57 DNA (de Villiers et al., 1989; Wu et al., 1993; Ogura et al., 1996). Occasionally, also HPV 16 and 18 DNA has been noted in malignant tumors of these sites (Furuta et al., 1992; Buchwald et al., 1997, 2001).

Thus, at these sites HPV 11, 57 and 6 (all low-risk viruses) seem to pose a higher risk for invasive proliferations in comparison to infections by these viruses at other locations. It seems that HPV 6 and 11 play a role in a small percentage of these tumors, and that HPV 16 is also found in a small number of additional biopsies of these cancers.

Several reports have described the presence of HPV 16 and 18 DNA in conjunctival dysplasias and invasive cancers (McDonnell et al., 1989; Saegusa et al., 1995; Scott et al., 2002; Moubayed et al., 2004). One group failed to confirm these findings, but reported HPV 6 and 11 DNA in a substantial percentage of conjunctival papillomas (Eng et al., 2002). One recent publication claimed a very high rate (86 %) of squamous cell carcinomas of the conjunctiva positive for epidermodysplasia verruciformis-related papillomavirus types (Ateenyi-Agaba et al., 2004). Related viruses (HPV 5, 20, and 23) were also found in an ocular syringoma (Assdoullina et al., 2000). The available results point to the need to expand the studies on ocular carcinomas for papillomavirus DNA. Most likely as the consequence of the ongoing AIDS epidemic, dysplastic lesions and epithelial tumors of the conjunctive account for approximately 2 % of all tumors in Tanzania (Moubayed et al., 2004). Although suggestive, further investigations are required before the involvement of HPV infections may be implied in the etiology of these tumors.

5.3.7.8 Cancer of the Larynx

Laryngeal papillomatosis is caused by HPV 11 and to a lesser degree also by HPV 6. It affects mainly children, but extends in some cases into adult age. Recurrent laryngeal papillomatosis may represent a life-threatening condition. Occasionally – though rarely – the lesions may descend into the bronchial tree, reveal dysplastic histology and convert into squamous cell carcinomas (reviewed in zur Hausen, 1977). Thus, carcinomas of the larynx, occurring predominantly at a higher age, emerged as a possible candidate for a papillomavirus etiology, although other factors such as smoking are also involved.

The first reports on the presence of papillomavirus in laryngeal cancers appeared in 1985 and 1986 (Abramson et al., 1985; Brandsma et al., 1986; Kahn et al., 1986; Scheurlen et al., 1986). Whereas three of these reports found HPV 16 DNA in the cancer biopsies, Kahn et al. described a novel HPV type (HPV 30) in a laryngeal carcinoma. In subsequent years a large number of positive reports were published, although some others failed to find HPV DNA in these tumors (Lindeberg and Krogdahl, 1999; for reviews, see Franceschi et al., 1996; Hobbs and Birchall, 2004). From published data it appears that the figure of 24% of laryngeal carcinomas positive for HPV (Franceschi et al., 1996) is too high, although substantial variations are reported in the literature. A figure of 10% or less is probably more realistic.

Although some of the HPV-positive laryngeal cancers contain HPV 11 or 6 DNA (Brandsma and Abramson, 1989; Zarod et al., 1988; Lie et al., 1996; Lin et al., 1997; Rady et al., 1998), the majority of positive tumors contained HPV 16 DNA.

Laryngeal carcinoma emerges as an additional type of cancer, where a subset of these tumors is linked mainly to high-risk papillomavirus infections, although a fraction appears to be due to the low-risk types HPV 11 and 6.

5.3.7.9 Cancer of the Esophagus

Cancer of the esophagus shows wide variations in its geographic distribution, and has been linked to a number of environmental risk factors, including alcohol consumption, smoking, consumption of very hot beverages, fermented fish, and other dietary sources of nitrosamines and micronutrients (Rogers et al., 1995; Castellsague et al., 1999, 2000; Onuk et al., 2002; Ke et al., 2002). The first reports which attempted to link papillomavirus infections to these malignancies were stimulated by the publication of Jarrett et al. (1978), which claimed an interaction of a specific papillomavirus infection with an environmental carcinogen in esophageal cancer of cattle. In 1982, Syrjänen et al. postulated a role for HPV in human esophageal cancers based on the histological detection of koilocytotic cells and immunoperoxidase staining of cells from esophageal papillomas for viral group-specific antigens.

During the following years a large number of remarkably controversial publications appeared, some claiming a high incidence of positive tumors, particularly in high-risk regions of China (Chang et al., 1990; Li et al., 2001; de Villiers et al., 2004 b), whereas other groups reported basically negative results (Loke et al., 1990; Polyak et al., 1998; Peixoto Guimaraes et al., 2001). The data were even controversial in different studies by the same group by analyzing samples from different geographic regions (Chang et al., 1991, 1992). Since in some additional studies novel HPV types were isolated from esophageal cancers and characterized (Togawa and Rustgi, 1995; West et al., 1996; de Villiers et al., 1999; Lavergne and de Villiers, 1999), the likelihood of inadvertent contaminations due to handling procedures should be extremely small.

In esophageal cancer of cattle linked to BPV 4 infections it appears that persistence of viral DNA is not required for the progression and maintenance of the malignant state (Campo et al., 1985), although C127 mouse cells transformed by BPV 4 DNA maintain amplified and rearranged copies of the BPV 4 genome (Smith and Campo, 1989).

In view of the large number of additional controversial manuscripts that have been published during the past 20 years, two conclusions can be drawn. First, clearly, papillomavirus infections occur within the human esophagus and we may not have identified all types affecting these tissues. Second, there exists an urgent need for broad-based experimental and epidemiologic studies to clarify the role of these infections in the etiology of esophageal cancers and their possible interaction with other environmental carcinogens.

5.3.8
Cutaneous Papillomavirus Infections and Skin Cancer

The first hints for a role of papillomavirus infections in cancers of the skin origi-nated from studies in patients with the rare hereditary disease epidermodysplasia verruciformis (EV) (reviewed in Jablonska and Majewski, 1994). Though rare, this condition occurs worldwide, starting frequently in the age group between 5 and 8 years. The lesions are frequently barely recognizable as papillomas, and usually form reddish plaques. Within the following 20 to 30 years, about one-half of these patients reveal progression of the lesions, initially as actinic keratoses and Bowenoid changes, but subsequently they may convert to squamous cell carcinomas. The tumors are commonly localized at light-exposed sites, such as the forehead, the dor-sal hand or on the arms of these patients.

The HPVs found in these lesions belong into the genus β of HPV, and comprise more than 20 different genotypes. The same patient frequently contains multiples of these virus types. Most of the squamous cell carcinomas contain HPV 5, but some harbor a closely related genotype HPV 8. Several other types (e.g., HPV 14, 17, 20, 47) have also been isolated from such tumors (reviewed in Orth, 2005). EV-type HPVs are widely spread in the general population and occur here without induction of apparent lesions (Antonsson et al., 2003).

Carcinomas in EV patients commonly contain high copy numbers of episomal HPV 5 DNA, which is also present in metastases derived from these tumors. Inter-estingly, most of the persisting viral genomes revealed some rearrangements or deletions (Ostrow et al., 1982; Yabe et al., 1989). Morphological transformation of murine C127 cells has been achieved with HPV-5. The transformed cells retained episomal copies of viral DNA (Watts et al., 1984). The *E6* gene of HPV 5, 8, and 47 also induced morphological changes in rat 3Y1 cells (Hiraiwa et al., 1993). Joint transfection of constructs containing the SV40 promoter/enhancer and HPV 8 *E7* or *E6* and *E7* genes and the activated *Ha-ras* gene resulted in tumorigenic transforma-tion of primary rat embryo fibroblasts (Nishikawa, 1994). In addition, mice trans-genic for the complete early region of HPV 8 under the control of the keratin-14 pro-moter developed in 91% single or multifocal papillomas and in 6% squamous cell carcinomas (Schaper et al., 2005). The cancer cells expressed *E2*, *E7* and *E6* genes. In benign lesions, HPV 5 DNA transcription is differentiation-dependent (Haller et al., 1995).

All of these data suggest that HPV 5 and 8 – and probably also the types 14, 17, 20, and 47 – possess oncogenic potential, specifically expressed in the rare hereditary condition of EV. It is interesting to note that the susceptibility to papillomavirus infections of EV patients seems to affect selectively members of the genus β, but not other HPV genera. Two genetic modifications have been described in EV patients mapping to the chromosome regions 2p21-p24 and 17q25 (Ramoz et al., 1999, 2002). Nonsense mutations were identified in two adjacent genes, *EVER1* and *EVER2*, that are associated with the disease. Their gene products seem to represent integral membrane proteins and are localized in the endoplasmic reticulum (Ramoz et al., 2002).

EV-like lesions have also been observed in immunosuppressed patients following organ transplantation (Lutzner et al., 1980; Gassenmeier et al., 1986; Rüdlinger et al., 1986). These patients, however, also develop warts caused by other types of HPV (Ingelfinger et al., 1977; Schneider et al., 1983). A different spectrum of HPV types in cutaneous and mucosal lesions emerged in HIV-infected and immuno-suppressed patients (Greenspan et al., 1988; Milburn et al., 1988). Oral warts were preferentially found to contain HPV 7, also known as "butcher's wart" virus.

Early studies on non-melanoma skin cancers were performed with specific probes of anogenital HPV types. By using consensus primers which cover a broad spectrum of HPV types the results changed substantially. A large number of different, in part novel, HPV types was found in benign and malignant lesions, initially in immuno-suppressed patients (Shamanin et al., 1994a, 1996; Berkhout et al., 1995, 2000; de Villiers et al., 1997). The use of different primer combinations and different sensi-tivities and specificities of methodological approaches seems to account for some re-ported discrepancies between individual studies. In squamous cell carcinomas of renal allograft recipients, the detection rate was particularly high, reaching up to 90% of all samples tested (de Villiers et al., 1997). In immunocompetent patients suffering from squamous cell carcinomas of the skin, most reports found a positive association with HPV infections (Boxman et al., 2000). The rate of positivity varied between 27% and 65 % (Shamanin et al., 1996; Harwood et al., 2000; Forslund et al., 2003; Iftner et al., 2003; Meyer et al., 2003). It should be noted, however, that even unaffected skin of immunocompetent individuals revealed a relatively high percent-age of HPV-positive samples, particularly when plucked hair or cutaneous tape-stripped biopsies were analyzed (Boxman et al., 1997, 2000; Astori et al., 1998; Fors-lund et al., 2004), although they were commonly less positive than squamous cell carcinomas. Most studies analyzing basal cell cancer biopsies found viral DNA in the range of normal skin biopsies.

Even serological results seem to point to a specific role for cutaneous HPV infec-tions in squamous cell cancer of the skin, since seroreactivity to five EV HPV types (5, 8, 15, 20, and 24) was significantly increased in patients with this malignancy (Feltkamp et al., 2003).

Although persuasive, the role of cutaneous HPV types in squamous cell carci-nomas is by no means settled. One obvious dilemma originates from quantitative evaluations of the viral copy number within positive cancers. In virtually all analyses it is far beyond one DNA copy per tumor cell. In addition, HPV positivity in swab samples from the top of these tumors was higher than in biopsied material (Forslund et al., 2004). Although HPV types 20, 23, 38, and two newly identified types were more prevalent in one series (de Villiers et al., 1997), this preponderance was less pronounced in other studies. Thus, the role of these viruses clearly does not seem to correspond to that of high-risk anogenital HPV, which commonly persist in higher copy numbers in each tumor cell.

A potential mechanistic explanation for these observations could originate from studies demonstrating an effect of specific cutaneous papillomavirus types in preventing apoptosis in damaged cells. In 1999, Purdie et al. reported that the promoter of a cutaneous HPV type (HPV 77) is stimulated by UV-irradiation and that this responsiveness is mediated through a consensus p53 binding site. Two publications during the year 2000 described the inhibition of UV-induced apoptosis by the E6 protein of several cutaneous papillomavirus types, and of HPV 18 (Jackson et al., 2000; Jackson and Storey, 2000). This appears to be mediated by an E6 deregulation of the p53-dependent transactivation of pro-apoptotic proteins upon UV-B irradiation (Giampieri et al., 2004). A postulated role of this effect in the development of squamous cell carcinomas of the skin finds some further support in the observation that reduced levels of apoptotic activity in squamous cell carcinomas of the skin, but not in basal cell carcinomas, correlate with the detection of cutaneous HPV (Jackson et al., 2002). In addition, the repair of UV-induced thymine dimers is compromised in cells expressing the E6 protein of HPV types 5 and 18 (Giampieri and Storey, 2004).

A tentative scheme of the indirect function by which cutaneous HPVs may contribute to the development of squamous cell carcinomas of the skin is illustrated in Figure 5.15. This scheme emphasizes a joint and synergistic function between persisting infections by these viruses of the skin and UV-exposure at sun-exposed sites. Sunburn episodes in the past, especially at the age of 13 to 20 years, were reported to be associated with an enhanced risk of EV-HPV DNA persistence (Termorshuizen et al., 2004).

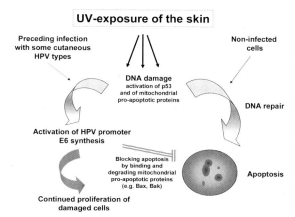

Fig. 5.15 Tentative scheme of the contribution of cutaneous papillomavirus infections to the development of squamous cell carcinomas. In non-infected cells, DNA damage is either repaired or leads to apoptosis. Specific HPV types prevent apoptosis due to interactions with proapoptotic proteins and permit continued proliferation of cells carrying UV-induced DNA modifications.

Interestingly, similar to high-risk HPV-induced high-grade and malignant lesions, both squamous cell carcinomas of the skin and also basal cell carcinomas frequently reveal mutations and functional inactivation of p16^{INK4} and p14^{ARF} (Soufir et al., 1999; Saridaki et al., 2000; Brown et al., 2004).

At least one more aspect of cutaneous papillomavirus infections deserves attention: HPV 38, a type relatively often found in squamous cell carcinomas of the skin, displays transforming properties. Its E7 protein inactivates the tumor suppressor pRb and induces loss of the pRb-mediated G$_1$/S transition control of the mitotic cycle. HPV 38 induces long-lasting proliferation of primary human keratinocytes and thus, seems to resemble to a certain degree high-risk anogenital HPV infections (Caldeira et al., 2003).

In summary, although a number of observations suggest that cutaneous papillomavirus infections may play a (probably indirect) role in squamous cell cancer of the skin, numerous questions remain unanswered, and the role of these viruses in tumorigenesis is clearly not resolved.

5.4
The Role of Cofactors

5.4.1
Non-Infectious Cofactors

5.4.1.1 Smoking

During the past two decades it has been suspected that, besides HPV, other factors might also interact in the etiology of anogenital cancers. Indeed, the first observations on a role of smoking in cervical cancer date back to the 1960s and 1970s (Naguib et al., 1966; Winkelstein, 1977, 1990). During the past 15 years, many studies have shown a significant association between smoking and cervical cancer or its precursor lesions (reviewed in Plummer et al., 2003). These studies were conducted by either adjusting for HPV infection or by excluding HPV-negative cases (reviewed by Haverkos et al., 2003). The majority of case-control and prospective studies revealed an excess risk for ever smoking of 2.17, for current smokers of 2.30, and for ex-smokers of 1.80 (Plummer et al., 2003). Smoke constituents and mutagenic factors in the vaginal mucus of smokers were detected as early as the 1980s (Sasson et al., 1985; Holly et al., 1986; Schiffman et al., 1987), and increased levels of DNA adducts were subsequently found in the cervix of smoking women (Ali et al., 1994). Prospective studies also revealed a prolonged duration of HPV infections and a lower rate of clearing these infections in present or former smokers, resulting in a significant increase in persisting HPV infections (Giuliano et al., 2002; Minkoff et al., 2004). These experimental and epidemiologic data support the concept that exogenous mutagens contribute and moderately elevate the risk for cervical cancer and its precursors in addition to HPV infection.

5.4.1.2 Hormones and Hormonal Contraceptive Use

In 1987, Gloss and colleagues described a sequence element in the promoter of HPV 16 which confers strong inducibility of the p97 promoter by dexamethasone. The same element was active in HeLa cells. Subsequently, other groups demonstrated the oncogenic transformation of primary cells with a combination of HPV 16 DNA and the activated form of the human *H-ras* oncogene or v-fos by the glucocorticoid hormone dexamethasone (Pater et al., 1988; Crook et al., 1988; Dürst et al., 1989). Progesterone and glucocorticoid response elements were found in high- (HPV 16 and 18) and low-risk (HPV 11) human papillomaviruses (Chan et al., 1989). The induction of the HPV 31 promoter is differentiation-dependent since monolayer cultures are insensitive to this treatment, whereas growth of infected cells in semisolid media results in promoter activation (Bromberg-White et al., 2003)

The potential carcinogenic effects of estrogens have been suspected and demonstrated experimentally for more than half a century (Emge et al., 1949; Kirkman and Bacon, 1950). 16-Alpha-hydroxyestrone has been recognized as one of the metabolic products of estrogen, forming covalent linkages with amino groups on proteins and nucleotides (Bucala et al., 1982; Bradlow et al., 1986). The most estrogen-sensitive cells at the transformation zone are at greatest risk for HPV-related cancers. Explants from the transformation zone are able to promote 16-α-hydroxylation of estradiol (Auborn et al., 1991). Since immortalization of cervical and foreskin epithelial cells by HPV 16 is greatly enhanced by 16-α-hydroxyestrone, Auborn and colleagues proposed a cooperative effect for cell transformation. Approximately 90% of cervical cancers arise at the periphery of the transformation zone. It should be noted that proliferating nondifferentiated cells almost reach the surface of the epithelial layer at these sites, and are therefore most easily infected. Thus, it appears that hormonal effects and the specific localization of infectable cells close to the surface probably contribute jointly to the high rate of cervical cancer in comparison to the low rate of penile cancer in males. Available data on the 16-α-hydroxylation of estrogens and the possible relationship to cervical neoplasias have been reviewed recently (de Villiers, 2003).

In HPV 18 transgenic mice, carrying the bacterial β-galactosidase gene under the control of the URR, estradiol and progesterone activated the viral URR (Michelin et al., 1997). A similar model of K14 HPV 16 transgenic mice demonstrated preferential neoplastic progression of the transformation zone by a combination of low-dose estrogen and low level of HPV oncogene expression (Elson et al., 2000). In these transgenic mice exposure to 17α-estradiol increased the proliferation of cervical and vaginal epithelial cells and carcinogenesis, accompanied by an up-regulation of E6/E7 oncogene expression (Arbeit et al., 1996). In HPV 16 transgenic mice, estrogen contributes to the onset, persistence, and malignant progression of cervical cancer (Brake and Lambert, 2005).

These experimental data are less clearly supported by epidemiologic studies (reviewed in de Villiers, 2003; Green et al., 2003; Smith et al., 2003). The latter have been conducted as retrospective case-control studies or as prospective studies in long-term contraceptive use in women. In women using oral contraceptives for more than 5–10 years, a slightly increased risk for cervical cancer was noted (Ylitalo et al., 1999; Hildesheim et al. 2001); this was confirmed in nine case-control studies from the International Agency for research of Cancer in Lyon (Franceschi, 2005). Other studies did not find any association with pre-neoplastic or malignant disease in current and long-term oral contraceptive users (Krüger-Kjaer et al., 1998; Lacey et al., 1999; Shapiro et al., 2003; Giuliano et al., 2004). Among prospective studies, one investigation reported a significantly increased risk for women who used oral contraceptives for more than 8 years (Deacon et al., 2000). In two other studies, data from current contraceptive users were analyzed and no increased risk was found for the incidence of cervical intraepithelial lesions (Moscicki et al., 2001; Castle et al., 2002).

Combined with the experimental data, these results point to a role of long-term hormonal contraceptive use in stimulating gene activity of persisting papillomavirus infections, and probably also by enhancing the duration of HPV persistence. This in turn seems to be responsible for the slightly elevated risk for pre-neoplastic lesions and their eventual malignant progression.

5.4.1.3 Parity

A number of reports have described an elevated risk for cervical cancer in multi-parous women; however, based on the few studies which analyzed only HPV-positive women the association remains inconsistent. Although some retrospective studies reported a significant association between multiparity and ASCUS (atypical squamous cells of unknown significance), squamous intraepithelial lesions and cancer (Kjaer et al., 1996; Hildesheim et al., 2001; Muñoz et al., 2002), other studies failed to confirm this (Krüger-Kjaer et al., 1998; Giuliano et al., 2004).

In view of the described effects of estrogens and progesterone, however, it is likely that multiparity will lead to an increased risk for pre-neoplastic and malignant lesions of the cervix in high-risk HPV-positive women.

5.4.1.4 Nutrients

The role of nutrition in cervical cancer development or cervical cancer prevention has been studied repeatedly. Some retrospective studies yielded controversial results. An inverse relationship between the consumption of vegetables and fruits and the risk for cervical cancer was reported from India (Rajkumar et al., 2003). A study analyzing a possible link between vitamins A, C, E, β-carotene, folate, and zinc and the risk for low- and high-grade intraepithelial lesions in Portland, USA, failed to reach significance (Wideroff et al., 1998). Higher levels of serum retinol seemed to show some protective effect for cervical intraepithelial neoplasias in one study (French et al., 2000), but a second investigation failed to demonstrate this effect (Ho et al., 1998). In the latter study, only vitamin C was associated with a significant reduced risk of disease. An elevated risk without statistical significance for cervical cancer has been reported for women with low serum and red blood cell levels of folic acid (Weinstein et al., 2001).

Among prospective studies no link between serum retinol and serum α-to-copherol and cervical cancer was noted in one investigation (Lehtinen et al., 1999), whereas a second study reported significant links between serum β-carotene and α-tocopherol with transient HPV infections in contrast to persistently HPV-infected women (Giuliano et al., 1997). The same group were unable to detect any association with serum folate, vitamin B_{12} or homocysteine (Sedjo et al., 2003). A protective ef-fect of cis-lycopene, high vegetable consumption and lutein intake was also reported (Sedjo et al., 2002 a,b).

Two Phase II clinical trials have been completed to study the effect of folic acid in cervical cancer prevention (Butterworth et al., 1992; Childers et al., 1995), but both failed to reveal any protective effect. Similarly, five Phase II/III trials on supplemen-tal β-carotene failed to reveal any significant effect (de Vet et al., 1991; Fairley et al., 1996; Romney et al., 1997; Mackerras et al., 1999; Keefe et al., 2001). One of three tri-als using all-*trans* retinoic acid reported a significant effect of three administrations of the compound on regression of CIN II lesions (Meyskens et al., 1994). In contrast, two other studies failed to demonstrate any effect (Follen et al., 2001; Alvarez et al., 2003).

As a baseline of these data, clear-cut evidence for a role of nutritional constituents in preventing premalignant or malignant cervical lesions is, at present, still missing.

5.4.2
Infectious Cofactors

5.4.2.1 Herpes viruses

Cytological and histological changes typical of herpes simplex virus (HSV) infec-tions, when frequently observed in women with cervical lesions, provided an early hint for the possible involvement of HSV type 2 (HSV-2) in cervical cancers (Naib et al., 1969). These initial suggestions were supported by data from early seroepidemi-ological studies conducted by three different groups (Rawls et al., 1969; Nahmias et al., 1970; Royston and Aurelian, 1970). These data seemed to be supported by the demonstration of an HSV fragment in only one cervical carcinoma biopsy (Frenkel et al., 1972), and studies which revealed the transforming properties of partially UV-inactivated HSV-2 for hamster cells (Duff and Rapp, 1971).

These positive findings were, however, not confirmed by other groups: zur Hausen et al. (1974 a,b) and Pagano (1975) were unable to detect HSV-2 DNA in cer-vical cancer biopsies. An early large seroepidemiologic prospective study also failed to confirm the previously reported positive data (Vonka et al. 1984 a,b).

The discovery of a mutagenic activity of HSV infections for host cell DNA and the ability of the virus to induce selective amplification of persisting polyoma- or papil-lomavirus DNA (Schlehofer and zur Hausen, 1982; Schlehofer et al., 1983; Schmitt et al., 1989; Heilbronn and zur Hausen, 1989; Clarke and Clements, 1991) permitted the interpretation of an indirect contribution of HSV infections to human carcinogenesis.

Even today, epidemiologic data on a possible role of HSV-2 in cervical cancer remain inconsistent and difficult to interpret. Indeed, two recently conducted large studies arrived at conflicting results. Lehtinen et al. (2002) pooled data and specimens from three population-based Nordic cohorts, containing a total population of more than 500 000 women. They found no difference in HSV-2 seroprevalence of cervical cancer cases and controls, even after adjustment for HPV 16/18/33 VLP antibodies and for cigarette smoking. A study conducted by Smith et al. (2002), which included data from seven case-control studies, reported a significant association of HSV-2 seroantibodies with squamous cell carcinoma of the cervix (odds ratio 2.2). However, by combining data on seroreactivity against HSV-2 in cases and controls obtained during the past 20 years, the majority of these studies failed to detect any significant association. Although some studies reported a high prevalence of HSV DNA in neoplastic cervical material by PCR technology (Koffa et al., 1995; Han et al., 1997), others failed to confirm these findings (Vecchione et al., 1994; Tran-Thanh et al., 2003; Yang et al., 2004).

Thus, although plausible due to a set of experimental data, a role for HSV infection in cervical neoplasias remains open and is, in all probability, at best marginal.

5.4.2.2 Chlamydia trachomatis

Chlamydia trachomatis represents a very common bacterial, sexually transmitted infection. These infections frequently remain asymptomatic and may persist for months or even years (Stamm, 1999; Peipert, 2003; Stephens, 2003). Chronic infection may result in pelvic inflammatory disease and squamous metaplasia.

Early suggestions for a possible role of chlamydial infections in cervical cancer date back to 1971 and the following decade (Alexander, 1973; Schachter et al., 1975; Kalimo et al., 1981). The present evidence is mainly based on seroepidemiologic and epidemiologic observations. Most of these studies reported a significant association of *Chlamydia* seropositivity and squamous cell carcinomas of the cervix. The two large epidemiologic studies analyzing also the role of HSV-2 in cervical cancer reported a significant increase of seropositivity in cervical carcinoma patients (Koskela et al., 2000; Smith, J.S., et al., 2004). Since 1991, more than 10 additional studies have been published supporting the seroepidemiologic evidence for an involvement of chlamydial infections in cervical cancer, though most also found high-risk HPV reactivity.

In addition to the serologic findings, *Chlamydia trachomatis* DNA in pre-diagnostic Pap smears was also associated with a subsequent risk for cervical cancer or low-grade squamous intraepithelial lesions (Wallin et al., 2002; Golijow et al., 2005). A mechanism by which chlamydial infections may contribute to cervical carcinogenesis has recently been suggested by Sillins et al. (2005). In their study, the most significant risk factor for the persistent presence of HPV DNA was a self-reported history of previous *Chlamydia trachomatis* infection. This raises the possibility that chlamydial infections facilitate HPV persistence and may thus contribute indirectly to cervical carcinogenesis.

5.4.2.3 Human Immunodeficiency Virus

Human immunodeficiency viruses (HIV) types 1 and 2 can be considered as the classical indirect carcinogens. Immunosuppression induced by these infections results in an increased incidence of tumors caused by other viruses [see Chapter 4, Sections 4.3.1 (EBV) and Section 4.4.1 (HHV-8)]. The majority of many epidemiological studies also indicate an increased incidence of precursor lesions of anogenital neoplasias in these patients (e.g., Sun et al., 1995; Palefsky, 1995, 1999; Jamieson et al., 2002; Strickler et al., 2005). This is supported by a number of reports on an increased incidence of cervical cancer in these patients (e.g., Goedert et al., 1998; Frisch et al., 2000 b; Dorucci et al., 2001; Mbulaiteye et al., 2003).

It is possible that the effect of HIV in cervical neoplasias is not solely mediated by the virus-induced immunosuppression, but may also be exerted by a co-activation of the HPV promoter by HIV *tat* (Vernon et al., 1993; Buonaguro et al., 1994). HIV infections emerge, however, as one of the important cofactors for cervical neoplasias.

5.4.2.4 Other Infections

A number of other viral and nonviral agents have been suspected of playing a role as cofactors in cervical carcinogenesis. Among the herpesvirus family, human cytomegalovirus, EBV, and human herpesvirus types 6 and 7 have been detected in cervical premalignant and malignant specimens (Young and Sixbey, 1988; Han et al., 1997; Chan et al., 2001). Neither these findings, nor reports on elevated antibody titers against the respective viruses, were confirmed in subsequent studies – which leaves the question open as to whether they play any role in cervical cancer. Cytomegalovirus has been shown in the past to effectively mediate the amplification of the human polyoma-type virus JC (Heilbronn et al., 1993), which points to similar properties of this virus as previously described for herpes simplex viruses. Studies on the role of cytomegalovirus infections on the amplification of HPV DNA are presently not available.

A few studies have reported an association of *Trichomonas vaginalis* infections with cervical neoplasia (Gram et al., 1992; Zhang and Begg, 1994; Viikki et al., 2000). Here, the reported detection of N-nitrosamines in the vaginal vault of women with trichmoniasis could provide some supportive evidence (Nunn et al., 1974; O'Farrell, 1989). The association was, however, not confirmed in other studies (Becker et al., 1994; Schiff et al., 2000; Watts et al., 2005). Similarly, bacterial vaginosis, *Neisseria gonorrhoeae*, *Treponema pallidum* and *Candida albicans* infections have been considered as cofactors in cervical carcinogenesis (reviewed in Rotkin, 1973). Recent studies did not provide supportive evidence, however.

Thus, to summarize this section, there exists conclusive evidence for the role of HIV infections as cofactors for HPV-mediated oncogenesis, and for chlamydial infections the role is suggestive but not proven. For HSV-2 infections, a possible role is at best marginal, but for all other anogenital infections the evidence remains inconclusive.

5.5
Preventive Vaccination

Initial attempts to vaccinate against papillomaviruses were made in animal models by using bovine papillomaviruses (Campo et al., 1993), canine oral papillomavirus (Suzich et al., 1995) or cotton-tail rabbit papillomavirus vaccines (Breitburd et al., 1995), and all of these proved to be highly successful. These and subsequent vaccines were based on an observation made by Salunke et al. (1986). This group demonstrated that purified polyoma virus structural proteins are able to self-assemble to virus-like particles (VLPs). The same was shown subsequently by Zhou et al. (1991, 1992) and Kirnbauer et al. (1992) for papillomavirus structural proteins L1 and L2 produced in vaccinia and yeast vector systems. Clinical trials were soon initiated with VLPs of HPV types 6, 11, 16, and 18, which indicated that VLP preparations were well tolerated and induced high titers of neutralizing antibodies, as well as T-cell responses (Zhang et al., 2000; Harro et al., 2001; Brown et al., 2001; Evans et al., 2001; Emeny et al., 2002). The titers usually exceeded those reached in natural infections by more than 40-fold.

A first double-blind study determined whether HPV 16 VLP vaccination prevented the respective infection and also premalignant lesions (Koutsky et al., 2002). Two groups, each including more than 750 HPV 16-negative women, aged 16 to 23 years, received three VLP vaccinations or placebo vaccinations over 6 months, respectively, and were analyzed initially after 17 months. During this period, 41 persistent HPV infections occurred in the placebo group, and none in the vaccinated group. Nine HPV 16-positive squamous intraepithelial lesions (SILs) occurred only in the placebo group, although in each of the two groups 22 lesions of non-HPV 16-associated SIL were observed. Six women of the vaccinated group and 27 among the placebo group acquired a transient HPV 16 infection, without developing SIL.

Two other studies have been published recently confirming and extending these results (Harper et al., 2004; Villa et al., 2005). The study by Harper and colleagues used a bivalent vaccine containing HPV 16 and 18 VLPs. Villa et al. (2005) used a quadrivalent vaccine containing in addition HPV 6 and HPV 11 VLPs. In these studies incident infections were prevented by more than 90%, and persistent infections by 100%.

These data are extremely encouraging and raise the hope that cervical cancer can be successfully prevented in the future. It will of course require long-term observations to demonstrate the preventive effect for cervical cancer, but the prevention of premalignant lesions caused by these high-risk HPVs strongly points into this direction.

At present, a number of additional attempts are being made to produce a cheap and efficient HPV vaccine. One of the most promising candidates is a capsomere vaccine produced in bacteria. L1 proteins, expressed in vesicular stomatitis virus vectors, have provided promising results in preclinical models (Roberts et al., 2004). Bacterially expressed L1 proteins assemble into pentameric structures, corresponding to capsomeres with neutralizing epitopes (Li et al., 1997). In canine oral papillomatosis this vaccine reveal an efficacy similar to that of VLP vaccines (Yuan et al., 2001). Moreover, it can also be applied intranasally, avoiding the use of syringes. The repeated use of syringes is difficult to avoid under conditions of poor hygiene, and bears the risk of transmitting other viral infections such as hepatitis viruses and HIV.

L1 and L2 proteins possess antigenic domains that crossreact with additional HPV types. Antibodies to these regions do not seem to react with VLPs, nor do they neutralize infection (Jenson et al., 1980; Christensen et al., 1990; Hines et al., 1994). Some studies indicate, however, that L2 antibodies neutralize homologous and heterologous HPV types (Kawana et al., 1999, 2003; Roden et al., 2000). Consequently, there is hope that vaccines may be developed which cover a broad spectrum of papillomavirus infections.

Additional attempts are being made to express viral structural proteins in plants, in Salmonella, in vaccinia virus, or to vaccinate with naked viral DNA or viral DNA vectored in various viral vector systems (adeno-associated virus, adenovirus, lentivirus), and these have shown some promising results (Dale et al., 2002; Liu et al., 2005; Berg et al., 2005). A chimeric hepatitis B/HPV16 E7 vaccine encoded by an adenovirus vector may even have a therapeutic application (Báez-Astúa et al., 2005). However, all of these products are currently only in the preclinical phase of testing.

5.6
Therapeutic Vaccination

Early attempts to develop vaccines which might also be effective therapeutically were made by linking a segment of the *E7* gene to the carboxy-terminus of L1 or L2 (Müller et al., 1997; Greenstone et al., 1998). Although preclinical studies demonstrated the induction of neutralizing antibodies to VLPs and T-cell responses to L1 and *E7*, a first clinical trial with these chimeric vaccines failed to reveal a convincing result (Kaufmann et al., 2001).

Since cervical carcinoma cells and high-grade intraepithelial lesions mainly express *E6* and *E7* genes, most studies have focused on eliciting cytotoxic T lymphocytes (CTLs) directed against these oncoproteins. Although preclinical trials in murine systems have been performed successfully (Da Silva et al., 2001; Preville et al., 2005), a number of clinical trials have not yet yielded very convincing results. HLA class I-restricted epitopes have been mapped for E6 and E7 (Kast et al., 1993; Beverley et al., 1994), and several clinical trials using these epitopes have been conducted. The inoculation of such vaccines into 15 HPV 16-positive, A-0201-positive cancer patients resulted in neither any CTL detection nor any measurable clinical effect (Ressing et al., 2000). Another trial was also unsuccessful (van Driel et al., 1999). However, a third report, in which the vaccine was applied to 18 women with high-grade intraepithelial lesions, recorded 10 CTL responses to the E7 peptide, with three of the women revealing a complete clinical regression (Muderspach et al., 2000). A prolongation of the epitope peptide seems to elicit a more effective CTL response than minimal epitopes, which can be further enhanced by admixture of dendritic cells, including an activating adjuvant (Zwaveling et al., 2002). The linkage of such a peptide to palmitic acid resulted in a CTL response in three out of 12 cervical cancer patients, and in a complete clinical response in one of these (Steller et al., 1998; Steller, 2002). These sets of data suggest that therapeutic vaccines might have some value in patients with premalignant lesions, but they are less likely to be effective in cancer patients. This is in line with previously discussed data, revealing the loss of antigen presentation in cervical carcinoma cells.

Recombinant vaccinia virus expressing mutated HPV 16 and 18 *E7* genes was applied to patients with advanced cervical cancer (Boursnell et al., 1996; Borysiewicz et al., 1996). Only one of the patients developed CTLs with a clinical remission. Among 29 patients with stage Ib or Ia, four developed CTLs and eight revealed serologic responses to the HPV proteins (Kaufmann et al., 2002). In more recent studies, the treatment of patients with intraepithelial neoplasias was found to be somewhat more successful: Baldwin et al. (2003) found some improvement in 83% of 12 treated patients, while Davidson et al. (2003) reported a reduction of high-grade vulvar intraepithelial lesions in diameter by at least 50% in eight out of 18 vaccinated women. Other viral vector systems (E7 or poly-epitope proteins) used in therapeutic approaches were recombinant adenoviruses (Tobery et al., 2003), adeno-associated virus (Liu et al., 2000), RNA-based poliovirus (van Kuppeveld et al., 2002), and alphavirus (Velders et al., 2001). Several of these systems are currently undergoing clinical trials.

In order to increase the immunogenicity of the E7 protein, this oncogene has been fused to the heat shock gene (coding for hsp 70) of *Mycobacterium tuberculosis* (Chen et al., 2000) or to hsp 65 of Bacillus Calmette-Guerin (Goldstone et al., 2002). This should stimulate immunogenicity via the Toll-like receptor 4. Among 14 patients with anogenital warts, three had a complete resolution and an additional 10 had a reduction in wart size. Such DNA vaccines were stimulated in their immunogenic potency by coadministration of a DNA-encoding serine protease inhibitor-6 (Kim et al., 2004). Inoculation of fusion protein of a mutated HPV 16 *E7* gene to the first 108 amino acids of *Haemophilus influenzae* protein D in patients with CIN III and CIN I elicited systemic specific immune responses (Hallez et al., 2004).

Peptide or protein pulsed dendritic cells are thought to be more effective in inducing anti-tumor CTLs than peptides alone (Schoell et al., 1999). In murine cells, E7-loaded dendritic cells transfected with BAK/BAX siRNA, to down-regulate these pro-apoptotic genes, resulted in a strong therapeutic effect (Peng et al., 2005). Monocytes from cancer patients differentiate into dendritic cells following admixture of IL-4 and granulocyte-macrophage colony stimulating factor (GM-CSF). Several smaller clinical studies have used this approach, though without any significant therapeutic effects (Steller et al., 1998; Santin et al., 1999, 2002; Ferrara et al., 2003; Adams et al., 2003).

Overall, the available data on immunotherapeutic interferences with specific viral antigens or epitopes seems promising for HPV-positive premalignant lesions, but less so for malignant tumors. In the latter cases, immunotherapeutic approaches may be more promising by targeting the modified expression of specific cellular proteins, as for instance p16^{INK4}.

5.7
Therapy

This section briefly summarizes some of the most commonly used treatments for HPV-linked mucocutaneous lesions. Surgical treatments include cryotherapy, electrocoagulation, laser surgery, and surgical excision. Cryotherapy usually provides aesthetically satisfying results and is only traumatic to a limited degree. In genital warts, it frequently requires several sessions. Freezing of the tissue results in the destruction of warts (Kouronis et al., 1999; Scala et al., 2002).

Laser surgery permits high-precision surgery which seals small blood vessels immediately. The results are usually excellent, with a very low postoperative morbidity. Similarly, photodynamic therapy by topical application of amino-levulinic acid with subsequent irradiation with light of different wavelengths, can be used for superficial lesions (Roberts and Cairnduff, 1995). The surgical removal of lesions is indicated in case of a limited number of lesions. Extensive intra-anal and vulvovaginal condylomata should be removed under general anesthesia (von Krogh et al., 2001). The surgical removal of malignant lesions will not be detailed at this point.

One special problem is posed by recurrent respiratory papillomatosis, which represents the most common benign neoplasm in the larynx of children (Kimberlin, 2004). It frequently leads to obstruction of the airways and respiratory distress, and even surgical removal cannot protect against multiple recurrences. At present, there is no truly effective therapy against this condition, although indole-3-carbinole, diindolylmethane, interferon and photodynamic therapies are used as additional modalities (Armbruster, 2002; Auborn, 2002).

A number of pharmacological therapies have been used to treat mucosal and cutaneous HPV-linked lesions. One such compound is cidofovir, an acyclic nucleoside phosphonate which specifically inhibits viral DNA polymerases. The reported activity against HPV lesions is surprising in view of the absence of virus-coded DNA-polymerases (Stragier et al., 2002). Close to 50% of lesions seem to be cleared by cidofovir treatment (Snoeck et al., 2001). Cidofovir is presently also used for the treatment of laryngeal papillomatosis, but the observed nephrotoxicity of the drug limits its systemic application (de Clerq, 2003).

Notably in the case of anogenital warts, cytodestruction has been achieved by the application of podophyllin resin, podophyllotoxin, salicylic acid, trichloroacetic acid, and cytostatic agents such as bleomycin and 5-fluorouracil. Podophyllin resin and its derivative podophyllotoxin induce tissue necrosis by blocking cell division and inhibiting microtubule assembly (Manso-Martinez, 1982). Gels of salicylic acid are commonly used for the treatment of non-genital warts (Rivera and Tyring, 2004).

Trichloroacetic acid has been used as an alternative to podophyllin. It induces tissue coagulation and seems to be effective in cervical condylomata acuminata (Menendez Velazquez et al., 1993). Bleomycin and 5-fluorouracil, both of which are mainly applied topically, have also been reported to result in excellent clearance rates (Munn et al., 1996; Syed et al., 2000; Swineheart et al., 1997).

Substantial hope is presently placed on immunomodulatory treatments, specifically on imidazoquinolines. Imiquimod and its homologues act through the activation of Toll-like receptors, and stimulates macrophages and other cells to secrete proinflammatory cytokines (interferon-α, TNF-α, IL-12). This induces a local Th-1 cell-mediated immune response and the production of cytotoxic effectors (Stanley, 2002). The topical use of imiquimod for up to 16 weeks was found to be effective and safe, with a low recurrence rate (Edwards et al., 1998; Cox et al., 2004).

All interferons possess anti-HPV activity. Topical, intralesional or systemic interferon application in some instances leads to partial or complete remission of respiratory papillomatosis, of cutaneous or anogenital warts, in condylomata acuminata in part also in combination with podophyllin (Weck et al., 1986). Interferon-α has been approved by the US Federal Drug Administration for the treatment of genital warts, but has dose-limiting side effects (Wiley et al., 2002).

Some hope is placed on RNA interference for treating cancers caused by viral infection, and here specifically on cervical cancer (Milner, 2003). Interfering RNA (RNAi), triggered by double-stranded RNA, permits gene silencing by targeting specific mRNA transcripts for degradation. Hutvagner et al. (2001) showed that short RNA duplexes, containing 19–22 nucleotides initiated RNAi in mammalian cells. In HPV-carrying cervical carcinoma cells the silencing of *E6* RNA had little effect, whereas the silencing of *E6* and *E7* and of *E7* alone resulted in apoptosis of the transfected cells (Jiang and Miller, 2002). One problem here for clinical use is the mode of application, though at present topical application promises the best results.

References

Abbate, E.A., Berger, J.M., and Botchan, M.R. The X-ray structure of the papillomavirus helicase in complex with its molecular matchmaker E2. *Genes Dev.* 18: 1981–1996, **2004**.

Abdel-Hady, E.S., Martin-Hirsch, P., Duggan-Keen, M., Stern, P.L., Moore, J.V., Corbitt, G., Kitchener, H.C., and Hampson, I.N. Immunological and viral factors associated with the response of vulval intraepithelial neoplasia to photodynamic therapy. *Cancer Res.* 61: 192–196, **2001**.

Abramson, A.L., Brandsma, J., Steinberg, B., and Winkler, B. Verrucous carcinoma of the larynx. Possible human papillomavirus etiology. *Arch. Otolaryngol.* 111: 709–715, **1985**.

Acevedo, C.M., Henriquez, M., Emmert-Buck, M.R., and Chuaqui, R.F. Loss of heterozygosity on chromosome arms 3p and 6q in microdissected adenocarcinomas of the uterine cervix and adenocarcinoma in situ. *Cancer* 94: 793–802, **2002**.

Adams, M., Navabi, H., Jasani, B., Man, S., Fiander, A., Evans, A.S., Donnonger, C., and Mason, M. Dendritic cell (DC) based therapy for cervical cancer: use of DC pulsed with tumour lysate and matured with a novel synthetic clinically non-toxic double stranded RNA analogue poly [I]:poly [C(12)U] (Ampligen R). *Vaccine* 21: 787–790, **2003**.

Aguilar-Lemarroy, A., Gariglio, P., Whitaker, N., Eichhorst, S., zur Hausen, H., Krammer, P.H., and Rösl, F. Restoration of p53 expression sensitizes human papillomavirus type 16 immortalized human keratinocytes to CD95-mediated apoptosis. *Oncogene* 21: 165–175, **2002**.

Albrechtsen, N., Dornreiter, I., Grosse, F., Kim, E., Wiesmüller, L. and Deppert, W. Maintenance of genomic integrity by p53: complementary roles for activated and non-activated p53. *Oncogene* 18: 7706–7717, **1999**.

Alexander, E.R. Possible etiologies of cancer of the cervix other than herpesvirus. *Cancer Res.* 33: 1485–1490, **1973**.

Ali, S., Astley, S. B., Sheldon, T.A., Peel, K.R., and Wells, M. Detection and measurement of DNA adducts in the cervix of smokers and non-smokers. *Int. J. Gynecol. Cancer* 4: 188–193, **1994**.

Alonso, L.G., Garcia-Alai, M.M., Smal, C., Centeno, J.M., Iacono, R., Castaño, E., Gualfetti, P., and de Prat-Gay, G. The HPV16 E7 viral oncoprotein self-assembles into defined spherical oligomers. *Biochemistry* 43: 3310–3317, **2004**.

Alunni-Fabbroni, M., Littlewood, T., Deleu, L., Caldeira, S., Giarre, M., Dell'Orco, M., and Tommasino, M. Induction of S phase and apoptosis by the human papillomavirus type 16 E7 protein are separable events in immortalized rodent fibroblasts. *Oncogene* 19: 2277–2285, **2000**.

Alvarez, R.D., Conner, M.G., Weiss, H., Klug, P.M., Niwas, S., Manne, U., Bacus, J., Kagan, V., Sexton, K.C., Grubbs, C.J., Eltoum, I.E., and Grizzle, W.E. The efficacy of 9-cis-retinoic acid (aliretinoin) as a chemopreventive agent for cervical dysplasia: results of a randomized double-blind clinical trial. *Cancer Epidemiol. Biomarkers Prev.* 12: 114–119, **2003**.

Alvarez-Salas, L.M., Arpawong, T.E., and DiPaolo, J.A. Growth inhibition of cervical tumor cells by antisense oligodeoxynucleotides directed to the human papillomavirus type 16 E6 gene. *Antisense Nucleic Acid Drug Dev.* 9: 441–450, **1999**.

Andersson-Ellström, A., Dillner, J., Hagmar, B., Schiller, J., and Forssman, L. No serological evidence for non-sexual spread of HPV 16. *Lancet* 344: 1435, **1994**.

Androphy, E.J., Lowy, D.R., and Schiller, J.T. Bovine papillomavirus E2 trans-acting gene product binds to specific sites in papillomavirus DNA. *Nature* 325: 70–73, **1987**.

Antinore, M.J., Birrer, M.J., Patel, D., Nader, L., and McCance, D.J. The human papillomavirus type 16 E7 gene product interacts with and trans-activates the AP1 family of transcription factors. *EMBO J.* 15: 1950–1960, **1996**.

Antonsson, A., Erfurt, C., Hazard, H., Holmgreen, V., Simon, M., Kataoka, A., Hossain, S., Hakangard, C., and Hansson, B.G. Prevalence and type spectrum of human papillomaviruses in healthy skin samples collected in three continents. *J. Gen. Virol.* 84: 1881–1886, **2003**.

Anwar, K., Naiki, H., Nakakuki, K., and Inuzuka, M. High frequency of human papillomavirus infection in carcinoma of the urinary bladder. *Cancer* 70: 1967–1973, **1992**.

Arbeit, J.M., Münger, K., Howley, P.M., and Hanahan, D. Neuroepithelial carcinomas in mice transgenic with human papillomavirus type 16 E6/E7 ORFs. *Am. J. Pathol.* 142: 1187–1197, **1993**.

Arbeit, J.M., Howley, P.M., and Hanahan, D. Chronic estrogen-induced cervical and vaginal squamous carcinogenesis in human papillomavirus type 16 transgenic mice. *Proc. Natl. Acad. Sci. USA* 93: 2930–2935, **1996**.

Armbruster, C. Novel treatments for recurrent respiratory papillomatosis. *Expert Opin. Investig. Drugs* 11: 1139–1148, **2002**.

Arroyo, M., Bagchi, S., and Raychaudhuri, P. Association of human papillomavirus type 16 E7 protein with the S-phase-specific E2F-cyclin A complex. *Mol. Cell. Biol.* 13: 6537–6546, **1993**.

Ascano, J.M., Beverly, L.J., and Capobianco, A.J. The C-terminal PDZ-ligand of JAGGED1 is essential for cellular transformation. *J. Biol. Chem.* 278: 8771–8779, **2003**.

Ashrafi, G.H., Haghshenas, M.R., Marchetti, B., O'Brien, P.M., and Campo, M.S. E5 protein of human papillomavirus type 16 selectively downregulates surface HLA class I. *Int. J. Cancer* 113: 276–283, **2005**.

Assadoullina, A., Bialasiewicz, A.A., de Villiers, E.-M., and Richard, G. Detection of HPV-20, HPV-23, and HPV-DL332 in a solitary eyelid syringoma. *Am. J. Ophthalmol.* 129: 99–101, **2000**.

Astori, G., Lavergne, D., Benton, C., Hock-mayr, B., Egawa, K., Garbe, C., and de Villi-ers, E.-M. Human papillomaviruses are commonly found in normal skin of immunocompetent hosts. *J. Invest. Derma-tol.* 110: 752–755, **1998**.

Ateenyi-Agaba, C., Weiderpass, E., Smet, A., Dong, W., Dai, M., Kahwa, B., Wabinga, H., Katongole-Mbidde, E., Franceschi, S., and Tommasino, M. Epidermodysplasia veruciformis human papillomavirus types and carcinoma of the conjunctiva: a pilot study. *Br. J. Cancer* 90: 1777–1779, **2004**.

Auborn, K.J. Therapy for recurrent respira-tory papillomatosis. *Antivir. Ther.* 7: 1–9, **2002**.

Auborn, K.J., Woodworth, C., DiPaolo, J.A., and Bradlow, H.L. The interaction between HPV infection and estrogen metabolism in cervical carcinogenesis. *Int. J. Cancer* 49: 867–869, **1991**.

Auster, A.S., and Joshua-Tor, L. The DNA-binding domain of human papillomavirus type 18 E1. Crystal structure, dimerization, and DNA binding. *J. Biol. Chem.* 279: 3733–3742, **2004**.

Avvakumov, N., Torchia, J., and Mymryk, J.S. Interaction of the HPV E7 proteins with the pCAF acetyltransferase. *Oncogene* 22: 3833–3841, **2003**.

Azar, K.K., Tani, M., Yasuda, H., Sakai, A., Inoue, M., and Sasagawa, T. Increased secretion patterns of interleukin-10 and tumor necrosis factor α in cervical squamous intraepithelial lesions. *Hum. Pathol.* 35: 1376–1384, **2004** .

Bachmann, A., Hanke, B., Zawatzky, R., Soto, U., van Riggelen, J., zur Hausen, H., and Rösl, F. Disturbance of tumor necrosis fac-tor α-mediated β interferon signaling in cervical carcinoma cells. *J. Virol.* 76: 280–291, **2002**.

Báez-Astúa, A., Herráez-Hernández, E., Garbi, N., Pasolli, H.A., Juárez, V., zur Hausen, H., and Cid-Arregui, A. Low-dose adenovirus vaccine encoding chimeric hepatitis B virus surface antigen-human papillomavirus type 16 E7 proteins induces enhanced E7-specific antibody and cyto-toxic T-cell response. *J. Virol.* 79: 12 807–12 817, **2005**.

Baksch, C., Wagenbach, N., Nonn, M., Leis-tritz, S., Stanbridge, E., Schneider, A., and Dürst, M. Microcell-mediated transfer of chromosome 4 into HeLa cells suppresses telomerase activity. *Genes Chromosomes Cancer* 31: 196–198, **2001** .

Balaram, P., Nalinakumari, K.R., Abraham, E., Balan, A., Hareendran, N.K., Bernard, H.U., Chan, S. Y. Human papillomaviruses in 91 oral cancers from Indian betel quid chewers – high prevalence and multiplicity of infections. *Int. J. Cancer* 61: 450–454, **1995**.

Baldwin, P.J. , van der Burg, S. H., Boswell, C.M., Offringa, R., Hickling, J.K., Dobson, J., Roberts, J.S., Latimer, J.A., Moseley, R.P., Coleman, N., Stanley, M.A., and Ster-ling, J.C. Vaccinia-expressed human papil-lomavirus 16 and 18 E6 and E7 as a ther-apeutic vaccination for vulval and vaginal intraepithelial neoplasia. *Clin. Cancer Res.* 9: 5205–5213, **2003**.

Balz, V., Scheckenbach, K., Gotte, K., Bockmühl, U., Petersen, I., and Bier, H. Is the p53 inactivation frequency in squamous cell carcinomas of the head and neck underestimated? Analysis of p53 exons 2–11 and human papillomavirus 16/18 E6 transcripts in 123 unselected tumor specimens. *Cancer Res.* 63: 1188–1191, **2003**.

Band, V., Zaychowski, D., Kulesa, V., and Sager, R. Human papillomavirus DNAs immortalize normal human mammary epithelial cells and reduce their growth fac-tor requirements. *Proc. Natl. Acad. Sci. USA* 87: 463–467, **1990**.

Band, V., De Caprio, J.A., Delmolino, L., Kulesa, V., and Sager, R. Loss of p53 pro-tein in human papillomavirus type 16 E6-immortalized human mammary epithelial cells. *J. Virol.* 65: 6671–6676, **1991**.

Barbosa, M.S., Lowy, D.R., and Schiller, J.T. Papillomavirus polypeptides E6 and E7 are zinc-binding proteins. *J. Virol.* 63: 1404–1407, **1989**.

Barnard, P. and McMillan, N.A. The human papillomavirus E7 oncoprotein abrogates signalling mediated by interferon-α. *Virology* 259: 305–313, **1999**.

Barzon, L., Pizzighella, S., Corti, L., Mengoli, C., and Palu, G. Vaginal dysplastic lesions in women with hysterectomy and receiving radiotherapy are linked to high-risk human papillomavirus. *J. Med. Virol.* 67: 401–405, **2002**.

Bauer, H.M., Hildesheim, A., Schiffman, M.H., Glass, A.G., Rush, B.B., Scott, D.R., Cadell, D.R., Kurman, R.J., and Manos, M.M. Determinants of genital human papillomavirus infection in low risk women in Portland, Oregon. *Sex. Transm. Dis.* 20: 274–278, **1993**.

Bauknecht, T., Angel, P., Royer, H.-D., and zur Hausen, H. Identification of a negative regulatory domain in the human papillomavirus type 18 promoter: Interaction with the transcriptional repressor YY1. *EMBO J.* 11: 4607–4617, **1992** .

Becker, T.M., Wheeler, C.M., McGough, N.S., Parmenter, C.A., Jordan, S. W., Stidley, C., McPherson, R.S., and Dorin, M.H. Sexually transmitted diseases and other risk factors for cervical dysplasia among southwestern Hispanics and non-Hispanic white women. *JAMA* 271: 1181–1188, **1994**.

Bedell, M.A., Jones, K.H., and Laimins, L.A. The E6-E7 region of human papillomavirus type 18 is sufficient for transformation of NIH 3T3 and rat-1 cells. *J. Virol.* 61: 3635–3640, **1987**.

Bedrosian, C.L. and Bastia, D. The DNA-binding domain of the HPV-16 E2 protein interaction with the viral enhancer: protein-induced DNA bending and role of the non-conserved core sequence in binding site affinity. *Virology* 174: 557–575, **1990**.

Bejui-Thivolet, F., Chardonnet, Y., and Patricot, L.M. Human papillomavirus type 11DNA in papillary squamous cell lung carcinoma. *Virchows Arch. A Pathol. Anat. Histopathol.* 417: 457–461, **1990**.

Berezutskaya, E. and Bagchi, S. The human papillomavirus E7 oncoprotein functionally interacts with the S4 subunit of the 26S proteasome. *J. Biol. Chem.* 272: 30135–30140, **1997**.

Berezutskaya, E., Yu, B., Morozow, A., Raychaudhuri, P., and Bagchi, S. Differential regulation of the pocket domains of the retinoblastoma family proteins by the HPV 16 E7 oncoprotein. *Cell Growth Differ.* 8: 1277–1286, **1997**.

Berg, M., Difatta, J., Hoiczyk, E., Schlegel, R., and Ketner, G. Viable adenovirus vaccine prototypes: high-level production of a papillomavirus capsid antigen from the major late transcriptional unit. *Proc. Natl. Acad. Sci. USA* 102: 4590–4595, **2005**.

Berkhout, R.J., Tieben, L.M., Smits, H.L., Bavinck, J.N., Vermeer, B.J., and ter Schegget, J. Nested PCR approach for detection and typing of epidermodysplasia verruciformis-associated human papillomavirus types in cutaneous cancers from renal transplant recipients. *J. Clin. Microbiol.* 33: 690–695, **1995**.

Berkhout, R.J., Bouwes Bavinck, J.N., and ter Schegget J. Persistence of human papillomavirus DNA in benign and (pre)malignant skin lesions from renal transplant recipients. *J. Clin. Microbiol.* 38: 2087–2096, **2000**.

Bernauer, H.S., Welkoborsky, H.J., Tilling, A., Amedee, R.G., and Mann, W.J. Inverted papillomas of the paranasal sinuses and the nasal cavity: DNA indices and HPV infection. *Am. J. Rhinol.* 11: 155–160, **1997**.

Beverley, P.C., Sadovnikova, E., Zhu, X., Hickling, J., Gao, L., Chain, B., Collins, S., Crawford, L., Vousden, K., and Stauss, H.J. Strategies for studying mouse and human immune responses to human papillomavirus type 16. *CIBA Found. Symp.* 187: 78–96, **1994**.

Bezerra, A.L., Lopes, A., Landman, G., Alencar, G.N., Torloni, H., and Villa, L.L. Clinicopathologic features and human papillomavirus DNA prevalence of warty and squamous cell carcinoma of the penis. *Am. J. Surg. Pathol.* 25: 673–678, **2001**.

Bischof, O., Nacerddine, K., and Dejean, A. Human papillomavirus oncoprotein E7 targets the promyelocytic leukemia protein and circumvents cellular senescence via the Rb and p53 tumor suppressor pathways. *Mol. Cell. Biol.* 25: 1013–1024, **2005**.

Bjorge, T., Dillner, J., Anttila, T., Engeland, A., Hakulinen, T., Jellum, E., Lehtinen, M., Luostarinen, T., Paavonen, J., Pukkala, E., Sapp, M., Schiller, J., Youngman, L., and Thoresen, S. Prospective seroepidemiological study of role of human papillomavirus in non-cervical anogenital cancers. *Br. Med. J.* 315: 646–649, **1997**.

Blachon, S. and Demeret, C. The regulatory E2 proteins of human genital papillomaviruses are pro-apoptotic. *Biochemie* 85: 813–819, **2003**.

Black, P.H., Hartley, J.W., Rowe, W.P., and Huebner, R.J. Transformation of bovine tissue culture cells by bovine papilloma virus. *Nature* 199: 1016–1018, **1963**.

Boccardo, E., Noya, F., Broker, T.R., Chow, L.T., and Villa, L.L. HPV-18 confers resistance to TNF-α in organotypic cultures of human keratinocytes. *Virology* 328: 233–243, **2004**.

Bodaghi, S., Yamanegi, K., Xiao, S. Y., Da Costa, M., Palefsky, J.M., and Zheng, Z.M. Colorectal papillomavirus infection in patients with colorectal cancer. *Clin. Cancer Res.* 11: 2862–2867, **2005**.

Boiron, M., Levy, J.P., Thomas, M., Friedmann, J.C., and Bernard, J. Some properties of bovine papilloma virus. *Nature* 201: 423–424, **1964**.

Boner, W., Taylor, E.R., Tsirimonaki, E., Yamane, K., Campo, M.S., and Morgan, I.M. A functional interaction between the human papillomavirus 16 transcription/replication factor E2 and the DNA damage response protein TopBP1. *J. Biol. Chem.* 277: 22 297–22 302, **2002**.

Bonnez, W., Elswick, R.K., Jr., Bailey-Farchione, A., Hallahan, D., Bell, R., Isenberg, R., Stoler, M.H., and Reichman, R.C. Efficacy and safety of 0.5% podofilox solution in the treatment and suppression of anogenital warts. *Am. J. Med* . 96: 420–425, **1994**.

Bonne-Andrea, C., Santucci, S., Clertant, P., and Tillier, F. Bovine papillomavirus E1 protein binds specifically DNA polymerase á but not replication protein A. *J. Virol.* 69: 2341–2350, **1995**.

Bontkes, H.J., Walboomers. J.M.M., Meijer, C.J.L.M., Helmerhorst, T.J.M., and Stern, P.L. Specific HLA class I down-regulation is an early event in cervical dysplasia associated with clinical progression. *Lancet* 351: 187–188, **1998** .

Bontkes, H.J., de Gruijl, T.D., van den Muysenberg, A.J., Verheijen, R.H., Stukart, M.J., Meijer, C.J.M., Scheper, R.J., Stacey, S. N., Duggan-Keen, M.F., Stern, P.L., Man, S., Borysiewicz, L.K., Walboomers, J.M. Human papillomavirus type 16 E6/E7-specific cytotoxic T lymphocytes in women with cervical neoplasia. *Int. J. Cancer* 88: 92–98, **2000**.

Borysiewicicz, L.K., Fiander, A., Nimako, M., Man, S., Wilkinson, G.W., Westmoreland, D., Evans, A.S., Adams, M., Stacey, S. N., Boursnell, M.E., Rutherford, E., Hickling, J.K., and Inglis, S. C. A recombinant vaccinia virus encoding human papil-

lomavirus types 16 and 18, E6 and E7 proteins as immunotherapy for cervical cancer. *Lancet* 347: 1523–1527, **1996**.

Bosch, F.X. and Muñoz, N. Human papillomavirus and cervical neoplasia: a critical review of the epidemiological evidence. In: *Human Papillomaviruses and Cervical Cancer*. IARC Scientific Publications. No. 94: p. 148, **1989**.

Bosch, F., Schwarz, E., Boukamp, P., Fusenig, N.E., Bartsch, D., and zur Hausen, H. Suppression in vivo of human papillomavirus type 18 E6-E7 gene expression in nontumorigenic HeLa-fibroblast hybrid cells. *J. Virol.* 64: 4743–4754, **1990**.

Bosch, F.X., Muñoz, N., de Sanjose, S., Izarzugaza, I., Gili, M., Viladiu, P., Tormo, M.J., Moreo, P., Ascunce, N., Gonzalez, L.C., et al. Risk factors for cervical cancer in Colombia and Spain. *Int. J. Cancer.* 52: 750–758, **1992**.

Bosch, F.X., Manos, M.M., Muñoz, N., Sherman, M., Jansen, A.M., Peto, J., Schiffman, M.H., Moreno, V., Kurman, R., Shah, K.V., and Int. Biol. Study Cervical Cancer (IBSCC) Study Group. Prevalence of human papillomavirus in cervical cancer: a worldwide perspective. *J. Natl. Cancer Inst.* 87: 796–802, **1995**.

Boshart, M. and zur Hausen, H. Human papillomaviruses in Buschke-Löwenstein tumors: physical state of the DNA and identification of a tandem duplication in the noncoding region of a human papillomavirus 6 subtype. *J. Virol.* 58: 963–966, **1986**.

Boshart, M., Gissmann, L., Ikenberg, H., Kleinheinz, A., Scheurlen, W., and zur Hausen, H. A new type of papillomavirus DNA, its presence in genital cancer and in cell lines derived from genital cancer. *EMBO J.* 3, 1151–1157, **1984** .

Bothner, B., Lewis, W.S., DiGiammarino, E.L., Weber, J.D., Bothner, S. J., and Kriwacki, R.W. Defining the molecular basis of Arf and Hdm2 interactions. *J. Mol. Biol.* 314: 263–277, **2001**.

Bourgault Villada, I., Moyal Barracco, M., Ziol, M., Chaboissier, A., Barget, N., Berville, S., Paniel, B., Jullian, E., Clerici, T., Maillere, B., and Guillet, J.G. Spontaneous regression of grade 3 vulvar intraepithelial neoplasia associated with human papillomavirus-16-specific CD4(+) and CD8(+)

T-cell responses. *Cancer Res.* **2004** 64: 8761–8766, **2004**.

Boursnell, M.E., Rutherford, E., Hickling, J.K., Rollinson, E.A., Munro, A.J., Rolley, N., McLean, C.S., Borysiewicz, L.K., Vousden, K., and Inglis, S. C. Construction and characterization of a recombinant vaccinia virus expressing human papillomavirus proteins for immunotherapy of cervical cancer. *Vaccine* 14: 1485–1494, **1996**.

Bouvard, V., Storey, A., Pim, D., and Banks, L. Characterization of the human papillomavirus E2 protein: evidence of trans-activation and trans-repression in cervical keratinocytes. *EMBO J.* 13: 5451–5459, **1994a**.

Bouvard, V., Matlashewski, G., Gu, Z.M., Storey, A., and Banks, L. The human papillomavirus type 16 E5 gene cooperates with the E7 gene to stimulate proliferation of primary cells and increases viral gene expression. *Virology* 203: 73–80, **1994b**.

Bouwes Bavinck, J.N. and Berkhout, R.J. HPV infections and immunosuppression. *Clin. Dermatol.* 15: 427–437, **1997**.

Boxman, I.L., Berkhout, R.J., Mulder, L.H., Wolkers, M.C., Bouwes Bavinck, J.N., Vermeer, B.J., and ter Schegget, J. Detection of human papillomavirus DNA in plucked hairs from renal transplant recipients and healthy volunteers. *J. Invest. Dermatol .* 108: 712–715, **1997**.

Boxman, I.L., Russell, A., Mulder, L.H., Bavinck, J.N., ter Schegget, J., and Green, A. Case-control study in a subtropical Australian population to assess the relation between non-melanoma skin cancer and epidermodysplasia verruciformis human papillomavirus DNA in plucked eyebrow hairs. The Nambour Skin Cancer Prevention Study Group. *Int. J. Cancer* 86: 118–121, **2000**.

Bradlow, H.L., Hershcopf, R.E., and Fishman, J.F. Oestradiol 16 alpha-hydroxylase: a risk marker for breast cancer. *Cancer Surv.* 5: 573–583, **1986**.

Brady, C.S., Bartholomew, J.S., Burt, D.J., Duggan-Keen, M.F., Glenville, S., Telford, N. Little, A.M., Davidson, J.A., Jimenez, P., Ruiz-Cabello, F., Garrido, F., and Stern, P.L. Multiple mechanisms underlie HLA dysregulation in cervical cancer. *Tissue Antigens* 55: 401–411, **2000**.

Brake, T. and Lambert, P.F. Estrogen contributes to the onset, persistence, and malignant progression of cervical cancer in a human papillomavirus-transgenic mouse model. *Proc. Natl. Acad. Sci. USA* 102: 2490–2495, **2005**.

Brandsma, J.L. and Abramson, A.L. Association of papillomavirus with cancers of the head and neck. *Arch. Otolaryngol. Head Neck Surg.* 115: 621–625, **1989**.

Brandsma, J.L., Steinberg, B.M., Abramson, A.L., and Winkler, B. Presence of human papillomavirus type 16 related sequences in verrucous carcinoma of the larynx. *Cancer Res.* 46: 2185–2188, **1986**.

Bratthauer, G.L., Tvassoli, F.A., and O'Leary, T.J. Etiology of breast carcinoma: no apparent role for papillomavirus types 6/11/16/18. *Pathol. Res. Pract.* 188: 384–386, **1992**.

Braun, L., Dürst, M., Mikumo, R., and Gruppuso, P. Differential response of non-tumorigenic and tumorigenic human papillomavirus type 16-positive epithelial cells to transforming growth factor beta 1. *Cancer Res.* 50: 7324–7332, **1990** .

Brehm, A., Miska, E.A., McCance, D.J., Reid, J.L., Bannister, A.J., and Kouzarides, T. Retinoblastoma protein recruits histone deacetylase to repress transcription. *Nature* 391: 597–601, **1998**.

Breitburd, F., Croissant, O., and Orth, G. Expression of human papillomavirus type 1 E4 gene products in warts. Cancer Cells. *Cold Spring Harbor Laboratory* 5: 115–122, **1987**.

Breitburd, F., Kirnbauer, R., Hubbert, N.L., Nonnenmacher, B., Trin-Dingh-Desmarquet, C., Orth, G., Schiller, J.T., and Lowy, D.R. Immunization with virus-like particles from cottontail rabbit papillomavirus (CRPV) can protect against experimental CRPV infection. *J. Virol.* 69: 3959–3963, **1995**.

Bromberg-White, J.L., Sen, E., Alam, S., Bodily, J.M., and Meyers, C. Induction of the upstream regulatory region of human papillomavirus type 31 by dexamethasone is differentiation dependent. *J. Virol.* 77: 10975–10983, **2003**.

Brooks, L.A., Sullivan, A., O'Nions, J., Bell, A., Dunne, B., Tidy, J.A., Evans, D.J., Osin, P., Vousden, K.H., Gusterson, B., Farrell, P.J., Storey, A., Gasco, M., Saka, T., and

Crook, T. E7 proteins from oncogenic human papillomavirus types transactivate p73: role in cervical intraepithelial neoplasia. *Br. J. Cancer* 86: 263–268, **2002**.

Brouchet, L., Valmary, S., Dahan, M., Didier, A., Galateau-Salle, F., Brousset, P., and Degano, B. Detection of oncogenic virus genomes and gene products in lung carcinoma. *Br. J. Cancer* 92: 743–746, **2005**.

Brown, D.R., Bryan, J.,T., Schroeder, J.M., Robinson, T.S., Fife, K.H., Wheeler, C.M., Barr, E., Smith, P.R., Chiacchierini, L., DiCello, A., and Jansen, K.U. Neutralization of human papillomavirus type 11 (HPV-11) by serum from women vaccinated with yeast-derived HPV-11 L1 virus-like particles: correlation with competitive radioimmunoassay titer. *J. Infect. Dis.* 184: 1183–1186, **2001**.

Brown, V.L., Harwood, C.A., Crook, T., Cronin, J.G., Kelsell, D.P., and Proby, C.M. p16INK4a and p14ARF tumor suppressor genes are commonly inactivated in cutaneous squamous cell carcinoma. *J. Invest. Dermatol.* 122: 1284–1292, **2004**.

Bryce, S. D., Morrison, V., Craig, N.J., Forsyth, N.R., Fitzsimmons, S. A., Ireland, H., Cuthbert, A.P., Newbold, R.F., and Parkinson, E.K. A mortality gene(s) for the human adenocarcinoma line HeLa maps to a 130-kb region of human chromosome 4q22-q23. *Neoplasia* 4: 544–550, **2002**.

Bubb, V., McCance, D.J., and Schlegel, R. DNA sequence of the HPV-16 E5 ORF and the structural conservation of its encoded protein. *Virology* 163: 243–246, **1988**.

Bucala, R., Fishman, J., and Cerami, A. Formation of covalent adducts between cortisol and 16 alpha-hydroxyestrone and protein: possible role in the pathogenesis of cortisol toxicity and systemic lupus erythematosus. *Proc. Natl. Acad. Sci. USA* 79: 3320–3324, **1982**.

Buchwald, C., Franzmann, M.B., Jacobsen, G.K., Juhl, B.R., and Lindeberg, H. Carcinomas occurring in papillomas of the nasal septum associated with human papilloma virus (HPV). *Rhinology* 35: 74–78, **1997**.

Buchwald, C., Lindeberg, H., Pedersen, B.L., and Franzmann, M.B. Human papilloma virus and p53 expression associated with sinonasal papillomas: a Danish epidemiological study. *Laryngoscope* 111: 1104–1110, **2001**.

Buonaguro, F.M., Tornesello, M.L., Buonaguro, L., Del Gaudio, E., Beth-Giraldo, E., and Giraldo, G. Role of HIV as cofactor in HPV oncogenesis: in vitro evidences of virus interactions. *Antibiot. Chemother.* 46: 102–109, **1994**.

Bussiere, D.E., Kong, X., Egan, D.A., Walter, K., Holzman, T.F., Lindh, F., Robins, T., and Giranda, V.L. Structure of the E2 DNA-binding domain from human papillomavirus serotype 31 at 2.4 A. *Acta Crystallogr. D. Biol. Crystallogr* . 54: 1367–1376, **1998**.

Butterworth, C.E., Jr., Hatch, K.D., Soong, S. J., Cole, P., Tamura, T., Sauberlich, H.E., Borst, M., Macaluso, M., and Baker, V. Oral folic acid supplementation for cervical dysplasia: a clinical intervention trial. *Am. J. Obstet. Gynecol.* 166: 803–809, **1992**.

Butz, K. and Hoppe-Seyler, F. Transcriptional control of human papillomavirus (HPV) oncogene expression: composition of the HPV type 18 upstream regulatory region. *J. Virol.* 67: 6476–6486, **1993**.

Butz, K., Denk, C., Ullmann, A., Scheffner, M., and Hoppe-Seyler, F. Induction of apoptosis in human papillomavirus-positive cancer cells by peptide aptamers targeting the viral E6 oncoprotein. *Proc. Natl. Acad. Sci. USA* 97: 6693–6697, **2000**.

Buyru, N., Budak, M., Yazici, H., and Dalay, N. p53 gene mutations are rare in human papillomavirus-associated colon cancer. *Oncol. Rep.* 10: 2089–2092, **2003**.

Byrne, J.C., Tsao, M.S., Fraser, R.S., and Howley, P.M. Human papillomavirus-11 DNA in a patient with chronic laryngotracheobronchial papillomatosis and metastatic squamous-cell carcinoma of the lung. *N. Engl. J. Med.* 317: 873–878, **1987**.

Caldeira, S., Zehbe, I., Accardi, R., Malanchi, I., Dong, W., Giarre, M., de Villiers, E.-M., Filotico, R., Boukamp, P., and Tommasino, M. The E6 and E7 proteins of the cutaneous human papillomavirus type 38 display transforming properties. *J. Virol.* 77: 2195–2206, **2003**.

Campo, M.S., Moar, M.H., Sartirana, M.L., Kennedy, I.M., and Jarrett, W.F. The presence of bovine papillomavirus type 4 DNA is not required for the progression to, or the maintenance of, the malignant state in cancers of the alimentary canal in cattle. *EMBO J.* 4: 1819–1825, **1985**.

Campo, M.S., Grindlay, G.J., O'Neil, B.W., Chandrachud, L.M., McGarvie, G.M., and Jarrett, W.F.H. Prophylactic and therapeutic vaccination against a mucosal papillomavirus. *J. Gen. Virol.* 74: 945–953, **1993**.

Carozzi, F., Lombardi, F.C., Zendron, P., Confortini, M., Sani, C., Bisanzi, S., Pontenani, G., and Ciatto, S. Association of human papillomavirus with prostate cancer: analysis of a consecutive series of prostate biopsies. *Int. J. Biol. Markers* 19: 257–261, **2004**.

Cartin, W. and Alonso, A. The human papillomavirus HPV 2 a E5 protein localizes to the Golgi apparatus and modulates signal transduction. *Virology* 314: 572–579, **2003**.

Castellsague, X., Muñoz, N., De Stefani, E., Victora, C.G., Castelletto, R., Rolon, P.A. and Quintana, M.J. Independent and joint effects of tobacco smoking and alcohol drinking on the risk of esophageal cancer in men and women. *Int. J. Cancer* 82: 657–664, **1999**.

Castellsague, X., Muñoz, N., De Stefani, E., Victora, C.G., Castelletto, R., and Rolon, P.A. Influence of mate drinking, hot beverages and diet on esophageal cancer risk in South America. *Int. J. Cancer* 88: 658–664, **2000**.

Castle, P.E., Wacholder, S., Lorincz, A.T., Scott, D.R., Sherman, M.E., Glass, A.G., Rush, B.B., Schussler, J.E., and Schiffman, M. A prospective study of high grade cervical neoplasia risk among human papillomavirus-infected women. *J. Natl. Cancer Inst.* 94: 1406–1414, **2002**.

Chan, P.K., Chan, M.Y., Li, W.W., Chan, D.P., Cheung, J.L., and Cheng, A.F. Association of β-herpesviruses with the development of cervical cancer: bystanders or cofactors. *J. Clin. Pathol.* 54: 48–53, **2001**.

Chan, W.K., Klock, G., and Bernard, H.U. Progesterone and glucocorticoid response elements occur in the long control regions of several human papillomaviruses involved in anogenital neoplasia. *J. Virol.* 63: 3261–3269, **1989**.

Chang, F., Syrjänen, S., Shen, Q., Ji, H.X., and Syrjänen, K. Human papillomavirus (HPV) DNA in esophageal precancer lesions and squamous cell carcinomas from China. *Int. J. Cancer* 45: 21–25, **1990**.

Chang, F., Janutuinen, E., Pikkarainen, P., Syrjänen, S., and Syrjänen, K. Esophageal squamous cell papillomas. Failure to detect human papillomavirus DNA by in situ hybridization and polymerase chain reaction. *Scand. J. Gastroenterol.* 26: 535–543, **1991**.

Chang, F., Syrjänen, S., Shen, Q., Wang, L., Wang, D., and Syrjänen, K. Human papillomavirus involvement in esophageal precancerous lesions and squamous cell carcinomas as evidenced by microscopy and different DNA techniques. *Scand. J. Gastroenterol* . 27: 553–563, **1992**.

Chellappan, S., Kraus, V.B., Kroger, B., Münger, K., Howley, P.M., Phelps, W.C., and Nevins, J.R. Adenovirus E1A, simian virus 40 tumor antigen, and human papillomavirus E7 protein share the capacity to disrupt the interaction between transcription factor E2F and the retinoblastoma gene product. *Proc. Natl. Acad. Sci. USA* 89: 4549–4553, **1992**.

Chen, C.H., Wang, T.L., Hung, C.F., Yang, Y., Young, R.A., Pardoll, D.M., and Wu, T.C. Enhancement of DNA vaccine potency by linkage of antigene gene to an HSP70 gene. *Cancer Res.* 60: 1035–1042, **2000**.

Chen, E.Y., Howley, P.M., Levinson, A.D., and Seeburg, P.H. The primary structure and genetic organization of the bovine papillomavirus type 1 genome. *Nature* 299: 529–534, **1982**.

Chen, J.J., Hong, Y., Rustamzadeh, E., Baleja, J.D., and Androphy, E.J. Identification of an α-helical motif sufficient for association with papillomavirus E6. *J. Biol. Chem.* 273: 13 537–13 544, **1998**.

Cheng, Y.W., Chiou, H.L., Sheu, G.T., Hsieh, L.L., Chen, T., Chen, C.Y., Su, J.M., and Lee, H. The association of human papillomavirus 16/18 infection with lung cancer among nonsmoking Taiwanese women. *Cancer Res.* 61: 2799–2803, **2001** .

Chiang, C.M., Ustav, M., Stenlund, A., Ho, T.F., Broker, T.R., and Chow, L.T. Viral E1 and E2 proteins support replication of homologous and heterologous papillomaviral origins. *Proc. Natl. Acad. Sci. USA* 89: 5799–5803, **1992**.

Childers, J.M., Chu, J., Voigt, L.F., Feigl, P., Tamimi, H.K., Franklin, E.W., Alberts, D.S., and Meyskens, F.L., Jr. Chemoprevention of cervical cancer with folic acid: a phase III Southwest Oncology Group Intergroup study. *Cancer Epidemiol. Biomarkers Prev.* 4: 155–159, **1995**.

Chin-Hong, P.V., Vittinghoff, E., Cranston, R.D., Buchbinder, S., Cohen, D., Colfax, G., Da Costa, M., Darragh, T., Hess, E., Judson, F., Koblin, B., Madison, M., and Palefsky, J.M. Age-Specific prevalence of anal human papillomavirus infection in HIV-negative sexually active men who have sex with men: the EXPLORE study. *J. Infect. Dis.* 190: 2070–2076, **2004**.

Chow, L.T. and Broker, T.R. Papillomavirus DNA replication. *Intervirology* 37: 150–158, **1994**.

Chow, L.T., Nasseri, M., Wollinski, S. M., and Broker, T.R. Human papillomavirus types 6 and 11 mRNAs from genital condylomata acuminata. *J. Virol.* 61: 2581–2588, **1987 a**.

Chow, L.T., Reilly, S. S., Broker, T.R., and Taichman, L.B. Identification and mapping of human papillomavirus type 1 RNA transcripts recovered from plantar warts and infected epithelial cell cultures. *J. Virol.* 61: 1913–1918, **1987 b**.

Christensen, N.D., Kreider, J.W., Cladel, N.M., and Galloway, D.A. Immunological cross-reactivity to laboratory-produced HPV-11 virions of polysera raised against bacterially derived fusion proteins and synthetic peptides of HPV-6 b and HPV-16 capsid proteins. *Virology* 175: 1–9, **1990**.

Ciccolini, F., Di Pasquale, G., Carlotti, F., Crawford, L., and Tommasino, M. Functional studies of E7 proteins from different HPV types. *Oncogene* 9: 2633–2638, **1994**.

Clark, M.A., Hartley, A., and Geh, J.I. Cancer of the anal canal. *Lancet Oncol.* 5: 149–157, **2004**.

Clarke, P. and Clements J.B. Mutagenesis occurring following infection with herpes simplex virus does not require virus replication. *Virology* 182: 597–606, **1991**.

Classon, M. and Dyson, N. p107 and p130: versatile proteins with interesting pockets. *Exp. Cell Res.* 264: 135–147, **2001**.

Conrad, M., Bubb, V.J., and Schlegel, R. The human papillomavirus type 6 and 16 E5 proteins are membrane-associated proteins which associate with the 16-kilodalton pore-forming protein. *J. Virol.* 67: 6170–6178, **1993**.

Cook, J.R., Hill, D.A., Humphrey, P.A., Pfeifer, J.D., and El-Mofty, S. K. Squamous cell carcinoma arising in recurrent respiratory papillomatosis with pulmonary involvement: emerging common pattern of clinical features and human papillomavirus serotype association. *Mod. Pathol.* 13: 914–918, **2000**.

Cox, J.T., Petry, K.U., Rylander, E., and Roy, M. Using imiquimod for genital warts in female patients. *J. Womens Health* 13: 265–271, **2004**.

Craven, S. E. and Bredt, D.S. PDZ proteins organize synaptic signaling pathways. *Cell* 93: 495–498, **1998**.

Crawford, L.V. and Crawford, E.M. A comparative study of polyoma and papilloma viruses. *Virology* 21: 258–263, **1963**.

Cripe, T.P., Haugen, T.H., Turk, J.P., Tabatabai, F., Schmid, P.G., Dürst, M., Gissmann, L., Roman, A., and Turek, L.P. Transcriptional regulation of the human papillomavirus-16 E6-E7 promoter by a keratinocyte-dependent enhancer, and by viral E2 trans-activator and repressor gene products: implications for cervical carcinogenesis. *EMBO J.* 6: 3745–3753, **1987**.

Critchlow, C.W. and Koutsky, L.A. Epidemiology of human papillomavirus infection. In: Midel, A. (Ed.), *Genital Warts. Human Papillomavirus Infection.* London, Edward Arnold Publ., pp. 53–81, **1995**.

Crook, T., Storey, A., Almond, N., Osborn, K., and Crawford, L. Human papillomavirus type 16 cooperates with activated ras and fos oncogenes in the hormone-dependent transformation of primary mouse cells. *Proc. Natl. Acad. Sci. USA* 85: 8820–8824, **1988**.

Crum, C.P., Ikenberg, H., Richart, R.M., and Gissmann, L. Human papillomavirus type 16 and early cervical neoplasia. *N. Engl. J. Med.* 310: 880–883, **1984**.

Csaszar, A. and Abel, T. Receptor polymorphisms and diseases. *Eur. J. Pharmacol.* 414: 9–22, **2001**.

Cubilla, A.L., Meijer, C.J.M., and Young, R.H. Morphological features of epithelial abnormalities and precancerous lesions of the penis. *Scand. J. Urol. Nephrol. Suppl.* 205: 215–219, **2000**.

Czerwenka, K., Heuss, F., Hosmann, J.W., Manavi, M., Lu, Y., Jelincic, D., and Kubista, E. Human papilloma virus DNA: a factor in the pathogenesis of mammary Paget's disease? *Breast Cancer Res. Treat.* 41: 51–57, **1996**.

Dahlgren, L., Dahlstrand, H.M., Lindquist, D., Hogmo, A., Bjornestal, L., Lindholm, J., Lundberg, B., Dalianis, T., and Munck-Wikland, E. Human papillomavirus is more common in base of tongue than in mobile tongue cancer and is a favorable prognostic factoring base of tongue cancer patients. *Int. J. Cancer* 112: 1015–1019, **2004**.

Dale, C.J., Liu, X.S., De Rose, R., Purcell, D.F., Anderson, J., Xu, Y., Leggatt, G.R., Frazer, I.H., and Kent, S. J. Chimeric human papilloma virus-simian/human immunodeficiency virus virus-like-particle vaccines: immunogenicity and protective efficacy in macaques. *Virology* 301: 176–187, **2002**.

Daling, J.R., Madeleine, M.M., Schwartz, S. M., Shera, K.A., Carter, J.J., McKnight, B., Porter, P.L., Galloway, D.A., McDougall, J.K., and Tamimi, H. A population-based study of squamous cell vaginal cancer: HPV and cofactors. *Gynecol. Oncol* . 84: 263–270, **2002**.

Damin, A.P.S., Karam, R., Zettler, C.G., Caleffi, M., and Alexandre, C.O.P. Evidence for an association of human papillomavirus and breast carcinomas. *Breast Cancer Res. Treat.* 84: 131–137, **2004**.

Daniel, B., Mukherjee, G., Seshadri, L., Vallikad, E., and Krishna, S. Changes in the physical state and expression of human papillomavirus type 16 in the progression of cervical intraepithelial neoplasia lesions analysed by PCR. *J. Gen. Virol.* 76: 2589–2593, **1995**.

Danos, O., Katinka, M., and Yaniv, M. Human papillomavirus 1a complete DNA sequence: a novel type of genome organization among papovaviridae. *EMBO J.* 1: 231–236, **1982**.

Da Silva, D.M., Eiben, G.L., Fausch, S. C., Wakabayashi, M.T., Rudolf, M.P., Velders, M.P., and Kast, W.M. Cervical cancer vaccines: emerging concepts and developments. *J. Cell Physiol.* 186: 169–182, **2001**.

Davidson, E.J., Boswell, C.M., Sehr, P., Pawlita, M., Tomlinson, A.E., McVey, R.J., Dobson, J., Roberts, J.S., Hickling, J., Kitchener, H.C., Stern, P.L. Immunological and clinical responses in women with vulval intraepithelial neoplasia vaccinated with a vaccinia virus encoding human papillomavirus 16/18 oncoproteins. *Cancer Res.* 63: 6032–6041, **2003**.

Davy, C.E., Jackson, D.J., Raj, K., Peh, W.L., Southern, S. A., Das, P., Sorathia, R., Laskey, P., Middleton, K., Nakahara, T., Wang, Q., Masterson, P.J., Lambert, P.F., Cuthill, S., Millar, J.B., and Doorbar, J. Human papillomavirus type 16 E1 E4-induced G2 arrest is associated with cytoplasmic retention of active Cdk1/cyclin B1 complexes. *J. Virol.* 79: 3998–4011, **2005**.

D'Costa, J., Saranath, D., Dedhia, P., Sanghvi, V., and Mehta, A.R. Detection of HPV-16 genome in human oral cancers and potentially malignant lesions from India. *Oral Oncol.* 34: 413–420, **1998**.

Deacon, J.M., Evans, C.D., Yule, R., Desai, M., Binns, W., Taylor, C., and Peto, J. Sexual behaviour and smoking as determinants of cervical HPV infection and of CIN3 among those infected: a case-control study nested within the Manchester cohort. *Br. J. Cancer* 83: 1565–1572, **2000**.

de Clercq, E. Clinical potential of the acyclic nucleoside phosphonates cidofovir, adefovir, and tenofovir in treatment of DNA virus and retrovirus infections. *Clin. Microbiol. Rev.* 16: 569–596, **2003**.

de Gruijl, T.D., Bontkes, H.J., Walboomers, J.M.M., Stukart, M.J., Doekhie, M.S., Remmink, A.J., Helmerhorst, T.J., Verheijen, R.H., Duggan-Keen, M.F., Stern, P.L., Meijer, C.J.M., and Scheper, R.J. Differential T helper cell responses to human papillomavirus type 16 E7 related to viral clearance or persistence in patients with cervical neoplasia: a longitudinal study. *Cancer Res.* 58: 1700–1706, **1998**.

Delius, H. van Ranst, M.A., Jenson, A.B., zur Hausen, H., and Sundberg, J.P. Canine oral papillomavirus genome sequence: a unique 1.5 kb intervening sequence between E2 and L2 open reading frames. *Virology* 204: 447–452, **1994**.

Dell, G., Wilkinson, K.W., Tranter, R., Parish, J., Leo Brady, R., and Gaston, K. Comparison of the structure and DNA-binding properties of the E2 proteins from an oncogenic and a non-oncogenic human papillomavirus. *J. Mol. Biol.* 334: 979–991, **2003**.

del Mar Pena, L.M. and Laimins, L.A. Differentiation-dependent chromatin rearrangement coincides with activation of human papillomavirus type 31 late gene expression. *J. Virol.* 75: 10005–10013, **2001**.

Delvenne, P., al-Saleh, W., Gilles, C., Thiry, A., and Boniver, J. Inhibition of growth of normal and human papillomavirus-transformed keratinocytes in monolayer and organotypic cultures by interferon-γ and tumor necrosis factor-α. *Am. J. Pathol.* 146: 589–598, **1995**.

Demeret, C., Desaintes, C.M.Y., and Thierry, F. Different mechanisms contribute to the E2-mediated transcriptional repression of human papillomavirus type 18 viral oncogenes. *J. Virol.* 71: 9343–9349, **1997**.

Deng, W., Jin, G., Lin, B.Y., Van Tine, B.A., Broker, T.R., and Chow, L.T. mRNA splicing regulates human papillomavirus type 11 E1 protein production and DNA replication. *J. Virol.* 77: 10 213–10 226, **2003**.

Deng, W., Lin, B.Y., Jin, G., Wheeler, C.G., Ma, T., Harper, J.W., Broker, T.R., and Chow, L.T. Cyclin/CDK regulates the nucleocytoplasmic localization of the human papillomavirus E1 DNA helicase. *J. Virol.* 78: 13 954–13 965, **2004**.

Denis, M., Chadee, K., and Matlashewski, G.J. Macrophage killing of human papillomavirus type 16-transformed cells. *Virology* 170: 342–345, **1989**.

Dennis, L.K. and Dawson, D.V. Meta-analysis of measures of sexual activity and prostate cancer. *Epidemiology* 13: 72–79, **2002**.

Deshpande, A., Nolan, J.P., White, P.S., Valdez, Y.E., Hunt, W.C., Peyton, C.L., and Wheeler, C.M. TNF-α promoter polymorphisms and susceptibility to human papillomavirus 16-associated cervical cancer. *J. Infect. Dis.* 191: 969–976, **2005**.

de Vet, H.C., Knipschild, P.G., Grol, M.E., Schouten, H.J., Sturmans, F. The role of beta-carotene and other dietary factors in the aetiology of cervical dysplasia: results of a case-control study. *Int. J. Epidemiol.* 20: 603–610, **1991** .

de Villiers, E.-M. Taxonomic classification of papillomaviruses. *Papillomavirus Rep.* 12: 57–63, **2001**.

de Villiers, E.-M. Relationship between steroid hormone contraceptives and HPV, cervical intraepithelial neoplasia and cervical carcinoma. *Int. J. Cancer* 103: 705–708, **2003**.

de Villiers, E.-M., Gissmann, L., and zur Hausen, H. Molecular cloning of viral DNA from human genital warts. *J. Virol.* 40: 932–935, **1981**.

de Villiers, E.-M. Hirsch-Behnam, A., von Knebel Doeberitz, C., and zur Hausen, H. Two newly identified human papillomavirus types (HPV 40 and 57) isolated from mucosal lesions. *Virology* 171: 248–259, **1989**.

de Villiers, E.-M., Lavergne, D., McLaren, K., and Benton, E.C. Prevailing papillomavirus types in non-melanoma carcinomas of the skin in renal allograft recipients. *Int. J. Cancer* 73: 356–361, **1997**.

de Villiers, E.-M., Lavergne, D., Chang, F., Syrjänen, K., Tosi, P., Cintorino, M., Santopietro, R., and Syrjänen, S. An interlaboratory study to determine the presence of human papillomavirus DNA in esophageal carcinoma from China. *Int. J. Cancer* 81: 225–228, **1999**.

de Villiers, E.-M., Fauquet, C., Broker, T.R., Bernard, H.-U., and zur Hausen, H. Classification of papillomaviruses. *Virology* 324: 17–27, **2004 a**.

de Villiers, E.-M., Gunst, K., Stein, H., and Scherübl, H. Esophageal squamous cell cancer in patients with head and neck cancer: prevalence of human papillomavirus DNA sequences. *Int. J. Cancer* 109: 253–258, **2004 b**.

de Villiers, E.-M., Sandstroem, R.E., zur Hausen, H., and Buck, C.E. Presence of papillomavirus sequences in condylomatous lesions of the mamillae and in invasive carcinoma of the breast. *Breast Cancer Res.* 7: R1–11, **2005**.

Dianzani, C., Bucci, M., Pierangeli, A., Calvieri, S., and Degener, A.M. Association of human papillomavirus type 11 with carcinoma of the penis. *Urology* 51: 1046–1048, **1998**.

Dickson, M.A., Hahn, W.C., Ino, Y., Ronfard, V., Wu, J.Y., Weinberg, R.A., Louis, D.N., Li, F.P., and Rheinwald, J.G. Human keratinocytes that express hTERT and also bypass a p16[INK4a]-enforced mechanism that limits life span become immortal yet retain normal growth and differentiation characteristics. *Mol. Cell. Biol.* 20: 1436–1447, **2000**.

Di Leonardo, A., Venuti, R., and Marcante, M.L. Human papillomavirus in breast cancer. *Breast Cancer Res. Treat.* 21: 95–100, **1992**.

Dillner, J., Knekt, P., Boman, J., Lehtinen, M., Af Geijersstam, V., Sapp, M., Schiller, J.,

Maatela, J., and Aromaa, A. Seroepidemiological association between human papillomavirus infection and risk of prostate cancer. *Int. J. Cancer* 75: 564–567, **1998**.

DiLorenzo, T.P., Tamsen, A., Abramson, A.L., and Steinberg, B.M. Human papillomavirus type 6a DNA in the lung carcinoma of a patient with recurrent laryngeal papillomatosis is characterized by a partial duplication. *J. Gen. Virol.* 73: 423–428, **1992**.

DiMaio, D., Guralski, D., and Schiller, J.T. Translation of open reading frame E5 of bovine papillomavirus is required for its transforming activity. *Proc. Natl. Acad. Sci. USA* 83: 1797–1801, **1986**.

Disbrow, G.L., Hanover, J.A., and Sclegel, R. Endoplasmic reticulum-localized human papillomavirus type 16 E5 protein alters endosomal pH but not trans-Golgi pH. *J. Virol.* 79: 5829–5846, **2005**.

Doorbar, J., Campbell, D., Grand, R.J.A., and Gallimore, P.H. Identification of the human papillomavirus-1a E4 gene products. *EMBO J.* 5: 355–362, **1986**.

Doorbar, J., Parton, A., Hartley, K., Banks, L., Crook, T., Stanley, M., and Crawford, L. Detection of novel splicing patterns in a HPV16-containing keratinocyte cell line. *Virology* 178: 254–262, **1990**.

Doorbar, J., Ely, S., Sterling, J., and Crawford, L. Specific interactions between HPV 16 E1-E4 and cytokeratin results in collapse of the epithelial cell intermediate filament network. *Nature* 352: 824–827, **1991**.

Doorbar, J., Elston, R.C., Napthine, S., Raj, K., Medcalf, E., Jackson, D., Coleman, N., Griffin, H.M., Masterson, P., Stacey, S., Mengistu, Y., and Dunlop, J. The E1E4 protein of human papillomavirus type 16 associates with a putative RNA helicase through sequences in its C terminus. *J. Virol.* 74: 10081–10095, **2000**.

Dorruci, M., Suligoi, B., Serraino, D., Tirelli, U., Rezza, G., the Italian HIV Seroconversion Study. Incidence of invasive cervical cancer in a cohort of HIV-seropositive women before and after the introduction of highly active antiretroviral therapy. *J. Acquir. Immune Defic. Syndr.* 26: 377–380, **2001**.

Dostatni, N., Thierry, F., and Yaniv, M. A dimmer of BPV-1 E2 containing a protease resistant core interacts with its DNA target. *EMBO J.* 7: 3807–3816, **1988**.

Dostatni, N., Lambert, P.F., Sousa, R., Ham, J., Howley, P.M., and Yaniv, M. The functional BPV-1 E2 trans-activating protein can act as a repressor by preventing formation of the initiation complex. *Genes Dev.* 5: 1657–1671, **1991** .

Duensing, S. and Münger, K. The human papillomavirus type 16 E6 and E7 oncoproteins independently induce numerical and structural chromosome instability. *Cancer Res.* 62: 7075–7082, **2002**.

Duensing, S. and Münger, K. Human papillomavirus type 16 E7 oncoprotein can induce abnormal centrosome duplication through a mechanism independent of inactivation of retinoblastoma protein family members. *J. Virol.* 77: 12331–12335, **2003**.

Duensing, S., Duensing, A., Flores, E.R., Do, A., Lambert, P.F., and Münger, K. Centrosome abnormalities and genomic instability by episomal expression of human papillomavirus type 16 in raft cultures of human keratinocytes. *J. Virol.* 75: 7712–7716, **2001**.

Duff, R. and Rapp, F. Properties of hamster embryo fibroblasts transformed in vitro after exposure to ultraviolet irradiated herpes simplex virus type 2. *J. Virol.* 8: 469–474, **1971**.

Dürst, M., Gissmann, L., Ikenberg, H., and zur Hausen, H. A papillomavirus DNA from a cervical carcinoma and its prevalence in cancer biopsy samples from different geographic regions. *Proc. Natl. Acad. Sci. USA* 80: 3812–3815, **1983** .

Dürst, M., Dzarlieva-Petrusevska, R.T., Boukamp, P., Fusenig, N.E., and Gissmann, L. Molecular and cytogenetic analysis of immortalized human primary keratinocytes obtained after transfection with human papillomavirus type 16 DNA. *Oncogene* 1: 251–256, **1987**.

Dürst, M., Gallahan, D., Jay, G., and Rhim, J.S. Glucocorticoid-enhanced neoplastic transformation of human keratinocytes by human papillomavirus type 16 and an activated ras oncogene. *Virology* 173: 767–771, **1989**.

Dürst, M., Bosch, F.X., Glitz, D., Schneider, A., and zur Hausen, H. Inverse relationship between human papillomavirus (HPV) type 16 early gene expression and cell differentiation in nude mouse epithelial cysts and tumors induced by HPV-positive human cell lines. *J. Virol.* 65: 796–804, **1991**.

Dürst, M., Glitz, D., Schneider, A., and zur Hausen, H. Human papillomavirus type 16 (HPV16) gene expression and DNA replication in cervical neoplasia: analysis by in situ hybridization. *Virology* 189: 132–140, **1992**.

Dyson, N., Howley, P.M., Münger, K., and Harlow, E. The human papilloma virus-16 E7 oncoprotein is able to bind to the retinoblastoma gene product. *Science* 243: 934–937, **1989**.

Dyson, N., Guida, P., Münger, K., and Harlow, E. Homologous sequences in adenovirus E1A and human papillomavirus E7 proteins mediate interaction with the same set of cellular proteins. *J. Virol.* 66: 6893–6902, **1992**.

Edmonds, C. and Vousden, K.H. A point mutational analysis of human papillomavirus type 16 E7 protein. *J. Virol.* 63: 2650–2656, **1989**.

Edwards, L., Ferenczy, A., Eron, L., Baker, D., Owens, M.L., Fox, T.L., Hougham, A.J., and Schmitt, K.A. Self-administered topical 5% imiquimod cream for external anogenital warts. HPV Study Group. Human Papilloma Virus. *Arch. Dermatol*. 134: 25–30, **1998**.

el-Deiry, W.S., Tokino, T., Velculescu, V.E., Levy, D.B., Parsons, R., Lin, D.M., Mercer, W.E., Kinzler, K.W.V., and Vogelstein, B. WAF1, a potential mediator of p53 tumor suppression. *Cell* 75: 817–825, **1993**.

El-Mofty, S. K. and Lu, D.W. Prevalence of human papillomavirus type 16 DNA in squamous cell carcinoma of the palatine tonsil, and not the oral cavity, in young patients: a distinct clinicopathologic and molecular disease entity. *Am. J. Surg. Pathol.* 27: 1463–1470, **2003**.

Elson, D.A., Riley, R.R., Lacey, A., Thordarson, G., Talamantes, F.J., and Arbeit, J.M. Sensitivity of the cervical transformation zone to estrogen-induced squamous carcinogenesis. *Cancer Res.* 60: 1267–1275, **2000**.

Elston, R.C., Naphtine, S., and Doorbar, J. The identification of a conserved binding motif within human papillomavirus type 16 E6 binding peptides E6AP and E6BP. *J. Gen. Virol.* 79: 371–374, **1998**.

Emeny, R.T., Wheeler, C.M., Jansen, K.U., Hunt, W.C., Fu, T.M., Smith, J.F., MacMullen, S., Esser, M.T., and Paliard, X. Priming of human papillomavirus type 11-specific humoral and cellular immune responses in college-aged women with a virus-like particle vaccine. *J. Virol.* 76: 7832–7842, **2002**.

Emge, L.A. Estrogen imbalance and uterine cancer. *Trans. Pac. Coast Obstet. Gynecol. Soc.* 17: 185–194, **1949**.

Enemark, E.J., Chen, G., Vaughn, D.E., Stenlund, A., and Joshua-Tor, L. Crystal structure of the DNA binding domain of the replication initiation protein E1 from papillomavirus. *Mol. Cell.* 6: 149–158, **2000**.

Enemark, E.J., Stenlund, A., and Joshua-Tor, L. Crystal structure of two intermediates in the assembly of the papillomavirus replication initiation complex. *EMBO J.* 21: 1487–1496, **2002**.

Eng, H.L., Lin, T.M., Chen, S.,Y., Wu, S. M., and Chen, W.J. Failure to detect human papillomavirus DNA in malignant epithelial neoplasms of conjunctiva by polymerase chain reaction. *Am. J. Clin. Pathol.* 117: 429–436, **2002**.

Euvrard, S., Chardonnet, Y., Pouteil-Noble, C., Kanitakis, J., Chignol, M.C., Thivolet, J., and Touraine, J.L. Association of skin malignancies with various and multiple carcinogenic human papillomaviruses in renal transplant recipients. *Cancer* 72: 2198–2206, **1993**.

Evans, T.G., Bonnez, W., Rose, R.C., Koenig, S., Demeter, L., Suzich, J.A., O'Brien, D., Campbell, M., White, W.I., Balsley, J., and Reichman, R.C. A phase 1 study of a recombinant virus-like particle vaccine against human papillomavirus type 11 in healthy adult volunteers. *J. Infect. Dis.* 183: 1485–1493, **2001**.

Eymin, B., Karayan, L., Seite, P., Brambilla, C., Brambilla, E., Larsen, C.J., and Gazzeri, S. Human ARF binds E2F1 and inhibits its transcriptional activity. *Oncogene* 20: 1033–1041, **2001**.

Fairley, C.K., Chen, S., Tabrizi, S. N., Leeton, K., Quinn, M.A., and Garland, S. M. The absence of genital human papillomavirus DNA in virginal women. *Int. J. STD AIDS* 3: 414–417, **1992**.

Fairley, C.K., Tabrizi, S. N., Chen, S., Baghurst, P., Young, H., Quinn, M., Medley, G., McNeill, J.J., and Garland, S. M. A randomized clinical trial of β-carotene vs. placebo for the treatment of cervical HPV infection. *Int. J. Gynecol. Cancer* 6: 225–230, **1996**.

Favre, M., Breitburd, F., Croissant, O., and Orth, G. Chromatin-like structures obtained after alkaline disruption of bovine and human papillomaviruses. *J. Virol.* 21: 1205–1209, 1977.

Favre-Bonvin, A., Reynaud, C., Kretz-Remy, C., and Jalinot, P. Human papillomavirus type 18 E6 protein binds the cellular PDZ protein TIP-2/GIPC, which is involved in transforming growth factor beta signaling and triggers its degradation by the proteasome. *J. Virol.* 79: 4229–4237, **2005**.

Feltkamp, M.C., Broer, R., di Summa, F.M., Struijk, L., van der Meijden, E., Verlaan, B.P., Westendorp, R.G., ter Schegget, J., Spaan, W.J., and Bouwes Bavinck, J.N. Seroreactivity to epidermodysplasia verruciformis-related human papillomavirus types is associated with nonmelanoma skin cancer. *Cancer Res.* 63: 2695–2700, **2003**.

Ferenczy, A., Bergeron, C., and Richart, R.M. Carbon dioxide laser energy disperses human papillomavirus desoxyribonucleic acid onto treatment fields. *Am. J. Obstet. Gynecol.* 163: 1271–1274, **1990**.

Fernández, L., Galán, Y., Jiménez, R., Guttiérrez, Á., Guerra, M., Pereda, C., Alonso, C., Riboli, E., Agudo, A., and González, C. Sexual behaviour, history of sexually transmitted diseases, and the risk of prostate cancer: a case-control study from Cuba. *Int. J. Epidemiol.* 34: 193–197, **2005**.

Ferrara, A., Nonn, M., Sehr, P., Schreckenberger, C., Pawlita, M., Dürst, M., Schneider, A., Kaufmann, A.M. Dendritic cell-based tumor vaccine for cervical cancer II: results of a clinical pilot study in 15 individual patients. *J. Cancer Res. Clin. Oncol.* 129: 521–530, **2003**.

Filippova, M., Parkhurst, L., and Duerksen-Hughes, P.J. The human papillomavirus E6 protein binds to Fas-associated death domain and protects cells from Fas-triggered apoptosis. *J. Biol. Chem.* 279: 25729–25744, **2004** .

Finbow, M.E. and Pitts, J.D. Is the gap-junction channel – the connexon – made of connexin or ductin? *J. Cell Sci.* 106: 123–132, **1993**.

Follen, M., Atkinson, E.N., Schottenfeld, D., Maplica, A., West, L., Lippman, S., Zou, C., Hittelman, W., Lotan, R., and Hong, W.K. A randomized clinical trial of 4-hydroxyphenylretinamide for high-grade squamous intraepithelial lesions of the cervix. *Clin. Cancer Res.* 7: 3356–3365, **2001**.

Forslund, O., Ly, H., Reid, C., and Higgins, G. A broad spectrum of human papillomavirus types is present in the skin of Australian patients with non-melanoma skin cancers and solar keratosis. *Br. J. Dermatol.* 149: 64–73, **2003**.

Forslund, O., Lindelof, B., Hradil, E., Nordin, P., Stenquist, B., Kirnbauer, R., Slupetzky, K., and Dillner, J. High prevalence of cutaneous human papillomavirus DNA on the top of skin tumors but not in 'stripped' biopsies from the same tumors. *J. Invest. Dermatol.* 123: 388–394, **2004**.

Fortunato, E.A. and Spector, D.H. p53 and RPA are sequestered in viral replication centers in the nuclei of cells infected with human cytomegalovirus. *J. Virol.* 72: 2033–2039, **1998**.

Foster, S. A., Wong, D.J., Barrett, M.T., and Galloway, D.A. Inactivation of p16 in human mammary epithelial cells by CpG island methylation. *Mol. Cell. Biol.* 18: 1793–1801, **1998**.

Fouret, P., Monceaux, G., Temam, S., Lacourreye, L. and St. Guily, J.L. Human papillomavirus in head and neck squamous cell carcinomas in nonsmokers. *Arch. Otolaryngol. Head Neck Surg.* 123: 513–516, **1997**.

Frame, M.C. Src in cancer: deregulation and consequences for cell behaviour. *Biochim. Biophys. Acta* 1602: 114–130, **2002**.

Franceschi, S. The IARC commitment to cancer prevention: the example of papillomavirus and cervical cancer. *Recent Results Cancer Res.* 166: 277–297, **2005**.

Franceschi, S., Muñoz, N., Bosch, X.F., Snijders, P.J., and Walboomers, J.M. Human papillomavirus and cancers of the upper aerodigestive tract: a review of epidemiological and experimental evidence. *Cancer Epidemiol. Biomarkers Prev.* 5: 567–75, **1996**.

French, A.L., Kirstein, L.M., Massad, L.S., Semba, R.D., Minkoff, H., Landesman, S., Palefsky, J., Young, M., Anastos, K., and Cohen, M.H. Association of vitamin A deficiency with cervical squamous intraepithelial lesions in human immunodeficiency virus-infected women. *J. Infect. Dis.* 182: 1084–1089, **2000**.

Frenkel, N., Roizman, B., Cassai, E., and Nahmias, A. A DNA fragment of herpes simplex 2 and its transcription in human cervical cancer tissue. *Proc. Natl Acad. Sci. USA* 69: 3784–3789, **1972**.

Friedmann, J.C., Lévy, J.-P., Lasneret, J., Thomas, M., Boiron, M., and Bernard, J. Induction de fibromes sous-cutanés chez le hamster doré par inoculation d'extraits acellulaires de papillomes bovines. *C. R. Hebd. Seances Acad. Sci. (Paris)* 257: 2328–2331, **1963**.

Frisch, M., Hjalgrim, H., Jaeger, A.B., and Biggar, R.J. Changing patterns of tonsillar squamous cell carcinoma in the United States. *Cancer Causes Control* 11: 489–495, **2000 a**.

Frisch, M., Biggar, R.J., and Goedert, J.J. Human papillomavirus-associated cancers in patients with human immunodeficiency virus infection and acquired immunodeficiency syndrome. *J. Natl. Cancer Inst.* 92: 1500–1510, **2000 b**.

Funk, J.O., Waga, S., Harry, J.B., Espling, E., Stillman, B., and Galloway D.A. Inhibition of CDK activity and PCNA-dependent DNA replication by p21 is blocked by interaction with the HPV-16 E7 oncoprotein. *Genes Dev.* 11: 2090–2100, **1997**.

Furuta, Y., Takasu, T., Asai, T., Shinohara, T., Sawa, H., Nagashima, K., and Inuyama, Y. Detection of human papillomavirus DNA in carcinomas of the nasal cavities and paranasal sinuses by polymerase chain reaction. *Cancer* 69: 353–357, **1992**.

Gaiotti, D., Chung, J., Iglesias, M., Nees, M., Baker, P.D., Evans, C.H., and Woodworth, C.D. Tumor necrosis factor-α promotes human papillomavirus (HPV) E6/E7 RNA expression and cyclin-dependent kinase activity in HPV-immortalized keratinocytes by a ras-dependent pathway. *Mol. Carcinog.* 27: 97–109, **2000**.

Garden, J.M., O'Banion, M.K., Shelnitz, M.S., Pinski, K.S., Bakus, A.D., Reichmann, M.E., and Sundberg, J.P. Papillomavirus in the vapor of carbon-dioxide laser-treated verrucae. *J. Am. Med. Assoc.* 259: 1299–1202, **1988**.

Gassenmaier, A., Fuchs, P., Schell, H., and Pfister, H. Papillomavirus DANN in warts of immunosuppressed renal allograft recipients. *Arch. Dermatol. Res.* 278: 219–223, **1986**.

Gewin, L., Myers, H., Kiyono, T., and Galloway, D.A. Identification of a novel telomerase repressor that interacts with the human papillomavirus type-16 E6/E6-AP complex. *Genes Dev.* 18: 2269–2282, **2004**.

Ghaderi, M., Nikitina, L., Peacock, C.S., Hjelmstrom, P., Hallmans, G., Wiklund, F., Lenner, P., Blackwell, J.M., Dillner, J., and Sanjeevi, C.B. Tumor necrosis factor α-11 and DR15-DQ6 (B*0602) haplotype increase the risk for cervical intraepithelial neoplasia in human papillomavirus 16 seropositive women in Northern Sweden. *Cancer Epidemiol. Biomarkers Prev.* 9: 1067–1070, **2000**.

Ghaderi, M., Nikitina Zake, L., Wallin, K., Wiklund, F., Hallmans, G., Lenner, P., Dillner, J., and Sanjeevi, C.B. Tumor necrosis factor α and MHC class I chain related gene A (MIC-A) polymorphisms in Swedish patients with cervical cancer. *Hum. Immunol.* 62: 1153–1158, **2001**.

Giampieri, S., and Storey, A. Repair of UV-induced thymine dimers is compromised in cells expressing the E6 protein from human papillomaviruses types 5 and 18. *Br. J. Cancer* 90: 2203–2209, **2004**.

Giampieri, S., Garcia-Escudero, R., Green, J., and Storey, A. Human papillomavirus type 77 E6 protein selectively inhibits p53-dependent transcription of proapoptotic genes following UV-B irradiation. *Oncogene* 23: 5864–5870, **2004**.

Gillison, M.L. Human papillomavirus-associated head and neck cancer is a distinct epidemiologic, clinical, and molecular entity. *Semin. Oncol.* 31: 744–754, **2004**.

Gillison, M.L., Koch, W.M., Capone, R.B., Spafford, M., Westra, W.H., Wu, L., Zahurak, M.L., Daniel, R.W., Shah, K.V., Viglione, M., Symer, D.E., and Sidransky, D. Evidence for a causal association between human papillomavirus and a subset of head and neck cancers. *J. Natl. Cancer Inst.* 92: 709–720, **2000**.

Giri, I., Danos, O., and Yaniv, M. Genomic structure of the cottontail rabbit (Shope) papillomavirus. *Proc. Natl. Acad. Sci. USA* 82: 1580–1584, **1985**.

Gissmann, L. and zur Hausen, H. Human papilloma virus DNA: physical mapping and genetic heterogeneity. *Proc. Natl. Acad. Sci. USA* 73: 1310–1313, **1976**.

Gissmann, L. and zur Hausen, H. Partial characterization of viral DNA from human genital warts (condylomata acuminata). *Int. J. Cancer* 25: 605–609, **1980**.

Gissmann, L. Pfister, H., and zur Hausen, H. Human papilloma viruses (HPV): characterization of four different isolates. *Virology* 76: 569–580, **1977**.

Gissmann, L., Diehl, V., Schultz-Coulon, H., and zur Hausen, H. Molecular cloning and characterization of human papilloma virus DNA derived from a laryngeal papilloma. *J. Virol.* 44: 393–400, **1982**.

Giuliano, A.R., Papenfuss, M., Nour, M., Canfield, L.M., Schneider, A., and Hatch, K. Antioxidant nutrients: associations with persistent human papillomavirus infection. *Cancer Epidemiol. Biomarkers Prev.* 6: 917–923, **1997**.

Giuliano, A.R., Sedjo, R.L., Roe, D.J., Harris, R., Baldwin, S., Papenfuss, M.R., Abrahamsen, M., and Inserra, P. Clearance of oncogenic human papillomavirus (HPV) infection: effect of smoking (United States). *Cancer Causes Control* 13: 839–845, **2002**.

Giuliano, A.R., Papenfuss, M., De Galaz, E.M., Feng, J., Abrahamsen, M., Denman, C., de Zapien, J.G., Navarro Henze, J.L., Garcia, F., and Hatch, K. Risk factors for squamous intraepithelial lesions (SIL) of the cervix among women residing at the US-Mexico border. *Int. J. Cancer.* 109: 112–118, **2004**.

Glaunsinger, B.A., Lee, S. S., Thomas, M., Banks, L., and Javier, R. Interactions of the PDZ-protein MAGI-1 with adenovirus E4-ORF1 and high-risk papillomavirus E6 oncoproteins. *Oncogene* 19: 5270–5280, **2000**.

Gloss, B., Bernard, H.-U., Seedorf, K., and Klock, G. The upstream regulatory region of the human papillomavirus-16 contains an E2 protein-independent enhancer which is specific for cervical carcinoma cells and regulated by glucocorticoid hormones. *EMBO J.* 6: 3735–3743, **1987**.

Goedert, J.J., Cote, T.R., Virgo, P., Scoppa, S. M., Kingma, D.W., Gail, M.H., Jaffe, E.S. and Biggar, R.J. Spectrum of AIDS-associated malignant disorders. *Lancet* 351: 1833–1939, **1998**.

Goldstone, S. E., Palefsky, J.Y., Winnett, M.T., and Neefe, J.R. Activity of HspE7, a novel immunotherapy, in patients with anogenital warts. *Dis. Colon Rectum* 45: 502–507, **2002**.

Golijow, C.D., Abba, M.C., Mouron, S. A., Laguens, R.M., Dulout, F.M. and Smith, J.S. *Chlamydia trachomatis* and human papillomavirus infections in cervical disease in Argentine women. *Gynecol. Oncol.* 96: 181–186, **2005** .

Gomperts, S. N. Clustering membrane proteins: It's all coming together with the PSD-95/SAP90 protein family. *Cell* 84: 659–662, **1996**.

González-Suárez, E., Samper, E., Ramírez, A., Flores, J.M., Martin-Caballero, J., Jorcano, J.L., and Blasco, M.A. Increased epidermal tumors and increased skin wound healing in transgenic mice overexpressing the catalytic subunit of telomerase, mTERT, in basal keratinocytes. *EMBO J.* 20: 2619–2630, **2001**.

Goodman, A. Primary vaginal cancer. *Surg. Oncol. Clin. N. Am.* 7: 347–361, **1998**.

Gram, I.T., Macaluso, M., Churchill, J., and Stalsberg, H. Trichomonas vaginalis (TV) and human papillomavirus (HPV) infection and the incidence of cervical intraepithelial neoplasia (CIN) grade III. *Cancer Causes Control* 3: 231–236, **1992**.

Green, J., Berrington de Gonzalez, A., Smith, J.S., Franceschi, S., Appleby, P., Plummer, M., and Beral, V. Human papillomavirus infection and use of oral contraceptives. *Br. J. Cancer* 88: 1713–1720, **2003**.

Greenhalgh, D.A., Wang, X.J., Rothnagel, J.A., Eckhardt, J.N., Quintanilla, M.I., Barber, J.L., Bundman, D.S., Longley, M.A., Schlegel, R., and Roop, D.R. Transgenic mice expressing targeted HPV-18 E6 and E7 oncogenes in the epidermis develop verrucous lesions and spontaneous, rasHa-activated papillomas. *Cell Growth Differ.* 5: 667–675, **1994**.

Greenspan, D.A., de Villiers, E.-M., Greenspan, J.S., de Souza, Y.G., and zur Hausen, H. Unusual HPV types in oral warts in association with HIV infection. *J. Oral Pathol.* 17: 482–488, **1988**.

Greenspan, D.L., Connolly, D.C., Wu, R., Lei, R.Y., Vogelstein, J.T., Kim, Y.T., Mok, J.E.,

Mu[ntilde]oz, N., Bosch, F.X., Shah, K.V., and Cho, K.R. Loss of FHIT expression in cervical carcinoma cell lines and primary tumors. *Cancer Res.* 57: 4692–4298, **1997**.

Greenstone, S. E., Nieland, J.D., de Visser, K.E., De Bruijn, M.L.H., Kirnbauer, R., Roden, R.B.S., Lowy, D.R., Kast, W.M., and Schiller, J.T. Chimeric papillomavirus virus-like particles elicit antitumor immunity against the E7 oncoprotein in an HPV16 tumor model. *Proc. Natl. Acad. Sci. USA* 95: 1800–1805, **1998**.

Grm, H.S. and Banks, L. Degradation of hDlg and MAGIs by human papillomavirus E6 is E6-AP-independent. *J. Gen. Virol.* 85: 2815–2819, **2004**.

Grossman, S. and Laimins, L.A. E6 protein of human papillomavirus type 18 binds zinc. *Oncogene* 4: 1089–1093, **1989**.

Grussendorf-Conen, E.I., Deutz, F.J., de Villiers, E.-M. Detection of human papillomavirus-6 in primary carcinoma of the urethra in men. *Cancer* 60: 1832–1835, **1987**.

Gu, Z., Pim, D., Labrecque, S., Banks, L., and Matlashewski, G. DNA damage induced p53 mediated transcription is inhibited by human papillomavirus type 18 E6. *Oncogene* 9: 629–633, **1994**.

Guillou, L., Sahli, R., Chaubert, P., Monnier, P., Cuttat, J.F., and Costa, J. Squamous cell carcinoma of the lung in a nonsmoking, nonirradiated patient with juvenile laryngotracheal papillomatosis. Evidence of human papillomavirus-11 DNA in both carcinoma and papillomas. *Am. J. Surg. Pathol.* 15: 891–898, **1991**.

Gutman, L.T., St. Claire, K.K., Everett, V.D., Ingram, D.L., Soper, J., Johnston, W.W., Mulvaney, G.G., and Phelps, W.C. Cervical-vaginal and intraanal human papillomavirus infection of young girls with external genital warts. *J. Infect. Dis* . 170: 339–344, **1994**.

Hafkamp, H.C., Speel, E.J., Haesevoets, A., Bot, F.J., Dinjens, W.N., Ramaekers, F.C., Hopman, A.H., and Manni, J.J. A subset of head and neck squamous cell carcinomas exhibits integration of HPV 16/18 DNA and overexpression of p16INK4A and p53 in the absence of mutations in p53 exons 5–8. *Int. J. Cancer* 107: 394–400, **2003**.

Haga, T., Kim, S. H., Jensen, R.H., Darragh, T., and Palefsky, J.M. Detection of genetic changes in anal intraepithelial neoplasia (AIN) of HIV-positive and HIV-negative men. *J. Acquir. Immune Defic. Syndr.* 26: 256–262, **2001**.

Halbert, C.L. and Galloway, D.A. Identification of the E5 open reading frame of human papillomavirus type 16. *J. Virol.* 62: 1071–1075, **1988**.

Haller, K., Stubenrauch, F., and Pfister, H. Differentiation-dependent transcription of the epidermodysplasia verruciformis-associated human papillomavirus type 5 in benign lesions. *Virology* 214: 245–255, **1995**.

Hallez, S., Simon, P., Maudoux, F., Doyen, J., Noel, J.C., Beliard, A., Capelle, X., Buxant, F., Fayt, I., Lagrost, A.C., Hubert, P., Gerday, C., Burny, A., Boniver, J., Foidart, J.M., Delvenne, P., and Jacobs, N. Phase I/II trial of immunogenicity of a human papillomavirus (HPV) type 16 E7 protein-based vaccine in women with oncogenic HPV-positive cervical intraepithelial neoplasia. *Cancer Immunol. Immunother.* 53: 642–650, **2004**.

Han, C.P., Tsao, Y.P., Sun, C.A., Ng, H.T., and Chen, S. L. Human papillomavirus, cytomegalovirus and herpes simplex virus infections for cervical cancer in Taiwan. *Cancer Lett.* 120: 217–221, **1997**.

Harper, J.W., Adami, G.R., Wei, N., Keymarsi, K., and Elledge, S. J. The p21 Cdk-interacting protein Cip1 is a potent inhibitor of G1 cyclin dependent kinases. *Cell* 75: 805–816, **1993**.

Harper, D.M., Franco, E.L., Wheeler, C.M., Ferris, D.G., Jenkins, D., Schuind, A., Zahaf, T., Innis, B., Naud, P., de Carvalho, N.S., Roteli-Martins, C.M., Teixeira, J., Blatter, M.M., Korn, A.P., Quint, W., and Dubin, G. and GlaxoSmithKline HPV Vaccine Study Group. Efficacy of a bivalent L1 virus-like particle vaccine in prevention of infection with human papillomavirus types 16 and 18 in young women: a randomised controlled trial. *Lancet* 364: 1757–1765, **2004**.

Harris, S. F. and Botchan, M.R. Crystal structure of the human papillomavirus type 18 E2 activation domain. *Science* 284: 1673–1677, **1999**.

Harris, M.O., Beck, J.C., Lancaster, W., Gregoire, L., Carey, T.E., and Bradford, C.R. The HPV 6 E6/E7 transforming genes are expressed in inverted papillomas. *Otolaryngol. Head Neck Surg.* 118: 312–318, **1998**.

Harro, C.D., Pang, Y.Y., Roden, R.B., Hildesheim, A., Wang, Z., Reynolds, M.J., Mast, T.C., Robinson, R., Murphy, B.R., Karron, R.A., Dillner, J., Schiller, J.T., and Lowy, D.R. Safety and immunogenicity trial in adult volunteers of a human papillomavirus 16 L1 virus-like particle vaccine. *J. Natl. Cancer Inst.* 93: 284–292, **2001**.

Hartley, K.A. and Alexander, K.A. Human TATA binding protein inhibits human papillomavirus type 11 DNA replication by antagonizing E1-E2 protein complex formation on the viral origin of replication. *J. Virol.* 76: 5014–5023, **2002** .

Harwood, C.A., Surentheran, T., McGregor, J.M., Spink, P.J., Leigh, I.M., Breuer, J., and Proby, C.M. Human papillomavirus infection and non-melanoma skin cancer in immunosuppressed and immunocompetent individuals. *J. Med. Virol.* 61: 289–297, **2000**.

Haverkos, H.W., Soon, G., Steckley, S. L., and Pickworth, W. Cigarette smoking and cervical cancer: Part I: a meta-analysis. *Biomed. Pharmacother.* 57: 67–77, **2003**.

Hawley-Nelson, P., Vousden, K.H., Hubbert, N.L., Lowy, D.R., and Schiller, J.T. HPV 16 E6 and E7 proteins cooperate to immortalize human foreskin keratinocytes. *EMBO J.* 8: 3905–3910, **1989**.

Hayes, R.B., Pottern, L.M., Strickler, H.D., Rabkin, C., Pope, V., Swanson, G.M., Greenberg, R.S., Schoenberg, J.B., Liff, J., Schwartz, A.G., Hoover, R.N., and Fraumeni, J.F., Jr. Sexual behaviour, STDs and risk of prostate cancer. *Br. J. Cancer* 82: 718–725, **2000**.

Heck, D.V., Yee, C.L., Howley, P.M., and Münger, K. Efficiency of binding the retinoblastoma protein correlates with the transforming capacity of the E7 oncoproteins of the human papillomaviruses. *Proc. Natl. Acad. Sci. USA* 89: 4442–4446, **1992**.

Hegde, R.S. The papillomavirus E2 proteins: structure, function, and biology. *Annu. Rev. Biophys. Biomol. Struct.* 31: 343–360, **2002**.

Hegde, R.S., Grossman, S. R., Laimins, L.A., and Sigler, P.B. Crystal structure at 1.7 A of the bovine papillomavirus-1 E2 DNA-binding domain bound to its DNA target. *Nature* 359: 505–512, **1992**.

Heilbronn, R. and zur Hausen, H. A subset of herpes simplex virus replication genes induces DNA amplification within the host cell genome. *J. Virol.* 63: 3683–3692, **1989**.

Heilbronn, R., Albrecht, I., Stephan, S., Bürkle, A., and zur Hausen, H. Human cytomegalovirus induces JC virus DNA replication in human fibroblasts. *Proc. Natl. Acad. Sci. USA* 90: 11406–11410, **1993**.

Heim, K., Widschwendter, A., Szedenik, H., Geier, A., Christensen, N.D., Bergant, A., Concin, N., and Höpfl, R. Specific serologic response to genital human papillomavirus types in patients with vulvar precancerous and cancerous lesions. *Am. J. Obstet. Gynecol.* 192: 1073–1083, **2005**.

Helt, A.M., Funk, J.O., and Galloway, D.A. Inactivation of both the retinoblastoma tumor suppressor and p21 by the human papillomavirus type 16 E7 oncoprotein is necessary to inhibit cell cycle arrest in human epithelial cells. *J. Virol.* 76: 10559–10568, **2002**.

Hemmati, P.G., Normand, G., Verdoodt, B., von Haefen, C., Hasenjäger, A., Guner, D., Wendt, J., Dörken, B., and Daniel, P.T. Loss of p21 disrupts p14ARF-induced G1 cell cycle arrest but augments p14ARF-induced apoptosis in human carcinoma cells. *Oncogene* 24: 4114–4128, **2005**.

Hemminki, K., Jiang, Y., and Dong, C. Second primary cancers after anogenital, skin, oral, esophageal, and rectal cancers: etiological links? *Int. J. Cancer* 93: 294–298, **2001**.

Hengstermann, A., Linares, L.K., Ciechanover, A., Whitaker, N.J., and Scheffner, M. Complete switch from Mdm2 to human papillomavirus E6-mediated degradation of p53 in cervical cancer cells. *Proc. Natl. Acad. Sci. USA* 98: 1218–1223, **2001**.

Herrero, R., Castellsague, X., Pawlita, M., Lissowska, J., Kee, F., Balaram, P., Rajkumar, T., Sridhar, H., Rose, B., Pintos, J., Fernandez, L., Idris, A., Sanchez, M.J., Nieto, A., Talamini, R., Tavani, A., Bosch, F.X., Reidel, U., Snijders, P.J., Meijer, C.J., Viscidi, R., Mu[ntilde]oz, N., Franceschi, S., IARC Multicenter Oral Cancer Study Group. Human papillomavirus and oral cancer: the International Agency for Research on Cancer multicenter study. *J. Natl. Cancer Inst.* 95: 1772–1783, **2003**.

Hildesheim, A. and Wang, S. S. Host and viral genetics and risk of cervical cancer: a review. *Virus Res.* 89: 229–240, **2002**.

Hildesheim, A., Herrero, R., Castle, P.E., Wacholder, S., Bratti, M.C., Sherman, M.E., Lorincz, A.T., Burk, R.D., Morales, J., Rodriguez, A.C., Helgesen, K., Alfaro, M., Hutchinson, M., Balmaceda, I., Greenberg, M., and Schiffman, M. HPV co-factors related to the development of cervical cancer: results from a population-based study in Costa Rica. *Br. J. Cancer* 84: 1219–1226, **2001**.

Hines, J.F., Ghim, S. J., Christensen, N.D., Kreider, J.W., Barnes, W.A., Schlegel, R., and Jenson, A.B. Role of conformational epitopes expressed by human papillomavirus major capsid proteins in the serologic detection of infection and prophylactic vaccination. *Gynecol. Oncol.* 55: 13–20, **1994**.

Hiraiwa, A., Kiyono, T., Segawa, K., Utsumi, K.R., Ohashi, M., and Ishibashi, M. Comparative study onE6 and E7 genes of some cutaneous and genital papillomaviruses of human origin for their ability to transform 3Y1 cells. *Virology* 192: 102–111, **1993**.

Hisada, M., Rabkin, C.S., Strickler, H.D., Wright, W.E., Christianson, R.E., and van den berg, B.J. Human papillomavirus antibody and risk of prostate cancer. *JAMA* 283: 340–341, **2000**.

Ho, G.Y.F., Palan, P.R., Basu, J., Romney, S. L., Kadish, A.S., Mikhail, M., Wassertheil-Smoller, S., Runowicz, C., and Burk, R.D. Viral characteristics of human papillomavirus infection and antioxidant levels as risk factors for cervical dysplasia. *Int. J. Cancer* 78: 594–599, **1998**.

Ho, G.Y.F., Studentsov, Y.Y., Bierman, R., and Burk, R.D. Natural history of human papillomavirus type 16 virus-like particle antibodies in young women. *Cancer Epidemiol. Biomarkers Prev.* 13: 110–116, **2004**.

Hobbs, C.G. and Birchall, M.A. Human papillomavirus infection in the etiology of laryngeal carcinoma. *Curr. Opin. Otolaryngol. Head Neck Surg.* 12: 88–92, **2004**.

Holly, E.A., Petrakis, N.L., Friend, N.F., Sarles, D.L., Lee, R.E., and Flander, L.B. Mutagenic mucus in the cervix of smokers. *J. Natl. Cancer Inst.* 76: 983–986, **1986**.

Holt, S. E., Schuller, G., and Wilson, V.G. DNA binding specificity of the bovine papillomavirus E1 protein is determined by sequences contained within an 18-base-pair inverted repeat element of the origin of replication. *J. Virol.* 68: 1094–1102, **1994**.

Hørding, U., Daugaard, S., Iversen, A.K., Knudsen, J., Bock, J.E., and Norrild, B. Human papillomavirus type 16 in vulvar carcinoma, vulvar intraepithelial neoplasia, and associated cervical neoplasia. *Gynecol. Oncol.* 42: 22–26, **1991**.

Horner, S. M., DeFilippis, R.A., Manuelidis, L., and DiMaio, D. Repression of the human papillomavirus E6 gene initiates p53-dependent, telomerase-independent senescence and apoptosis in HeLa cervical carcinoma cells. *J. Virol.* 78: 4063–4073, **2004**.

Huang, F.Y., Kwok, Y.K., Lau, E.T., Tang, M.H., Ng, T.Y., Ngan, H.Y. Genetic abnormalities and HPV status in cervical and vulvar squamous cell carcinomas. *Cancer Genet. Cytogenet.* 157: 42–48, **2005**.

Hubbert, N.L., Sedman, S. A. and Schiller, J.T. Human papillomavirus type 16 E6 increases the degradation rate of p53 in human keratinocytes. *J. Virol.* 66: 6237–6241, **1992**.

Huh, K.-W., DeMasi, J., Ogawa, H., Nakatani, Y., Howley, P.M., and Münger, K. Association of the human papillomavirus type 16 E7 oncoprotein with the 600-kDa retinoblastoma protein-associated factor, p600. *Proc. Natl. Acad. Sci. USA* 102: 11 492–11 497, **2005**.

Huibregste, J.M., Scheffner, M.M., and Howley, P.M. A cellular protein mediates association of p53 with the E6 oncoprotein of human papillomavirus types 16 or 18. *EMBO J.* 10: 4129–4135, **1991**.

Huibregtse, J.M., Scheffner, M., and Howley, P.M. Cloning and expression of the cDNA for E6-AP, a protein that mediates the interaction of the human papillomavirus E6 oncoprotein with p53. *Mol. Cell. Biol.* 13: 775–784, **1993**.

Huibregtse, J.M., Scheffner, M., Beaudenon, S., and Howley, P.M. A family of proteins structurally and functionally related to the E6-AP ubiquitin-protein ligase. *Proc. Natl. Acad Sci USA* 92: 2563–2567, **1995**.

Hutvagner, G., McLachlan, J., Pasquinelli, A.E., Balint, E., Tuschl, H., and Zamore,

P.D. A cellular function for the RNA-interference enzyme Dicer in the maturation of the let-7 small temporal RNA. *Science* 293: 834–838, **2001**.

Hwang, E.-S., Nottoli, T., and DiMaio, D. The HPV 16 E5 protein: expression, detection, and stable complex formation with transmembrane proteins in COS cells. *Virology* 211: 227–233, **1995**.

IARC, *Human Papillomaviruses*, Monograph 90, in press, **2006**.

Iftner, A., Klug, S. J., Garbe, C., Blum, A., Stancu, A., Wilczynski, S. P., and Iftner, T. The prevalence of human papillomavirus genotypes in nonmelanoma skin cancers of nonimmunosuppressed individuals identifies high-risk genital types as possible risk factors. *Cancer Res.* 63: 7515–7519, **2003**.

Ikenberg, H., Gissmann, L., Gross, G., Grussendorf-Conen, E.-I., and zur Hausen, H. Human papillomavirus type-16-related DNA in genital Bowen's disease and in Bowenoid papulosis. *Int. J. Cancer* 32: 563–565, **1983**.

Ikenberg, H., Runge, M., Goppinger, A., and Pfleiderer, A. Human papillomavirus DNA in invasive carcinoma of the vagina. *Obstet. Gynecol.* 76: 432–438, **1990**.

Ingelfinger, J.R., Grupe, W.E., Topor, M., and Levey, R.H. Warts in a pediatric transplant population. *Dermatologica* 155: 7–12, **1977**.

Ishiji, T., Lace, M.J., Parkkinen, S., Anderson, R.D., Haugen, T.H., Cripe, T.P., Xiao, J.H., Davidson, I., Chambon, P., and Turek, L.P. Transcriptional enhancer factor (TEF)-1 and its cell-specific co-activator activate human papillomavirus-16 E6 and E7 oncogene transcription in keratinocytes and cervical carcinoma cells. *EMBO J.* 11: 2271–2281, **1992**.

Jablonska, S. and Majewski, S. Epidermodysplasia verruciformis: immunological and clinical aspects. *Curr. Topics Microbiol. Immunol.* 186: 157–175, **1994**.

Jablonska, S., Dabrowski, J., and Jakubowicz, K. Epidermodysplasia verruciformis as a model in studies on the role of papovaviruses in oncogenesis. *Cancer Res.* 32: 583–589, **1972**.

Jackson, S. and Storey, A. E6 proteins from diverse cutaneous HPV types inhibit apoptosis in response to UV damage. *Oncogene* 19: 592–598, **2000**.

Jackson, S., Harwood, C., Thomas, M., Banks, L., and Storey, A. Role of Bak in UV-induced apoptosis in skin cancer and abrogation by HPV E6 proteins. *Genes Dev.* 14: 3065–3073, **2000**.

Jackson, S., Ghali, L., Harwood, C., and Storey, A. Reduced apoptotic levels in squamous but not basal cell carcinomas correlates with detection of cutaneous human papillomavirus. *Br. J. Cancer* 87: 319–323, **2002**.

Jamieson, D.J., Duerr, A., Burk, R., Klein, R.S., Paramsothy, P., Schuman, P., Cu-Uvin, S., Shah, K: HIV Epidemiology Research Study (HERS) Group. *Am. J. Obstet. Gynecol.* 186: 21–27, **2002**.

Jarrard, D.F., Sarkar, S., Shi, Y., Yeager, T.R., Magrane, G., Kinoshita, H., Nassif, N., Meisner, L., Newton, M.A., Waldman, F.M., and Reznikoff, C.A. p16/pRb pathway alterations are required for bypassing senescence in human prostate epithelial cells. *Cancer Res.* 59: 2957–2964, **1999**.

Jarrett, W.F., McNeil, P.E., Grimshaw, W.T., Selman, I.E., and McIntiyre, W.I. High incidence area of cattle cancer with a possible interaction between an environmental carcinogen and a papilloma virus. *Nature* 274: 215–217, **1978** .

Jenson, A.B., Rosenthal, J.D., Olson, C., Pass, F., Lancaster, W.D., and Shah, K.V. Immunologic relatedness of papillomaviruses from different species. *J. Natl. Cancer Inst.* 64: 495–500, **1980**.

Jewers, R.J., Hildebrandt, P., Ludlow, J.W., Kell, B., and McCance, D.J. Regions of human papillomavirus type 16 E7 oncoprotein required for immortalization of human keratinocytes. *J. Virol.* 66: 1329–1335, **1992**.

Jiang, M. and Milner, J. Selective silencing of viral gene expression in HPV-positive human cervical carcinoma cells treated with siRNA, a primer of RNA interference. *Oncogene* 21: 6041–6048, **2002**.

Jones, D.L., Alani, R.M., and Münger, K. The human papillomavirus E7 oncoprotein can uncouple cellular differentiation and proliferation in human keratinocytes by abrogating p21Cip1-mediated inhibition of cdk2. *Genes Dev.* 11: 2101–2111, **1997**.

Kabsch, K., Mossadegh, N., Kohl, A., Komposch, G., Schenkel, J., Alonso, A., and Tomakidi, P. The HPV-16 E5 protein inhibits TRAIL- and FasL-mediated apoptosis in human keratinocyte raft cultures. *Intervirology* 47: 48–56, **2004**.

Kadish, A.S., Ho, G.Y.F., Burk, R.D., Wang, Y., Romney, S. L., Ledwidge, R., and Angeletti, R.H. Lymphoproliferative responses to human papillomavirus (HPV) type 16 proteins E6 and E7: outcome of HPV infection and associated neoplasia. *J. Natl. Cancer Inst.* 89: 1285–1293, **1997**.

Kahn, T., Schwarz, E., and zur Hausen, H. Molecular cloning and characterization of the DNA of a new human papillomavirus (HPV 30) from a laryngeal carcinoma. *Int. J. Cancer* 37: 61–65, **1986**.

Kahn, T., Turazza, E., Ojeda, R., Bercovich, A., Stremlau, A., Lichter, P., Poustka, A., Grinstein, S., and zur Hausen, H. Integration of human papillomavirus type 6 a DNA in a tonsillar carcinoma: chromosomal localization and nucleotide sequence of the genomic target region. *Cancer Res.* 54: 1305–1312, **1994**.

Kalantari, M., Calleja-Macias, I.E., Tewari, D., Hagmar, B., Lie, K., Barrera-Saldana, H.A., Wiley, D.J., and Bernard, H.U. Conserved methylation patterns of human papillomavirus type 16 DNA in asymptomatic infection and cervical neoplasia. *J. Virol.* 78: 12 762–12 772, **2004**.

Kalimo, K., Terho, P., Honkonen, E., Gronroos, M., and Halonen, P. *Chlamydia trachomatis* and herpes simplex IgA antibodies in cervical secretions of patients with cervical atypia. *Br. J. Obstet. Gynaecol.* 88: 1130–1134, **1981**.

Kalinski, P., Hilkens, C.M., Wierenga, E.A., and Kapsenberg, M.L. T-cell priming by type-1 and type-2 polarized dendritic cells: the concept of a third signal. *Immunol. Today* 20: 561–567, **1999**.

Kanao, H., Enomoto, T., Ueda, Y., Fujita, M., Nakashima, R., Ueno, Y., Miyatake, T., Yoshizaki, T., Buzard, G.S., Kimura, T., Yoshino, K., and Murata, Y. Correlation between p14(ARF)/p16(INK4A) expression and HPV infection in uterine cervical cancer. *Cancer Lett.* 213: 31–37, **2004**.

Kanda, T., Watanabe, S., Zanma, S., Sato, H., Furuno, A., and Yoshiike, K. Human papillomavirus type 16 E6 proteins with glycine substitution for cysteine in the metal-binding motif. *Virology* 185: 536–543, **1991**.

Kang, M.K. and Park, N.H. Conversion of normal to malignant phenotype: telomere shortening, telomerase activation, and genomic instability during immortalization of human oral keratinocytes. *Crit. Rev. Oral Biol. Med.* 12: 38–54, **2001** .

Kao, W.H., Beaudenon, S. L., Talis, A.L., Huibregste, J.M., and Howley, P.M. Human papillomavirus type 16 E6 induces self-ubiquitination of the E6AP ubiquitin-protein ligase. *J. Virol.* 74: 6408–6417, **2000**.

Kashima, H.K., Shah, F., Lyles, A., Glackin, R., Muhammad, N., Turner, L., Van Zandt, S., Whitt, S., and Shah, K.V. A comparison of risk factors in juvenile-onset and adult-onset recurrent papillomatosis. *Laryngoscope* 102: 9–13, **1992 a**.

Kashima, H.K., Kessis, T.D., Hruban, R.H., Wu, T.C., Zinreich, S. J., and Shah, K.V. Human papillomavirus in sinonasal papillomas and squamous cell carcinoma. *Laryngoscope* 102: 973–976, **1992 b**.

Kast, W.M., Brandt, R.M., Drijfhout, J.W., and Melief, C.J. Human leukocyte antigen-A2.1 restricted candidate cytotoxic T lymphocyte epitopes of human papillomavirus type 16 E6 and E7 proteins identified by using the processing-defective human cell line T2. *J. Immunother.* 14: 115–120, **1993**.

Kaufmann, A.M., Nieland, J., Schinz, M., Nonn, M., Gabelsberger, J., Meissner, H., Müller, R.T., Jochmus, I., Gissmann, L., Schneider, A., and Dürst, M. HPV16 L1E7 chimeric virus-like particles induce specific HLA-restricted T cells in humans after in vitro vaccination. *Int. J. Cancer.* 92: 285–93, **2001**.

Kaufmann, A.M., Stern, P.L., Rankin, E.M., Sommer, H., Nuessler, V., Schneider, A., Adams, M., Onon, T.S., Bauknecht, T., Wagner, U., Kroon, K., Hickling, J., Boswell, C.M., Stacey, S. N., Kitchener, H.C., Gillard, J., Wanders, J., Roberts, J.S., and Zwierzina, H. Safety and immunogenicity of TA-HPV, a recombinant vaccinia virus expressing modified human papillomavirus (HPV)-16 and HPV-18 E6 and E7 genes, in women with progressive cervical cancer. *Clin. Cancer Res.* 8: 3676–3685, **2002** .

Kawana, K., Yoshikawa, H., Taketani, Y., Yoshiike, K., and Kanda, T. Common neutralization epitope in minor capsid protein L2 of human papillomavirus types

16 and 6. *J. Virol.* 73: 6188–6190, **1999**.

Kawana, K., Yasugi, T., Kanda, T., Kino, N., Oda, K., Okada, S., Kawana, Y., Nei, T., Takada, T., Toyoshima, S., Tsuchiya, A., Kondo, K., Yoshikawa, H., Tsutsumi, O., and Taketani, Y. Safety and immunogenicity of a peptide containing the cross-neutralization epitope of HPV16 L2 administered nasally in healthy volunteers. *Vaccine* 21: 4256–4260, **2003**.

Kaur, P. and McDougall, J.K. Characterization of primary human keratinocytes transformed by human papillomavirus type 18. *J. Virol.* 62: 1917–1924, **1988**.

Ke, L., Yu, P., and Zhang, Z.X. Novel epidemiologic evidence for the association between fermented fish sauce and esophageal cancer in South China. *Int. J. Cancer* 99: 424–426, **2002**.

Ke, L.D., Adler-Storthz, K., Mitchell, M.F., Clayman, G.L., and Chen, Z. Expression of human papillomavirus E7mRNA in human oral and cervical neoplasia and cell lines. *Oral Oncol.* 35: 415–20, **1999**.

Keating, P., Cromme, F., Duggan-Keen, M., Snijders, P.J.F., Walboomers, J.M.M., Hunter, R.D., Dyer, P.A., and Stern, P.L. Frequency of down-regulation of individual HLA-A and -B alleles in cervical carcinomas in relation to TAP-1 expression. *Br. J. Cancer* 72: 405–411, **1995**.

Keefe, K.A., Schell, M.J., Brewer, C., McHale, M., Brewster, W., Chapman, J.A., Rose, G.S., McMeeken, D.S., Lagerberg, W., Peng, Y.M., Wilczynski, S. P., Anton-Culver, H., Meyskens, F.L., and Berman, M.L. A randomized, double-blind, Phase III trial using oral β-carotene supplementation for women with high grade cervical intraepithelial neoplasia. *Cancer Epidemiol. Biomarkers Prev.* 10: 1029–1035, **2001**.

Kelley, M.L., Keiger, K.E., Lee, C.J., and Huibregtse, J.M. The global transcriptional effects of the human papillomavirus E6 protein in cervical carcinoma cell lines are mediated by the E6AP ubiquitin ligase. *J. Virol.* 79: 3737–3747, **2005**.

Kerley, S. W., Persons, D.L., and Fishback, J.L. Human papillomavirus and carcinoma of the urinary bladder. *Mod. Pathol.* 4: 316–319, **1991**.

Kern, S. E., Kinzler, K.W., Bruskin, A., Jarosz, D., Friedman, P., Prives, C., and Vogelstein, B. Identification of p53 as a sequence-specific DNA-binding protein. *Science* 252: 1708–1711, **1991**.

Kessis, T.D., Conolly, D.C., Hedrick, L., and Cho, K.R. Expression of HPV16 E6 or E7 increases integration of foreign DNA. *Oncogene* 13: 427–431, **1996**.

Key, T. Risk factors for prostate cancer. *Cancer Surv.* 23: 63–77, **1985**.

Kim, M.S., Shin, K.H., Baek, J.H., Cherrick, H.M., and Park, N.H. HPV-16, tobacco-specific N-nitrosamine, and N-methyl-N'-nitro-N-nitrosoguanidine in oral carcinogenesis. *Cancer Res.* 53: 4811–4816, **1993**,

Kim, T.W., Hung, C.F., Boyd, D.A., He, L., Lin, C.T., Kaiserman, D., Bird, P.I., and Wu, T.C. Enhancement of DNA vaccine potency by coadministration of a tumor antigen gene and DNA encoding serine protease inhibitor-6. *Cancer Res.* 64: 400–405, **2004**.

Kimberlin, D.W. Current status of antiviral therapy for juvenile-onset recurrent respiratory papillomatosis. *Antiviral Res.* 63: 141–151, **2004**.

Kirkman, H. and Bacon, R.L. Malignant renal tumors in male hamsters (*Cricetus auratus*) treated with estrogen. *Cancer Res.* 10: 122–124, **1950**.

Kirkpatrick, A., Bidwell, J., van den Brule, A.J., Meijer, C.J.M., Pawade, J., and Glew, S. TNFα polymorphism frequencies in HPV-associated cervical dysplasia. *Gynecol. Oncol.* 92: 675–679, **2004**.

Kirnbauer, R., Booy, F., Cheng, N., Lowy, D.R., and Schiller, J.T. Papillomavirus L1 major capsid protein self-assembles into virus-like particles that are highly immunogenic. *Proc. Natl. Acad. Sci. USA* 89: 12180–12184, **1992**.

Kiyabu, M.T., Shibata, D., Arnheim, N., Martin, W.J., and Fitzgibbons, P.L. Detection of human papillomavirus in formalin-fixed, invasive squamous carcinomas using polymerase chain reaction. *Am. J. Surg. Pathol.* 13: 221–224, **1989** .

Kiyono, T., Hiraiwa, A., Fujita, M., Hayashi, Y., Akiyama, T., and Ishibashi, M. Binding of high risk human papillomavirus E6 oncoproteins to the human homologue of the Drosophila discs large tumor suppressor protein. *Proc. Natl. Acad. Sci. USA* 94: 11612–11616, **1997**.

Kiyono, T., Foster, S. A., Koop, J.I., McDougall, J.K., Galloway, D.A., and Klingelhutz, A.J. Both Rb/p16INK4a inactivation and telomerase activity are required to immortalize human epithelial cells. *Nature* 396: 84–88, **1998**.

Kjaer, S. K. van den Brule, A.J.C., Bock, J.E., Poll, P.A., Engholm, G., Sherman, M.E., Walboomers, J.M.M., and Meijer, C.J.L. Human papillomavirus – the most significant risk determinant of cervical intraepithelial neoplasia. *Int. J. Cancer* 65: 601–606, **1996**.

Klaes, R., Woerner, S. M., Ridder, R., Wentzensen, N., Dürst, M., Schneider, A., Lotz, B., Melsheimer, P., and von Knebel Doeberitz, M. Detection of high-risk cervical intraepithelial neoplasia and cervical cancer by amplification of transcripts derived from integrated papillomavirus oncogenes. *Cancer Res.* 59: 6132–6126, **1999**.

Kleine, K., König, G., Kreuzer, J., Komitowski, D., zur Hausen, H., and Rösl, F. The effect of the JE (MCP-1) gene, which encodes monocyte chemoattractant protein-1, on the growth of HeLa cells and derived somatic-cell hybrids in nude mice. *Mol. Carcinog.* 14: 179–189, **1995**.

Kleine-Lowinski, K., Gillitzer, R., Kühne-Heid, R., and Rösl, F. Monocyte-chemo-attractant-protein-1 (MCP-1)-gene expression in cervical intra-epithelial neoplasias and cervical carcinomas. *Int. J. Cancer* 82: 6–11, **1999**.

Kleine-Lowinski, K., Rheinwald, J.G., Fichorova, R.N., Anderson, D.J., Basile, J., Münger, K., Daly, C.M., Rösl, F., and Rollins, B.J. Selective suppression of monocyte chemoattractant protein-1 expression by human papillomavirus E6 and E7 oncoproteins in human cervical epithelial and epidermal cells. *Int. J. Cancer* 107: 407–415, **2003**.

Klingelhutz, A.J., Foster, S. A., and McDougall, J.K. Telomerase activation by the E6 gene product of human papillomavirus type 16. *Nature* 380: 79–82, **1996**.

Klug, A. and Finch, J.T. Structure of viruses of the papilloma-polyoma type. I. Human wart virus. *J. Mol. Biol.* 11: 403–423, **1965**.

Klussmann, J.P., Gultekin, E., Weissenborn, S. J., Wieland, U., Dries, V., Dienes, H.P.,

Eckel, H.E., Pfister, H.J., and Fuchs, P.G. Expression of p16 protein identifies a distinct entity of tonsillar carcinomas associated with human papillomavirus. *Am. J. Pathol.* 162: 747–753, **2003**.

Knight, G.L., Grainger, J.R., Gallimore, P.H., and Roberts, S. Cooperation between different forms of the human papillomavirus type 1 E4 protein to block cell cycle progression and cellular DNA synthesis. *J. Virol.* 78: 13 920–13 933, **2004**.

Ko, L.J. and Prives, C. p53: puzzle and paradigm. *Genes Dev.* 10: 1054–1072, **1996**.

Koffa, M., Koumantakis, E., Ergazaki, M., Tsatsanis, C., and Spandidos, D.A. Association of herpesvirus infection with the development of genital cancer. *Int. J. Cancer* 63: 58–62, **1995**.

König, C., Roth, J., and Dobbelstein, M. Adenovirus type 5 E4orf3 protein relieves p53 inhibition by E1B-55-kilodalton protein. *J. Virol.* 73: 2253–2262, **1999**.

Koopman, L.A., Corver, W.E., van der Slik, A.R., Giphart, M.J., and Fleuren, G.J. Multiple genetic alternations cause frequent and heterogeneous human histocompatibility leukocyte antigen class I loss in cervical cancer. *J. Exp. Med.* 191: 961–976, **2000**.

Koppikar, P., de Villiers, E.M., and Mulherkar R. Identification of human papillomaviruses in tumors of the oral cavity in an Indian community. *Int. J. Cancer* 113: 946–950, **2005**.

Koskela, P., Anttila, P., Bjorge, T., Brunsvig, A., Dillner, J., Hakama, M., Hakulinen, T., Jellum, E., Lehtinen, M., Lenner, P., Luostarinen, T., Pukkula, E., Saikku, P., Thoresen, S., Youngman, L., and Paavonen, J. *Chlamydia trachomatis* infection as a risk factor for invasive cervical cancer. *Int. J. Cancer* 85: 35–39, **2000**.

Koskinen, W.J., Chen, R.W., Leivo, I., Makitie, A., Back, L., Kontio, R., Suuronen, R., Lindqvist, C., Auvinen, E., Molijn, A., Quint, W.G., Vaheri, A., and Aaltonen, L.M. Prevalence and physical status of human papillomavirus in squamous cell carcinomas of the head and neck. *Int. J. Cancer* 107: 401–406, **2003**.

Kouronis, G., Iatrakis, G., Diakakis, I., Sakellaropoulos, G., Ladopoulos, I., and Prapa, Z. Treatment results of liquid nitrogen cryotherapy on selected pathologic changes of the uterine cervix. *Clin. Exp. Obstet. Gynecol.* 26: 115, **1999**.

Koutsky, L.A., Galloway, D.A., and Holmes, K.K. Epidemiology of genital human papillomavirus infection. *Epidemiol. Rev.* 10: 122–163, **1988**.

Koutsky, L.A., Ault, K.A., Wheeler, C.M., Brown, D.R., Barr, E., Alvarez, F.B., Chiacchierine, L.M., Jansen, K.U. Proof of Principle Study Investigators. A controlled trial of a human papillomavirus type 16 vaccine. *N. Engl. J. Med.* 347: 1645–1651, **2002**.

Kreimer, A.R., Clifford, G.M., Boyle, P., and Franceschi, S. Human papillomavirus types in head and neck squamous cell carcinomas worldwide: a systematic review. *Cancer Epidemiol. Biomarkers Prev.* 14: 467–475, **2005**.

Krivak, T.C., McBroom, J.W., Seidman, J., Venzon, D., Crothers, B., MacKoul, P.J., Rose, G.S., Carlson, J.W., and Birrer, M.J. Abnormal fragile histidine triad (FHIT) expression in advanced cervical carcinoma: a poor prognostic factor. *Cancer Res.* 61: 4382–4385, **2001**.

Krüger-Kjaer, S., van den Brule, A.J., Svare, E.I., Engholm, G., Sherman, M.E., Poll, P.A., Walboomers, J.M., Bock, J.E., and Meijer, C.J. Different risk factor patterns for high-grade and low-grade intraepithelial lesions on the cervix among HPV-positive and HPV-negative young women. *Int. J. Cancer* 76: 613–619, **1998**.

Kuerbitz, S. J., Plunkett, B.S., Walsh, W.V., and Kastan, M.B. Wild-type p53 is a cell cycle checkpoint determinant following irradiation. *Proc. Natl. Acad. Sci. USA* 89: 7491–7495, **1992**.

Kutler, D.I., Auerbach, A.D., Satagopan, J., Giampietro, P.F., Batish, S. D., Huvos, A.G., Goberdhan, A., Shah, J.P., and Singh, B. High incidence of head and neck squamous cell carcinoma in patients with Fanconi anemia. *Arch. Otolaryngol. Head Neck Surg.* 129: 106–112, **2003**a.

Kutler, D.I., Wreesmann, V.B., Goberdhan, A.,. Ben-Porat, L., Satagopan, J., Ngai, I., Huvos, A.G., Giampietro, P., Levran, O., Pujara, K., Diotti, R., Carlson, D., Huryn, L.A., Auerbach, A.D., and Singh, B. Human papillomavirus DNA and p53 polymorphism in squamous cell carcinomas from Fanconi anemia patients. *J. Natl. Cancer Inst.* 95: 1718–1721, **2003**b.

Kyo, S., Inoue, M., Hayasaka, N., Inoue, T., Yutsudo, M., Tanizawa, O., and Hakura, A. Regulation of early gene expression of human papillomavirus type 16 by inflammatory cytokines. *Virology* 200: 130–139, **1994**.

Lacey, J.V., Jr., Brinton, L.A., Abbas, F.M., Barnes, W.A., Gravitt, P.E., Greenberg, M.D., Greene, S. M., Hadjimichael, O.C., McGowan, L., Mortel, R., Schwartz, P.E., Silverberg, S. G., and Hildesheim, A. Oral contraceptives as risk factors for cervical adenocarcinomas and squamous cell carcinomas. *Cancer Epidemiol. Biomarkers Prev.* 8: 1079–1085, **1999**.

Lam, E.W., Morris, J.D., Davies, R., Crook, T., Watson, R.J., and Vousden, K.H. HPV 16 E7 oncoprotein deregulates B-myb expression: correlation with targeting of p107/E2F complexes. *EMBO J.* 13: 871–878, **1994**.

Lambert, P.F., Pan, H., Pitot, H.C., Liem, A., Jackson, M., and Griep, A.E. Epidermal cancer associated with expression of human papillomavirus type 16 E6 and E7 oncogenes in the skin of transgenic mice. *Proc. Natl. Acad. Sci. USA* 90: 5583–5587, **1993**.

Lappalainen, K., Urtti, A., Jaaskelainen, I., Syrjänen, K., and Syrjänen, S. Cationic liposomes mediated delivery of antisense oligonucleotides targeted to HPV 16 E7mRNA in CaSki cells. *Antiviral Res.* 23: 119–130, **1994**.

La Thangue, N.B. DRTF1/E2F: an expanding family of heterodimeric transcription factors implicated in cell-cycle control. *Trends Biochem. Sci.* 19: 108–114, **1994**.

Lavergne, D. and de Villiers, E.-M. Papillomavirus in esophageal papillomas and carcinomas. *Int. J. Cancer* 80: 682–684, **1999**.

Lechner, M.S. and Laimins, L.A. Inhibition of p53 DNA binding by human papillomavirus E6 proteins. *J. Virol.* 68: 4262–4273, **1994**.

Lee, S. S., Weiss, R.S., and Javier, E.T. Binding of human virus oncoproteins to hDlg/SAP97, a mammalian homolog of the *Drosophila* discs large tumor suppressor protein. *Proc. Natl. Acad. Sci. USA* 94: 6670–6675, **1997** .

Lee, S. S., Glaunsinger, B., Mantovani, F., Banks, L., and Javier, R.T. Multi-PDZ domain protein MUPP1 is a cellular target for both adenovirus E4-ORF1 and high risk papillomavirus type 18 E6 proteins. *J. Virol.* 74: 9680–9693, **2000** .

Leechanachai, P., Banks, L., Moreau, F., and Mathlashewski, G. The E5 gene from human papillomavirus type 16 is an oncogene which enhances growth factor-mediated signal transduction to the nucleus. *Oncogene* 7: 19–25, **1992**.

Lehtinen, M., Luostarinen, T., Youngman, L.D., Anttila, T., Dillner, J., Hakulinen, T., Kosekela, P., Lenner, P., and Hallmans, G. Low levels of serum vitamin A and E in blood and subsequent risk for cervical cancer: interaction with HPV seropositivity. *Nutr. Cancer* 34: 229–234, **1999**.

Lehtinen, M., Koskela, P., Jellum, E., Bloigu, A., Anttila, T., Hallmans, G., Luukkaala, T., Thoresen, S., Youngman, L., Dillner, J., and Hakama, M. Herpes simplex virus and risk of cervical cancer: a longitudinal, nested case-control study in the Nordic countries. *Am. J. Epidemiol.* 156: 687–692, **2002**.

Lele, S. M., Pou, A.M., Ventura, K., Gatalica, Z., and Payne, D. Molecular events in the progression of recurrent respiratory papillomatosis to carcinoma. *Arch. Pathol. Lab. Med.* 126: 1184–1188, **2002**.

Leptak, C., Ramon y Cajal, S., Kulke, R., Horwitz, B.H., Riese D.J., II, Dotto, G.P., and DiMaio, D. Tumorigenic transformation of murine keratinocytes by the E5 genes of bovine papillomavirus type 1 and human papillomavirus type 16. *J. Virol.* 65: 7078–7083, **1991**.

Li, M., Cripe, T.P., Estes, P.A., Lyon, M.K., Rose, R.C., and Garcea, R.L. Expression of the human papillomavirus type 11 L1 capsid protein in *Escherichia coli*: characterization of protein domains involved in DNA binding and capsid assembly. *J. Virol.* 71: 2988–2995, **1997**.

Li, R., Yang, L., Fouts, E., and Botchan, M.R. Site-specific DNA-binding proteins important for replication and transcription have multiple activities. *Cold Spring Harbor Symp. Quant. Biol.* 58: 403–413, **1993**.

Li, S. L., Kim, M.S., Cherrick, H.M., Doniger, J., and Park, N.H. Sequential combined tumorigenic effect of HPV-16 and chemical carcinogens. *Carcinogenesis* 13: 1981–1987, **1992**.

Li, T., Lu, Z.M., Chen, K.N., Guo, M., Xing, H.P., Mei, Q, Yang, H.H., Lechner, J.F.,

and Ke, Y. Human papillomavirus type 18 is an important infectious factor in the high incidence of esophageal cancer in Anyang area of China. *Carcinogenesis* 22: 929–934, **2001**.

Lie, E.S., Karlsen, F., and Holm, R. Presence of human papillomavirus in squamous cell laryngeal carcinomas. A study of thirty-nine cases using polymerase chain reaction and in situ hybridization. *Acta Otolaryngol.* 116: 900–905, **1996** .

Lin, B.Y., Makhov, A.M., Griffith, J.D., Broker, T.R., and Chow, L.T. Chaperone proteins abrogate inhibition of the human papillomavirus (HPV) E1 replicative helicase by the HPV E2 protein. *Mol. Cell. Biol.* 22: 6592–6604, **2002**.

Lin, D., Shields, M.T., Ullrich, S. J., Appella, E., and Mercer, W.E. Growth arrest induced by wild-type p53 protein blocks cells prior to or near the restriction point in late G1 phase. *Proc. Natl. Acad. Sci. USA* 89: 9210–9214, **1992**.

Lin, K.Y., Westra, W.H., Kashima, H.K., Mounts, P., and Wu, T.C. Coinfection of HPV-11 and HPV-16 in a case of laryngeal squamous papillomas with severe dysplasia. *Laryngoscope* 107: 942–947, **1997**.

Lindeberg, H. and Krogdahl, A. Laryngeal cancer and human papillomavirus: HPV is absent in the majority of laryngeal carcinomas. *Cancer Lett.* 146: 9–13, **1999**.

Lindel, K., Beer, K.T., Laissue, J., Greiner, R.H., and Aebersold, D.M., Human papillomavirus positive squamous cell carcinoma of the oropharynx: a radiosensitive subgroup of head and neck carcinoma. *Cancer* 92: 805–813, **2001**.

Little, A.M. and Stern, P.L. Does HLA type predispose some individuals to cancer? *Mol. Med. Today* 5: 337–342, **1999**.

Liu, D.W., Tsao, Y.P., Kung, J.T., Ding, Y.A., Sytwu, H.K., Xiao, X., and Chen, S. L. Recombinant adeno-associated virus expressing human papillomavirus type 16 E7 peptide DNA fused with heat shock protein DNA as a potential vaccine for cervical cancer. *J. Virol.* 74: 2888–2894, **2000**.

Liu, D.W., Chang, J.L., Tsao, Y.P., Huang, C.W., Kuo, S. W., and Chen, S. L. Co-vaccination with adeno-associated virus vectors encoding human papillomavirus 16 L1 proteins and adenovirus encoding murine GM-CSF can elicit strong and prolonged neutralizing antibody. *Int. J. Cancer*. 113: 93–100, **2005**.

Liu, X., Yuan, H., Fu, B., Disbrow, G.L., Apolinario, T., Tomaic, V., Kelley, M.L., Baker, C.C., Huibregtse, J., and Schlegel, R. The E6AP ubiquitin ligase is required for transactivation of the hTERT promoter by human papillomavirus E6 oncoprotein. *J. Biol. Chem*. 280: 10807–10816, **2005**.

Liu, Y., Chen, J.J., Gao, Q., Dalal, S., Hong, Y., Mansur, C.P., Band, V., and Androphy, E.J. Multiple functions of human papillomavirus type 16 E6 contribute to the immortalization of mammary epithelial cells. *J. Virol*. 73: 7297–7307, **1999**.

Liu, Y., Klimberg, V.S., Andrews, N.R., Hicks, C.R., Peng, H., Chiriva-Internati, M., Henry Tilman, R., and Hermonat, P.L. Human papillomavirus DNA is present in a subset of unselected breast cancers. *J. Hum. Virol*. 4: 329–334, **2001**.

Livingstone, L.R., White, A., Sprouse, J., Livanos, E., Jacks, T., and Tlsty, T.D. Altered cell cycle arrest and gene amplification potential accompany loss of wild-type p53. *Cell* 70: 923–935, **1992**.

Loke, S. L., Ma, L., Wong, M., Srivastava, G., Lo, I., and Bird, C.C. Human papillomavirus in oesophageal squamous cell carcinoma. *J. Clin. Pathol*. 43: 909–912, **1990**.

Longworth, M.S. and Laimins, L.A. Pathogenesis of human papillomaviruses in differentiating epithelia. *Microbiol. Mol. Biol*. 68: 362–372, **2004a**.

Longworth, M.S and Laimins, L.A. The binding of histone deacetylases and the integrity of zinc finger – like motifs of the E-7 protein are essential for the life cycle of human papillomavirus type 31. *J. Virol*. 78: 3533–3541, **2004 b**.

Löning, T., Ikenberg, H., Becker, J., Gissmann, L., Hoepfer, I., and zur Hausen, H. Analysis of oral papillomas, leukoplakias, and invasive carcinomas for human papillomavirus type related DNA. *J. Invest. Dermatol*. 84: 417–20, **1985**.

Loo, Y.M. and Melendy, T. Recruitment of replication protein A by the papillomavirus E1 protein and modulation by single-stranded DNA. *J. Virol*. 78: 1605–1615, **2004**.

Lu, Z., Hu, X., Li, Y., Zheng, L., Zhou, Y., Jiang, H., Ning, T., Basang, Z., Zhang, C.,

and Ke, Y. Human papillomavirus 16 E6 oncoprotein interferences with insulin signaling pathway by binding to tuberin. *J. Biol. Chem*. 279: 35664–35 670, **2004**.

Lüscher-Firzlaff, J.M., Westendorf, J.M., Zwicker, J., Burkhardt, H., Henriksson, M., Müller, R., Pirollet, F., and Lüscher, B. Interaction of the fork head domain transcription factor MPP2 with the human papilloma virus 16 E7 protein: enhancement of transformation and transactivation. *Oncogene* 18: 5620–5630, **1999**.

Lutzner, M., Croissant, O., Ducasse, M.F., Kreis, H., Crosnier, J., and Orth, G. A potentially oncogenic human papillomavirus (HPV-5) found in two renal allograft recipients. *J. Invest. Dermatol*. 75: 353–356, **1980**.

Mack, D.H. and Laimins, L.A. A keratinocyte-specific transcription factor, KRF-1, interacts with AP-1 to activate expression of human papillomavirus type 18 in squamous epithelial cells. *Proc. Natl. Acad. Sci. USA* 88: 9102–9106, **1991**.

Magnusson, P.K. and Gyllensten, U.B. Cervical cancer risk: is there a genetic component? *Mol. Med. Today* 6: 146–148, **2000**.

Mackerras, D., Irwig, L., Simpson, J.M., Weisberg, E., Cardona, M., Webster, F., Walton, L., and Ghersi, D. Randomized double-blind trial of β-carotene and vitamin C in women with minor cervical abnormalities. *Br. J. Cancer* 79: 1448–1453, **1999**.

Mai, K.T., Yazdi, H.M., Bertrand, M.A., LeSaux, N., and Catheart, L.L. Bilateral primary ovarian squamous cell carcinoma with human papilloma virus infection and vulvar and cervical intraepithelial neoplasia. *Am. J. Surg. Pathol*. 20: 767–772, **1996**.

Malanchi, I., Accardi, R., Diehl, F., Smet, A., Androphy, E., Hoheisel, J., and Tommasino, M. Human papillomavirus type 16 promotes retinoblastoma protein phosphorylation and cell cycle progression. *J. Virol*. 78: 13769–13778, **2004**.

Malcles, M.H., Cueille, N., Mechali, F., Coux, O., and Bonne-Andrea, C. Regulation of bovine papillomavirus replicative helicase e1 by the ubiquitin-proteasome pathway. *J. Virol*. 76: 11350–11358, **2002**.

Malejczyk, J., Malejczyk, M., Kock, A., Urbanski, A., Majewski, S., Hunzelmann, N.,

Jablonska, S., Orth, G., and Luger, T.A. Autocrine growth limitation of human papillomavirus type 16-harbouring keratinocytes by constitutively released tumor necrosis factor-α. *J. Immunol.* 149: 2702–2708, **1992**.

Maloney, K.E., Wiener, J.S., and Walther, P.J. Oncogenic human papillomaviruses are rarely associated with squamous cell carcinoma of the bladder: evaluation by differential polymerase chain reaction. *J. Urol.* 151: 360–364, **1994** .

Mannhardt, B., Weinzimer, S. A., Wagner, M., Fiedler, M., Cohen, P., Jansen-Dürr, P., and Zwerschke, W. Human papillomavirus type 16 E7 oncoprotein binds and inactivates growth-inhibitory insulin-like growth factor binding protein 3. *Mol. Cell. Biol.* 20: 6483–6495, **2000**.

Manolaraki, M.M., Arvanitis, D.A., Sourvinos, G., Sifakis, S., Koumantakis, E., and Spandidos, D.A. Frequent loss of heterozygosity in chromosomal region 9pter-p13 in tumor biopsies and cytological material of uterine cervical cancer. *Cancer Lett.* 176: 175–181, **2002**.

Manolitsas, T.P., Lanham, S. A., Hitchcock, A., and Watson, R.H. Synchronous ovarian and cervical squamous intraepithelial neoplasia: an analysis of the HPV status. *Gynecol. Oncol.* 70: 428–431, **1998**.

Manso-Martinez, R. Podophyllotoxin poisoning of microtubules at steady state: effect of substoichiometric and superstoichiometric concentrations of drug. *Mol. Cell. Biochem.* 45: 3–11, **1982**.

Mantovani, F. and Banks, L. The human papillomavirus E6 protein and its contribution to malignant progression. *Oncogene* 20: 7874–7887, **2001**.

Marks, P., Rifkind, R.A., Richon, V.M., Breslow, R., Miller, T., and Kelly, W.K. Histone deacetylases and cancer: causes and therapies. *Nat. Rev. Cancer* 1: 194–202, **2001**.

Martelli, F., Hamilton, T., Silver, D.P., Sharpless, N.E., Bardeesy, N., Rokas, M., DePinho, R.A., Livingston, D.M., and Grossman, S. R. p19ARF targets certain E2F species for degradation. *Proc. Natl. Acad. Sci. USA* 98: 4455–4460, **2001**.

Martin, L.G., Demers, G.W., and Galloway, D.A. Disruption of the G1/S transition in human papillomavirus type 16 E7-expressing human cells is associated with altered regulation of cyclin E. *J. Virol.* 72: 975–985, **1998**.

Massimi, P., Pim, D., Storey, A., and Banks, L. HPV-16 E7 and adenovirus E1a complex formation with TATA box binding protein is enhanced by casein kinase II phosphorylation. *Oncogene* 12: 2325–2330, **1996**.

Massimi, P., Pim, D., and Banks, L. Human papillomavirus type 16 E7 binds to the conserved carboxy-terminal region of the TATA box binding protein and this contributes to E7 transforming activity. *J. Gen. Virol.* 78: 2607–2613, **1997** .

Massimi, P., Pim, D., Bertoli, C., Bouvard, V., and Banks, L. Interaction between the HPV-16 E2 transcriptional activator and p53. *Oncogene* 18: 7748–7754, **1999**.

Matsukura, T. and Sugase, M. Identification of genital human papillomaviruses in cervical biopsy specimens: segregation of specific virus types in specific clinicopathological lesions. *Int. J. Cancer* 61: 13–22, **1995**.

Matsukura, T., Koi, S., and Sugase, M. Both episomal and integrated forms of human papillomavirus type 16 are involved in invasive cervical cancers. *Virology* 172: 63–72, **1989**.

Mbutlaiteye, S. M., Biggar, R.J., Goedert, J.J., and Engels, E.A. Immune deficiency and risk for malignancy among persons with AIDS. *J. Acquir. Immune Defic. Syndr.* 32: 527–533, **2003**.

McDonnell, J.M., Mayr, A.J., and Martin, W.J. DNA of human papillomavirus type 16 in dysplastic and malignant lesions of the conjunctiva and cornea. *N. Engl. J. Med.* 320: 1442–1446, **1989**.

McIntyre, M.C., Ruesch, M.N., and Laimins, L.A. Human papillomavirus E7 oncoproteins bind a single form of cyclin E in a complex with cdk2 and p107. *Virology* 215: 73–82, **1996**.

Melchers, W., de Mare, S., Kuitert, S., Galama, J., Walboomers, J., and van den Brule, A.J.C. Human papillomavirus and cutaneous warts in meat handlers. *J. Clin. Microbiol.* 31: 2547–2549, **1993**.

Mellin, H., Friesland, S., Lewensohn, R., Dalianis, T., and Munck-Wikland, E., Human papillomavirus (HPV) DNA in tonsillar cancer: clinical correlates, risk of relapse, and survival. *Int. J. Cancer* 89: 300–304, **2000**.

Mellin, H., Dahlgren, L., Munck-Wikland, E., Lindholm, J., Rabbani, H., Kalantari, M., and Dalianis, T. Human papillomavirus type 16 is episomal and a high viral load may be correlated to better prognosis in tonsillar cancer. *Int. J. Cancer.* 102: 152–158, **2002**.

Melsheimer, P., Vinokurova, S., Wentzensen, N., Bastert, G., and von Knebel Doeberitz, M. DNA aneuploidy and integration of human papillomavirus type 16 E6/E7 oncogenes in intraepithelial neoplasia and invasive squamous cell carcinoma of the cervix uteri. *Clin. Cancer Res.* 10: 3059–3063, **2004**.

Menendez Velazquez, J.F., Gonzalez Sanchez, J.L., Rodriguez de Santiago, J.D., Muñoz Reyes, R., and Baibn Uriza, R. [The treatment of cervical human papillomavirus (HPV) infection with trichloroacetic acid] (in Spanish). *Ginecol. Obst. Mex.* 61: 48–51, **1993**.

Mevorach, R.A., Cos, L.R., di Sant'Agnese, P.A., and Stoler, M. Human papillomavirus type 6 in grade I transitional cell carcinoma of the urethra. *J. Urol.* 143: 126–128, **1990**.

Meyer, T., Arndt, R., Nindl, I., Ulrich, C., Christophers, E., and Stockfleth, E. Association of human papillomavirus infections with cutaneous tumors in immunosuppressed patients. *Transpl. Int.* 16: 146–153, **2003**.

Meyerson, M., Counter, C.M., Eaton, E.N., Ellisen, L.W., Steiner, P., Caddle, S. D., Ziaugra, L., Beijersbergen, R.L., Davidoff, M.J., Liu, Q., Bacchetti, S., Haber, D.A., and Weinberg, R.A. hEST2, the putative human telomerase catalytic subunit gene, is up-regulated in tumor cells and during immortalization. *Cell* 90: 785–795, **1997**.

Meyskens, F.L., Jr., Surwit, E., Moon, T.E., Childers, J.M., Davis, J.R., Dorr, R.T., Johnson, C.S., and Alberts, C.S. Enhancement of regression of cervical intraepithelial neoplasia II (moderate dysplasia) with topically applied all-trans-retinoic acid: a randomized trial. *J. Natl. Cancer Inst.* 86: 539–343, **1994**.

Michelin, D., Gissmann, L., Street, D., Potkul, R.K., Fisher, S., Kaufmann, A.M., Qiao, L., Schreckenberger, C. Regulation of human papillomavirus type 18 in vivo: effects of estrogen and progesterone in transgenic mice. *Gynecol. Oncol.* 66: 202–208, **1997**.

Milburn, P.B., Brandsma, J.L., Goldsman, C.I., Teplitz, E.D., and Heilman, E.I. Disseminated warts and evolving squamous cell carcinomas in a patient with acquired immunodeficiency syndrome. *J. Am. Acad. Dermatol.* 19: 401–405, **1988** .

Milner, J. RNA interference for treating cancers caused by viral infection. *Expert Opin. Biol. Ther.* 3: 459–467, **2003**.

Minkoff, H., Feldman, J.G., Strickler, H.D., Watts, D.H., Bacon, M.C., Levine, A., Palefsky, J.M., Burk, R., Cohen, M.H., and Anastos, K. Relationship between smoking and human papillomavirus infections in HIV-infected and -uninfected women. *J. Infect. Dis.* 189: 1821–1828, **2004**.

Moran, E. and Mathews, M.B. Multiple functional domains in the adenovirus E1A gene. *Cell* 48: 177–178, **1987**.

Mork, J., Lie, A.K., Glattre, E., Hallmans, G., Jellum, E., Koskela, P., Möller, B., Pukkala, E., Schiller, J.T., Youngman, L., Lehtinen, M., and Dillner, J. Human papillomavirus infection as a risk factor for squamous-cell carcinoma of the head and neck. *N. Engl. J. Med.* 344: 1125–1131, **2001**.

Moscicki, A.B., Palefsky, J., Gonzales, J., and Schoolnik, G.K. Human papillomavirus infection in sexually active adolescent females: prevalence and risk factors. *Pediatr. Res.* 28: 507–513, **1990**.

Moscicki, A.B., Ellenberg, J.H., Vermund, S. H., Holland, C.A., Darragh, T., Crowley-Nowick, P.A., Levin, L., and Wilson, C.M. Prevalence of and risks for cervical human papillomavirus infection and squamous intraepithelial lesions in adolescent girls: impact of infection with human immunodeficiency virus. *Arch. Pediatr. Adolesc. Med.* 154: 127–34, **2000**.

Moscicki, A.B., Hills, N., Shiboski, S., Powell, K., Jay, N., Hanson, E., Miller, S., Clayton, L., Farhat, S., Broering, J., Darragh, T., and Palefsky, J. Risks for incident human papillomavirus infection and low-grade squamous intraepithelial lesion development in young females. *JAMA* 285: 2995–3002, **2001**.

Moubayed, P., Mwakyoma, H., and Schneider, D.T. High frequency of human papillomavirus 6/11, 16, and 18 infections in precancerous lesions and squamous cell carcinoma of the conjunctiva in subtropical Tanzania. *Am. J. Clin. Pathol.* 122: 938–943, **2004**.

Mouret, S., Sauvaigo, S., Peinnequin, A., Favier, A., Beani, J.C., and Leccia, M.T. E6* oncoprotein expression of human papillomavirus type-16 determines different ultraviolet sensitivity related to glutathione and glutathione peroxidase antioxidant defence. *Exp. Dermatol.* 14: 401–410, **2005**.

Moy, R.L., Eliezri, Y.D., Nuovo, G.J., Zitelli, J.A., Bennett, R.G., and Silverstein, S. Human papillomavirus type 16 DNA in periungual squamous cell carcinomas. *JAMA* 261: 2669–2673, **1989**.

Muderspach, L., Wilczynski, S., Roman, L., Bade, L., Felix, J., Small, L.A., Kast, W.M., Fascio, G., Marty, V., and Weber, J. A phase I trial of a human papillomavirus (HPV) peptide vaccine for women with high grade cervical and vulvar intraepithelial neoplasia who are HPV 16 positive. *Clin. Cancer Res.* 6: 3406–3416, **2000**.

Müller, M., Zhou, J., Reed, T.D., Rittmüller, C., Burger, A., Gabelsberger, J., Braspenning, J., and Gissmann, L. Chimeric papillomavirus-like particles. *Virology* 234: 93–111, **1997**.

Münger, K., Phelps, W.C., Bubb, V., Howley, P.M., and Schlegel, R. The E6 and E7 genes of the human papillomavirus type 16 are necessary and sufficient for transformation of primary human keratinocytes. *J. Virol.* 63: 4417–4423, **1989**.

Münger, K., Baldwin, A., Edwards, K.M., Hayakawa, H., Nguyen, C.L., Owens, M., Grace, M., and Huh, K.W. Mechanisms of human papillomavirus-induced oncogenesis. *J. Virol.* 78: 11451–11460, **2004**.

Munn, S. E., Higgins, E., Marshall, M., and Clement, M. A new method of intralesional bleomycin therapy in the treatment of recalcitrant warts. *Br. J. Dermatol.* 135: 969–971, **1996**.

Muñoz, N., Bosch, F.X., de Sanjosé, S., Tafur, L., Izarzugaza, I., Gili, M., Viladiu, P., Navarro, C., Martos, C., Asunce, N., et al. The causal link between human papillomavirus and invasive cervical cancer: a population-based case-control study in Columbia and Spain. *Int. J. Cancer* 52: 743–749, **1992**.

Muñoz, N., Franceschi, S., Bosetti, C., Moreno, V., Herrero, R., Smith, J.S., Shah, K.V., Meijer, C.J.L. and Bosch, F.F. Role of parity and human papillomavirus in cervical cancer: the IARC multicentral case-control study. *Lancet* 359: 1093–1101, **2002**.

Nagpal, J.K., Patnaik, S., and Das, B.R. Prevalence of high-risk human papilloma virus types and its association with P53 codon 72 polymorphism in tobacco addicted oral squamous cell carcinoma (OSCC) patients of Eastern India. *Int. J. Cancer* 97: 649–653, **2002**.

Naguib, S. M., Lundin, F.E., Jr., and Davis, H.J. Relation of various epidemiologic factors to cervical cancer as determined by a screening program. *Obstet. Gynecol.* 28: 451–459, **1966**.

Nahmias, A.J., Josey, W.E., Naib, Z.M., Luce, C.F., and Guest, B.A. Antibodies to Herpesvirus hominis types 1 and 2 in humans. II. Women with cervical cancer. *Am. J. Epidemiol.* 91: 547–552, **1970**.

Naib, Z.M., Nahmias, A.J., Josey, W.E., and Kramer, J.H. Genital herpetic infection: association with cervical dysplasia and carcinoma. *Cancer* 23: 940–945, **1969**.

Nakagawa, S. and Huibregtse, J.M. Human scribble (vartul) is targeted for ubiquitin-mediated degradation by the high risk papillomavirus E6 proteins and the E6AP ubiquitin-protein ligase. *Mol. Cell. Biol.* 20: 8244–8253, **2000**.

Nakahara, T., Nishimura, A., Tanaka, M., Ueno, T., Ishimoto, A., and Sakai, H. Modulation of the cell division cycle by human papillomavirus type 18 E4. *J. Virol.* 76: 10914–10920, **2002**.

Nakamura, T.M., Morin, G.B., Chapman, K.B., Weinrich, S. L., Andrews, W.H., Lingner, J., Harley, C.B., and Cech, T.R. Telomerase catalytic subunit homologs from fission yeast and human. *Science* 277: 955–959, **1997**.

Nandakumar, A., Gupta, P.C., Gangadharan, P., Visweswara, R.N., and Parkin, D.M. Geographic pathology revisited: Development of an atlas of cancer in India. *Int. J. Cancer* 116: 740–754, **2005**.

Neary, K., Horwitz, B.H., and DiMaio, D. Mutational analysis of open reading frame E4 of bovine papillomavirus type 1. *J. Virol.* 61: 1248–1252, **1987**.

Neill, S. M., Lessana-Leibowitch, M., Pelisse, M., and Moyal-Barracco, M. Lichen sclerosus, invasive squamous cell carcinoma, and human papillomavirus. *Am. J. Obstet. Gynecol.* 162: 1633–1634, **1990**.

Nguyen, D.X., Westbrook, T.F., and McCance, D.J. Human papillomavirus type 16 E7 maintains elevated levels of the cdc25A tyrosine phosphatase during deregulation of cell cycle arrest. *J. Virol.* 76: 619–632, **2002**.

Nguyen, M.L., Nguyen, M.M., Lee, D., Griep, A.E., and Lambert, P.F. The PDZ ligand domain of the human papillomavirus type 16 E6 protein is required for E6's induction of epithelial hyperplasia in vivo. *J. Virol.* 77: 6957–6964, **2003** .

Nie, J., McGill, M.A., Dermer, M., Dho, S. E., Wolting, C.D., and McGlade, C.J. LNX functions as a RING type E3 ubiquitin ligase that targets the cell fate determinant Numb for ubiquitin-dependent degradation. *EMBO J.* 21: 93–102, **2002** .

Niedergang, F., Didierlaurent, A., Kraehenbühl, J.P., and Sirard, J.C. Dendritic cells: the host Achilles' heel for mucosal pathogens? *Trends Microbiol.* 12: 79–88, **2004**.

Niedobitek, G., Pitteroff, S., Herbst, H., Shepherd, P., Finn, T., Anagnostopoulos, I., and Stein, H. Detection of human papillomavirus type 16 DNA in carcinomas of the palatine tonsil. *J. Clin. Pathol.* 43: 918–921, **1990**.

Nishikawa, T. [Experimental study on carcinogenesis by human papillomavirus type 8 E7 gene] Article in Japanese. *Hokkaido Igaku Zasshi* 69: 563–573, **1994**.

Noel, J.C., Vandenbossche, M., Peny, M.O., Sassine, A., de Dobbeleer, G., Schulman, C.C., and Verhest, A. Verrucous carcinoma of the penis: importance of human papillomavirus typing for diagnosis and therapeutic decision. *Eur. Urol.* 22: 83–85, **1992**.

Nunn, J.R., Harington, J.S., Allsobrook, A.J., Du Plessis, L.S., and Nunn, A.J. N-nitrosamines in the human vaginal vault. *S. Afr. Med. Sci.* 39: 179–182, **1974**.

O'Connor, M. and Bernard, H.-U. Oct-1 activates the epithelial-specific enhancer of human papillomavirus type 16 via a synergistic interaction with NF1 at a conserved composite regulatory site. *Virology* 207: 77–88, **1995**.

Oda, H., Kumar, S., and Howley, P.M. Regulation of the Src family tyrosine kinase Blk through E6AP-mediated ubiquitination. *Proc. Natl. Acad. Sci. USA* 96: 9557–9562, **1999**.

O'Farrell, N. N-nitrosamines, trichomoniasis and cervical cancer. *S. Afr. Med. J.* 75: 247–248, **1989**.

Ogura, H., Fukushima, K., and Watanabe, S. A high prevalence of human papillomavirus DNA in recurrent nasal papillomas. *J. Med. Microbiol.* 45: 162–166, **1996**.

O'Leary, J., Landers, R., Crowley, M., Healy, I., O'Donovan, M., Healy, V., Kealy, W.F., Hogan, J., and Doyle, CT. Human papillomavirus and mixed epithelial tumors of the endometrium. *Hum. Pathol.* 29: 309–310, **1998**.

Olson, C., Pamukcu, A.M., Brobst, D.F., Kowalczyk, T., Satter, E.J., and Price, J.M. A urinary bladder tumor induced by a bovine cutaneous papilloma agent. *Cancer Res.* 19: 779–782, **1959**.

Onuk, M.D., Oztopuz, A., and Memik, F. Risk factors for esophageal cancer in eastern Anatolia. *Hepatogastroenterology* 49: 1290–1292, **2002**.

Oriel, J.D. Natural history of genital warts. *Br. J. Vener. Dis.* 47: 1–13, **1971**.

Orth, G. Human papillomaviruses associated with epidermodysplasia verruciformis in non-melanoma skin cancers: guilty or innocent? *J. Invest. Dermatol.* 125: xii – xiii, **2005**.

Orth, G., Favre, M., and Croissant, O. Characterization of a new type of human papillomavirus that causes skin warts. *J. Virol.* 24: 108–120, **1977**.

Orth, G., Jablonska, S., Favre, M., Jarzabek-Chorzelska, M., and Rzesa, G. Characterization of two types of human papillomaviruses in lesions of epidermodysplasia verruciformis. *Proc. Natl. Acad. Sci. USA* 75: 1537–1541, **1978**.

Orth, G., Jablonska, S., Jarzabek-Chorzelska, M., Obalek, S., Rzesa, G., Favre, M., and Croissant, O. Characteristics of the lesions and risk of malignant conversion associated with the type of the human papillomavirus involved in epidermodysplasia verruciformis. *Cancer Res.* 39: 1074–1082, **1979**.

Ostrow, R.S., Bender, M., Niimura, M., Seki, T., Kawashima, M., Pass, F., and Faras, A.J. Human papillomavirus DANN in cutaneous primary and metastasized squamous cell carcinomas from patients with epidermodysplasia verruciformis. *Proc. Natl. Acad. Sci. USA* 79: 1634–1638, **1982**.

Ostrow, R.S., Manias, D.A., Fong, W.J., Zachow, K.R., and Faras, A.J. A survey of human cancers for papillomavirus DNA by filter hybridization. *Cancer* 59: 429–434, **1987**.

Ostrow, R.S., LaBresh, K.V., and Faras, A.J. Characterization of the complete RhPV1 genomic sequence and an integration locus from a metastatic tumor. *Virology* 181: 424–429, **1991**.

Pagano, J.S. Diseases and mechanisms of persistent DNA virus infection: latency and cellular transformation. *J. Infect. Dis.* 132: 209–223, **1975**.

Palefsky, J.M. Human papillomavirus-associated malignancies in HIV-positive men and women. *Curr. Opin. Oncol.* 7: 437–441, **1995**.

Palefsky, J.M. Anal squamous intraepithelial lesions: relation to HIV and human papillomavirus infection. *J. Acquir. Immune Defic. Syndr.* 21, Suppl 1: S42–S48, **1999**.

Palefsky, J.M., Holly, E.A., Gonzales, J., Berline, J., Ahn, D.K., and Greenspan, J.S. Detection of human papillomavirus DNA in anal intraepithelial neoplasia and anal cancer. *Cancer Res.* 51: 1014–1019, **1991**.

Pan, W., Datta, A., Adami, G.R., Raychaudhuri, P., and Bagchi, S. P19ARF inhibits the functions of the HPV16 E7 oncoprotein. *Oncogene* 22: 5496–5503, **2003**.

Park, J.S., Kim, E.J., Kwon, H.J., Hwang, E.S., Namkoong, S. E., and Um, S. J. Inactivation of interferon regulatory factor-1 tumor suppressor protein by HPV E7 oncoprotein. Implications for the E7-mediated immune evasion mechanism in cervical carcinogenesis. *J. Biol. Chem.* 275: 6764–6769, **2000**.

Parkin, D.M., Bray, F., Ferlay, J., and Pisani, P. Global cancer statistics, 2002. *CA Cancer J. Clin.* 55: 74–108, **2005**.

Patel, D., Huang, S. M., Baglia, L.A., and McCance, D.J. The E6 protein of human papillomavirus type 16 binds to and inhibits co-activation by CBP and p300. *EMBO J.* 18: 5061–5072, **1999**.

Patel, D., Incassati, A., Wang, N., and McCance, D.J. Human papillomavirus type

16 E6 and E7 cause polyploidy in human keratinocytes and up-regulation of G2-M-phase proteins. *Cancer Res.* 64: 1299–1306, **2004**.

Pater, M.M., Hughes, G.A., Hyslop, D.E., Nakshatri, H., and Pater, A. Glucocorticoid-dependent oncogenic transformation by type 16 but not type 11 human papilloma virus DNA. *Nature* 335: 832–835, **1988**.

Paz, I.B., Cook, N., Odom-Maryon, T., Xie, Y., and Wilczynski, S. P. Human papillomavirus (HPV) in head and neck cancer. An association of HPV 16 with squamous cell carcinoma of Waldeyer's tonsillar ring. *Cancer* 79: 595–604, **1997**.

Peipert, J.F. Clinical practice. Genital chlamydial infections. *N. Engl. J. Med.* 349: 2424–2430, **2003**.

Peixoto Guimaraes, D., Hsin Lu, S., Snijders, P., Wilmotte, R., Herrero, R., Lenoir, G., Montesano, R., Meijer, C.J.M., Walboomers, J., and Hainaut, P. Absence of association between HPV DNA TP53 codon 72 polymorphism, and risk of oesophageal cancer in a high risk area of China. *Cancer Lett.* 162: 231–235, **2001**.

Peng, S., Kim, T.W., Lee, J.H., Yang, M., He, L., Hung, C.F., and Wu, T.C. Vaccination with dendritic cells transfected with BAK and BAX siRNA enhances antigen-specific immune responses by prolonging dendritic cell life. *Hum. Gene Ther.* 16: 584–593, **2005**.

Pett, D., Alazawi, W.O., Roberts, I., Dowen, S., Smith, D.I., Stanley, M.A., and Coleman, N. Acquisition of high level chromosomal instability is associated with integration of human papillomavirus type 16 in cervical keratinocytes. *Cancer Res.* 64: 1359–1368, **2004**.

Pfister, H. and zur Hausen, H. Characterization of proteins of human papilloma virus (HPV) and antibody response to HPV 1. *Med. Microbiol. Immunol.* 166: 13–19, **1978**.

Phelps, W.C., and Howley, P.M. Transcriptional trans-activation by the human papillomavirus type 16 E2 gene product. *J. Virol.* 61: 1630–1638, **1987**.

Phelps, W.C., Yee, C.L., Münger, K., and Howley, P.M. Functional and sequence similarities between HPV16 E7 and adenovirus E1A. *Curr. Top. Microbiol. Immunol.* 144: 153–166, **1989**.

Phelps, W.C., Münger, K., Yee, C.L., Barner, J.A., and Howley, P.M. Structure-function analysis of the human papillomavirus type 16 E7 oncoprotein. *J. Virol.* 66: 2418–2427, **1992**.

Phillips, A.C. and Vousden, K.H. Analysis of the interaction between human papillomavirus type 16 E7 and the TATA-binding protein, TBP. *J. Gen. Virol.* 78: 905–909, **1997**.

Piboonniyom, S. O., Duensing, S., Swilling, N.W., Hasskarl, J., Hinds, P.W., and Münger, K. Abrogation of the retinoblastoma tumor suppressor checkpoint during keratinocyte immortalization is not sufficient for induction of centrosome-mediated genomic instability. *Cancer Res.* 63: 476–483, **2003**.

Pilotti, S., Donghi, R., D'Amato, L., Giarola, M., Longoni, A., Della Torre, G., De Palo, G., Pierotti, M.A., and Rilke, F. HPV detection and p53 alteration in squamous cell verrucous malignancies of the lower genital tract. *Diagn. Mol. Pathol* . 2: 248–256, **1993**.

Pim, D., Collins, M., and Banks, L. Human papillomavirus type 16 E5 gene stimulates the transforming activity of the epidermal growth factor receptor. *Oncogene* 7: 27–32, **1992**.

Pim, D., Massimi, P., and Banks, L. Alternatively spliced HPV-18 E6* protein inhibits E6 mediated degradation of p53 and suppresses transformed cell growth. *Oncogene* 15: 257–264, **1997**.

Pins, M.R., Young, R.H., Crum, C.P., Leach, I.H., and Scully, R.E. Cervical squamous cell carcinoma in situ with intraepithelial extension to the upper genital tract and invasion of tubes and ovaries: report of a case with human papilloma virus analysis. *Int. J. Gynecol. Pathol.* 16: 272–278, **1997**.

Pirisi, L., Yasumoto, S., Feller, M., Doniger, J., and DiPaolo, J.A. Transformation of human fibroblasts and keratinocytes with human papillomavirus type 16 DNA. *J. Virol.* 61: 1061–1066, **1987**.

Plummer, M., Herrero, R., Franceschi, S., Meijer, C.J.M., Snijders, P., Bosch, F.X., de Sanjosé, S., and Muñoz, N. IARC multicentre Cervical Cancer Study Group. Smoking and cervical cancer: pooled analysis of the IARC multi-centric case-control study. *Cancer Causes Control* 14: 805–814, **2003**.

Poetsch, M., Lorenz, G., Bankau, A., and Kleist, B. Basaloid in contrast to non-basaloid head and neck squamous cell carcinomas display aberrations especially in cell control genes. *Head Neck* 25: 904–910, **2003**.

Polyak, M., Cerar, A., and Seme, K. Human papillomavirus infection in esophageal carcinomas: a study of 121 lesions using multiple broad-spectrum polymerase chain reactions and literature review. *Hum. Pathol.* 29: 266–271, **1998**.

Preville, X., Ladant, D., Timmerman, B., and Leclerc, C. Eradication of established tumors by vaccination with recombinant *Bordetella pertussis* adenylate cyclase carrying the human papillomavirus 16 E7 oncoprotein. *Cancer Res.* 65: 641–649, **2005**.

Prusty, B.K. and Das, B.C. Constitutive activation of transcription factor AP-1 in cervical cancer and suppression of human papillomavirus (HPV) transcription and AP-1 activity in HeLa cells by curcumin. *Int. J. Cancer* 113: 951–960, **2005**.

Purdie, K.J., Pennington, J., Proby, C.M., Khalaf, S., de Villiers, E.-M., Leigh, I.M., and Storey, A. The promoter of a novel human papillomavirus (HPV77) associated with skin cancer displays UV responsiveness, which is mediated through a consensus p53 binding sequence. *EMBO J.* 18: 5359–5369, **1999**.

Pyeon, D., Lambert, P.F., and Ahlquist, P. Production of infectious human papillomavirus independently of viral replication and epithelial cell differentiation. *Proc. Natl. Acad. Sci. USA* 192: 9311–9316, **2005**.

Quelle, D.E., Zindy, F., Ashmun, R.A. and Sherr, C.J. Alternative reading frames of the INK4a tumor suppressor gene encode two unrelated proteins capable of inducing cell cycle arrest. *Cell* 83: 993–1000, **1995**.

Rabson, M.S., Yee, C., Yang, Y.C., and Howley, P.M. Bovine papillomavirus type 1 3'-early region: transformation and plasmid maintenance functions. *J. Virol.* 60: 626–634, **1986**.

Rady, P.L., Schnadig, V.J., Weiss, R.L., Hughes, T.K., and Tyring, S. K. Malignant transformation of recurrent respiratory papillomatosis associated with integrated human papillomavirus type 11 DNA and mutation of p53. *Laryngoscope* 108: 735–740, **1998**.

Raj, K., Berguerand, S., Southern, S., Doorbar, J., and Beard, P. E1 empty set E4 protein of human papillomavirus type 16 associates with mitochondria. *J. Virol.* 78: 7199–7207, **2004**.

Rajkumar, T., Sridhar, H., Balaram, P., Vaccarella, S., Gajalakshmi, V., Nandakumar, A., Ramdas, K., Jayshree, R., Muñoz, N., Herrero, R., Franceschi, S., and Weiderpass, E. Oral cancer in Southern India: the influence of body size, diet, infections and sexual practices. *Eur. J. Cancer Prev.* 12: 135–143, **2003**.

Ramoz, N., Rueda, L.A., Bouadjar, B., Favre, M., and Orth, G. A susceptibility locus for epidermodysplasia verruciformis, an abnormal predisposition to infection with the oncogenic human papillomavirus type 5, maps to chromosome 17qter in a region containing the psoriasis locus. *J. Invest. Dermatol.* 112: 259–263, **1999**.

Ramoz, N. Rueda, L.A., Boudjar, B., Montoya, L.S., Orth, G., and Favre, M. Mutations in two adjacent novel genes are associated with epidermodysplasia verruciformis. *Nat. Genet.* 32: 579–581, **2002**.

Rao, P.H., Arias-Pulido, H., Lu, X.Y., Harris, C.P., Vargas, H., Zhang, F.F., Narayan, G., Schneider, A., Terry, M.B., and Murty, V.V. Chromosomal amplifications, 3q gain and deletions of 2q33-q37 are the frequent t genetic changes in cervical carcinomas. *BMC Cancer* 4: 5, **2004**.

Rasmussen, K.A. Verrucae plantares; symptomatology and epidemiology. *Acta Derm. Venereol.* 38 (suppl. 39): 1–146, **1958**.

Rawls, W.E., Tompkins, W.A.F., and Melnick, J.L. The association of herpesvirus type 2 and carcinoma of the uterine cervix. *Am. J. Epidemiol.* 89: 547–554, **1969**.

Rector, A., Tachezy, R., van Doorslaer, K., MacNamara, T., Burk, R.D., Sundberg, J.P., and Van Ranst, M. Isolation and cloning of papillomavirus from a North American porcupine by using multiply primed rolling-circle amplification: the Erethizon dorsatum papillomavirus type 1. *Virology* 331: 449–456, **2005**.

Respler, D.S., Jahn, A., Pater, A., and Pater, M.M. Isolation and characterization of papillomavirus DNA from nasal inverting (schneiderian) papillomas. *Acta Otol. Rhinol. Laryngol.* 96: 170–173, **1987**.

Ressing, M.E., van Driel, W.J., Brandt, R.M., Kenter, G.G., de Jong, J.H., Bauknecht, T., Fleuren, G.J., Hoogerhout, P., Offringa, R., Sette, A., Celis, E., Grey, H., Trimbos, B.J., Kast, W.M., and Melief, C.J. Detection of T helper responses, but not of human papillomavirus-specific cytotoxic T lymphocyte responses, after peptide vaccination of patients with cervical carcinoma. *J. Immunother.* 23: 255–266, **2000**.

Reznikoff, C.A., Yeager, T.R., Belair, C.D., Savelieva, E., Puthenveettil, J.A., and Stadler, W.M. Elevated p16 at senescence and loss of p16 at immortalization in human papillomavirus 16 E6, but not E7, transformed human uroepithelial cells. *Cancer Res.* 56: 2886–2890, **1996**.

Riethdorf, S., Neffen, E.F., Cviko, A., Löning, T., Crum, C.P., and Riethdorf, L. p16INK4A expression as biomarker for HPV 16-related vulvar neoplasias. *Hum. Pathol.* 35: 1477–1483, **2004**.

Rivera, A. and Tyring, S. K. Therapy of cutaneous human papillomavirus infections. *Dermatol. Ther.* 17: 441–448, **2004**.

Roberts, A., Reuter, J.D., Wilson, J.H., Baldwin, S., and Rose, J.K. Complete protection from papillomavirus challenge after a single vaccination with a vesicular stomatitis virus vector expressing high levels of L1 protein. *J. Virol.* 78: 3196–3199, **2004**.

Roberts, D.J. and Cairnduff, F. Photodynamic therapy of primary skin cancer: a review. *Br. J. Plast. Surg.* 48: 360–370, **1995**.

Roberts, S., Ashmole, I., Johnson, G.D., Kreider, J.W., and Gallimore, P.H. Cutaneous and mucosal human papillomavirus E4 proteins form intermediate filament-like structures in epithelial cells. *Virology* 197: 176–187, **1993**.

Roden, R.B., Yutzy, W.H., IV, Fallon, R., Inglis, S., Lowy, D.R., and Schiller, J.T. Minor capsid protein of human genital papillomaviruses contains subdominant, cross-neutralizing epitopes. *Virology* 270: 254–257, **2000**.

Rogers, M.A., Vaughan, T.L., Davis, S., and Thomas, D.B. Consumption of nitrate, nitrite, and nitrosodimethylamine and the risk of upper aerodigestive tract cancer. *Cancer Epidemiol. Biomarkers Prev.* 4: 29–36, **1995**.

Romanczuk, H. and Howley, P.M. Disruption of either the E1 or E2 regulatory gene of human papillomavirus type 16 increases viral immortalization capacity. *Proc. Natl. Acad. Sci. USA* 89: 3159–3163, **1992**.

Romney, S. L., Ho, G.Y.F., Palan, P.R., Basu, J., Kadish, A.S., Klein, S., Mikhail, M., Hagan, R.J., Chang, C.J., and Burk, R.D. Effects of β-carotene and other factors on outcome of cervical dysplasia and human papillomavirus infection. *Gynecol. Oncol.* 65: 483–492, **1997**.

Ronco, L.V., Karpova, A.Y., Vidal, M., and Howley, P.M. Human papillomavirus 16 E6 oncoprotein binds to interferon regulatory factor-3 and inhibits its transcriptional activity. *Genes Dev.* 12: 2061–2072, **1998**.

Rorke, E.A. Antisense human papillomavirus (HPV) E6/E7 expression, reduced stability of epidermal growth factor, and diminished growth of HPV-positive tumor cells. *J. Natl. Cancer Inst.* 89: 1243–1246, **1997**.

Rosas-Acosta, G., Langereis, M.A., Deyrieux, A., and Wilson, V.G. Proteins of the PIAS family enhance the sumoylation of the papillomavirus E1 protein. *Virology* 331: 190–203, **2005**.

Rosenblatt, K.A., Wicklund, K.G., and Stanford, J.L. Sexual factors and the risk of prostate cancer. *Am. J. Epidemiol.* 12: 1152–1158, **2001**.

Rosenblatt, K.A., Carter, J.J., Iwasaki, L.M., Galloway, D.A., and Stanfords, J.L. Serologic evidence of human papillomavirus 16 and 18 infections and risk of prostate cancer. *Cancer Epidemiol. Biomarkers Prev.* 12: 763–768, **2003** .

Rosenfeld, W.D., Vermund, S. H., Wentz, S. J., and Burk, R.D. High prevalence rate of human papillomavirus infection and association with abnormal Papanicolaou smears in sexually active adolescents. *Am. J. Dis. Child.* 143: 1443–1447, **1989**.

Rösl, F., Lengert, M., Albrecht, J., Kleine, K., Zawatzky, R., Schraven, B., and zur Hausen, H. Differential regulation of the JE gene encoding the monocyte chemoattractant protein (MCP-1) in cervical carcinoma cells and derived hybrids. *J. Virol.* 68: 2142–2150, **1994**.

Rotkin, I.D. A comparison review of key epidemiological studies in cervical cancer related to current searches for transmissible agents. *Cancer Res.* 33: 1353–1367, **1973**.

Rous, P. and Beard, J.W. Carcinomatous changes in virus-induced papillomas of the skin of the rabbit. *Proc. Soc. Exp. Biol. Med.* 32: 578–580, **1934**.

Rous, P. and Kidd, J. G. The carcinogenic effect of a papillomavirus on the tarred skin of rabbits. I. Description of the phenomenon. *J. Exp. Med.* 67: 399–422, **1938**.

Rous, P. and Friedewald, W.F. The effect of chemical carcinogens on virus-induced rabbit papillomas. *J. Exp. Med.* 79: 511–537, **1944**.

Routes, J.M., Morris, K., Ellison, M.C., and Ryan, S. Macrophages kill human papillomavirus type 16 E6-expressing tumor cells by tumor necrosis factor α- and nitric oxide-dependent mechanisms. *J. Virol.* 79: 116–123, **2005** .

Royston, I. and Aurelian, L. The association of genital herpesvirus with cervical atypia and carcinoma in situ. *Am. J. Epidemiol.* 91: 531–538, **1970**.

Rüdlinger, R., Smith, I.W., Bunney, M.H., and Hunter, J.A. Human papillomavirus infections in a group of renal transplant recipients. *Br. J. Dermatol.* 115: 681–692, **1986**.

Rufforny, I., Wilkinson, E.J., Liu, C., Zhu, H., Buteral, M., and Massoll, N.A. Human papillomavirus infection and p16(INK4a) protein expression in vulvar intraepithelial neoplasia and invasive squamous cell carcinoma. *J. Low. Genit. Tract. Dis.* 9: 108–113, **2005**.

Ruhul Quddus, M., Xu, C., Steinhoff, M.M., Zhang, C., Lawrence, W.D., and Sung, C.J. Simplex (differentiated) type VIN: absence of p16INK4 supports its weak association with HPV and its probable precursor role in non-HPV related vulvar squamous cancers. *Histopathology* 46: 718–720, **2005**.

Rylander, E., Ruusuvaara, L., Almströmer, M.W., Evander, M., and Wadell, G. The absence of vaginal human papillomavirus type 16 DNA in women who have not experienced sexual intercourse. *Obstet. Gynecol.* 83: 735–737, **1994**.

Saegusa, M., Takano, Y., Hashimura, M., Okayasu, I., and Shgiga, J. HPV type 16 in conjunctival and junctional papilloma, dysplasia, and squamous cell carcinoma. *J. Clin Pathol.* 48: 1106–1110, **1995**.

Salunke, D.M., Caspar, D.L., and Garcea, R.L. Self-assembly of purified polyomavirus capsid protein VP1. *Cell* 46: 895–904, **1986**.

Sanders, C.M. and Maitland, N.J. Kinetic and equilibrium studies of the human papillomavirus type 16 transcription regulatory protein E2 interacting with core enhancer elements. *Nucleic Acids Res.* 22: 4890–4897, **1994**.

Sano, T., Masuda, N., Oyama, T., and Nakajima, T. Overexpression of p16 and p14ARF is associated with human papillomavirus infection in cervical squamous cell carcinoma and dysplasia. *Pathol. Int.* 52: 375–383. **2002**.

Santin, A.D., Hermonat, P.L., Ravaggi, A., Chiriva-Internati, M., Zhan, D., Pecorelli, S., Parham, G.P., and Cannon, M.J. Induction of human papillomavirus-specific CD4(+) and CD8(+) lymphocytes by E7-pulsed autologous dendritic cells in patients with human papillomavirus type 16- and 18-positive cervical cancer. *J. Virol.* 73: 5402–5410, **1999**.

Santin, A.D., Bellone, S., Gokden, M., Cannon, M.J., and Parkham, G.P. Vaccination with HPV-18 E7-pulsed dendritic cells in a patient with metastatic cervical cancer. *N. Engl. J. Med.* 346: 1752–1753, **2002**.

Saridaki, Z., Koumantaki, E., Liloglou, T., Sourvinos, G., Papadopoulos, O., Zoras, O., and Spandidos, D.A. High frequency of loss of heterozygosity on chromosome region 9p21-p22 but lack of p16INK4a/p19ARF mutations in Greek patients with basal cell carcinoma of the skin. *J. Invest. Dermatol.* 115: 719–725, **2000**.

Sasagawa, T., Kondoh, G., Inoue, M., Yutsudo, M., Hakura, A. Cervical/vaginal dysplasias of transgenic mice harbouring human papillomavirus type 16 E6-E7 genes. *J. Gen. Virol.* 75: 3057–3065, **1994**.

Sasson, I.M., Haley, N.J., Hoffmann, D., Wynder, E.L., Hellberg, D., and Nilsson, S. Cigarette smoking and neoplasia of the uterine cervix: smoke constituents in cervical mucus. *N. Engl. J. Med.* 312: 315–316, **1985**.

Sayhan, N., Yazici, H., Budak, M., Bitisik, O., and Dalay, N. p53 codon 72 genotypes in colon cancer. Association with human papillomavirus infection. *Res. Commun. Mol. Path. Pharmacol.* 109: 25–34, **2001**.

Scala, M., Bonelli, G., Gipponi, M., Margarino, G., and Muzza, A. Cryosurgery plus adjuvant systemic alpha2-interferon for HPV-associated lesions. *Anticancer Res.* 22: 1171–1176, **2002**.

Schachter, J., Hill, E.C., King, E.B., Coleman, V.R., Jones, P., and Meyer, K.F. Chlamydial infection in women with cervical dysplasia. *Am. J. Obstet. Gynecol.* 123: 753–757, **1975**.

Schaper, I.D., Marcuzzi, G.P., Weissenborn, S. J., Kasper, H.U., Dries, V., Smyth, N., Fuchs, P., and Pfister, H. Development of skin tumors in mice transgenic for early genes of human papillomavirus type 8. *Cancer Res.* 65: 1394–1400, **2005**.

Scheffner, M., Werness, B.A., Huibregtse, J.M., Levine, A.J., and Howley, P.M. The E6 oncoprotein encoded by human papillomavirus types 16 and 18 promotes the degradation of p53. *Cell* 63: 1129–1136, **1990**.

Scheurlen, W., Stremlau, A., Gissmann, L., Hohn, D., Zenner, H.P., and zur Hausen, H. Rearranged HPV 16 molecules in an anal and in a laryngeal carcinoma. *Int. J. Cancer* 38: 671–676, **1986**.

Schiff, M., Becker, T.M., Masuk, M., van Asselt-King, L., Wheeler, C.M., Altobelli, K.K., North, C.Q., and Nahmias, A.J. Risk factors for cervical intraepithelial neoplasia in southwestern American Indian women. *Am. J. Epidemiol.* 152: 716–726, **2000**.

Schiffman, M.H., Haley, N.J., Felton, J.S., Andrews, A.W., Kaslow, R.A., Lancaster, W.D., Kurman, R.J., Brinton, L.A., Lannom, L.B., and Hoffmann, D. Biochemical epidemiology of cervical neoplasia: measuring cigarette constituents in the cervix. *Cancer Res.* 47: 3886–3888, **1987**.

Schiffman, M.H., Bauer, H.M., Hoover, R.N., Glass, A.G., Cadell, D.M., Rush, B.B., Scott, D.R., Sherman, M.E., Kurman, R.J., and Wacholder, S. Epidemiologic evidence showing that human papillomavirus infection causes most cervical intraepithelial neoplasia. *J. Natl. Cancer Inst.* 85: 958–964, **1993**.

Schiller, J.T., Vass, W.C., Vousden, K., and Lowy, D.R. E5 open reading frame of bovine papillomavirus type 1 encodes a transforming gene. *J. Virol.* 57: 1–6, **1986**.

Schilling, B., De-Medina, T., Syken, J., Vidal, M., and Münger, K. A novel human DnaJ protein, hTid-1, a homolog of the *Drosophila* tumor suppressor protein Tid56, can interact with the human papillomavirus type 16 E7 oncoprotein. *Virology* 247: 74–85, **1998**.

Schlegel, R., Phelps, W.C., Zhang, Y.L., and Barbosa, M. Quantitative keratinocyte assay detects two biological activities of human papillomavirus DNA and identifies viral types associated with cervical carcinoma. *EMBO J.* 7: 3181–3187, **1988**.

Schlehofer, J.R. and zur Hausen, H. Induction of mutations within the host cell genome by partially inactivated herpes simplex virus type 1. *Virology* 122: 471–475, **1982**.

Schlehofer, J.R., Gissmann, L., Matz, B., and zur Hausen, H. Herpes simplex virus induced amplification of SV40 sequences in transformed Chinese hamster embryo cells. *Int. J. Cancer* 32: 99–103, **1983**.

Schmitt, A., Harry, J.B., Rapp, B., Wettstein, F.O., and Iftner, T. Comparison of the properties of the E6 and E7 genes of low- and high-risk cutaneous papillomaviruses reveals strongly transforming and high Rb-binding activity of the low risk human papillomavirus type 1. *J. Virol.* 68: 7051–7059, **1994**.

Schmitt, J., Schlehofer, J.R., Mergener, K., Gissmann, L., and zur Hausen, H. Amplification of bovine papillomavirus DNA by N-methyl-N'-nitro-N-nitrosoguanidine, ultraviolet-irradiation, or infection with herpes simplex virus. *Virology* 172: 73–81, **1989**.

Schneider, V., Kay, S., and Lee, H.M. Immunosuppression as a high-risk factor in the development of condyloma acuminatum and squamous neoplasia of the cervix. *Acta Cytol.* 27: 220–224, **1983**.

Schneider-Gädicke, A., Kaul, S., Schwarz, E., Gausepohl, H., Frank, R., and Bastert, G. Identification of the human papillomavirus type 18 E6 and E6 proteins in nuclear protein fractions from human cervical carcinoma cells grown in the nude mouse or in vitro. *Cancer Res.* 48: 2969–2974, **1988**.

Schoell, W.M., Mirhashemi, R., Liu, B., Janicek, M.F., Podack, E.R., Penalver, M.A., and Averette, H.E. Generation of tumor-specific cytotoxic T lymphocytes by stimulation with HPV type 16 E7 peptide-pulsed dendritic cells: an approach to immunotherapy of cervical cancer. *Gynecol. Oncol.* 74: 448–455, **1999**.

Schwartz, S. M., Daling, J.R., Doody, D.R., Wipf, G.C., Carter, J.J., Madeleine, M.M., Mao, E.J., Fitzgibbons, E.D., Huang, S., Beckmann, A.M., McDougall, J.K., and Galloway, D.A. Oral cancer risk in relation to sexual history and evidence of human papillomavirus infection. *J. Natl. Cancer Inst.* 90: 1626–1636, **1998**.

Schwartz, S. R., Yueh, B., McDougall, J.K., Daling, J.R., and Schwartz, S. M., Human papillomavirus infection and survival in oral squamous cell cancer: a population-based study. *Otolaryngol. Head Neck Surg.* 125: 1–9, **2001**.

Schwarz, E., Freese, U.K., Gissmann, L., Mayer, W., Roggenbuck, B., and zur Hausen, H. Structure and transcription of human papillomavirus sequences in cervical carcinoma cells. *Nature* 314: 111–114, **1985**.

Scott, I.U., Karp, C.L., and Nuovo, G.J. Human papillomavirus 16 and 18 expression in conjunctival intraepithelial neoplasia. *Ophthalmology* 109: 542–547, **2002**.

Seavey, S. E., Holubar, M., Saucedo, L.J., and Perry, M.E. The E7 oncoprotein of human papillomavirus type 16 stabilizes p53 through a mechanism independent of p19(ARF). *J. Virol.* 73: 7590–7598, **1999**.

Sedjo, R.L., Inserra, P., Abrahamsen, M., Harris, R.B., Roe, D.J., Baldwin, S., and Giuliano, A.R. Human papillomavirus persistence and nutrients involved in the methylation pathway among a cohort of young women. *Cancer Epidemiol. Biomarkers Prev* . 11: 353–359, **2002a**.

Sedjo, R.L., Roe, D.J., Abrahamsen, M., Harris, R.B., Craft, N., Baldwin, S., and Giuliano, A.R. Vitamin A, carotenoids, and risk of persistent oncogenic human papillomavirus infection. *Cancer Epidemiol. Biomarkers Prev.* 11: 876–884, **2002b**.

Sedjo, R.L., Fowler, B.M., Schneider, A., Henning, S. M., Hatch, K., and Giuliano, A.R. Folate, vitamin B12, and homocysteine status: findings of no relation between human papillomavirus persistence and cervical dysplasia. *Nutrition* 19: 497–502, **2003**.

Sedman, S. A., Barbosa, M.S., Vass, W.C., Hubbert, N.L., Haas, J.A., Lowy, D.R., and Schiller, J.T. The full-length E6 protein of human papillomavirus type 16 has transforming and trans-activating activities and cooperates with E7 to immortalize keratinocytes in culture. *J. Virol.* 65: 4860–4866, **1991**.

Seo, Y.S., Müller, F., Lusky, M., Gibbs, E., Kim, H.Y., Phillips, B., and Hurwitz, J. Bovine papillomavirus (BPV)-encoded E2 protein enhances binding of E1 protein to the BPV replication. *Proc. Natl. Acad. Sci. USA* 90: 2865–2869, **1993** .

Serth, J., Panitz, F., Paeslack, U., Kuczyk, M., and Jonas, U. Increased levels of human papillomavirus DNA in a subset of prostate cancers. *Cancer Res.* 59: 823–825, **1999**.

Shamanin, V., Glover, M., Rausch, C., Proby, C., Leigh, I.M., zur Hausen, H., and de Villiers, E.-M. Specific types of human papillomavirus found in benign proliferations and carcinomas of the skin in immunosuppressed patients. *Cancer Res.* 54: 4610–4613, **1994 a**.

Shamanin, V., Delius, H., and de Villiers, E.-M. Development of a broad spectrum PCR assay for papillomaviruses and its application in screening lung cancer biopsies. *J. Gen. Virol.* 75: 1149–1156, **1994 b**.

Shamanin, V., zur Hausen, H., Lavergne, D., Proby, C.M., Leigh, I.M., Neumann, C., Hamm, H., Goos, M., Haustein, U.-F., Jung, E.G., Plewig, G., Wolff, H., and de Villiers, E.-M. Human papillomavirus infections in nonmelanoma skin cancers from renal transplant recipients and non-immunosuppressed patients. *J. Natl. Cancer Inst.* 88: 802–811, **1996**.

Shapiro, S., Rosenberg, L., Hoffman, M., Kelly, J.P., Cooper, D.D., Carrara, H., Denny, L.E., du Toit, G., Allan, B.R., Stander, I.A., and Williamson, A.L. Risk of invasive cancer of the cervix in relation to the use of injectable progestogen contraceptives and combined estrogen/progestogen oral contraceptives (South Africa). *Cancer Causes Control.* 14: 485–495, **2003**.

Sherr, C.J. Tumor surveillance via the ARF-p53 pathway. *Genes Dev.* 12: 2984–2991, **1998**.

Sherwood, J.B., Carlson, J.A., Gold, M.A., Chou, T.Y., Isacson, C., and Talerman, A. Squamous metaplasia of the endometrium associated with HPV 6 and 11. *Gynecol. Oncol.* 66: 141–145, **1997**.

Shiboski, C.H., Schmidt, B.L., and Jordan, R.C. Tongue and tonsil carcinoma: increasing trends in the U.S. population ages 20–44 years. *Cancer* 103: 1843–1849, **2005**.

Sillins, I., Ryd, W., Strand, A., Wadell, G., Tornsberg, S., Hansson, B.G., Wang, X., Arnheim, L., Dahl, V., Bremell, D., Persson, K., Dillner, J., and Rylander, E. Chlamydia trachomatis infection and persistence of human papillomavirus. *Int. J. Cancer* 116: 110–115, **2005**.

Sisk, E.A., Soltys, S. G., Zhu, S., Fisher, S. G., Carey, T.E., and Bradford, C.R. Human papillomavirus and p53 mutational status as prognostic factors in head and neck carcinoma. *Head Neck* 24: 841–849, **2002**

Six, E.M., Ndiaye, D., Sauer, G., Laabi, Y., Athman, R., Cumano, A., Brou, C., Israel, A., and Logeat, F. The notch ligand Delta1 recruits Dlg1 at cell-cell contacts and regulates cell migration. *J. Biol. Chem.* 279: 55 818–55 826, **2004**.

Slansky, J.E. and Farnham, P.J. Introduction to the E2F family: protein structure and gene regulation. *Curr. Top. Microbiol. Immunol.* 208: 1–30, **1996**.

Smith, E.M., Hoffman, H.T., Summersgill, K.S., Kirchner, H.L., Turek, L.P., and Haugen, T.H. Human papillomavirus and risk of oral cancer. *Laryngoscope* 108: 1098–1103, **1998**.

Smith, E.M., Ritchie, J.M., Summersgill, K.F., Klussmann, J.P., Lee, J.H., Wang, D., Haugen, T.H. and Turek, L.P. Age, sexual behaviour and human papillomavirus infection in oral cavity and oropharyngeal cancers. *Int. J. Cancer* 108: 766–772, **2004**.

Smith, J.S., Herrero, R., Bosetti, C., Mu[ntilde]oz, N., Bosch, F.X., Eluf-Neto, J., Castellsague, X., Meijer, C.J.M., van den Brule, A.J., Franceschi, S., Ashley, R. International Agency for Research on Cancer (IARC) Multicentric Cervical Cancer Study Group. Herpes simplex virus-2 as a human papillomavirus cofactor in the etiology of invasive cervical cancer. *J. Natl. Cancer Inst.* 94: 1604–1613, **2002**.

Smith, J.S., Green, J., Berrington de Gonzalez, A., Appleby, P., Peto, J., Plummer, M., Franceschi, S., and Beral, V. Cervical cancer and use of hormonal contraceptives: a systematic review. *Lancet* 361: 1159–1167, **2003**.

Smith, J.S., Bosetti, C., Mu[ntilde]oz, N., Herrero, R., Bosch, F.X., Eluf-Neto, J., Meijer, C.J.M., van den Brule, A.J., Franceschi, S., and Peeling, R.W. Chlamydia trachomatis and invasive cervical cancer: a pooled analysis of the IARC multicentric case-control study. *Int. J. Cancer* 111: 431–439, **2004**.

Smith, K.T. and Campo, M.S. Amplification of specific DNA sequences in C127 mouse cells transformed by bovine papillomavirus type 4. *Oncogene* 4: 409–413, **1989**.

Snijders, P.J., Cromme, F.V., van den Brule, A.J., Schrijnemakers, H.F., Snow, G.B., Meijer, C.J., and Walboomers, J.M. Prevalence and expression of human papillomavirus in tonsillar carcinomas, indicating a possible viral etiology. *Int. J. Cancer* . 51: 845–50, **1992**.

Snijders, P.J., Steenbergen, R.D., Top, B., Scott, S. D., Meijer, C.J., and Walboomers, J.M. Analysis of p53 status in tonsillar carcinomas associated with human papillomavirus. *J. Gen. Virol.* 75: 2769–2775, **1994**.

Snoeck, R., Bossens, M., Parent, D., Delaere, B., Degreef, H., Van Ranst, M., Noel, J.C., Wulfsohn, M.S., Rooney, J.F., Jaffe, H.S., and De Clercq, E. Phase II double-blind, placebo-controlled study of the safety and efficacy of cidofovir topical gel for the treatment of patients with human papillomavirus infection. *Clin. Infect. Dis.* 33: 597–602, **2001**.

Song, S., Pitot, H.C., and Lambert, P.F. The human papillomavirus type 16 E6 gene alone is sufficient to induce carcinomas in transgenic animals. *J. Virol.* 73: 5887–5893, **1999**.

Soto, U., Das, B.C., Lengert, M., Finzer, P., zur Hausen, H., and Rösl, F. Conversion of HPV 18 positive non-tumorigenic HeLa-fibroblast hybrids to invasive growth involves loss of TNF-α mediated repression of viral transcription and modification of the AP-1 transcription complex. *Oncogene* 18: 3187–3198, **1999**.

Soto, U., Denk, C., Finzer, P., Hutter, K.J., zur Hausen, H., and Rösl, F. Genetic complementation to non-tumorigenicity in cervical-carcinoma cells correlates with alterations in AP-1 composition. *Int. J. Cancer* 86: 811–817, **2000** .

Soufir, N., Moles, J.P., Vilmer, C., Moch, C., Verola, O., Rivet, J., Tesniere, A., Dubertret, L., and Basset-Seguin, N. P16 UV mutations in human skin epithelial tumors. *Oncogene* 18: 5477–5481, **1999**.

Stamm, W. *Chlamydia trachomatis* infections of the adult. In: Holmes, K.K. (Ed.), *Sexually Transmitted Diseases*. 3rd edn., McGraw-Hill, New York, pp. 407–422, **1999**.

Stanley, M.A. Imiquimod and the imidazoquinolones: mechanism of action and therapeutic potential. *Clin. Exp. Dermatol.* 27: 571–577, **2002**.

Stark, L.A., Arends, M.J., McLaren, K.M., Benton, E.C., Shahidullah, H., Hunter, J.A., and Bird, C.C. Prevalence of human papillomavirus DNA in cutaneous neoplasms from renal allograft recipients supports a possible viral role in tumour promotion. *Br. J. Cancer* 69: 222–229, **1994**.

Steenbergen, R.D., Hermsen, M.A., Walboomers, J.M., Joenje, H., Arwert, F., Meijer, C.J., and Snijders, P.J. Integrated human papillomavirus type 16 and loss of heterozygosity at 11 q22 and 18 q21 in an oral carcinoma and its derivative cell line. *Cancer Res.* 55: 5465–5471, **1995**.

Steller, M.A. Cervical cancer vaccines: progress and prospects. *J. Soc. Gynecol. Investig.* 9: 254–264, **2002**.

Steller, M.A., Gurski, K.J., Murakami, M., Daniel, R.W., Shah, K.V., Celis, E., Sette, A., Trimble, E.L., Park, R.C., and Marincola, F.M. Cell-mediated immunological responses in cervical and vaginal cancer patients immunized with a lapidated epitope of human papillomavirus type 16 E7. Clin. *Cancer Res.* 4: 2103–2109, **1998**.

Stephens, R.S. The cellular paradigm of chlamydial pathogenesis. *Trends Microbiol.* 11: 44–51, **2003**.

Stern, P.L. Immune control of human papillomavirus (HPV) associated anogenital disease and potential for vaccination. *J. Clin. Virol.* 32: S72–S82, **2005**.

Stoler, M.H., Mills, S. E., Gersell, D.J., and Walker, A.N. Small-cell neuroendocrine carcinoma of the cervix. A human papillomavirus type 18-associated cancer. *Am. J. Surg. Pathol.* 15: 28–32, **1991**.

Stoler, M.H., Rhodes, C.R., Whitbeck, A., Wolinsky, S. M., Chow, L.T., and Broker, T.R. Human papillomavirus type 16 and 18 gene expression in cervical neoplasias. *Hum. Pathol.* 23: 117–128, **1992**.

Stoppler, M.C., Straight, S. W., Tsao, G., Schlegel, R., and McCance, D.J. The E5 gene of HPV-16 enhances keratinocyte immortalization by full-length DNA. *Virology* 223: 251–254, **1996**.

Storey, A. and Banks, L. Human papillomavirus type 16 E6 gene cooperates with EJ-ras to immortalize primary mouse cells. *Oncogene* 8: 919–924, **1993**.

Stott, F.J., Bates, S., James, M.C., McConnell, B.B., Strarborg, M., Brookes, S., Palmero, I., Ryan, K., Hara, E., Vousden, K.H., and Peters, G. The alternative product from the human CDKN2A locus, p14(ARF), participates in a regulatory feedback loop with p53 and MDM2. *EMBO J.* 17: 5001–5014, **1998**.

Stragier, I., Snoeck, R., de Clercq, E., Van Den Ord, J.J., Van Ranst, M., and De Greef, H. Local treatment of HPV-induced skin lesions by Cidofovir. *J. Med. Virol.* 67: 241–245, **2002**.

Straight, S. W., Hinkle, P.M., Jewers, R.J., and McCance, D.J. The E5 oncoprotein of human papillomavirus type 16 transforms fibroblasts and effects the downregulation of the epidermal growth factor receptor in keratinocytes. *J. Virol.* 67: 4521–4532, **1993**.

Strauss, M.J., Shaw, E.W., Bunting, H., and Melnick, J.L. Crystalline virus-like particles from skin papillomas characterized by intranuclear inclusion bodies. *Proc. Soc. Exp. Biol. Med.* 72: 46–50, **1949**.

Stremlau, A., Gissmann, L., Ikenberg, H., Stark, M., Bannasch, P., and zur Hausen, H. Human papillomavirus type 16 related DNA in an anaplastic carcinoma of the lung. *Cancer* 55: 1737–1740, **1985**.

Strickler, H.D. and Goedert, J. Sexual behaviour and evidence for an infectious cause of prostate cancer. *Epidemiol. Rev.* 23: 144–151, **2001**.

Strickler, H.D., Burk, R.D., Fazzari, M., Anastos, K., Minkoff, H., Massad, L.S., Hall, C., Bacon, M., Levine, A.M., Watts, D.H., Silverberg, M.J., Xue, X., Schlecht, N.F., Melnick, S., and Palefsky, J.M. Natural history and possible reactivation of human papillomavirus in human immunodeficiency virus-positive women. *J. Natl. Cancer Inst.* 97: 577–86, **2005**.

Strome, S. E., Savva, A., Brissett, A.E., Gostout, B.S., Lewis, J., Clayton, A.C., McGovern, R., Weaver, A.L., Persing, D., and Kasperbauer, J.L. Squamous cell carcinoma of the tonsils: a molecular analysis of HPV associations. *Clin. Cancer Res.* 8: 1093–1100, **2002**.

Stubenrauch, F., Lim, H.B., and Laimins, L.A. Differential requirements for conserved E2 binding sites in the life cycle of oncogenic human papillomavirus type 31. *J. Virol.* 72: 1071–1077, **1998**.

Sun, S., Thorner, L., Lentz, M., MacPherson, P., and Botchan, M. Identification of a 68 kilodalton nuclear ATP-binding phosphoprotein encoded by bovine papillomavirus type 1. *J. Virol.* 64: 5093–5105, **1990**.

Sun, X.W., Ellerbrock, T.V., Lungu, O., Chiasson, M.A., Bush, T.J., and Wright, T.C., Jr. Human papillomavirus infection in human immunodeficiency virus-seropositive women. *Obstet. Gynecol.* 85: 680–686, **1995**.

Suprynowicz, F.A., Disbrow, G.L., Simic, V., and Schlegel, R. Are transforming properties of the bovine papillomavirus E5 protein shared by E5 from high risk human papillomavirus type 16? *Virology* 332: 102–113, **2005**.

Suzich, J.A., Ghim, S. J., Palmer-Hill, F.J., White, W.I., Tamura, J.K., Bell, J.A., Newsome, J.A., Jenson, A.B., and Schlegel, R. Systemic immunization with papillomavirus L1 protein completely prevents the development of viral mucosal papillomas. *Proc. Natl. Acad. Sci. USA* 92: 11553–11557, **1995**.

Sverdrup, F. and Khan, S. A. Replication of human papillomavirus (HPV) DNAs supported by the HPV type 18 E1 and E2 proteins. *J. Virol.* 68: 505–509, **1994**.

Swineheart, J.M., Sperling, M., Phillips, S., Kraus, S., Gordon, S., McCarty, J.M., Webster, G.F., Skinner, R., Korey, A., and Orenberg. E.K. Intralesional fluorouracil/epinephrine injectable gel for management of condylomata acuminata. A phase 3 clinical study. *Arch. Dermatol.* 133: 67–73, **1997**.

Syed, T.A., Qureshi, Z.A., Ahmad, S. A., and Ali, S. M. Management of intravaginal warts in women with 5-fluorouracil (1%) in vaginal hydrophilic gel: a placebo-controlled double-blind study. *Int. J. STD AIDS* 11: 371–374, **2000** .

Syrjänen, K., Pyrhönen, S., Aukee, S., and Koskela, E. Squamous cell papilloma of the esophagus: a tumor probably caused by human papilloma virus. *Diagn. Histopathol.* 5: 291–296, **1982**.

Syrjänen, K., Syrjänen, S., Lamberg, M., Pyrhönen, S., and Nuutinen, J. Morphological and immunohistochemical evidence suggesting human papillomavirus (HPV) involvement in oral squamous cell carcinogenesis. *Int. J. Oral Surg.* 12: 418–424, **1983**.

Syrjänen, S., Happonen, R.P., Virolainen, E., Siivonen, L., and Syrjänen, K. Detection of human papillomavirus (HPV) structural antigens and DNA types in inverted papillomas and squamous cell carcinomas of the nasal cavities and paranasal sinuses. *Acta Otolaryngol.* 104: 334–341, **1987**.

Szabo, I., Sepp, R., Nakamoto, K., Maeda, M., Sakamoto, H., and Uda, H. Human papillomavirus not found in squamous and large cell lung carcinomas by polymerase chain reaction. *Cancer* 73: 2740–2744, **1994**.

Tao, W. and Levine, A.J. P19(ARF) stabilizes p53 by blocking nucleo-cytoplasmic shuttling of MdM2. *Proc. Natl. Acad. Sci. USA* 96: 6937–6941, **1999**.

Taylor, E.R., Dornan, E.S., Boner, W., Connolly, J.A., McNair, S., Kannouche, P., Lehmann, A.R., and Morgan, I.M. The fidelity of HPV16 E1/E2-mediated DNA replication. *J. Biol. Chem.* 278: 52 223–52 230, **2003**.

Taylor, M.L., Mainous, A.G., III, and Wells, B.J. Prostate cancer and sexually transmitted diseases: a meta-analysis. *Fam. Med.* 37: 506–512, **2005**.

Termorshuizen, F., Feltkamp, M.C., Struijk, L., de Gruijl, F.R., Bavinck, J.N., and van Loveren, H. Sunlight exposure and (sero)prevalence of epidermodysplasia verruciformis-associated human papillomavirus. *J. Invest. Dermatol.* 122: 1456–1462, **2004**.

Thierry, F., Benotmane, M.A., Demeret, C., Mori, M., Teissier, S., and Desaintes, C. A genomic approach reveals a novel mitotic pathway in papillomavirus carcinogenesis. *Cancer Res.* 64: 895–903, **2004**.

Thomas, M. and Banks, L. Human papillomavirus (HPV) E6 interactions with Bak are conserved amongst E6 proteins from high and low risk HPV types. *J. Gen. Virol.* 80: 1513–1517, **1999**.

Thomas, M., Lévy, J.-P., Tanzer, J., Boiron, M., and Bernard, J. Transformation in vitro de cellules de peau de veaux embryonnaire sous l'action d'extraits acellulaires de papillomes bovines. *Compt. Rend. Acad. Sci. (Paris)* 257: 2155–2158, **1963**.

Thyrell, L., Dangfeldt, O., Zhivotovsky, B., Pokroskaja, K., Wang, Y., Einhorn, S., and Grander, D. The HPV-16 E7 oncogene sensitizes malignant cells to IFN-α-induced apoptosis. *J. Interferon Cytokine Res.* 25: 63–72, **2005** .

Tindle R.W. and Frazer I.H. Immune response to human papillomaviruses and the prospects for human papillomavirus-specific immunisation. *Curr. Top. Microbiol. Immunol.* 186: 217–253, **1994**.

Tinsley, J.M., Fisher, C., and Searle, P.F. Abnormalities of epidermal differentiation associated with expression of the human papillomavirus type 1 early region in transgenic mice. *J. Gen. Virol.* 73: 1251–1260, **1992**.

Tobery, T.W., Smith, J.F., Kuklin, N., Skulsky, D., Ackerson, C., Huang, L., Chen, L., Cook, J.C., McClemments, W.L., and Jansen, K.U. Effect of vaccine delivery system on the induction of HPV 16 L1-specific humoral and cell-mediated immune responses in immunized rhesus macaques. *Vaccine* 21: 1539–1547, **2003**.

Todd, R.W., Roberts, S., Mann, C.H., Luesley, D.M., Gallimore, P.H., and Steele, J.C. Human papillomavirus (HPV) type 16-specific CD8+ T cell responses in women with high grade vulvar intraepithelial neoplasia. *Int. J. Cancer* 108: 857–862, **2004**.

Togawa, K. and Rustgi, A.K. A novel papillomavirus sequence based on L1 general primers. *Virus Res.* 36: 293–297, **1995**.

Tommasino, M., Adamczewski, J.P., Carlotti, F., Barth, C.F., Manetti, R., Contorni, M., Cavalieri, F., Hunt, T., and Crawford, L. HPV 16 E7 protein associates with the protein kinase p33CDK2 and cyclin A. *Oncogene* 8: 195–202, **1993**.

Tong, X. and Howley, P.M. The bovine papillomavirus E6 oncoprotein interacts with paxillin and disrupts the actin cytoskeleton. *Proc. Natl. Acad. Sci. USA* 94: 4412–4417, **1997**.

Tran-Thanh, D., Provencher, D., Koushik, A., Duarte-Freanco, E., Kessous, A., Drouin, P., Wheeler, C.M., Dubuc-Lissoir, J., Gauthier, P., Allaire, G., Vauclair, R., DiPaolo, J.A., Gravitt, P., Franco, E., and Coutlee, F. Herpes simplex virus type II is not a cofactor in cancer of the uterine cervix. in cancer of the uterine cervix. *Am. J. Obstet. Gynecol.* 188: 129–134, **2003**.

Tsutsui, T., Kumakura, S., Yamamoto, A., Kanai, H., Tamura, Y., Kato, T., Anpo, M., Tahara, A., and Barrett, J.C. Association of p16(INK4a) and pRb inactivation with immortalization of human cells. *Carcinogenesis* 23: 2111–2117, **2002**.

Tugizov, S., Berline, J., Herrera, R., Penaranda, M.E., Nakagawa, M., and Palefsky, J. Inhibition of human papillomavirus type 16 E7 phosphorylation by the S100 MRP-8/14 protein complex. *J. Virol.* 79: 1099–1112, **2005**.

Ustav, M. and Stenlund, A. Transient replication of BPV-1 requires two viral polypeptides encoded by the E1 and E2 open reading frames. *EMBO J.* 10: 449–457, **1991**.

Ustav, M., Ustav, E., Szymanski, P., and Stenlund, A. Identification of the origin of replication of bovine papillomavirus and characterization of the viral origin recognition factor E1. *EMBO J.* 10: 4321–4329, **1991**.

Valle, G.F. and Banks, L. The human papillomavirus (HPV)-6 and HPV-16 E5 proteins co-operate with HPV-16 E7 in the transformation of primary rodent cells. *J. Gen. Virol.* 76: 1239–1245, **1995**.

van der Burg, S. H., Ressing, M.E., Kwappenberg, K.M., de Jong, A., Straathof, K., de Jong, J. Geluk, A., van Meijgaarden, K.E., Franken, K.L., Ottenhoff, T.H., Fleuren, G.J., Kenter, G., Melief, C.J., and Offringa, R. Natural T-helper immunity against human papillomavirus type 16 (HPV 16) E7-derived peptide epitopes in patients with HPV16-positive cervical lesions: identification of 3 human leukocyte antigen class II-restricted epitopes. *Int. J. Cancer* 91: 612–618, **2001**.

van Driel, W.J., Ressing, M.E., Kenter, G.G., Brandt, R.M., Krul, E.J., van Rossum, A.B., Schuuring, E., Offringa, R., Bauknecht, T., Tamm-Hermelink, A., van Dam, P.A., Fleuren, G.J., Kast, W.M., Melief, C.J., and Trimbos, J.B. Vaccination with HPV 16 peptides of patients with advanced cervical carcinoma: clinical evaluation of phase I-II trial. *Eur. J. Cancer* 35: 946–952, **1999**.

van Houten, V.M., Snijders, P.J., van den Brekel, M.W., Kummer, J.A., Meijer, C.J., van Leeuwen, B., Denkers, F., Smeele, M.E., Snow, G.B., and Brakenhoff, R.H. Biological evidence that human papillomaviruses are etiologically involved in a subgroup of head and neck squamous cell carcinomas. *Int. J. Cancer* 93: 232–235, **2001**.

van Kuppeveld, F.J., de Jong, A., Dijkman, H.B., Andino, R., and Melchers, W.J. Studies towards the potential of poliovirus as a vector for the expression of HPV 16 viruslike particles. *FEMS Immunol. Med. Microbiol.* 34: 201–208, **2002** .

van Ranst, M., Fuse, A., Fiten, P., Beuken, E., Pfister, H., Burk, R.D., and Opdenakker, G. Human papillomavirus type 13 and pygmy chimpanzee papillomavirus type 1: comparison of the genome organizations. *Virology* 190: 587–596, **1992** .

van Riggelen, J., Buchwalter, G., Soto, U., De-Castro Arce, J., zur Hausen, H., Wasylyk, B., and Rösl, F. Loss of net as repressor leads to constitutive increased c-fos transcription in cervical cancer cells. *J. Biol. Chem.* 280: 3286–3294, **2005**.

Vecchione, A., Cermele, C., Giovagnoli, M.R., Valli, C., Alimandi, M., Carico, E., Esposito, D.L., Mariani-Costantini, R., and French, D. p53 expression and genetic evidence for viral infection in intraepithelial neoplasia of the uterine cervix. *Gynecol. Oncol.* 55: 343–348, **1994**.

Veeraraghavalu, K., Pett, M., Kumar, R.V., Nair, P., Rangarajan, A., Stanley, M.A., and Krishna, S. Papillomavirus-mediated neoplastic progression is associated with reciprocal changes in JAGGED1 and manic fringe expression linked to notch activation. *J. Virol.* 78: 8687–8700, **2004**.

Velders, M.P., McElhiney, S., Cassetti, M.C., Eiben, G.L., Higgins, T., Kovacs, G., Elmishad, A.G., Kast, W.M., and Smith, L.R. Eradication of established tumors by vaccination with Venezuelan equine encephalitis virus replicon particles delivering human papillomavirus 16 E7 RNA. *Cancer Res.* 61: 7861–7877, **2001**.

Veldman, T., Liu, X., and Schlegel, R. Human papillomavirus E6 and Myc proteins associate in vivo and bind to and cooperatively activate the telomerase reverse transcriptase promoter. *Proc. Natl. Acad. Sci. USA* 100: 8211–8216, **2003** .

Vernon, S. D., Hart, C.E., Reeves, W.C., and Icenogle, J.P. The HIV-1 tat protein enhances E2-dependent human papillomavirus 16 transcription. *Virus Res.* 27 : 133–145, **1993**.

Vieira, K.B., Goldstein, D.J., and Villa, L.L. Tumor necrosis factor α interferes with the cell cycle of normal and papillomavirus-immortalized human keratinocytes. *Cancer Res.* 56: 2452–2457, **1996**.

Viikki, M., Pukkala, E., Nieminen, P., and Hakama, M. Gynaecological infections as risk determinants of subsequent cervical neoplasia. *Acta Oncol.* 39: 1–5, **2000**.

Villa, L.L., Vieira, K.B., Pei, X.F., and Schlegel, R. Differential effect of tumor necrosis factor on proliferation of primary human keratinocytes and cell lines containing human papillomavirus types 16 and 18. *Mol. Carcinog.* 6: 5–9, **1992**.

Villa, L.L., Costa, R.L., Petta, C.A., Andrade, R.P., Ault, K.A., Giuliano, A.R., Wheeler, C.M., Koutsky, L.A., Malm, C., Lehtinen, M., Skjeldestad, F.E., Olsson, S. E., Steinwall, M., Brown, D.R., Kurman, R.J., Ronnett, B.M., Stoler, M.H., Ferenczy, A., Harper, D.M., Tamms, G.M., Yu. J., Lupinacci, L., Railkar, R., Taddeo, F.J., Jansen, K.U., Esser, M.T., Sings, H.L., Saah, A.J., and Barr, E. Prophylactic quadrivalent human papillomavirus (types 6, 11, 16, and 18) L1 virus-like particle vaccine in young women: a randomised double-blind placebo-controlled multicentre phase II efficacy trial. *Lancet Oncol.* 6: 271–278, **2005**.

Viscidi, R.P., Schiffman, R., Hildesheim, A., Herrero, R., Castle, P.E., Bratti, M.C. Rodriguez, A.C., Sherman, M.E., Wang, S., Clayman, B., and Burk, R.D. Seroreactivity of human papillomavirus (HPV) types 16, 18 or 31 and risk of subsequent HPV infection: results from a population-based study in Costa Rica. *Cancer Epidemiol. Biomarkers Prev.* 13: 324–327, **2004**.

Vogt, M., Butz, K., Dymalla, S., Semzow, J., and Hoppe-Seyler, F. Inhibition of Bax activity is crucial for the antiapoptotic function of the human papillomavirus E6 oncoprotein. *Oncogene* **2006**. doi: 10.1038/sj.onc.1 209 429.

Vonka, V., Kanka, J., Jelinek, J., Subrt, I., Suchanek, A., Havrankova, A., Vachal, M., Hirsch, I., Domorazkova, A., Zavadova, H., et al. Prospective study on the relationship between cervical neoplasia and herpes simplex type-2 virus. I. Epidemiological characteristics. *Int. J. Cancer* 33: 49–60, **1984a**.

Vonka, V., Kanka, J., Hirsch, I., Zavadova, H., Krcmar, M., Suchankova, A., Rezacova, D., Broucek, J., Press, M., Domorazkova, E.,

Svoboda, B., Havrankova, A., and Jelinek, J. Prospective study on the relationship between cervical neoplasia and herpes simplex type-2 virus. II. Herpes simplex type-2 antibody presence in sera taken at enrollment. *Int. J. Cancer* 33: 61–66, **1984b**.

von Knebel Doeberitz, M., Rittmüller, C., Glitz, D., zur Hausen, H., and Dürst, M. Inhibition of tumorigenicity by cervical cancer cells in nude mice by HPV 18 E6-E7 anti-sense RNA. *Int. J. Cancer* 51: 831–834, **1992**.

von Knebel Doeberitz, M., Rittmüller, C., Aengeneyndt, F., Jansen-Dürr, P., and Spitkovsky, D. Reversible repression of papillomavirus oncogene expression in cervical carcinoma cells: consequences for the phenotype and E6-p53 and E7-pRB interactions. *J. Virol.* 68: 2811–2821, **1994**.

von Krogh, G. Management of anogenital warts (condylomata acuminata). *Eur. J. Dermatol.* 11: 598–603, **2001**.

Wallin, K.L., Wiklund, F., Luostarinen, T., Angstrom, T., Anttila, T., Bergman, F., Hallmans, G., Ikaheimo, I., Koskela, P., Lehtinen, M., Stendahl, U., Paavonen, J., and Dillner, J. A population-based prospective study of *Chlamydia trachomatis* infection and cervical carcinoma. *Int. J. Cancer* 101: 371–374, **2002**.

Wang, H.Y., Lee, D.A., Peng, G., Guo, Z., Li, Y., Kiniwa, Y.L., Shevach, E.M., and Wang, R.F. Tumor-specific human CD4+ regulatory T cells and their ligands: implications for immunotherapy. *Immunity* 20: 107–118, **2004**.

Wang, J., Sampath, A., Raychaudhuri, P., and Bagchi, S. Both Rb and E7 are regulated by the ubiquitin proteasome pathway in HPV-containing cervical tumor cells. *Oncogene* 20: 4740–4749, **2001**.

Wang, J.L., Zheng, B.Y., Li, X.D., Angstrom, T., Lindstrom, M.S., and Wallin, K.L. Predictive significance of the alterations of p16INK4A, p14ARF, p53, and proliferating cell nuclear antigen expression in the progression of cervical cancer. *Clin Cancer Res.* 10: 2407–2414, **2004**.

Wang, Q., Griffin, H., Southern, S., Jackson, D., Martin, A., McIntosh, P., Davy, C., Masterson, P.J., Walker, P.A., Laskey, P., Omary, M.B., and Doorbar, J. Functional analysis of the human papillomavirus type 16 E1 = E4 protein provides a mechanism for in vivo and in vitro keratin filament reorganization. *J. Virol.* 78: 821–833, **2004**.

Wang, Y., Coulombe, R., Cameron, D.R., Thauvette, L., Massariol, M.J., Amon, L.M., Fink, D., Titolo, S., Welchner, E., Yoakim, C., Archambault, J., and White, P.W. Crystal structure of the E2 transactivation domain of human papillomavirus type 11 bound to a protein interaction inhibitor. *J. Biol. Chem.* 279: 6978–6985, **2004**.

Watts, D.H., Fazarri, M., Minkoff, H., Hillier, S. L., Sha, B., Glesby, M., Levine, A.M., Burk, R.D., Palefsky, J.M., Moxley, M., Ahdieh-Grant, L., and Strickler, H.D. Effects of bacterial vaginosis and other genital infections on human papillomavirus natural history among HIV infected and uninfected women. *J. Infect. Dis.* 191: 1129–1139, **2005**.

Watts, S. L., Phelps, W.C., Ostrow, R.S., Zachow, K.R., and Faras, A.J. Cellular transformation by human papillomavirus DNA in vitro. *Science* 225: 634–636, **1984**.

Wazer, D.E., Liu, X.L., Chu, Q., Gao, Q., and Band, V. Immortalization of distinct human mammary epithelial cell types by papilloma virus 16 E6 or E7. *Proc. Natl. Acad. Sci. USA* 92: 3687–3691, **1995**.

Weck, P.K., Brandsma, J.L., and Whisnant, J.K. Interferons in the treatment of human papillomavirus diseases. *Cancer Metastasis Rev.* 5: 139–165, **1986**.

Weinstein, S. J., Ziegler, R.G., Frongillo, E.A., Jr., Colman, N., Sauberlich, H.E., Brinton, L.A., Hamman, R.F., Levine, R.S., Mallin, K., Stolley, P.D., and Bisogni, C.A. Low serum and red blood cell folate are moderately, but nonsignificantly associated with increased cervical cancer in US women. *J. Nutr.* 131: 2040–2048, **2001**.

Weintraub, S. J., Chow, K.N., Luo, R.X., Zhang, S. H., He, S., and Dean, D.C. Mechanism of active transcriptional repression by the retinoblastoma protein. *Nature* 375: 812–815, **1995**.

Wentzensen, N., Vinokurova, S., and von Knebel Doeberitz, M. Systematic review of genomic integration sites of human papillomavirus genomes in epithelial dysplasia and invasive cancer of the female lower genital tract. *Cancer Res.* 64: 3878–84, **2004**.

Werness, B.A., Levine, A.J., and Howley, P.M. Association of human papillomavirus types 16 and 18 E6 proteins with p53. *Science* 248: 76–79, **1990**.

West, A.B., Soloway, G.N., Lizarraga, G., Tyrrell, L., and Longley, J.B. Type 73 human papillomavirus in esophageal squamous cell carcinoma: a novel association. *Cancer* 77: 2440–2444, **1996**.

Westenend, P.J., Stoop, J.A., and Hendriks, J.G. Human papillomaviruses 6/11, 16/18 and 31/33/51 are not associated with squamous cell carcinoma of the urinary bladder. *Br. J. Urol. Int.* 88: 198–201, **2001**.

White, A.E., Livanos, E.M., and Tlsty, T.D. Differential disruption of genomic integrity and cell cycle regulation in normal human fibroblasts by the HPV oncoproteins. *Genes Dev.* 8: 666–677, **1994**.

Wideroff, L., Potischman, N., Glass, A.G., Greer, C.E., Manos, M.M., Scott, D.R., Burk, R.D., Sherman, M.E., Wacholder, S., and Schiffman, M. A nested case-control study on dietary factors and the risk of incident cytological abnormalities of the cervix. *Nutr. Cancer* 30: 130–136, **1998**.

Wiener, J.S. and Walther, P.J. A high association of oncogenic human papillomaviruses with carcinomas of the female urethra: polymerase chain reaction-based analysis of multiple histological types. *J. Urol.* 151: 49–53, **1994**.

Wiener, J.S., Liu, E.T., and Walther, P.J. Oncogenic human papillomavirus type 16 is associated with squamous cell cancer of the male urethra. *Cancer Res.* 52: 5018–5023, **1992**.

Wiest, T., Schwarz, E., Enders, C., Flechtenmacher, C., Bosch, F.X. Involvement of intact HPV16 E6/E7 gene expression in head and neck cancers with unaltered p53 status and perturbed pRb cell cycle control. *Oncogene.* 21: 1510–1517, **2002**.

Wilcock, D. and Lane, D.P. Localization of p53, retinoblastoma and host replication proteins at sites of viral replication in herpes-infected cells. *Nature* 349: 429–431, **1991**.

Wilczynski, S. P., Oft, M., Cook, N., Liao, S. Y., and Iftner, T. Human papillomavirus type 6 in squamous cell carcinoma of the bladder and cervix. *Hum. Pathol.* 24: 96–102, **1993**.

Wilczynski, S. P., Lin, B.T., Xie, Y., and Paz, I.B. Detection of human papillomavirus DNA and oncoprotein overexpression are associated with distinct morphological patterns of tonsillar squamous cell carcinoma. *Am. J. Pathol.* 152: 145–156, **1998**.

Wiley, D.J., Douglas, J., Beutner, K., Cox, T., Fife, K., Moscicki, A.B., and Fukumoto, L. External genital warts: Diagnosis, treatment, and prevention. *Clin. Infect. Dis.* 35 (Suppl. 2), S210–S224, **2002**.

Wilson, R., Fehrmann, F., and Laimins LA. Role of the E1–E4 protein in the differentiation-dependent life cycle of human papillomavirus type 31. *J. Virol.* 79: 6732–6740, **2005**.

Winkelstein, W., Jr. Smoking and cancer of the uterine cervix: hypothesis. *Am. J. Epidemiol.* 106: 257–259, **1977**.

Winkelstein, W., Jr. Smoking and cervical cancer – current status: a review. *Am. J. Epidemiol.* 131: 945–957, **1990**.

Wise-Draper, T.M., Allen, H.V., Thobe, M.N., Jones, E.E., Habash, K.B., Münger, K., and Wells, S. I. The human DEK proto-oncogene is a senescence inhibitor and an upregulated target of high-risk human papillomavirus E.7. *J. Virol.* 79: 14 319–14 317, **2005**.

Wistuba, I.I., Montellano, F.D., Milchgrub, S., Virmani, A.K., Behrens, C., Chen, H., Ahmadian, M., Nowak, J.A., Muller, C., Minna, J.D., and Gazdar, A.F. Deletions of chromosome 3p are frequent and early events in the pathogenesis of uterine cervical carcinoma. *Cancer Res.* 57: 3154–3158, **1997**.

Woodworth, C.D., Notario, V., and DiPaolo, J.A. Transforming growth factor β 1 and 2 transcriptionally regulate human papillomavirus (HPV) type 16 early gene expression in HPV-immortalized human genital epithelial cells. *J. Virol.* 64: 4767–4775, **1990**.

Woodworth, C.D., McMullin, E., Iglesias, M., and Plowman, G.D. Interleukin 1 α and tumor necrosis factor α stimulate autocrine amphiregulin expression and proliferation of human papillomavirus-immortalized and carcinoma-derived cervical epithelial cells. *Proc. Natl. Acad. Sci. USA* 92: 2840–2844, **1995**.

Wrede, D., Lugmani, Y.A., Coombes, R.C., and Vousden, K.H. Absence of HPV 16 and 18 DNA in breast cancer. *Br. J. Cancer* 65: 891–894, **1992**.

Wu, T.C., Trujillo, J.M., Kashima, H.K., and Mounts, P. Association of human papillomavirus with nasal neoplasia. *Lancet* 341: 522–524, **1993**.

Xiong, Y., Hannon, G.J., Zhang, H., Casso, D., Kobayashi, R., and Beach, D. p21 is a universal inhibitor of cyclin kinases. *Nature* 366: 701–704, **1993**.

Xiong, Y., Kuppuswamy, D., Li, Y., Livanos, E.M., Hixon, M., White, A., Beach, D., and Tlsty, T.D. Alteration of cell cycle kinase complexes in human papillomavirus E6- and E7-expressing fibroblasts precedes neoplastic transformation. *J. Virol.* 70: 999–1008, **1996**.

Xu, H., Lu, D.W., El-Mofty, S. K., and Wang, H.L. Metachronous squamous cell carcinomas evolving from independent oropharyngeal and pulmonary squamous papillomas: association with human papillomavirus 11 and lack of aberrant p53, Rb, and p16 protein expression. *Hum. Pathol.* 35: 1419–1422, **2004**.

Yabe, Y., Tanimura, Y., Sakai, A., Hitsumoto, T., and Nohara, N. Molecular characteristics and physical state of human papillomavirus DNA change with progressing malignancy: studies in a patient with epidermodysplasia verruciformis. *Int. J. Cancer* 43: 1022–1028, **1989**.

Yang, L., Mohr, I., Fouts, E., Lim, D.A., Nohaile, M., and Botchan, M. The E1 protein of bovine papillomavirus 1 is an ATP-dependent DNA helicase. *Proc. Natl. Acad. Sci. USA* 90: 5086–5090, **1993**.

Yang, Y.Y., Koh, L.W., Tsai, J.H., Tsai, C.H., Wong, E.F., Lin, S. J., and Yang, C.C. Correlation of viral factors with cervical cancer in Taiwan. *J. Microbiol. Immunol. Infect.* 37: 282–287, **2004**.

Yamamoto, A., Kumakura, S., Uchida, M., Barrett, J.C., and Tsutsui, T. Immortalization of normal human embryonic fibroblasts by introduction of either the human papillomavirus type 16 E6 or E7 gene alone. *Int. J. Cancer* 106: 301–309, **2003**.

Yasumoto, S., Burkhardt, A.L., Doniger, J., and DiPaolo, J.A. Human papillomavirus type 16 DNA-induced malignant transformation of NIH 3T3 cells. *J. Virol.* 57: 572–577, **1986**.

Yee, C., Krishnan-Hewlett, I., Baker, C.C., Schlegel, R., and Howley, P.M. Presence and expression of human papillomavirus sequences in human cervical carcinoma cell lines. *Am. J. Pathol.* 119: 361–366, **1985**.

Yin, Y., Tainsky, M.A., Bischoff, F.Z., Strong, L.C., and Wahl, G.M. Wild-type p53 restores cell cycle control and inhibits gene amplification in cells with mutant p53 alleles. *Cell* 70: 937–948, **1992**.

Ylitalo, N., Sorensen, P., Josefsson, A., Frisch, M., Sparen, P., Ponten, J., Gyllensten, U., Melbye, M., and Adami, H.O. Smoking and oral contraceptives as risk factors for cervical carcinoma in situ. *Int. J. Cancer.* 81: 357–365, **1999**.

Youde, S. J., Dunbar, P.R., Evans, E.M., Fiander, A.N., Borysiewicz, L.K., Cerundolo, V., Man, S. Use of fluorogenic histocompatibility leucocyte antigen A*0201/HPV 16 E7 peptide complexes to isolate rare human cytotoxic T-lymphocyte-recognizing endogenous human papillomavirus antigens. *Cancer Res.* 60: 365–371, **2000**.

Young, L.S. and Sixbey, J.W. Epstein-Barr virus and epithelial cells: a possible role for the virus in the development of cervical carcinoma. *Cancer Surv.* 7: 507–518, **1988**.

Yu, Y., Morimoto, T., Sasa, M., Okazaki, K., Harada, Y., Fujiwara, T., Irie, Y., Takahashi, E., Anigami, A., and Izumi, K. Human papillomavirus type 33 DNA in breast cancer in Chinese. *Breast Cancer* 7: 33–36, **2000**.

Yuan, H., Estes, P.A., Chen, Y., Newsome, J., Olcese, V.A., Garcea, R.L., and Schlegel, R. Immunization with a pentameric L1 fusion protein protects against papillomavirus infection. *J. Virol.* 75: 7848–7853, **2001**.

Zaki, S. R., Judd, R., Coffield, L.M., Greer, P., Rolston, F., and Evatt, B.L. Human papillomavirus infection and anal carcinoma. Retrospective analysis by in situ hybridization and the polymerase chain reaction. *Am. J. Pathol.* 140: 1345–1355, **1992**.

Zarod, A.P., Rutherford, J.D., and Corbitt, G. Malignant progression of laryngeal papilloma associated with human papilloma virus type 6 (HPV-6) DNA. *J. Clin. Pathol.* 41: 280–283, **1988**.

Zerfass, K., Schulze, A., Spitkovsky, D., Friedman, V., Henglein, B., and Jansen-Dürr, P. Sequential activation of cyclin E and cyclin A gene expression by human papillomavirus type 16E7 through sequences necessary for transformation. *J. Virol.* 69: 6389–6399, **1995**.

Zerfass-Thome, K., Zwerschke, W., Mannhardt, B., Tindle, R., Botz, J.W., and Jansen-Dürr, P. Inactivation of the cdk inhibitor p27KIP1 by the human papillomavirus type 16 E7 oncoprotein. *Oncogene* 13: 2323–2330, **1996**.

Zhang, B., Spandau, D.F., and Roman, A. E5 protein of human papillomavirus type 16 protects human foreskin keratinocytes from UV B-irradiation-induced apoptosis. *J. Virol.* 76: 220–231, **2002**.

Zhang, B., Li, P., Brahmi, Z., Dunn, K.W., Blum, J.S., and Roman, A. The E5 protein of human papillomavirus type 16 perturbs MHC class II maturation in human foreskin keratinocytes treated with interferon-ã. *Virology* 310: 100–108, **2003**.

Zhang, L.F., Zhou, J., Chen, S., Cai, L.L., Bao, Q.Y., Zheng, F.Y., Lu, J.Q., Padmanabha, J., Hengst, K., Malcolm, K., and Frazer, I.H. HPV6 b virus like particles are potent immunogens without adjuvant in man. *Vaccine* 18: 1051–1058, **2000**.

Zhang, Z.F. and Begg, C.B. Is *Trichomonas vaginalis* a cause of cervical neoplasia? Results from a combined analysis of 24 studies. *Int. J. Epidemiol.* 23: 682–690, **1994**.

Zhao, J., Bilsland, A., Jackson, K., and Keith, W.N. MDM2 negatively regulates the human telomerase RNA gene promoter. *BMC Cancer* 5: 6, **2005**.

Zhou, J., Sun, X.Y., Stenzel, D.J., and Frazer, I.H. Expression of vaccinia recombinant HPV 16 L1 and L2 ORF proteins in epithelial cells is sufficient for assembly of HPV virion-like particles. *Virology* 185: 251–257, **1991**.

Zhou, J., Sun, X.Y., Davies, H., Crawford, L., Park, D., and Frazer, I.H. Definition of linear antigenic regions of the HPV 16 L1 capsid protein using synthetic virion-like particles. *Virology* 189: 592–599, **1992**.

Zimmermann, H., Degenkolbe, R., Bernard, H.U., and O'Connor, M.J. The human papillomavirus type 16 E6 oncoprotein can down-regulate p53 activity by targeting the transcriptional coactivator CBP/p300. *J. Virol.* 73: 6209–6219, **1999** .

zur Hausen, H. Oncogenic herpes viruses. *Biochim. Biophys. Acta* 417: 25–53, **1975**.

zur Hausen, H. Condylomata acuminata and human genital cancer. *Cancer Res.* 36: 794, **1976**.

zur Hausen, H. Human papilloma viruses and their possible role in squamous cell carcinomas. *Curr. Top. Microbiol. Immunol.* 78: 1–30, **1977**.

zur Hausen, H. Genital papillomavirus infections. In: Rigby, P.W.J. and Wilkie, N.M. (Eds.), *Viruses and Cancer.* Cambridge University Press, pp. 83–90, **1986 a**.

zur Hausen, H. Intracellular surveillance of persisting viral infections: Human genital cancer resulting from failing cellular control of papillomavirus gene expression. *Lancet* 2: 489–491, **1986 b**.

zur Hausen, H. Papillomaviruses as carcinomaviruses. In: Klein, G. (Ed.), *Advances in Viral Oncology.* Raven Press, New York, Vol. 8, pp. 1–26, **1989 a**.

zur Hausen, H. Papillomavirus in anogenital cancer: the dilemma of epidemiologic approaches. *J. Natl. Cancer Inst.* 81: 1680–1682, **1989 b**.

zur Hausen, H. Papillomavirus infections – a major cause of human cancers. *Biochim. Biophys. Acta Rev. Cancer* 1288: F55–F78, **1996**.

zur Hausen, H., Meinhof, W., Scheiber, W., and Bornkamm, G.W. Attempts to detect virus-specific DNA in human tumors. I. Nucleic acid hybridizations with complementary RNA of human wart virus. *Int. J. Cancer* 13: 650–656, **1974 a**.

zur Hausen H., Schulte-Holthausen, H., Wolf, H., Dörries, K., and Egger, H. Attempts to detect virus-specific DNA in human tumors. II. Nucleic acid hybridizations with complementary RNA of human herpes group viruses. *Int. J. Cancer* 13: 657–664, **1974 b**.

zur Hausen, H., Gissmann, L., Steiner, W. Dippold, W., and Dreger, J. Human papilloma viruses and cancer. *Bibl. Haematol.* 43: 569–571, **1975**.

Zwaveling, S., Ferreira Mota, S. C., Nouta, J., Johnson, M., Lipford, G.B., Offringa, R., van der Burg, S. H., and Melief, C.J. Established human papillomavirus type 16-expressing tumors are effectively eradicated following vaccination with long peptides. *J. Immunol.* 169: 350–358, **2002**.

6
Hepadnaviruses

6.1
Hepatitis B

6.1.1
Historical Aspects

Hepatitis B virus (HBV) causes acute and chronic infections of the liver, resulting in part in fulminant liver failure, cirrhosis, and also in hepatocellular carcinoma (HCC). According to data provided by the International Agency for Research on Cancer (IARC, 1994), over 300 million people are estimated to be chronically infected worldwide, and between 250 000 and 1 000 000 die annually from HBV-associated disease.

The detection of the responsible virus has an interesting history. The recognition of hepatitis B as an infection primarily transmitted by parenteral inoculation of human serum causing an acute infection with jaundice dates back to the 1930s (Findlay and MacCallum, 1937). A widespread epidemic of hepatitis among US military troops in 1942 resulted in the acceptance of a high risk of the use of pooled and dried human plasma or after blood transfusion (Morgan and Williamson, 1943; Beeson, 1944). In 1947, the designations "hepatitis B" for "serum hepatitis", and "hepatitis A" for acute infectious hepatitis were coined (MacCallum, 1947). During the 1950s and 1960s, the seroepidemiologic relationship between hepatitis A and hepatitis B was investigated (Murray et al., 1954; Murray, 1955; Krugman et al., 1967), and later, in 1965, Blumberg et al. described a "new" antigen in the blood of an Australia aborigine ("Australia antigen") which formed a precipitin line with a serum obtained from a multiply transfused hemophiliac. Shortly thereafter, the relationship of this antigen to serum hepatitis was recognized (Blumberg et al., 1967, 1969; Prince, 1968). In 1970, 42-nm particles were described by Dane et al., which were suspected to represent hepatitis B particles. In 1973, an endogenous DNA-dependent DNA polymerase was found within the core of these particles (Kaplan et al., 1973). The genome was identified as a small, circular, partially double-stranded DNA (Robinson and Greenman, 1974; Robinson, 1977).

Early reports on a possible role of HBV infections in hepatocellular cancer appeared as early as the 1950s (Payet et al., 1956). Additional early epidemiological studies further reported a role of chronic hepatitis B infections in HCC development

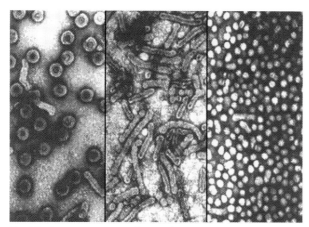

Fig. 6.1 Hepatitis B virus. Left: typical 42-nm particles containing an outer HB surface antigen (HBs) envelope, Center: filamentous forms of 20 nm diameter particles. Right: 20 nm particles. (Reprinted from VIRUS TAXONOMY, Eighth Report of the International Committee on Taxonomy of Viruses, Vol 1, Fauquet, C.M., et al. (Eds.), Part II – The DNA and RNA Reverse Transcribing Viruses, Hepadnaviridae, 373. Copyright 2005, with permission from Elsevier and courtesy of W. Gerlich.)

(Prince et al., 1970; Vogel et al., 1970; Denison et al., 1971; Sankalé et al., 1971; Teres et al., 1971; Nishioka et al., 1973; Trichopoulos et al., 1975; Larouzé et al., 1976). In 1981, Beasley et al. presented clear-cut epidemiologic evidence for a role of hepatitis B in HCC. In a prospective study conducted in government employees in Taiwan, these authors noted an increase in relative risk for HCC by a factor of 103 of hepatitis B carriers in comparison to negative individuals.

Typical hepatitis B particles are illustrated in Figure 6.1.

6.1.2
Epidemiology and Clinical Symptoms

In Western societies the majority of HBV cases are observed in age groups between 20 and 40 years, whereas in developing countries, infection occurs frequently during the perinatal period. There exist remarkable differences between males and females in liver cancers presently linked to HBV or hepatitis C virus (HCV) infections (Parkin et al., 2005) (Fig. 6.2), the percentage of males suffering from these cancers being approximately two-fold that of females.

There exists also a wide variation in the geographic prevalence of HBV infections, largely corresponding to that of HCCs (Fig. 6.3). The Asia-Pacific region and Africa tend to have the highest prevalence of hepatitis B infection worldwide (Lin, X., et al., 2005).

The mode of infection transmission depends on age: the infection of neonates – particularly those born to persistently infected mothers – reveals in 85 % of cases a

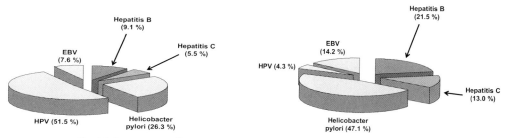

Fig. 6.2 Percentages of hepatitis B and C virus infections on the incidence of liver cancer in relation to other virus-linked human cancers in male (left) and female (right) patients. EBV: Epstein–Barr virus; HPV: human papillomavirus.

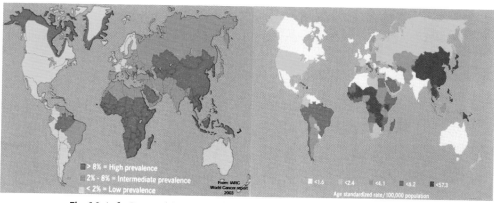

Fig. 6.3 Left: Geographic pattern of the prevalence of hepatitis B virus infections. Right: Geographic pattern of the prevalence of hepatocellular carcinoma. (World Cancer Report, Stewart, B.W. and Kleihues, P. (editors), Lyon, France: IARC Press, 2003 and Vaccines, Immunization and Biologicals, WHO 2000.)

chronic carrier state (Mitsuda et al., 1989). The risk for infection during later childhood increases among children whose siblings have already acquired the infection (Whittle et al., 1990). Contaminated needles, tattooing, syringes and acupuncture equipment have been clearly identified as important sources of infection (Kent et al., 1988). In adulthood, sexual transmission (Szmuness, 1975; reviewed in Atkins and Nolan, 2005) and parenteral infections appear to play the major role. Among homosexual men the rate of infection is commonly high and depends on the number of sexual partners (Alter et al., 1989; Rosenblum et al., 1992; Osmond et al., 1993). Intravenous drug users are at an especially high risk (Alter et al., 1990; Polakoff, 1990; Struve, 1992). Infection in developed as well as in developing countries is frequently facilitated by a low socioeconomic status (Szmuness et al. 1978a; Toukan, 1987).

For chronic infections the age of infection appears to play the prevailing role. This accounts in particular for neonates, where up to 100% of these children develop a chronic carrier state (Beasley et al., 1977; Wong et al., 1984). Among immunocompetent adults this occurs only in 0.5 to 3% of subjects (Pol, 2005).

The source of the infectious virus is commonly blood, but other secretions and excretions also contribute to infections; among these are included semen, saliva (Ward et al., 1972; Heathcote et al., 1974; Villlarejos et al., 1974; Karayiannis et al., 1985; Davison et al., 1987), vaginal secretions, and menstrual blood (Mosley, 1975). Tears and breast milk have also been recorded as containing infectious HBV. In addition, all other biological fluids from infected patients may be considered as potentially infectious. There exist indirect modes of transmission in renal dialysis units, through common use of fomates such as towels, razors and toothbrushes, as well as by acupuncture needles and medical instruments.

Hepatitis B infections occur throughout the world. Particularly high rates of infection are recorded in developing countries and under conditions of poor hygiene. The highest rates of chronic HBV carriers have been reported from China, Africa, Oceania and the South Pacific, the Middle East, and certain areas in South America (Sobeslavsky, 1975; Szmuness, 1975; Gust et al., 1978; Szmuness et al., 1978b).

There is no seasonal spreading of the infection and no typical epidemics, except under circumstances of transfusions with contaminated blood or by needle sharing of drug abusers (Maynard et al., 1976). In endemic areas the pattern of transmission is different in comparison to the Western world: in the former, most infections occur as maternal – neonatal transmissions, whereas in the latter group mainly adolescent children or young adults become infected (Szmuness et al., 1978a).

Asymptomatic infection with hepatitis B occurs in slightly more than 50% of cases, where no medical intervention is required. Between 80% and 85% of infected newborns, however, become chronic carriers if infection occurred during their first 2–3 months of life (Okada et al., 1976; Beasley et al., 1977; Shiraki et al., 1977; Lee et al., 1978). Generally, symptomatic cases occur after a latency period of 3–4 months. The clinical course and diagnosis of acute and fulminant hepatitis B have been described in detail previously (e.g., Zuckerman and Zuckerman, 2000), and will not be described here. In Western societies, chronic infections develop in up to 5% of infected people (IARC, 1994). Infection may result in not only a symptomatic but also an asymptomatic course. The incidence of chronic infections is higher in men than in women. Hepatitis B leads more frequently to asymptomatic infections of children than in adults, and affects particularly immunosuppressed patients (McMahon et al., 1985; Taylor et al., 1988; Edmunds et al., 1993). Viral persistence is accompanied by inflammatory reactions in the liver, necrosis of liver cells and frequently with integration of the hepatitis B genome into liver cell DNA (De Franchis et al., 1993). Continued replication of HBV results in serious problems for the infected patient: primarily benign lobular hepatitis, severe chronic active hepatitis and liver cirrhosis (Fattovich et al., 1990). The presence of HBV DNA in the serum represents a particular risk factor for the development of cirrhosis (Fattovich et al., 1991).

6.1.3
Taxonomy and Viral Genome Structure

Human hepatitis B virus belongs to the family of Hepadnaviridae, which comprises a growing number of mammalian and avian members. Mammalian viruses related to HBV have been isolated from woodchucks (Summers et al., 1978) and Beechey ground squirrels (Marion et al., 1980). In particular, the woodchuck virus was found to be an effective carcinogen in its native host. Additional isolates have been obtained from chimpanzees, gorillas, orangutans and gibbons (Starkman et al., 2003). It is interesting to note that the HBV variants found in orangutans were interspersed with variants from southerly distributed gibbon species (*Hylobates agilis* and *Hylobates moloch*), which occupy overlapping habitats. Gibbons from mainland Asia are phylogenetically distinct. Also in chimpanzees there seems to exist a geographical rather than a subspecies distribution of HBV variants.

Avian hepadnaviruses have been isolated from ducks (Mason et al., 1980), herons (Sprengel et al., 1988), snow geese (Chang et al., 1999), various types of additional exotic ducks and geese (Guo et al., 2005), storks (Pult et al., 2001), and cranes (Prassolov et al., 2003). There exists evidence for an interspecies spread of heron hepatitis B viruses among different species and subspecies of herons (Lin, L., et al., 2005). Phenotypic mixing has been observed of rodent, but not avian, hepadnavirus surface proteins into human HBV particles (Gerhardt and Bruss, 1995). Clearly, the family of hepadnaviruses is widely spread among mammalian and avian species. It is likely that additional virus types belonging to this family will emerge in the future. A phylogenetic tree of human and animal hepadnaviruses is illustrated in Figure 6.4.

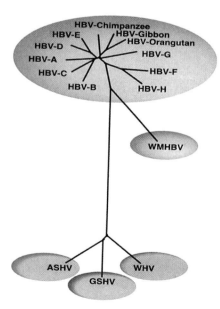

Fig. 6.4 Phylogenetic tree of human and animal hepadnaviruses. ASHV: Arctic ground squirrel hepatitis virus; GSHV: Ground squirrel hepatitis virus; WHV: woodchuck hepatitis virus; WMHBV: Woolly monkey hepatitis B virus. (Reprinted from VIRUS TAXONOMY, Eighth Report of the International Committee on Taxonomy of Viruses, Vol 1, Fauquet, C.M., Mayo, M.A., Maniloff, J., Desselberger, U. and Ball, L.A. (Eds.), Part II – The DNA and RNA Reverse Transcribing Viruses, Hepadnaviridae, 382. Copyright 2005, with permission from Elsevier.)

Eight different genotypes of human hepatitis B viruses (A–H) have been identified (Kao et al., 2000b; Kidd-Ljunggren et al., 2002; Shibayama et al., 2005). Their
differentiation is mainly based on comparative and phylogenetic analyses of the S
region. A sequence divergence of more than 8% of the entire genome, consisting of
approximately 3200 base pairs, is commonly used to differentiate between the individual HBV genotypes (Okamoto et al., 1988). The genotypes differ in geographic
prevalence: genotype A has been preferentially found in Northwest Europe, sub-
Saharan Africa, India and the United States (reviewed in Akuta and Kumada, 2005).
Genotypes B and C are more often found in south-east Asia, Japan and Oceania, and
genotype D mainly in Mediterranean countries. Genotype E seems to be restricted to
Africa, and F to Central and South America. The geographic prevalences of genotypes G and H have not yet been determined. Although not confirmed in all other
studies (Sumi et al., 2003; Yuen et al., 2003), case-control studies suggested that
genotype C is associated with more severe liver disease and a more rapid progression to cirrhosis and liver cancer (Kao and Chen, 2000; Sumi et al., 2003; Chan et
al., 2004). Since cirrhosis is more frequently induced by genotype C infections, the
latter suggestion gains some probability. This is further supported by a prospective
longitudinal cohort study of chronic hepatitis B patients in Hong Kong (Chan et al.,
2004).

The structure of hepatitis B virus DNA is shown in Figure 6.5. The 42-nm particle
is surrounded by a phospholipid bilayer envelope which harbors the surface antigens and encloses the nucleocapsid. Depending on the initiation site of transcription, three different sizes of surface proteins of 24, 32, and 39 kDa are produced; the
small surface protein (S-antigen) is most abundantly formed. The largest surface antigen form represents the binding site for host cell attachment. The infected cells
form large quantities of 22-nm particles consisting of surface proteins (mainly the

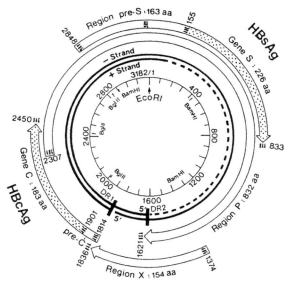

Fig. 6.5 Structure of the he-
patitis B DNA and transcripts
originating from the genome.
(Reproduced from Kao, J.-H.
and Chen, D.-C. Overview of
hepatitis B and C viruses. In:
Goedert, J.J. (Ed.), *Infectious
Causes of Cancer* . Humana
Press, pp. 313–330, 2000 a.
With permission.)

small form of S-antigen) and lipids which immunologically correspond to antigens expressed at the surface of infectious 42-nm particles. The core open reading frame (ORF) (nucleotides 1814 to 2450) contains a precore and a core region. The truncated precore protein is designated as e-antigen and can be demonstrated at the surface of infected cells and in the peripheral blood (Schlicht and Schaller, 1989; Hilleman, 2003). An ORF for 832 amino acids encodes the viral polymerase. The X-protein consisting of 154 amino acids is essential for viral infectivity and represents a transcriptional activator (Ganem and Schneider, 2001).

The genome of HBV consists of partially double-stranded DNA. For replication, the viral nucleocapsid is transported to the nucleus where the relaxed plus-strand is completed to a covalently bound closed circle and subsequently forms a supercoil. RNA transcription follows within the nucleus. The RNA is transported into the cytoplasm and translated into viral proteins. The assembled nucleocapsid takes up one strand of viral RNA where it is packaged. The viral polymerase reverse transcribes the minus-strand DNA, followed by an incomplete synthesis of the positive strand. Budding of the particle occurs from the endoplasmic reticulum where it acquires the lipid envelope with the embedded surface antigens. The reverse transcription of viral RNA without proofreading has a high probability for mutational events. Mutants in the core promoter may lead to enhanced viral replication and within the core and surface antigens to altered antigenicity of the virus (reviewed in Baumert et al., 2005). Mutations in the polymerase gene may confer resistance to antivirals.

6.1.4
Viral Gene Products and Functions

6.1.4.1 Core Antigen

The reading frame for the core antigen contains a pre-core and the core region. The pre-core protein represents a truncated form of the core protein, and is released as a soluble protein on the surface of infected host cells and into the blood stream (Schlicht and Schaller, 1989). It is designated as e-antigen. The regions of the pre-core and core protein are divided in a segment of redundant nucleotide sequences that imparts the common antigenic specificity to the e-antigen and core antigens (Milich et al., 1990; Hilleman, 2003). The HBV core protein contains 183 to 185 amino acids, depending on the subtype. Phosphorylation and dephosphorylation events seem to contribute to intracellular and extracellular forms of the core protein (Pugh and Summers, 1989; Mabit and Schaller, 2000). Phosphorylation precedes the HBS RNA encapsidation (Gazina et al., 2000).

6.1.4.2 Polymerase

The viral polymerase functions as a DNA polymerase and as reverse transcriptase. At about 90 kDa, it represents the largest protein produced by the HBV genome. There exists a structural similarity of the HBV polymerase to the corresponding domain of the of HIV reverse transcriptase (Das et al., 2001). Upon infection of sus-ceptible cells, within the nucleus the relaxed positive strand is completed and forms a covalently bonded closed-circle supercoil. Subsequently, full-length strands of RNA are transcribed, which are packaged into the assembled capsid, where the RNA is reversely transcribed by the viral polymerase to form the viral minus-strand. The incomplete positive strand is synthesized within the nucleocapsid. It is possible to separate the polymerase domains responsible for initiation of DNA replication and for reverse transcriptase activity (Beck and Nassal, 2001).

6.1.4.3 HB X Antigen

A typical ORF coding for the X-protein is only present in mammalian hepad-naviruses, and is either missing or present in a highly divergent form in avian hepadnaviruses (Chang et al., 2001). Since the latter commonly do not induce liver tumors, this led to the suspicion that HBx might play a role in carcinoma induction by animal hepadnaviruses. A comprehensive review on the present knowledge of features and functions of hepatitis B X gene products has been published by Bou-chard and Schneider (2004).

The *HBx* gene codes for a protein of 154 amino acids with a molecular mass of about 17.5 kDa. Its amino- and carboxy-terminal regions contain presumptive heli-cal domains and a potential coiled-coil motif (Kodoma et al., 1985; Colgrove et al., 1989). The 50 amino-terminal amino acids seem to contain a negative regulatory el-ement, since their deletion activates HBx transcriptional functions (Murakami et al., 1994). HBx is mainly found in the cytoplasm, but also reaches the nucleus (Doria et al., 1995; Sirma et al., 1998; Hoare et al., 2001).

In woodchucks, a gene corresponding to HBx is essential for the replication of woodchuck hepatitis virus (WHV) (Chen et al., 1993; Zoulim et al., 1994). In human HBV infections, the role of HBx is less clear, although it augments HBV infection and viral persistence (Melegari et al., 1998; Bouchard et al., 2001; Xu et al., 2002). The X protein stimulates transcription of various cellular transcription elements, usually containing binding sites for NF-κB, AP-1 and -2, c-EBP, ATF-CREB or cal-cium-activated factor NF-AT (Faktor and Shaul, 1990; Maguire et al., 1991; Lucito and Schneider, 1992; Williams and Andrisani, 1995; Lara-Pezzi et al., 1999). HBx also stimulates RNA polymerase I-, II- and III-dependent promoters (Aufiero and Schneider, 1990; Wang et al., 1998). It acts, however, also as a suppressor for other genes. This has been suggested for p21[WAF] (Ahn et al., 2001). Its transcriptional ac-tivity seems to be repressed by HBx-mediated down-regulation of Sp1, which regu-lates the activity of p21 [WAF].

HBx does not bind DNA directly, but binds to some components essential for basal transcription. Its interaction with the ZIP-region of CREB seems to be re-sponsible for the HBx-mediated activation of CREB-dependent transcription (Ma-guire et al., 1991; Williams and Andrisani, 1995).

The cytoplasmic HBx activates the extracellular signal-regulated kinases (ERKs), the stress-activated protein kinases/NH$_2$-terminal-Jun kinases, and the p38 kinase

(Benn et al., 1996; Tarn et al., 2001, 2002). HBx also activates indirectly the Ras-pathway by activating nonreceptor tyrosine kinases of the Src-family (Klein and Schneider, 1997; Lee and Yun, 1998; Tarn et al., 2002). This results in modifications of cellular adherens functions (Lara-Pezzi et al., 2001). The activation of Src kinases stimulates the HBV replication in established liver cell lines by 5- to 20-fold (Klein et al., 1999; Bouchard et al., 2001). Some functions of the HBV X protein are summarized in Figure 6.6.

Conflicting reports describe the potential interaction of HBx with p53. Although a direct binding has been reported (Feitelson et al., 1993; Wang et al., 1994; Truant et al., 1995), these results have not been confirmed in other studies (Puisieux et al., 1995; Su et al., 2000). Thus, this field still requires further analyses. The binding to the transcription factor CREB and other b-ZIP transcription factors, however, is firmly established (Maguire et al., 1991; Barnabas et al., 1997; Andrisani and Barnabas, 1999; Choi et al., 1999).

One study showed that HBx inhibits nucleotide excision repair (Jia et al., 1999). The interaction of HBx with the DNA repair proteins DDB1 and DDB2, as revealed by in-vitro and in-vivo studies, seems to be of particular importance (Becker et al., 1998; Sitterlin et al., 2000; Bergametti et al., 2002), although the immediate functional consequences are not entirely clear. Transgenic mice expressing HBx do not reveal an increased rate of spontaneous mutations (Madden et al., 2000). The hepatocytes of the same animals, however, are more sensitive to low levels of chemical mutagens (Madden et al., 2001; Zhu et al., 2004). Although not a primary mutagen, HBx seems to contribute to mutagenic functions of other carcinogens.

Induction of apoptosis by HBx has been controversial. In HBx-transgenic mice, two reports noted increased apoptotic rates in hepatocytes (Terradillos et al., 1997, 2002), whereas another report failed to confirm this observation (Madden et al., 2000). Similarly, several authors reported that HBx blocks apoptosis induced by tumor necrosis factor α (TNF-α), Fas, p53, or transforming growth factor-B (TGF-β) (Elmore et al., 1997; Shih et al., 2000; Pan et al., 2001). On the other hand, HBx expression independent of HBV replication was described as promoting apoptosis in various cell types (Chirillo et al., 1997; Su et al., 2001; Kim and Seong, 2003; Shirakata and Koike, 2003). It is very difficult to reconcile these diverging studies at

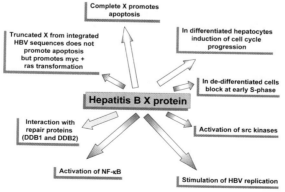

Fig. 6.6 Some functions of the hepatitis B X protein.

this stage. It seems to be important, however, that HBx expressed from replicating HBV genomes in cultured cells results in hypersensitivity to cell killing by TNF-α. This hypersensitivity requires a step involving HBx activation of c-Jun terminal kinase and Myc (Su et al., 2001; Kim and Seong, 2003; Bouchard and Schneider, 2004). Primary mouse hepatocytes are sensitized by HBx to ethanol and TNF-α-induced apoptosis by a caspase-3-dependent mechanism (Kim et al., 2005). In this respect, it is of interest that the differentiation stage of cells plays a role in determining HBx-dependent cell cycle progression (Lee et al., 2002). HBx-expressing differentiated hepatocytes proceed through G_1, S and G_2/S, concomitant with the induction of cyclins D1, A, and B and Cdc2. In HBx-positive dedifferentiated cells, the cells enter G_1 and S-phase, but do not proceed further.

In summary, HBx clearly represents a pleiotropic protein, the individual functions of which still remain at best enigmatic.

6.1.5
Pathogenesis and Immune Interactions

The pathogenesis of HBV infections is complex and involves innate and adaptive immune responses. The virus, in addition, has evolved mechanisms to induce immunotolerance, immune exhaustion and suppression, and immune escape through mutation, modification of the antigenic phenotype, molecular mimicry and others (Tai et al., 2002; Favoreel et al., 2003; Alcami, 2003; Vanlandschoot and Leroux-Roels, 2003).

Usually HBV DNA becomes detectable in the blood circulation within one month following primary infection, but remains at relatively low level of 10^2–10^4 genome equivalents per mL for up to 6 weeks (Rehermann and Nascimbeni, 2005). Subsequently, viral DNA, HbeAg, and HbsAg reach peak titers before specific antibodies arise (Hollinger, 1987). An elevated level of serum alanine amino-transferase which starts to rise approximately 10–15 weeks after primary infection is an indication for T-cell-mediated liver injury. The primary events contributing to liver injury and clearance of HBV infection are mediated by cytotoxic T lymphocytes (CTLs) (Bertoletti and Maini, 2000; Rehermann, 2000). Infected cells are destroyed by MHC class I-restricted CD8 + CTLs (Chisari and Ferrari, 1995). The aggressiveness of this response determines the outcome of the infection. A weak cell-mediated immune response commonly results in a persistent viral carrier state, initially clinically unapparent, but ending frequently in chronic active liver disease (Hilleman, 2003). Proinflammatory cytokines, such as interferon-α, interleukin (IL)-12, and IL-18, contribute as innate immune response to the outcome of the infection (Ferrari et al., 1987; Bertoletti et al., 1997). In mice transgenic for the entire HBV genome, transfer of CTLs or of their cytokines (interferon-γ, TNF-α, IL-2), abolishes virus replication and gene expression (Guidotti et al., 1996, 1999; Guidotti and Chisari, 1999; Thimme et al., 2003).

Clinical recovery results in life-long protective immunity, sometimes even in spite of traceable amounts of persisting virus in the blood. Under chemotherapy and severe immunosuppression, reactivation of the infection may even occur (Kawatani,

2001). Allografts from previously HBV-positive patients may lead to HBV transmission in immunosuppressed transplant recipients (Chazouilleres et al., 1994).

Tolerance against HBV antigens may arise as the consequence of in-utero infections (Milich et al., 1990, 1998; Wang and Zhu, 2000). The resultant absence of CTLs prevents clearance of the infected host cells and results in persistent HBV infection. The still immature immune system in perinatal and prenatal infections emerges as the main reason for the high percentage of HBV persistence in infections acquired during this period. Non-responsiveness to viral antigens may also arise from mutations within viral genes: in one investigation, 34 mutations were recorded in the pre-core/core gene, 12 in the polymerase sequence, and nine in the pre-S/S region (Brunetto et al., 1999). These represented in part genetic transitions, insertions, transversions, and deletions. It is likely that a substantial diversity of viral genotypes exists within individual infected liver cells and within the total liver. Interestingly, in this study the X gene was not mutated.

Hepatitis B virus infection also interacts directly with innate immune responses. The HBS core antigen inhibits the transcription of human interferon-β gene by interacting with regulatory DNA sequences 5' to the coding sequence of the interferon-β gene (Twu and Schloemer, 1989; Whitten et al., 1991). The viral polymerase gene, specifically its terminal domain, has also been described as inhibiting the responses to interferons α and ã (Foster et al., 1991). Subsequent studies showed that the HBV capsid protein of defective particles associated with chronic hepatitis B selectively inhibited induction of the MxA protein by suppressing and interacting directly with the MxA promoter (Rosmorduc et al., 1999). The MxA protein represents an interferon-inducible GTPase with antiviral activity against several viruses. HBV-encoded pre-core/core proteins blocked the MxA expression by affecting the interferon-stimulated response elements 2 and 3, upstream of the putative start codon of the MxA promoter (Fernandez et al., 2003).

6.1.6
Role in Hepatocellular Carcinoma

6.1.6.1 HBx Transgenic Mice and HCCs

Although an early report found no evidence for a role of HBx in transgenic mice (Lee et al., 1990), a number of subsequent studies reported a positive correlation of HBx expression and liver cancer in these animals. A construct including the HBx coding region as well as the HBV enhancer I region, the X gene promoter, and the HBV polyadenylation signal induced liver tumors directly linked to HBx expression (Kim et al., 1991; Yu et al., 1999). Particularly high levels of HBx expression resulted in a high rate of liver cancer in male mice (Koike et al., 1994).

Several authors have described a higher susceptibility of HBx-transgenic mice for chemical carcinogens (Slagle et al., 1996; Madden et al., 2001; Zhu et al., 2004). These groups suggest that HBx expression is not sufficient for carcinogenesis, but the *HBx* gene may rather act like a tumor promoter. On a similar line, expression of c-myc driven by WHV virus regulatory sequences in HBx-transgenic mice shortened the average tumor latency by 2–3 months (Terradillos et al., 1997; Lakhtakia et al., 2003). Again, these data seem to support a tumor promoter function of HBx. Knock-in experiments resulting in integration of the *HBx* gene into the p21^{WAF} locus resulted within 18 months in HCCs (Wang et al., 2004). One interesting observation made in the latter study was a high up-regulation of the estrogen receptor-β selectively in tumor tissues of male p21-HbsAg mice, providing suggestive genetic evidence that HbsAg might represent the factor explaining the higher prevalence of HCCs in males when compared to females.

Mutations within the X gene region involving nucleotides 1762(T)/1764(A), which are considered as markers for liver cancer development, have been described in HBV genomes derived from the plasma of patients with HCCs (Kuang et al., 2004). Within tumors from patients of Qidong in the Peoples Republic of China, 74.3% carried a double mutation at nucleotides 1762 (T) and 1764 (A). Four of six plasma samples from such patients were also positive. This mutation appears to have also some predictive value, since more than 50% of patients with liver cancer revealed this mutation several years prior to the detection of HCCs.

C-terminal truncation of HBx results in enhanced transformability of murine cells upon co-transfection with ras or myc constructs (Paterlini-Brechot et al., 2000, 2003), and reveals the biological impact of natural C-terminal deletions of hepatitis B virus X protein in HCC tissues (Tu et al., 2001).

6.1.6.2 HBS Transgenic Mice and HCCs

A first report appeared in 1990, describing hepatocarcinogenesis due to chronic liver cell injury in hepatitis B S antigen (HbsAg) transgenic mice (Dunsford et al., 1990). Within 4 months these animals developed chronic hepatitis, followed sequentially by the development of regenerative nodules and oval hyperplasia. Liver adenomas developed at 8 months of age, and carcinomas at 12 months. By 20 months, 100% of the animals had developed hepatocellular cancer. Within the same year another report described transgenic mice containing a single copy of HbsAg which revealed an elevated susceptibility to carcinogen-induced hepatocarcinogenesis (Dragani et al., 1990). Interestingly, in carcinogen-induced liver tumors expression of the HbsAg was inhibited, apparently due to de novo methylation of the S region (Farza et al., 1994). The synergistic effect between HbsAg-transgenic mice and chemical carcinogens was soon confirmed for aflatoxin and diethylnitrosamine (Sell et al., 1991). At least in these experimental mouse models, p53 and pRb mutations have not been found, possibly indicating an early stage of hepatocarcinogenesis (Pasquinelli et al., 1992). The development of liver cancer in HbsAg-transgenic mice depends on the level of expression of the transgene (Huang and Chisari, 1995).

TGF-α drastically accelerates hepatocarcinogenesis when overexpressed in TGF-α transgenic mice (Jhappan et al., 1990). Overexpression of this factor in hepatocytes in transgenic mice is sufficient to induce enhanced hepatocyte proliferation and HCCs (Jakubczak et al., 1997). Mice which were bitransgenic for TGF-α and HbsAg revealed a dramatically accelerated appearance of HCCs (Jakubczak et al., 1997).

HCCs in HBV-positive patients also show elevated expression levels of TGF-α (Hsia et al., 1994). Hepatitis B preS1, as part of large HbsAg, activates the transcription of TGF-α and may thus contribute to liver carcinogenesis (Ono et al., 1998). Mutants of the preS1 or preS2-regions cause oxidative stress and DNA damage (Hsieh et al., 2004). Since such mutants are found in late and non-replicative stages of HBV infection, this seems to indicate that preS1/S2 mutants induce oxidative stress and mutations in hepatocytes in late stages of HBV infection. This is shown schematically in Figure 6.7.

Oxidative stress in turn negatively regulates hepatitis B virus gene expression and viral replication (Zheng and Yen, 1994).

In acute HBV infections the small HbsAg is the major form that constitutes the envelope of the virion. In the chronic phase, the large form becomes dominant. Several truncated forms with a partially deleted pre-S region have been identified. Two of these contribute to two distinct histological patterns labeled as "ground glass hepatocyte" types I and II (Fan et al., 2000, 2001). Type I reveals an inclusion-like pattern of HbsAg which is deleted in the pre-S1 promoter region (Hsieh et al., 2004), whereas type II is deleted of nucleotides 4–57 in the pre-S2 region and contains a point mutation at the start codon. This results in a substantial decrease in the synthesis of small and middle surface antigens. In both types, HbsAg accumulates in the endoplasmic reticulum. In particular, type II is highly correlated with cirrhotic

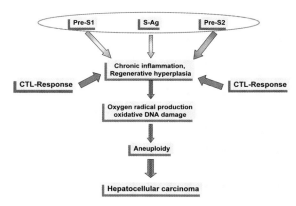

Fig. 6.7 Putative functions of HBs-antigens in the development of hepatocellular carcinomas.

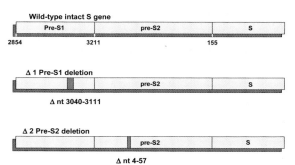

Fig. 6.8 Schematic outline of pre-S1 and pre-S2 deletions. (Modified from Hsieh, Y.H., et al., 2004.)

progression and HCC. This pre-S2 mutant also up-regulates cyclin A expression and induces nodular proliferation of hepatocytes (Wang et al., 2005). It emerges only in the late non-replicative phase of chronic HBV infection, and becomes the dominant gene product in hepatocytes (Hsieh et al., 2004). Both, pre-S1 and pre-S2 induce reactive oxygen species (ROS) in cells of the human liver cell line Huh-7 (Wang et al., 2003), though pre-S2 triggers a higher level of oxidative DNA damage. The two mutated S-antigen forms are outlined schematically in Figure 6.8.

Mutations in the X-linked *Hprt* gene in cells carrying the pre-S1 or pre-S2 mutant *HBS* genes are 4.5 to 6.2 times higher than in cells overexpressing the wild-type HbsAg (Hsieh et al., 2004). Thus, these two pre-S mutants reveal properties reminiscent of well-characterized oncogenes. Chromosomal imbalances occur already in cirrhotic nodules (Yeh et al., 2001).

6.1.7
Interaction of Hepatitis B Infection with Chemical Carcinogens (Aflatoxins and Alcohol)

A number of studies point to an interaction of HBV infections in hepatocarcinogenesis with chemical compounds that may induce liver damage upon repeated exposure (Wogan, 1992; Chen et al., 1997; Yu et al., 2000).

6.1.7.1 Alcohol

HCCs linked to alcohol consumption commonly occur after an initial development of liver cirrhosis. The main metabolite of alcohol, acetaldehyde, causes hepatocellular injury, which leads to increased oxidative stress and thus damages DNA (reviewed in Voigt, 2005). Alcohol, in addition, causes abnormalities in DNA methylation and may inactivate tumor suppressor genes. These effects of alcohol contribute to cancer development in chronically HBV-infected patients.

6.1.7.2 Aflatoxin

Early investigations on a synergistic role of aflatoxin exposure and concurrent HBV infections (reviewed in Kew, 2003) appeared from Swaziland (Peers et al., 1987) and China's Guangxi Province (Yeh et al., 1989). The authors of both studies concluded that simultaneous exposure to these agents was an important determinant for geographic variations in the incidence of liver cancer in these two regions. In transgenic mice, overexpressing the large polypeptide of HBV, the feeding of aflatoxin B1 resulted in rapid hepatocyte dysplasia and HCCs in comparison to unexposed littermates (Sell et al., 1991). Similarly, the feeding of hepatitis virus-infected woodchucks with aflatoxin B1 resulted in synergistic hepatocarcinogenesis (Bannasch et al., 1995). Four epidemiologic studies found a striking multiplicative carcinogenic effect of both agents (Ross et al., 1992; Qian et al., 1994; Wang et al., 1996; Lunn et al.,

1997). One study in Taiwan analyzed tumor tissue of HBV-infected patients by histochemical staining for aflatoxin B_1-N^7-guanine adducts and found that the positive patients were on average 10 years younger than those with adduct-negative cancers (Chen et al., 1992).

Approximately 60% of HCC patients from areas with high exposure to aflatoxin B1 reveal a guanine to thymine transversion at the third base of codon 249 of the *p53* gene (Hsu et al., 1991; Bressac et al., 1991). This was subsequently confirmed in epidemiologic studies in regions with high and low aflatoxin exposure (Ozturk, 1991; Eaton and Gallagher, 1994). There were some inconsistent reports, however. In Taiwan, in a first study codon 249 arginine to serine mutations were found in HbsAg-positive patients (Lunn et al., 1997), and in a second study in 36.3% of HBV-infected patients with liver cancer as compared to 11.7% of cancer patients without HBV markers (Wang et al., 1996). A meta-analysis of 49 published studies also failed to demonstrate any interaction between HBV and aflatoxin B_1 (Stern et al., 2001). In spite of these reports, there appears to be sufficient evidence for a synergistic interaction between persistent HBV infection and aflatoxin uptake in carcinogenesis. Whether the codon 249 transversion in *p53* of hepatocellular cancer patients originates indeed from aflatoxin exposure, or represents a marker of specific HBV infections, remains to be established.

The mechanism of interaction between HBV and aflatoxins is only partially understood: in HBV transgenic mouse lineages, specific cytochrome P450s (CYP 1A and CYP 2A5) are induced in association with liver injury (Kirby et al., 1994; Chemin et al., 1996, 1999; Chomarat et al., 1998). These effects were absent in lineages where liver injury was not associated with HBV transgene expression and occurred only in HBs, but not in HBx transgenic lineages (Chomarat et al., 1998; Chemin et al., 1999). Further studies are required to assess the significance of these observations.

Concomitant infection with hepatitis C virus which may occur within the same hepatocyte (Rodríguez-Íñigo et al., 2005) and diabetes mellitus are being discussed as additional risk factors (for reviews, see Hassan et al., 2002; Raimondo et al., 2005).

6.1.8
Mechanism of HBV-Mediated Oncogenesis

The previous sections have described specific functions of HBx and HbsAg in relation to events leading to liver cancer. A number of reports have speculated on a role of HBV DNA integration as cause of hepatocarcinogenesis. Integrated HBV sequences are found in approximately 80% of HBV-positive cancers (Brechot et al., 2000). The *HBx* gene is the most common ORF integrated into the host cell genome, where it becomes frequently mutated and rearranged (Huo et al., 2001). The integrated sequences possess a diminished ability to function as a transcriptional co-transactivator and as an NF-κB pathway activator. Yet, they are still able to bind to p53 and to abrogate p53-mediated apoptosis. In view of the fact that 20% of HBV-positive hepatocellular cancers are negative for HBV DNA integration, these observations may point to an auxiliary function of integrated HBx in malignant progression, although they do not support an essential role of this event.

A critical role for the integrational site of HBV DNA within the host cell genome has also been envisaged. Early observations claimed a rate of about 90% of integrated sequences in HBV-positive liver cancers, some of them without expression of HBsAg (Paterlini and Brechot, 1991). In contrast to observations made with WHV, no common integration site has been discovered. In some instances, however, integration has been noted in genes involved in cell proliferation, such as cyclin A2 (Wang et al., 1990), the retinoic acid receptor and steroid receptor genes (Dejean et al., 1986), in *SERCA1* and *TRAP1* genes (Graef et al., 1994; Pineau et al., 1996; Chami et al., 2000; Gozuacik et al., 2001), and into the human telomerase gene (Paterlini-Brechot et al., 2003). It should be of interest that a HBV pre-S-retinoic acid receptor beta chimera transforms erythrocytic progenitor cells *in vitro* (Garcia et al., 1993). Possibly related to this observation, the retinoid X receptor RXR alpha binds to and trans-activates the HBV enhancer (Huan and Siddiqui, 1992).

If one tries to summarize the available data, three prime factors appear to influence hepatocarcinogenesis in chronically HBV-infected patients: primarily functions of two viral genes, *HBx* and *HBs*, and in the latter case particularly mutated pre-S2, consistently act as mutagens by inducing oxidative stress within the infected cells and negatively interfering with DNA excision repair. These functions are in part initiated, augmented and amplified by the interaction of cytokines of CTLs. This chronic process of induced mutational events should eventually lead to necrotic changes and cirrhosis, and finally to the selection of clones with increased proliferative potential and invasive growth properties. The latency period, commonly in the order of 40 to 50 years after primary HBV infection, would find an explanation in this process, requiring a number of genetic modifications. The rare HCCs that arise already in childhood might find a reasonable explanation in pre-existing genetic modifications.

Based on these considerations, HBV-mediated carcinogenesis can be considered as a predominantly indirect process. On rare occasions, however, insertional mutagenesis may contribute more directly to cancer development.

6.1.9
Prevention and Control of HBV-Mediated Infections

6.1.9.1 Prevention

The discovery of HbsAg in the blood of infected carriers (Blumberg et al., 1967) paved the way for the development of hepatitis B vaccines. Initially, viral antigen was used and purified from the blood of HBs carriers (Buynak et al., 1976; Hilleman et al., 1983). This represented a major achievement in view of the absence of any suitable tissue culture system for virus propagation, and the lack of a neutralization test. Following the demonstration of the absence of infectious virus from the vaccine preparation in chimpanzees, and also of a protective effect against a HBV virus challenge, the clinical trials were commenced in 1975. Double-blind controlled clinical studies proved the protective efficacy of the vaccine (Szmuness et al., 1981; Francis et al., 1982), and the plasma-derived vaccine was licensed in 1981, representing the first licensed viral subunit vaccine. Subsequently, with the advance of technology, recombinant yeast and bacterial expression systems were developed and the yeast antigen vaccine was licensed in 1986 as the first recombinant vaccine (McAleer et al., 1984; Hilleman, 1987).

Application of the vaccine within hours after birth protected 75–80% of infants born to HBV-positive mothers that otherwise would become viral carriers in 80–90% of cases (for a review, see Hilleman, 2003). Follow-up surveillance studies were conducted in Gambia, China, Italy, Taiwan, and Alaska (MacMahon and Wainwright, 1993; Kao and Chen, 2002). The vaccine has been clearly successful in preventing persisting HBV infections and in preventing fulminant hepatitis cases. The present follow-up is too short to arrive at strong conclusions concerning the preventive effect of this vaccine for HCCs, although a trend towards a reduction of this cancer has already become apparent in Taiwan (Kao and Chen, 2002).

It seems that approximately 5% of the overall population possesses a genetically encoded HLA constitution that precludes the development of an adequate T-cell response (Desombere et al., 1998). In addition, mutations in the surface antigen of HBV may occur, particularly in position 145 of the S-antigen, changing a loop in the protein against which the antibody is directed. This may result in children who become "immune carriers" (Carman et al., 1990; Wallace and Carman, 1997; He et al., 2001; Torresi, 2002).

The perspective of global application of this vaccine – which in all likelihood can be considered as a vaccine against a specific type of cancer – bears substantial promise for the future control of a common human cancer. If combined with another anticancer vaccine directed against high-risk papillomaviruses, it would probably protect against the development of a second common malignancy, cancer of the cervix (Báez-Astúa et al., 2005).

6.1.9.2 **Therapy**

Two chemotherapeutic drugs have been licensed to treat hepatitis B infections. These are the nucleoside analogues lamivudine and adefovir. Both drugs are relatively nontoxic, although some kidney toxicity has been reported (for reviews, see Nguyen and Wright, 2001; Chen et al., 2002; Pramoolsinsup, 2002; Conjeevaram and Lok, 2003; Jain and Fung, 2003). Some therapeutic successes have been achieved with both drugs, although mutations in the virus may lead to the development of drug resistance.

Interferon α has been a longstanding option for the treatment of hepatitis B, though the effectiveness of this treatment is limited, even when combined with chemotherapy (Hilleman, 2003). The activity of interferon can be increased to some extent by covalent linkage of a polyethylene moiety (pegylated interferon) (Hui et al., 2005; Maillard and Gollan, 2005).

Novel approaches, the use of single-stranded anti-sense DNA oligonucleotides, of ribozymes, small interfering RNA, and the use of double-stranded RNA for interferon induction have not yet reached routine clinical application, and may be useful after solving the problems of their application (reviewed in Hilleman, 2003). The same appears to account for therapeutic vaccines which still require further research.

In general, success in the treatment of persistent HBV infections is still very limited and requires future attention of both basic and clinical research.

References

Ahn, J.Y., Chung, E.Y., Kwun, H.J., and Jang, K.L. Transcriptional repression of p21(waf1) promoter by hepatitis B virus X protein via a p53-independent pathway. *Gene* 275: 163–168, **2001**.

Akuta, N. and Kumada, H. Influence of hepatitis B virus genotypes on the response to antiviral therapies. *J. Antimicrob. Chemother.* 55: 139–142, **2005**.

Alcami, A. Viral mimicry of cytokines, chemokines and their receptors. *Nat. Rev. Immunol.* 3: 36–50, **2003**.

Alter, M.J., Coleman, P.J., Alexander, W.J., Kramer, E., Miller, J.K., Mandel, E., Hadler, S. C., and Margolis, H.S. Importance of heterosexual activity in the transmission of hepatitis B and non-A, non-B hepatitis. *JAMA* 262: 1201–1205, **1989**.

Alter, M.J., Hadler, S. C., Margolis, H.S., Alexander, W.J., Hu, P.Y., Judson, F.N., Mares, A., Miller, J.K., and Moyer, L.A. The changing epidemiology of hepatitis B in the United States. Need for alternative vaccination strategies. *JAMA* 263: 1218–1222, **1990**.

Andrisani, O. and Barnabas, S. The transcriptional function of the hepatitis B virus X protein and its role in hepatocarcinogenesis. *Int. J. Oncol.* 15: 373–379, **1999**.

Atkins, M. and Nolan, M. Sexual transmission of hepatitis B. *Curr. Opin. Infect. Dis.* 18: 67–72, **2005**.

Aufiero, B. and Schneider, R.J. The hepatitis B virus X-gene product trans-activates both RNA polymerase II and III promoters. *EMBO J.* 9: 497–504, **1990**.

Báez-Astúa, A., Herraez-Hernandez, E., García Garbi, N., Pasolli, H.A., Juarez, V., zur Hausen, H., and Cid-Arregui, A. Low-dose adenoviral vaccine encoding chimeric hepatitis B virus surface antigen-human papillomavirus type 16 E7 proteins induces enhanced E7-specific antibody and cytotoxic T cell responses. *J. Virol.*, 79: 12807–12817, **2005**.

Bannasch, P., Khoshkhou, N.I., Hacker, H.J., Radaeva, S., Mrozek, M., Zillmann, U., Kopp-Schneider, A., Haberkorn, U., Elgas, M., Tolle, T., et al. Synergistic hepatocarcinogenic effect of hepadnaviral infection and dietary aflatoxin B_1 in woodchucks. *Cancer Res.* 55: 3318–3330, **1995**.

Barnabas, S., Hai, T., and Andrisani, O.M. The hepatitis B virus X protein enhances the DNA binding potential and transcription efficacy of bZip transcription factors. *J. Biol. Chem.* 272: 20684–20690, **1997**.

Baumert, T.F., Barth, H., and Blum, H.E. Genetic variants of hepatitis B virus and their clinical relevance. *Minerva Gastroenterol. Dietol.* 51: 95–108, **2005**.

Beasley, R.P., Trepo, C., Stevens, C.E., and Szmuness, W. The e antigen and vertical transmission of hepatitis B surface antigen. *Am. J. Epidemiol.* 105: 94–98, **1977**.

Beasley, R.P., Hwang, L.Y. Lin, C.-C., and Chien, C.-S. Hepatocellular carcinoma and hepatitis B virus. A prospective study of 22 707 men in Taiwan. *Lancet* 2: 1129–1133, **1981**.

Beck, J. and Nassal, M. Reconstitution of a functional duck hepatitis B virus replication initiation complex from separate reverse transcriptase domains expressed in Escherichia coli. *J. Virol.* 75: 7410–7419, **2001**.

Becker, S. A., Lee, T.-H., Butel, J.S., and Slagle, B.L. Hepatitis B virus X protein interferes with cellular DNA repair. *J. Virol.* 72: 266–272, **1998**.

Beeson, P.B. Jaundice occurring one to four months after transfusion of blood or plasma: report of seven cases. *JAMA* 121: 1332–1334, **1944**.

Benn, J., Su, F., Doria, M., and Schneider, R.J. Hepatitis B virus HBx protein induces transcription factor AP-1 by activation of extracellular signal-regulated and c-Jun N-terminal mitogen-activated protein kinases. *J. Virol.*: 70: 4978–4985, **1996**.

Bergametti, F., Sitterlin, D., and Transy, C. Turnover of hepatitis B virus X protein is regulated by damaged DNA-binding complex. *J. Virol.* 76: 6495–6501, **2002**.

Bertoletti, A. and Maini, M.K. Protection or damage: a dual role for the virus-specific cytotoxic T lymphocyte response in hepatitis B and C infection? *Curr. Opin. Immunol.* 12: 403–408, **2000**.

Bertoletti, A., D'Elios, M.M., Boni, C., De Carli, M., Zignego, A.L., Durazzo, M., Missale, G., Penna, A., Fiaccadori, F., Del Prete, G., and Ferrari, C. Different cytokine profiles of intrahepatic T cells in chronic hepatitis B and hepatitis C virus infections. *Gastroenterology* 112: 193–199, **1997**.

Blumberg, B.S., Alter, H.J., and Visnich, S. A "new" antigen in leukaemia sera. *JAMA* 191: 541–546, **1965**.

Blumberg, B.S., Gerstley, B.J., Hungerford, D.A., London, W.T., and Sutnick, A.I. A serum antigen (Australia antigen) in Down's syndrome, leukemia, and hepatitis. *Ann. Intern. Med.* 66: 924–931, **1967**.

Blumberg, B.S., Sutnick, A.I., and London, W.T. Australia antigen and hepatitis. *JAMA* 207: 1895–1896, **1969**.

Bouchard, M.J. and Schneider, R.J. The enigmatic X gene of hepatitis B virus. *J. Virol.* 78: 12 725–12 734, **2004**.

Bouchard, M.J., Wang, L.H., and Schneider, R.J. Calcium signaling by HBx protein in hepatitis B virus DNA replication. *Science* 294: 2376–2378, **2001**.

Brechot, C., Gozuacik, D., Murakami, Y., and Paterlini-Brechot, P. Molecular bases for the development of hepatitis B virus (HBV) related hepatocellular carcinoma (HCC). *Semin. Cancer Biol.* 10: 211–231, **2000**.

Bressac, B., Kew, M.C., Wands, J.R., and Ozturk, M. Selective G to T mutations of p53 gene in hepatocellular carcinoma from southern Africa. *Nature* 350: 429–430, **1991**.

Brunetto, M.R., Rodriguez, U.A., and Bonino, F. Hepatitis B virus mutants. *Intervirology* 42: 69–80, **1999**.

Buynak, E.B., Roehm, R.R., Tytell, A.A., Bertland, A.U., II, Lampson, G.P., and Hilleman, M.R. Vaccine against human hepatitis B. *JAMA* 235: 2832–2834, **1976**.

Carman, W.F., Zanetti, A.R., Karayiannis, P., Waters, J., Manzillo, G., Tanzi, E., Zuckerman, A.J., and Thomas, H.C. Vaccine-induced escape mutant of hepatitis B virus. *Lancet* 336: 325–329, **1990**.

Chami, M., Gozuacik, D., Saigo, K., Capiod, T., Falson, P., Lecoeur, H., Urashima, T., Beckmann, J., Gougeon, M.L., Claret, M., le Maire, M., Brechot, C., and Paterlini-Brechot, P. Hepatitis B virus related insertional mutagenesis implicates SER-CA1 gene in the control of apoptosis. *Oncogene* 19: 2877–2886, **2000**.

Chan, H.L.-Y., Hui, A.Y., Wong, M.L., Tse, A.M.-L., Hung, L.C.-T., Wong, V.W.-S., and Sung, J.J.-Y. Genotype C hepatitis B virus infection is associated with an increased risk for hepatocellular carcinoma. *Gut* 53: 1494–1498, **2004** .

Chang, S. F., Netter, H.J., Bruns, M., Schneider, R., Frölich, K., and Will, H. A new avian hepadnavirus infecting snow geese (*Anser aerulescens*) produces a significant fraction of virions containing single-stranded DNA. *Virology* 262: 39–54, **1999**.

Chang, S. F., Netter, H.J., Hildt, E., Schuster, R., Schaefer, S., Hsu, Y.C., Rang, A., and Will, H. Duck hepatitis B virus expresses a regulatory HBx-like protein from a hidden open reading frame. *J. Virol.* 75: 161–170, **2001**.

Chazouilleres, O., Mamish, D., Kim, M., Carey, K., Ferrell, L., Roberts, J.P., Ascher, N.L., and Wright, T.L. 'Occult' hepatitis B virus as source of infection in liver transplant recipients. *Lancet* 343: 142–146, **1994**.

Chemin, I., Takahashi, S., Belloc, C., Lang, M.A., Ando, K., Guidotti, L.G., Chisari, F.V., and Wild, C.P. Differential induction of carcinogen metabolizing enzymes in a transgenic mouse model of fulminant hepatitis. *Hepatology* 24: 649–659, **1996**.

Chemin, I., Ohgaki, H., Chisar, F.V., and Wild, C.P. Altered expression of hepatic carcinogen metabolizing enzymes with liver injury in HBV transgenic mouse lineages expressing various amounts of hepatitis B surface antigen. *Liver* 19: 81–87, **1999**.

Chen, C.J., Zhang, Y.J., Lu, S. N., and Santella, R.M. Aflatoxin B_1-DNA adducts in smeared liver tumor tissue from patients with hepatocellular carcinoma patients. *Hepatology* 16: 1150–1155, **1992**.

Chen, C.J., Yu, M.W., and Liaw, Y.F. Epidemiological characteristics and risk factors of hepatocellular carcinoma. *J. Gastroenterol. Hepatol.* 12: S294–S308, **1997**.

Chen, H., Kaneko, S., Girones, R., Anderson, R.W., Hornbuckle, W.E., Tennant, B.C., Cote, P.J., Gerin, J.L., Purcell, R.H., and Miller, R.H. The woodchuck hepatitis virus X gene is important for establishment of virus infection in woodchucks. *J. Virol.* 67: 1218–1226, **1993**.

Chen, R.Y.M., Desmond, P.V., and Locarnini, S. A. Emerging therapies of hepatitis B and C. *J. Gastroenterol. Hepatol.* 17 (Suppl.): S471–S481, **2002**.

Chirillo, P., Pagano, S., Natoli, G., Puri, P.L., Burgio, V.L., Balsano, C., and Levrero, M. The hepatitis B virus X gene induces p53-mediated cell death. *Proc. Natl. Acad. Sci. USA* 94: 8162–8167, **1997**.

Chisari, F.V. and Ferrari, C. Hepatitis B virus immunopathogenesis. *Annu. Rev. Immunol.* 13: 29–60, **1995**.

Choi, B.H., Park, G.T., and Rho, H.M. Interaction of hepatitis B viral X protein and CCAAT/enhancer-binding protein α synergistically activates the hepatitis B viral enhancer II/pregenomic promoter. *J. Biol. Chem.* 274: 2858–2865, **1999**.

Chomarat, P., Rice, J.M., Slagle, B.L., and Wild, C.P. Hepatitis B virus-induced liver injury and altered expression of carcinogen metabolising enzymes: the role of the HBx protein. *Toxicol. Lett.* 102: 595–601, **1998**.

Colgrove, R., Simon, G., and Ganem, D. Transcriptional activation of homologous and heterologous genes of the hepatitis B virus X gene product in cells permissive for viral replication. *J. Virol.* 63: 4019–4026, 1989.

Conjeevaram, H.S. and Lok, A.S. -F. Management of chronic hepatitis B. *J. Hepatol.* 38 (Suppl.): S90–S103, **2003**.

Dane, D.S., Cameron, C.H., and Briggs, M. Virus-like particles in serum of patients with Australia-antigen-associated hepatitis. *Lancet* I: 695–698, **1970**.

Das, K., Xiong, X., Yang, H., Westland, C.E., Gibbs, C.S., Sarafianos, S. G., and Arnold, E. Molecular modeling and biochemical characterization reveal the mechanism of hepatitis B virus polymerase resistance to lamivudine (3 TC) and emtricitabine (FTC). *J. Virol.* 75: 4771–4779, **2001**.

Davison, F., Alexander, G.J.M., Trowbridge, R., Fagan, E.A., and Williams, R. Detection of hepatitis B virus DNA in spermatozoa, urine, saliva, and leucocytes of chronic HBsAg carriers. A lack of relationship with serum markers of replication. *Hepatology* 4: 37–44, **1987**.

De Franchis, R., Meucci, G., Vecchi, M., Tatarella, M., Colombo, M., Del Ninno, E., Rumi, M.G., Donato, M.F., and Ronchi, G. The natural history of asymptomatic hepatitis B surface antigen carriers. *Ann. Intern. Med.* 118: 191–194, **1993**.

Dejean, A., Bougueleret, L., Grzeschik, K.H., and Tiollais, P. Hepatitis B virus DNA integration in a sequence homologous to v-erb-A and steroid receptor genes in a hepatocellular carcinoma. *Nature* 322: 70–72, **1986**.

Denison, E.K., Peters, R.L., and Reynolds, T.B. Familial hepatoma with hepatitis-associated antigen. *Ann. Intern. Med.* 74: 391–394, **1971**.

Desombere, I., Willems, A., and Leroux-Roels, G. Response to hepatitis B vaccine: multiple HLA genes are involved. *Tissue Antigens* 51: 593–604, **1998**.

Doria, M., Klein, N., Lucito, R., and Schneider, R.J. Hepatitis B virus HBx protein is a dual specificity cytoplasmic activator of Ras and nuclear activator of transcription factors. *EMBO J.* 14: 4747–4757, **1995**.

Dragani, T.A., Manenti, G., Farza, H., Della Porta, G., Tiollais, P., and Pourcel, C. Transgenic mice containing hepatitis B virus sequences are more susceptible to carcinogen-induced hepatocarcinogenesis. *Carcinogenesis* 11: 953–956, **1990**.

Dunsford, H.A., Sell, S., and Chisari, F.V. Hepatocarcinogenesis due to chronic liver cell injury in hepatitis B virus transgenic mice. *Cancer Res.* 50: 3400–3407, **1990**.

Eaton, D.L. and Gallagher, E.P. Mechanisms of aflatoxin carcinogenesis. *Annu. Rev. Pharmacol. Toxicol.* 34: 135–172, **1994**.

Edmunds, W.J., Medley, G.F., Nokes, D.J., Hall, A.J., and Whittle, H.C. The influence of age on the development of the hepatitis

B carrier state. *Proc. Biol. Sci.* 253: 197–201, **1993**.

Elmore, L.W., Hancock, A.R., Chang. S. F., Wang, X.W., Chang, S., Callahan, C.P., Geller, D.A., Will, H., and Harris, C.C. Hepatitis B virus X protein and p53 tumor suppressor interactions in the modulation of apoptosis. *Proc. Natl. Acad. Sci. USA* 94: 14707–14712, **1997**.

Faktor, O. and Shaul, Y. The identification of hepatitis B virus X gene responsive elements reveals functional similarity of X and HTLV-I tax. *Oncogene* 5: 867–872, **1990**.

Fan, Y.-F., Lu, C.-C., Chang, Y.-C., Chang, T.-T., Lin, P.-W., Lei, H.-Y., and Su, I.-J. Identification of a pre-S2 mutant in hepatocytes expressing a novel marginal pattern of surface antigen in advanced disease of chronic hepatitis B virus infection. *J. Gastroenterol. Hepatol.* 15: 519–528, **2000**.

Fan, Y.-F., Lu, C.-C., Chen, W.-C., Yao, W.-J., Wang, H.-C., Chang, T.-T., Lei, H.-Y., Shiau, A.-L., and Su, I.-J. Prevalence and significance of hepatitis B virus (HBV) pre-S mutants in serum and liver at different replicative stages of chronic HBV infection. *Hepatology* 33: 277–286, **2001**.

Farza, H., Dragani, T.A., Metzler, T., Manenti, G., Tiollais, P., Della Porta, G., and Pourcel, C. Inhibition of hepatitis B virus surface antigen gene expression in carcinogen-induced liver tumors from transgenic mice. *Mol. Carcinog.* 9: 185–192, **1994**.

Fattovich, G., Brollo, L., Alberti, A., Realdi, G., Pontisso, P., Giustina, G., and Ruol, A. Spontaneous reactivation of hepatitis B virus infection in patients with chronic type B hepatitis. *Liver* 10: 141–146, **1990**.

Fattovich, G., Brollo, L., Giustina, G., Noventa, F., Pontisso, P., Alberti, A., Realdi, G., and Ruol, A. Natural history and prognostic factors for chronic hepatitis type B. *Gut* 32: 294–298, **1991**.

Favoreel, H.W., Van de Walle, G.R., Nauwynck, H.J., and Pensaert, M.B. Virus complement evasion strategies. *J. Gen. Virol.* 84: 1–15, **2003**.

Feitelson, M., Zhu, M., Duan, L.X., and London, W.T. Hepatitis B x antigen and p53 are associated in vitro and in liver tissues from patients with primary hepatocellular carcinoma. *Oncogene* 8: 1109–1117, **1993**.

Fernandez, M., Quiroga, J.A., and Carreno, V. Hepatitis B virus downregulates the human interferon-inducible MxA promoter through direct interaction of pre-core/core proteins. *J. Gen. Virol.* 84: 2073–2082, **2003**.

Ferrari, C., Penna, A., Giuberti, T., Tong, M.J., Ribera, E., Fiaccadori, F., and Chisari, F.V. Intrahepatic, nucleocapsid antigen-specific T cells in chronic active hepatitis B. *J. Immunol.* 139: 2050–2058, **1987**.

Findlay, G.M. and MacCallum, F.O. Note on acute hepatitis and yellow fever immunization. *Trans. R. Soc. Trop. Med. Hyg.* 31: 297–308, **1937**.

Foster, G.R., Ackrill, A.M., Goldin, R.D., Kerr, I.M., Thomas, H.C., and Stark, G.R. Expression of the terminal protein region of hepatitis B virus inhibits cellular responses to interferons α and γ and double-stranded RNA. *Proc. Natl. Acad. Sci. USA* 88: 2888–2892, **1991**.

Francis, D.P., Haller, S. C., Thompson, S. E., Maynard, J.E., Ostrow, D.G., and Altman, N. The prevention of hepatitis B with vaccine. Report of the Centers for Disease Control Multi-Center Efficacy Trial among Homosexual Men. *Ann. Intern. Med* . 97: 362–366, **1982**.

Ganem, D. and Schneider, R.J. Hepadnaviridae: viruses and their replication. In: Knipe, D.M., and Howley, P.M. (Eds.), *Field's Virology*. 4th edition, Lippincott, Williams and Wilkins, Philadelphia, Chapter 86: 2971–3036, **2001**.

Garcia, M., de Thé, H., Tiollais, P., Samarut, J., and Dejean, A. A hepatitis B virus pre-S-retinoic acid receptor beta chimera transforms erythrocytic progenitor cells in vitro. *Proc. Natl. Acad. Sci. USA.* 90: 89–93, **1993**.

Gazina, E.V., Fielding, J.E., Lin, B., and Anderson, D.A. Core protein phosphorylation modulates pregenomic RNA encapsidation to different extents in human and duck hepatitis B viruses. *J. Virol.* 74: 4721–4728, **2000**.

Gerhardt, E., and Bruss, V. Phenotypic mixing of rodent but not avian hepadnavirus surface proteins into human hepatitis B virus particles. *J. Virol.* 69: 1201–1208, **1995**.

Gozuacik, D., Murakami, Y., Saigo, K., Chami, M., Mugnier, C., Lagorce, D., Okanoue, T., Urashima, T., Brechot, C., and Paterlini-Brechot, P. Identification of human cancer related genes by naturally occurring hepatitis B virus DNA tagging. *Oncogene* 20: 6233–6240, **2001**.

Graef, E., Caselmann, W.H., Wells, J., and Koshy, R. Insertional activation of mevalonate kinase by hepatitis B virus DNA in a human hepatoma cell line. *Oncogene* 9: 81–87, **1994**.

Guidotti, L.G., Ishikawa, T., Hobbs, M.V., Matzke, B., Schreiber, R., and Chisari, F.V. Intracellular inactivation of the hepatitis B virus by cytotoxic T lymphocytes. *Immunity* 4: 25–36, **1996**.

Guidotti, L.G. and Chisari, F.V. Cytokine-induced viral purging – role in viral pathogenesis. *Curr. Opin. Microbiol.* 2: 388–391, **1999**.

Guidotti, L.G., Rochford, R., Chung, J., Shapiro, M., Purcell, R., and Chisari, F.V. Viral clearance without destruction of infected cells during acute HBV infection. *Science* 284: 825–829, **1999**.

Guo, H., Mason, W.S., Aldrich, C.E., Saputelli, J.R., Miller, D.S., Jilbert, A.R., and Newbold, J.E. Identification and characterization of avihepadnaviruses isolated from exotic anseriformes maintained in captivity. *J. Virol.* 79: 2729–2742, **2005**.

Gust, I.D., Dimitrakakis, M., and Zimmet, P. Studies on hepatitis B surface antigen and antibodies in Nauru. I. Distribution among Nauruans. *Am. J. Trop. Med. Hyg.* 27: 1030–1036, **1978**.

Hassan, M.M., Hwang, L.Y., Hatten, C.J., Swaim, M., Li, D., Abbruzzese, J.L., Beasley, P., and Patt, Y.Z. Risk factors for hepatocellular carcinoma: synergism of alcohol with viral hepatitis and diabetes mellitus. *Hepatology* 36: 1206–1213, **2002**.

He, C., Nomura, F., Itoga, S., Isobe, K., and Nakai, T. Prevalence of vaccine-induced escape mutants of hepatitis B virus in the adult population of China: a prospective study in 176 restaurant employees. *J. Gastroenterol. Hepatol.* 16: 1373–1377, **2001**.

Heathcote, J., Cameron, C.H., and Dane, D.S. Hepatitis-B antigen in saliva and semen. *Lancet* I: 71–73, **1974**.

Hilleman, M.R. Yeast recombinant hepatitis B vaccine. *Infection* 15: 3–7, **1987**.

Hilleman, M.R. Critical overview and outlook: pathogenesis, prevention, and treatment of hepatitis and hepatocarcinoma caused by hepatitis B virus. *Vaccine* 21: 4626–4649, **2003**.

Hilleman, M.R., McAleer, W.J., Buynak, E.B., and McLean, A.A. The preparation and safety of hepatitis B vaccine. *J. Infect.* 7 (Suppl.1): 3–8, **1983**.

Hoare, J., Henkler, F., Dowling, J.J., Errington, W., Goldin, R.D., Fish, D., and McGarvery, M.J. Subcellular localization of the X protein of HBV infected hepatocytes. *J. Med. Virol.* 64: 419–426, **2001**.

Hollinger, F.B. Serologic evaluation of viral hepatitis. *Hosp. Pract.* 22: 101–114, **1987**.

Hsia, C.C., Thorgeirsson, S. S., and Tabor, E. Expression of hepatitis B surface and core antigens and transforming growth factor-alpha in "oval cells" of the liver in patients with hepatocellular carcinoma. *J. Med. Virol.* 43: 216–221, **1994**.

Hsieh, Y.H., Su, I.J.., Wang, H.C., Chang, W.W., Lei, H.Y., Lai, M.D., Chang, W.T., and Huang, W. Pre-S mutant surface antigens in chronic hepatitis B virus infection induce oxidative stress and DNA damage. *Carcinogenesis* 25: 2023–2032, **2004**.

Hsu, I.C., Metcalf, R.A., Sun, T., Welsh, J.A., Wang, N.J., and Harris, C.C. Mutational hotspot in the p53 gene in human hepatocellular carcinomas. *Nature* 350: 427–428, **1991**.

Huan, B. and Siddiqui, A. Retinoid X receptor RXR alpha binds to and trans-activates the hepatitis B virus enhancer. *Proc. Natl. Acad. Sci. USA.* 89: 9059–9063, **1992**.

Huang, S. N. and Chisari, F.V. Strong, sustained hepatocellular proliferation precedes hepatocarcinogenesis in hepatitis B surface antigen transgenic mice. *Hepatology* 21: 620–626, **1995**.

Hui, A.Y., Chan, H.L., Cheung, A.Y., Cooksley, G., and Sung, J.J. Systematic review: treatment of chronic hepatitis B infection by pegylated interferon. *Aliment. Pharmacol. Ther.* 22: 519–528, **2005**.

Huo, T.I., Wang, X.W., Forgues, M. Wu, C.G., Spillare, E.A., Giannini, C., Brechot, C., and Harris, C.C.. Hepatitis B virus X mutants derived from human hepatocellular carcinoma retain the ability to abrogate p53-induced apoptosis. *Oncogene* 20: 3620–3628, **2001**.

IARC Monographs on the Evaluation of Carcinogenic Risks to Humans. *Hepatitis Viruses.* Volume 59, **1994**.

IARC World Cancer Report, Stewart, B.W. and Kleihues, P (Eds.), IARC Press, **2003**.

Jain, A.B. and Fung, J.J. Advances in hepatitis B virus infection. *Transpl. Proc.* 35: 342–344, **2003**.

Jakubczak, J.L., Chisari, F.V., and Merlino, G. Synergy between transforming growth factor α and hepatitis B virus surface antigen in hepatocellular proliferation and carcinogenesis. *Cancer Res.* 57: 3606–3611, **1997**.

Jhappan, C., Stahle, C., Harkins, R.N., Fausto, N., Smith, G.H., and Merlino, G.T. TGF alpha overexpression in transgenic mice induces liver neoplasia and abnormal development of the mammary gland and pancreas. *Cell* 61: 1137–1146, **1990**.

Jia, L., Wang, X.W., and Harris, C.C. Hepatitis B virus x protein inhibits nucleotide excision repair. *Int. J. Cancer* 80: 875–879, **1999**.

Kao, J.-H. and Chen, D.-C. Overview of hepatitis B and C viruses. In: Goedert, J.J. (Ed.), *Infectious Causes of Cancer*. Humana Press, pp. 313–330, **2000**.

Kao, J.-H. and Chen, D.-S. Global control of hepatitis B virus infection. *Lancet Infect. Dis.* 2: 395–403, **2002**.

Kao, J.-H., Chen. P.J., Lai, M.Y., and Chen, D.S. Hepatitis B genotypes correlate with clinical outcomes in patients with hepatitis B. Gastroenterology 118: 554–559, **2000**.

Kaplan, P.M., Greenman, R.L., Gerin, J.L., Purcell, R.H., and Robinson, W.S. DNA polymerase associated with human hepatitis B antigen. *J. Virol.* 13: 995–1005, **1973**.

Karayiannis, P., Novick, D.M., Lok, A.S., Fowler, M.J., Monjardino, J., and Thomas, H.C. Hepatitis B virus DNA in saliva, urine, and seminal fluid of carriers of hepatitis B e antigen. *Br. Med. J. (Clin. Res. Ed.)* 290: 1853–1855, **1985** .

Kawatani, T., Suou, T., Tajima, F., Ishiga, K., Omura, H., Endo, A., Ohmura, H., Ikuta, Y., Idobe, Y., and Kawasaki, H. Incidence of hepatitis virus infection and severe liver dysfunction in patients receiving chemotherapy for hematologic malignancies. *Eur. J. Haematol.* 67: 45–50, **2001**.

Kent, G.P., Brondum, J., Keenlyside, R.A., LaFazia, L.M., and Denman Scott, H. A large outbreak of acupuncture-associated hepatitis B. *Am. J. Epidemiol.* 127: 591–598, **1988**.

Kew, M.C. Synergistic interaction between aflatoxin B1 and hepatitis B virus in hepatocarcinogenesis. *Liver Int.* 23: 405–409, **2003**.

Kidd-Ljunggren, K., Miyakawa, Y., and Kidd, A.H. Genetic variability in hepatitis B viruses. *J. Gen. Virol.* 83: 1267–1280, **2002**.

Kim, C.M., Koike, K., Saito, I., Miyamura, T., and Jay, G. HBx gene of hepatitis B virus induces liver cancer in transgenic mice. *Nature* 351: 317–320, **1991**.

Kim, K.H. and Seong, B.L. Pro-apoptotic function of HBV X protein is mediated by interaction with c-FLIP and enhancement of death-inducing signal. *EMBO J.* 22: 2104–2116, **2003**.

Kim, W.H., Hong, F., Jaruga, B., Zhang, Z.S., Fan, S. J., Liang, T.J., and Gao, B. Hepatitis B virus X protein sensitizes primary mouse hepatocytes to ethanol and TNF-α-induced apoptosis by a caspase-3-dependent mechanism. *Cell. Mol. Immunol* . 2: 40–48, **2005**.

Kirby, G.M., Chemin, I., Montesano, R., Chisari, F.V., Lang, M.A., and Wild, C.P. Induction of specific cytochrome P450s involved in aflatoxin B1 metabolism in hepatitis B virus transgenic mice. *Mol. Carcinog.* 11: 74–80, **1994**.

Klein, N.P. and Schneider R.J. Activation of Src family kinases by hepatitis B virus HBx protein and coupled signaling to Ras. *Mol. Cell. Biol.* 17: 6427–6436, **1997**.

Klein, N.P., Bouchard, M., Wang, L.-H., Kobarg, C., and Schneider, R.J. Src kinases involved in hepatitis B virus replication. *EMBO J.* 18: 5019–5027, **1999**.

Kodama, K., Ogasawara, N., Yoshikawa, H., and Murakami, S. Nucleotide sequence of a cloned woodchuck hepatitis virus genome: evolutional relationship between hepadnaviruses. *J. Virol.* 56: 978–986, **1985**.

Koike, K., Moriya, K., Iino, S., Yotsuyanagi, H., Endo, Y., Miyamura, T., and Kurokawa, K. High level expression of hepatitis B virus HBx gene and hepatocarcinogenesis in transgenic mice. *Hepatology* 19: 810–819, **1994**.

Krugman, S., Giles, J.P., and Hammond, J. Infectious hepatitis. Evidence for two distinctive clinical, epidemiological and immunological types of infection. *JAMA* 200: 365–373, **1967**.

Kuang, S. Y., Jackson, P.E., Wang, J.B., Lu, P.X., Munoz, A., Qian, G.S., Kensler, T.W., and Groopman, J.D. Specific mutations of hepatitis B virus in plasma predict liver cancer development. *Proc. Natl. Acad. Sci. USA.* 101: 3575–3580, **2004**.

Lakhtakia, R., Kumar, V., Reddi, H., Mathur, M., Dattagupta, S., and Panda, S. K. Hepatocellular carcinoma in hepatitis B 'x' transgenic mouse model: a sequential pathological evaluation. *J. Gastroenterol. Hepatol.* 18: 80–91, **2003**.

Lara-Pezzi, E., Armesilla, A.L., Majano, P.L., Redondo, J.M., and Lopez-Cabrera, M. The hepatitis B virus X protein activates nuclear factor of activated T cells (NF-AT) by a cyclosporin A-sensitive pathway. *EMBO J.* 17: 7066–7077, **1998**.

Lara-Pezzi, E.., Roche, S., Andrisani, O., Sanchez-Madrid, F., and Lopez-Cabrera, M. The hepatitis B virus HBx protein induces adherens junction disruption in a src-dependent manner. *Oncogene* 20: 3323–3331, **2001**.

Larouzé, B., Saimot, G., Lustbader, E.D., London, W.T., Werner, B.G., and Payet, M., Host responses to hepatitis-B infection in patients with primary hepatic carcinomas and their families: A case/control study in Senegal, West Africa. *Lancet* II: 534–538, **1976**.

Lee, A.K.Y., Ip, H.M.H. and Wong, V.C.W. Mechanisms of maternal-fetal transmission of hepatitis B virus. *J. Infect. Dis.* 138: 668–671, **1978**.

Lee, S., Tarn, C., Wang, W.H., Chen, S., Hullinger, R.L., and Andrisani, O.M. Hepatitis B virus X protein differentially regulates cell cycle progression in X-transforming versus nontransforming hepatocyte (AML12) cell lines. *J. Biol. Chem.* 277: 8730–8740, **2002**.

Lee, T.H., Finegold, M.J., Shen, R.F., DeMayo, J.L., Woo, S. L., and Butel, J.S. Hepatitis B virus transactivator X protein is not tumorigenic in transgenic mice. *J. Virol.* 64: 5939–5947, **1990**.

Lee, Y.H. and Yun, Y. HBx protein of hepatitis B virus activates Jak1-STAT signaling. *J. Biol. Chem.* 273: 25 510–25 515, **1998**.

Lin, L., Prassolov, A., Funk, A., Quinn, L., Hohenberg, H., Frolich, K., Newbold, J., Ludwig, A., Will, H., Sirma, H., and Steinbach, F. Evidence from nature: interspecies spread of heron hepatitis B viruses. *J. Gen. Virol.* 86: 1335–1342, **2005**.

Lin, X., Robinson, N.J., Thursz, M., Rosenberg, D.M., Weild, A., Pimenta, J.M., and Hall, A.J. Chronic hepatitis B virus infection in the Asia-Pacific region and Africa: review of disease progression. *J. Gastroenterol. Hepatol.* 20: 833–843, **2005**.

Lucito, R. and Schneider, R.J. Hepatitis B virus X protein activates transcription factor NF-κB without a requirement for protein kinase C. *J. Virol.* 66: 983–991, **1992**.

Lunn, R.M., Zhang, Y.-J., Wang, L.-Y., Chen, C.J., Lee, P.H., Lee, C.S., Tsai, W.Y., and Santella, R.M. p53 mutations, chronic hepatitis B infection, and aflatoxin exposure in hepatocellular carcinoma in Taiwan. *Cancer Res.* 57: 3471–3477, **1997**.

Mabit, H. and Schaller, H. Intracellular hepadnavirus nucleocapsids are selected for secretion by envelope protein-independent membrane binding. *J. Virol.* 74: 11 472–11 478, **2000**.

MacCallum, F.O. Homologous serum jaundice. *Lancet* II: 691–692, **1947**.

MacMahon, B.J. and Wainwright, R.B. Protective efficacy of hepatitis B vaccines in infants, children and adults. In: Ellis, R.W. (Ed.) *Hepatitis B Vaccines in Clinical Practice.* New York, Marcel Dekker, pp. 243–261, **1993**.

Madden, C.R., Finegold, M., and Slagle, B. Expression of hepatitis B virus X protein does not alter the accumulation of spontaneous mutations in transgenic mice. *J. Virol.* 74: 5266–5272, **2000**.

Madden, C.R., Finegold, M., and Slagle, B. Hepatitis B virus X protein acts as a tumor promoter in development of diethylnitrosamine-induced preneoplastic lesions. *J. Virol.* 75: 3851–3858, **2001**.

Maguire, H.F., Hoeffler, J.P., and Siddiqui, A. HBV X protein alters the DNA binding specificity of CREB and ATF-2 by protein-protein interactions. *Science* 252: 842–844, **1991**.

Maillard, M.E. and Gollan, J.L. Emerging therapeutics for chronic hepatitis B. *Annu. Rev. Med.* 57: 155–166, **2005**.

Marion, P.L., Oshiro, L.S., Regnery, D.C., Scullard, G.H., and Robinson, W.S. . A virus in Beechey ground squirrels that is related to hepatitis B virus of humans. *Proc. Natl. Acad. Sci. USA* 77: 2941–2945, **1980**.

Mason, W.S., Seal, G., and Summers, J. Virus of Pekin ducks with structural and biological relatedness to human hepatitis B virus. *J. Virol.* 36: 829–836, **1980**.

Maynard, J.E., Bradley, D.W., Hornbeck, C.L., Fields, R.M., Doto, I.L., and Hollinger, F.B. Preliminary serologic studies of antibody to hepatitis A virus in populations in the United States. *J. Infect. Dis.* 134: 528–530, **1976**.

McAleer, W.J., Buynak, E.B., Maigetter, R.Z., Wampler, D.E., Miller, W.J., and Hilleman, M.R. Human hepatitis B vaccine from recombinant yeast. *Nature* 307: 178–180, **1984**.

McMahon, B.J., Alward, W.L.M., Hall, D.B., Heyward, W.L., Bender, T.R., Francis, D.P., and Maynard, J.E. Acute hepatitis B virus infection: relation of age to the clinical expression of disease and subsequent development of the carrier state. *J. Infect. Dis.* 151: 599–603, **1985**.

Melegari, M., Scaglioni, P.P., and Wands, R.J. Cloning and characterization of a novel hepatitis B virus x binding protein that inhibits viral replication. *J. Virol.* 72: 1737–1743, **1998**.

Milich, D.R., Jones, J.E., Hughes, J.L., Price, J., Raney, A.K., and McLachlan, A. Is a function of the secreted hepatitis B e antigen to induce immunologic tolerance in utero? *Proc. Natl. Acad. Sci. USA* 87: 6599–6603, **1990**.

Milich, D.R., Chen, M.K., Hughes, J.L., and Jones, J.E. The secreted hepatitis B precore antigen can modulate the immune response to the nucleocapsid: a mechanism for persistence. *J. Immunol.* 160: 2013–2021, **1998**.

Mitsuda, T., Yokota, S., Mori, T., Ibe, M., Ookawa, N., Shimizu, H., Aihara, Y., Kosuge, K., and Matsuyama, S. Demonstration of mother-to-infant transmission of hepatitis B virus by means of polymerase chain reaction. *Lancet* II: 886–888, **1989**.

Morgan, H.W. and Williamson, D.A.J. Jaundice following administration of human blood products. *Br. Med. J.* 1: 750–753, **1943**.

Mosley, J.W. The epidemiology of viral hepatitis: an overview. *Am. J. Med. Sci.* 270: 253–270, **1975**.

Murakami, S., Cheong, J., and Kaneko, S. Human hepatitis virus X gene encodes a regulatory domain that represses transactivation of X protein. *J. Biol. Chem.* 269: 15118–15123, **1994**.

Murray, R. Viral hepatitis. *Bull. NY. Acad. Med.* 31: 341–358, **1955**.

Murray, R., Ratner, F., Diefenbach, W.C.L., and Geller, H. Effect of storage at room temperature on infectivity of icterogenic plasma. *JAMA* 155: 13–15, **1954**.

Nguyen, M.H., and Wright, T.L. Therapeutic advances in the management of hepatitis B and hepatitis C. *Curr. Opin. Infect. Dis.* 14: 593–601, **2001**.

Nishioka, K., Hirayama, T., Sekine, T., Okochi, K., Mayumi, M., Jueilow, S., Chen-Hui, L., and Tong-Min, L. Australia antigen and hepatocellular carcinoma. *GANN Monogr. Cancer Res.* 14: 167–175, **1973**.

Okada, K., Kamiyama, I., Inomata, M., Imai, M., and Miyakawa, Y. E antigen and anti-e in the serum of asymptomatic carrier mothers as indicators of positive and negative transmission of hepatitis B virus to their infants. *N. Engl. J. Med.* 294: 746–749, **1976**.

Okamoto, H., Tsuda, F., Sakugawa, H., Sastrosoewignjo, R.I., Imai, M., Miyakawa, Y., and Mayumi, M. Typing hepatitis B virus by homology in nucleotide sequence: comparison of surface antigen subtypes. *J. Gen. Virol.* 69: 2575–2583, **1988**.

Ono, M., Morisawa, K., Nie, J., Ota, R., Taniguchi, T., Saibara, T., and Onishi, S. Transactivation of transforming growth factor α gene by hepatitis B virus preS1. *Cancer Res.* 58: 1813–1816, **1998**.

Osmond, D.H., Charlebois, E., Sheppard, H.W., Page, K., Winkelstein, W., Moss, A.R., and Rheingold, A. Comparison of risk factors for hepatitis C and hepatitis B virus infection in homosexual men. *J. Infect. Dis.* 167: 66–71, **1993**.

Ozturk, M. p53 mutation in hepatocellular carcinoma after aflatoxin exposure. *Lancet.* 338: 1356–1359, **1991**.

Pan, J., Duan, L.X., Sun, B.S., and Feitelson, M.A. Hepatitis B virus X protein protects against anti-Fas-mediated apoptosis in human liver cells by inducing NF-κB. *J. Gen. Virol.* 82: 171–182, **2001**.

Parkin, D.M., Bray, F., Ferlay, J., and Pisani, P. Global cancer statistics, **2002**. *CA Cancer J. Clin.* 55: 74–108, **2005**.

Pasquinelli, C., Bhavani, K., and Chisari, F.V. Multiple oncogenes and tumor suppressor genes are structurally and functionally intact during hepatocarcinogenesis in hepatitis B virus transgenic mice. *Cancer Res.* 52: 2823–2829, **1992** .

Paterlini, P. and Brechot, C. The detection of hepatitis B virus (HBV) in HbsAg negative individuals with primary liver cancer. *Dig. Dis. Sci.* 36: 1122–1129, **1991**.

Paterlini-Brechot, P., Vona, G., and Brechot, C. Circulating tumorous cells in patients with hepatocellular carcinoma. Clinical impact and future directions. *Semin. Cancer Biol.* 10: 241–249, **2000**.

Paterlini-Brechot, P., Saigo, K., Murakami, Y., Chami, M., Gozuacik, D., Mugnier, C., Lagorce, D., and Brechot, C. Hepatitis B virus-related insertional mutagenesis occurs frequently in human liver cancers and recurrently targets human telomerase gene. *Oncogene.* 22: 3911–3916, **2003**.

Payet, M., Camain, R., and Pene, P. Primary cancer of the liver. Critical study of 240 cases [in French]. *Rev. Int. Hepatol.* 6: 1–86, **1956**.

Peers, F., Bosch, X., Kaldor, J., Linsell, A., and Pluijmen, M. Aflatoxin exposure, hepatitis B virus infection and liver cancer in Swaziland. *Int. J. Cancer* 39: 545–553, **1987**.

Pineau, P., Marchio, A., Terris, B., Mattei, M.G., Tu, Z.X., Tiollais, P., and Dejean, A. A t(3;8) chromosomal translocation associated with hepatitis B virus integration involves the carboxypeptidase N locus. *J. Virol.* 70: 7280–7284, **1996**.

Pol, S. Epidemiology and natural history of hepatitis B. [Article in French] *Rev. Prat.* 55: 599–606, **2005**.

Polakoff, S. Acute viral hepatitis B, reported to the Public Health Laboratory Service. *J. Infect.* 20: 163–168, **1990**.

Pramoolsinsup, C. Management of viral hepatitis B. *J. Gastroenterol. Hepatol.* 17 (Suppl.): S125–S145, **2002**.

Prassolov, A., Hohenberg, H., Kalinina, T., Schneider, C., Cova, L., Krone, O., Frölich, K., Will, H., and Sirma, H. New hepatitis B virus of cranes that has an unexpected broad host range. *J. Virol.* 77: 1964–1976, **2003**.

Prince, A.M. An antigen detected in the blood during the incubation period of serum hepatitis. *Proc. Natl. Acad. Sci. USA* 60: 814–821, **1968**.

Prince, A.M., Leblanc, L., Krohn, K., Masseyeff, R. and Alpert, M.E.S. H. antigen and chronic liver disease. *Lancet* 2: 717–718, **1970**.

Pugh, J.C. and Summers, J.W. Infection and uptake of duck hepatitis B virus by duck hepatocytes maintained in the presence of dimethyl sulfoxide. *Virology* 172: 564–572, **1989**.

Puisieux, A., Ji, J., Guillot, C., Legros, Y., Soussi, T., Isselbacher, K., and Ozturk, M. p53-mediated cellular response to DNA damage in cells with replicative hepatitis B virus. *Proc. Natl. Acad. Sci. USA* 92: 1342–1346, **1995**.

Pult, I., Netter, H.J., Bruns, M., Prassolov, A., Sirma, H., Hohenberg, H., Chang, S. F., Frolich, K., Krone, O., Kaleta, E.F., and Will, H. Identification and analysis of a new hepadnavirus in white storks. *Virology* 289: 114–128, **2001**.

Qian, G.S., Ross, R.K., Yu, M.C., Yuan, J.M., Gao, Y.T., Henderson, B.E., Wogan, G.N., and Groopman, J.D. A follow-up study of urinary markers of aflatoxin exposure and liver cancer risk in Shanghai, People's Republic of China. *Cancer Epidemiol. Biomarkers Prev.* 3: 3–10, **1994**.

Raimondo, G., Cacciamo, G., and Saitta, C. Hepatitis B virus and hepatitis C virus co-infection: additive players in chronic liver disease? *Ann. Hepatol.* 4: 100–106, **2005**.

Rehermann, B. Intrahepatic T cells in hepatitis B: viral control versus liver cell injury. *J. Exp. Med.* 191: 1263–1268, **2000**.

Rehermann, B. and Nascimbeni, M. Immunology of hepatitis B virus and hepatitis C virus infection. *Nat. Rev. Immunol.* 5: 215–229, **2005**.

Robinson, W.S., The genome of hepatitis B virus. *Annu. Rev. Microbiol.* 31: 357–377, **1977**.

Robinson, W.S. and Greenman, R.L. DNA polymerase in the core of the human hepatitis B virus candidate. *J. Virol.* 13: 1231–1236, **1974**.

Rodríguez-Íñigo, J., Bartholomé, J., Ortiz-Movilla, N., Platero, C., López-Alcorocho, J.M., Pardo, M., Castillo, I., and Carreño, V. Hepatitis C virus (HCV) and hepatitis B virus (HBV) can coinfect the same hepatocyte in the liver of patients with chronic HCV and occult HBV infection. *J. Virol.* 79: 15578–15581, **2005**.

Rosenblum, L., Darrow, W., Witte, J., Cohen, J., French, J., Gil, P.S., Potterat, J., Sikes, K., Reich, R., and Hadler, S. Sexual practices in the transmission of hepatitis B virus and prevalence of delta virus infection in female prostitutes in the United States. *JAMA* 267: 2477–2481, **1992**.

Rosmorduc, O., Sirma, H., Soussan, P., Gordien, E., Lebon, P., Horisberger, M., Brechot, C., and Kremsdorf, D. Inhibition of interferon-inducible MxA protein expression by hepatitis B virus capsid protein. *J. Gen. Virol.* 80: 1253–1262, **1999**.

Ross, R.K., Yuan, J.M., Yu, M.C., Wogan, G.N., Qian, G.S., Tu, J.T., Groopman, J.D., Gao, Y.T., and Henderson, B.E. Urinary aflatoxin biomarkers and the risk of hepatocellular carcinoma. *Lancet* 339: 943–946, **1992**.

Sankalé, M., Seck, I., Linhard, J., Thaim, A.-A., Wane, A.-B., Diebolt, G., and Poll-Gouater, A. L'antigène Australie au cours de le cirrhose et du cancer primitive du foie chez l'Africain de Dakar. *Bull. Soc. Med. Afr. Noire Lang. fr.* 16: 167–171, **1971**.

Schlicht, H.-J. and Schaller, H. The secretory core protein of human hepatitis B virus is expressed on the cell surface. *J. Virol.* 63: 5399–5404, **1989**.

Sell, S., Hunt, J.M., Dunsford, H.A., and Chisari, F.V. Synergy between hepatitis B virus expression and chemical hepatocarcinogens in transgenic mice. *Cancer Res.* 51: 1278–1285, **1991**.

Shibayama, T., Masuda, G., Ajisawa, A., Hiruma, K., Tsuda, F., Nishizawa, T., Takahashi, M., and Okamoto, H. Characterization of seven genotypes (A to E, G and H) of hepatitis B virus recovered from Japanese patients infected with human immunodeficiency virus type 1. *J. Med. Virol.* 76: 24–32, **2005**.

Shih, W.-L., Kuo, M.-L., Chuang, S. -E., Cheng, A.-L., and Doong, S. -L. Hepatitris B virus X protein inhibits transforming growth factor-β-induced apoptosis through the activation of phophatidylinositol 3-kinase pathway. *J. Biol. Chem.* 275: 25858–25864, **2000**.

Shiraki, K., Yoshihara, N., Kawana, T., Yasui, H., and Sakurai, M. Hepatitis B surface antigen and chronic hepatitis in infants born to asymptomatic carrier mothers. *Am. J. Dis. Child.* 131: 644–647, **1977**.

Shirakata, Y. and Koike, K. Hepatitis B virus X protein induces cell death by causing loss of mitochondrial membrane potential. *J. Biol. Chem.* 278: 22071–22078, **2003**.

Sirma, H., Weil, R., Rosmorduc, O., Urban, S., Israel, A., Kremsdorf, D., and Brechot, C. Cytosol is the prime compartment of hepatitis B virus X protein where it colocalizes with the proteasome. *Oncogene* 16: 2051–2063, **1998**.

Slagle, B.L., Lee, T.H., Medina, D., Finegold, M.J., and Butel, J.S. Increased sensitivity to the hepatocarcinogen diethylnitrosoamine in transgenic mice carrying the hepatitis B X gene. *Mol. Carcinog.* 15: 261–269, **1996**.

Sitterlin, D., Bergametti, F., Tiollais, P., Tennant, B.C., and Transy, C. Correct binding of viral X protein to UVDDB-p127 cellular protein is critical for efficient infection by hepatitis B viruses. *Oncogene* 19: 4427–4431, **2000** .

Sobeslavsky, O. The program of the World Health Organization in the international surveillance of viral hepatitis B. *Am. J. Med. Sci.* 270: 283–285, **1975**.

Sprengel, R., Kaleta, E.F., and Will, H. Isolation and characterization of a hepatitis B virus endemic in herons. *J. Virol.* 62: 3832–3839, **1988**.

Starkman, S. E., MacDonald, D.M., Lewis, J.C., Holmes, E.C., and Simmonds, P. Geographic and species association of hepatitis B virus genotypes in non-human primates. *Virology.* 314: 381–393, **2003**.

Stern M.C., Umbach, D.M., Yu, M.C., London, S. J., Zhang, Z.-Q., and Taylor, J.A. Hepatitis B, aflatoxin B$_1$, and p53 codon 249 mutation in hepatocellular carcinoma from Guangxi, People's Republic of China, and meta-analysis of existing studies. *Cancer Epidemiol. Biomarkers Prev.* 10: 617–625, **2001**.

Struve, J. Hepatitis B virus infection among Swedish adults: aspects on seroepidemiology, transmission and vaccine response. *Scand. J. Infect. Dis. Suppl.* 82: 1–57, **1992**.

Su, Q., Schröder, C.H., Otto, G., and Bannasch, P. Overexpression of p53 protein is not directly related to hepatitis B X protein expression and is associated with neoplastic progression in hepatocellular carcinomas rather than hepatic preneoplasia. *Mutat. Res.* 462: 365–380, **2000**.

Su, Q., Theodosis, O.N., and Schneider, R.J. Role of NF-κB and myc proteins in apoptosis induced by hepatitis B virus HBx protein. *J. Virol.* 75: 215–225, **2001**.

Sumi, H., Yokosuka, O., Seki, N., Arai, M., Imazeki, F., Kurihara, T., Kanda, T., Fukai, K., Kato, M., and Saisho, H. Influence of hepatitis B virus genotypes on the progression of chronic type B liver disease. *Hepatology* 37: 19–26, **2003**.

Summers, J., Smolec, J.M., and Snyder, R. A virus similar to human hepatitis B virus associated with hepatitis and hepatoma in woodchucks. *Proc. Natl. Acad. Sci. USA* 75: 4533–4537, **1978**.

Szumness, W. Recent advances in the study of the epidemiology of hepatitis B. *Am. J. Pathol.* 81: 629–649, **1975**.

Szmuness, W., Harley, E.J., Ikram, H., and Stevens, C.E. Sociodemographic aspects of the epidemiology of hepatitis B. In: Vyas, G.N., Cohen, S. N., and Schmidt, R. (Eds.), *Viral Hepatitis.* Philadelphia, Franklin Institute Press, pp. 297–320, **1978 a**.

Szmuness, W., Stevens, C.E., Ikram, H., Much, M.I., Harley, E.J., and Hollinger, F.B. Prevalence of hepatitis B virus infection and hepatocellular carcinomas in Chinese-Americans. *J. Infect. Dis.* 137: 822–829, **1978 b**.

Szmuness, W., Stevens, C.E., Zang, E.A., Harley, E.J., and Keller, A. A controlled clinical trial of the efficacy of hepatitis B vaccine (Heptavax B): a final report. *Hepatology* 1: 377–385, **1981**.

Tai, P.-C., Suk, F.-M., Gerlich, W.H., Neurath, A.R., and Shih, C. Hypermodification and immune escape of an internally deleted middle-envelope (M) protein of frequent and predominant hepatitis B virus variants. *Virology* 292: 44–58, **2002**.

Tarn, C., Lee, S., Hu, Y., Ashendel, C., and Andrisani, O.M. Hepatitis B virus X protein differentially activates RAS-RAF-MAPK and JNK pathways I X-transforming versus non-transforming AML12 hepatocytes. *J. Biol. Chem.* 276: 34 671–34 680, **2001**.

Tarn, C., Zou, L., Hullinger, R.L., and Andrisani, O.M. Hepatitis B virus X protein activates the p38 mitogen-activated protein kinase pathway in dedifferentiated hepatocytes. *J. Virol.* 76: 9763–9772, **2002**.

Taylor, J.E., Stevens, C.E., de Cordoba, S. R., and Rubinstein, P. Hepatitis B virus and human immunodeficiency virus: possible interactions. In: Zuckerman, A.J. (Ed.), *Viral Hepatitis and Liver Disease.* Alan R. Liss, New York, pp. 198–200, **1988**.

Teres, J., Guardia, J., Bruguera, M., and Rodes, J. Hepatitis-associated antigen and hepatocellular carcinoma. *Lancet* 2: 215, **1971**.

Terradillos, O., Billet, O., Renard, C.-A., Levy, R., Molina, T., Briand, P., and Buendia, M.A. The hepatitis B virus X gene potentiates c-myc-induced liver carcinogenesis in transgenic mice. *Oncogene* 14: 395–404, **1997**.

Terradillos, O., de La Coste, A., Pollicino, T., Neuveut, C., Sitterlin, H., Lecoeur, H., Gougeon, M.L., Kahn, A., and Buendia, M.A. The hepatitis B virus X protein abrogates Bcl-2-mediated protection against Fas apoptosis in the liver. *Oncogene* 21: 377–386, **2002**.

Thimme, R., Wieland, S., Steiger, C., Ghrayeb, J., Reimann, K.A., Purcell, R.H., and Chisari, F.V. CD8(+) T cells mediate viral clearance and disease pathogenesis during acute hepatitis B virus infection. *J. Virol.* 77: 68–76, **2003** .

Torresi, J. The virological and clinical significance of mutations in the overlapping envelope and polymerase genes of hepatitis B virus. *J. Clin. Virol.* 25: 97–106, **2002**.

Toukan, A.U. Hepatitis B virus infection in urban residents of Jordan with particular reference to socioeconomic factors. *Trop. Gastroenterol.* 8: 161–166, **1987**.

Trichopoulos, D., Violaki, M., Sparros, L., and Xirouchaki, E. Epidemiology of hepatitis B and primary hepatic carcinoma. *Lancet* II: 1038–1039, **1975**.

Truant, R., Antunovic, J., Greenblatt, J., Prives, C., and Cromlish, J.A. Direct interaction of hepatitis B virus HBx protein with p53 leads to inhibition by Hbx of p53 response element-directed transactivation. *J. Virol.* 69: 1851–1859, **1995**.

Tu, H., Bonura, C., Giannini, C., Mouly, H., Soussan, P., Kew, M., Paterlini-Brechot, P., Brechot, C., and Kremsdorf, D. Biological impact of natural COOH-terminal deletions of hepatitis B virus X protein in hepatocellular carcinoma tissues. *Cancer Res.* 61: 7803–7810, **2001**.

Twu, J.S. and Schloemer, R.H. Transcription of the human β interferon gene is inhibited by hepatitis B virus. *J. Virol.* 63: 3065–3071, **1989**.

Vanlandschoot, P. and Leroux-Roels, G. Viral apoptotic mimicry: an immune evasion strategy developed by the hepatitis B virus? *Trends Immunol.* 24: 144–147, **2003**.

Villarejos, V.M., Visona, K.A., Gutierrez, A., and Rodriguez, A. Role of saliva, urine, and feces in transmission of type B hepatitis. *N. Engl. J. Med.* 291: 1375–1378, **1974**.

Vogel, C.L., Anthony, P.P., Mody, N., and Barker, L.F. Hepatitis-associated antigen in Ugandan patients with hepatocellular carcinoma. *Lancet* 2: 621–624, 1970.

Voigt, M.D. Alcohol in hepatocellular cancer. *Clin. Liver Dis.* 9: 151–169, **2005**.

Wallace, L.A., and Carman, W.F. Surface gene variation of HBV: scientific and medical relevance. *Viral Hepatol. Rev.* 3: 5–16, **1997**.

Wang, H.-C., Wu, H.-C., Chen, C.-F., Fausta, U., Lei, H.-Y., and Su, I.J. Different types of ground glass hepatocytes in chronic hepatitis B virus infection contain specific pre-S mutants that may induce endoplasmic reticulum stress. *Am. J. Path .* 163: 2441–2449, **2003**.

Wang, H.C., Chang, W.T., Chang, W.W., Wu, H.C., Huang, W., Lei, H.Y., Lai, M.D., Fausto, N., and Su, I.J. Hepatitis B virus pre-S2 mutant upregulates cyclin A expression and induces nodular proliferation of hepatocytes. *Hepatology* 41: 761–770, **2005**.

Wang, H.-D., Yuh, C.-H., Dang, C.V., and Johnson, D.L. The hepatitis B virus X protein increases the cellular level of TATA-binding protein which mediates transactivation of RNA polymerase III genes. *Mol. Cell. Biol.* 15: 6720–6728, **1995**.

Wang, H.-D., Trivedi, A., and Johnson, D.L. Regulation of RNA polymerase I-dependent promoters by the hepatitis B virus X protein via activated Ras and TATA-binding protein. *Mol. Cell Biol.* 18: 7086–7094, **1998**.

Wang, J., Chenivesse, X., Henglein, B., and Brechot, C. Hepatitis B virus integration in a cyclin A gene in a hepatocellular carcinoma. *Nature* 343: 555–557, **1990**.

Wang, J.-S. and Zhu, Q.R. Infection of the fetus with hepatitis B e antigen via the placenta. *Lancet* 355: 989, **2000**.

Wang, L.-Y., Hatch, M., Chen, C.-J., Levin, B., You, S. L., Lu, S. N., Wu, M.H., Wu, W.P., Wang, L.W., Wang, Q., Huang, G.T., Yang, P.M., Lee, H.S., and Santella, R.M. Aflatoxin exposure and risk of hepatocellular carcinoma in Taiwan. *Int. J. Cancer* 67: 620–625, **1996**.

Wang, X.W., Forrester, K., Yeh, H., Feitelson, M.A., Gu, J., and Harris, C.C. Hepatitis B virus X protein inhibits p53 sequence-specific DNA binding, transcriptional activity, and association with transcription factor ERCC3. *Proc. Natl. Acad. Sci. USA* 91. 2230–2234, **1994**.

Wang, Y., Cui, F., Lu, Y., Li, C., Xu, X., Deng, C., Wang, D., Sun, Y., Hu, G., Lang, Z., Huang, C., and Yang, X. HBsAg and HBx knocked into the p21 locus causes hepatocellular carcinoma in mice. *Hepatology* 39: 318–324, **2004**.

Ward, R., Borchert, P., Wright, A., and Kline, E. Hepatitis B antigen in saliva and mouth washings. *Lancet* II: 726–729, **1972**.

Whitten, T.M., Quets, A.T., and Schloemer, R.H. Identification of the hepatitis B virus factor that inhibits expression of the β interferon gene. *J. Virol.* 65: 4699–4704, **1991**.

Whittle, H.C., Inskip, H., Bradley, A.K., McLaughlan, K., Shenton, F., Lamb, W., Eccles, J., Baker, B.A., and Hall, A.J. The pattern of childhood hepatitis B infection in two Gambian villages. *J. Infect. Dis.* 161: 1112–1115, **1990** .

Williams, J.S. and Andrisani, O.M. The hepatitis B virus X protein targets the basic region-leucine zipper domain of CREB. *Proc. Natl. Acad. Sci. USA* 92: 3819–3823, **1995**.

Wogan, G.N. Aflatoxins as risk factors for hepatocellular carcinoma in humans. *Cancer Res.* 52: 2114s–2118s, **1992**.

Wong, V.C., Ip, H.M., Reesink, H.W., Lelie, P.N., Reerink-Brongers, E.E., Yeung, C.Y., and Ma, H.K. Prevention of the HBsAg carrier state in newborn infants of mothers who are chronic carriers of HBsAg and HBeAg by administration of hepatitis-B vaccine and hepatitis-B immunoglobulin. Double-blind randomised placebo-controlled study. *Lancet* 1: 921–926, **1984**.

Yeh, F.-S., Yu, M.C., Mo, C.-C., Luo, S., Tong, M.J., and Henderson, B.E. Hepatitis B virus, aflatoxins, and hepatocellular carcinoma in southern Guangxi, China. *Cancer Res.* 49: 2506–2509, **1989**.

Yeh, S. -H., Chen, P.-J., Shau, W.Y., Chen, Y.-W., Lee, P.-H., Chen, J.-T., and Chen, D.-S. Chromosomal allelic imbalance evolving from liver cirrhosis to hepatocellular carcinoma. *Gastroenterology* 121: 699–709, **2001**.

Yu, D.Y., Moon, H.B., Son, J.K., Jeong, S., Yu, S. L., Yoon, H., Han, Y.M., Lee, C.S., Park, J.S., Lee, C.H., Hyun, B.H., Murakami, S., and Lee, K.K. Incidence of hepatocellular carcinoma in transgenic mice expressing the hepatitis B virus X-protein. *J. Hepatol.* 31: 123–132, **1999**.

Yu, M.C., Yuan, J.M., Govindarajan, S., and Ross, R.K. Epidemiology of hepatocellular carcinoma. *Can. J. Gastroenterol.* 14: 703–709, **2000**.

Yuen, M.F., Sablon, E., Yuan, H.J. Wong, D.K., Hui, C.K., Wong, B.C., Chan, A.O., and Lai, C.L. Significance of hepatitis B virus genotype in acute exacerbation, HbeAg seroconversion, cirrhosis-related complications, and hepatocellular carcinoma. *Hepatology* 37: 19–26, **2003**.

Xu, Z., Yen, T.S., Wu, L., Madden, C.R., Tan, W., Slagle, B.L., and Ou, J.H. Enhancement of hepatitis B virus replication by its X protein in transgenic mice. *J. Virol.* 76: 2579–2584, **2002**.

Zheng, Y.W. and Yen, T.S. Negative regulation of hepatitis B virus gene expression and replication by oxidative stress. *J. Biol. Chem.* 269: 8857–8862, **1994**.

Zhu, H., Wang, Y., Chen, J., Cheng, G., and Xue, J. Transgenic mice expressing hepatitis B virus X protein are more susceptible to carcinogen induced hepatocarcinogenesis. *Exp. Mol. Pathol.* 76: 44–50, **2004**.

Zoulim, F., Saputelli, J., and Seeger, C. Woodchuck hepatitis virus X protein is required for viral infection in vivo. *J. Virol.* 68: 2026–2030, **1994**.

Zuckerman, J.N. and Zuckerman, A.J. Current topics in hepatitis *Br. J. Infect.* 41: 130–136, **2000**.

7

Flaviviruses

7.1
Hepatitis C Virus

7.1.1
History

During the 1970s it became clear that a specific form of post-transfusion hepatitis could be caused by an unidentified agent, clearly different from hepatitis A and B (Feinstone et al., 1975). Prior to 1983, this unidentified agent had been transmitted experimentally to chimpanzees (Tabor et al., 1983). The first sequences of this putative agent were cloned and reported in 1989 (Choo et al., 1989), and subsequent studies showed the virus to be widely spread among human populations, to cause acute and chronic hepatitis infections, and also to have links with hepatocellular carcinoma (HCC) (for a review, see Hoofnagle, 2002).

It has been estimated that, globally, more that 170 million people are currently infected with hepatitis C virus (HCV) (Alter and Seeff, 2000). Since acute infections are frequently asymptomatic, early diagnosis is often difficult (Chisari, 2005). Approximately 70% of HCV-infected persons acquire a persistent and chronic infection, commonly associated with serious liver disease, such as liver cirrhosis and HCC. Today, HCV infections are the most common indication for liver transplantation, accounting for 40–50 % of liver transplants (Brown, 2005).

7.1.2
Epidemiology

High rates of HCV seropositivity have been noted in Japan, Spain, Hungary, Saudi Arabia, and Southern Italy (van der Poel, 1994). In Egypt, up to 19.2% of blood donors were found to be HCV-positive (Saeed et al., 1991; Hibbs et al., 1993). Seropositivity increases with age. In children the rate is commonly very low; for example, in rural Egypt 2.3% of children aged 1–5 years were positive, while in children aged 6–10 years the rate increased to 5.8%, and in those aged 15 years it was 9.7% (Hibbs et al., 1993).

Anti-HCV antibodies are often observed in family members of HCV-positive patients, suggesting intrafamilial transmission (Kiyosawa et al., 1990). About 10%

Infections Causing Human Cancer. Harald zur Hausen
Copyright © 2006 WILEY-VCH Verlag GmbH & Co. KGaA, Weinheim
ISBN: 3-527-31056-8

of infected mothers transmit the infection to their babies (Lin et al., 1994; Ohto et al., 1994). Predominant risk factors for HCV transmission are discussed in Section 7.1.4.

Hepatocellular carcinoma often develops in cirrhotic livers, but it may also arise in noncirrhotic organs. This cancer commonly arises two to four decades after the primary HCV infection (Liang and Heller, 2004), its occurrence being linked to a number of environmental, dietary and lifestyle factors, including alcohol consumption, aflatoxin exposure and, in particular, HCV infection (El-Serag, 2001). In addition, male gender, hepatitis B virus co-infection, household contact, acupuncture, tattooing- and transfusion-related HCV-transmission, and needle-sharing by injecting drug users predispose to a higher risk (Kao and Chen, 2000; Seeff, 2002).

Six major genotypes and more than 50 subgenotypes of HCV have been identified (Simmonds, 2004). These differ substantially not only in their geographic distribution, but also in the clinical course of the disease and in their response to therapy (Feld and Hoofnagle, 2005). Genotypes are defined here as differing from each other by 30–50% at the nucleotide level, whereas subtypes show differences of 10–30% (Bukh et al., 1995; Simmonds et al., 2005). Different isolates of the same subtype may differ by 5 to 15% (Hoofnagle, 2002). Genotype 1a is most common in Northern Europe and in the United States, while genotype 1b represents the most common form worldwide (El-Serag and Mason, 1999). Genotypes 2a and 2b also show a worldwide distribution, but are particularly common in Japan and in Northern Italy. Genotype 3 prevails in India, and genotype 4 is mainly found in Africa and the Middle East. The other genotypes 5 and 6 are rare, although 5 is more common in South Africa and 6 in Hong Kong and south-east Asia. A phylogenetic tree indicating areas of higher prevalence of the respective genotypes is shown in Figure 7.1.

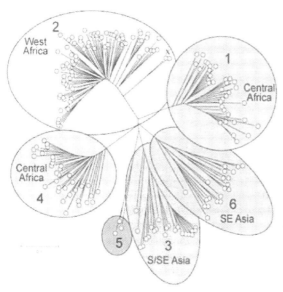

Fig. 7.1 Phylogenetic tree of hepatitis C virus genotypes and subtypes, together with indications of the prevalence of the respective infections. (Reprinted from Simmonds et al., *Consensus proposals for a unified system of nomenclature of hepatitis C virus genotypes.* Hepatology 42, 2005. With permission of Wiley-Liss, Inc, a subsidiary of John Wiley & Sons, Inc.)

The studies conducted to date indicate that HCV infections have been present for a long time in parts of Africa and Asia, and that the transmission pattern there has been different from that in Western and other non-tropical countries (Simmonds et al., 2005). Tattooing, skin scarifications, sexual contacts and pre- and perinatal transmissions seem to be the prime factors for transmission in some of the tropical areas. Blood transfusions, the use of nonsterilized needles and sharing of injection equipment most likely contributed to the spread of HCV infections in industrialized countries (Simmonds, 2001; Ndjomou et al., 2003). HCV genotype 1 appears to be most frequent among blood donors, hemophiliacs and hemodialysis patients, whereas genotype 3 was frequently found in cirrhotic patients and injecting drug users (Oliveira et al., 1999).

7.1.3
Viral Genome Structure, Transcription, Translation, Gene Functions, and Taxonomy

The HCV genome consists of 9.6 kb uncapped linear single-stranded RNA with positive polarity. Untranslated regions occur 5' and 3' which contain control elements for translation and replication (Sarnow, 2003; Lindenbach and Rice, 2005; Chisari, 2005). An uninterrupted open reading frame (ORF) codes for a single polyprotein of 3010 or 3011 amino acids, subsequently processed into structural and nonstructural proteins, cleaved by viral and host cell proteases (Lohmann et al., 1996; Penin et al., 2004). An outline of the HCV genome structure and derived proteins is shown in Figure 7.2.

Translation of viral RNA occurs entirely in the cytoplasm and depends on an internal ribosome entry site (IRES) located 5' in the genome (Spahn et al., 2001). The IRES sequence binds the 40S ribosomal subunit directly and induces mRNA-bound conformation in this subunit. After recruitment of the eukaryotic initiation factor eIF-3 and the ternary complex Met-tRNA-eIF-2-GTP, the 48S intermediate is formed which transits into the translationally active 80S complex (Ji et al., 2004; Otto and Pu-

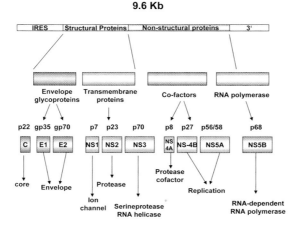

Fig. 7.2 Genomic structure of the hepatitis C virus genome and derived proteins cleaved by viral and cellular proteases.

glisi, 2004; Lindenbach and Rice, 2005). The translated large viral polyprotein is subsequently cleaved into 10 proteins: a basic core protein; two glycoproteins E1 and E2 and a small membrane protein; and p7, which probably functions as an ion channel (Griffin et al., 2003; Pavlovic et al., 2003). Additional nonstructural proteins NS2, NS3, NS4A, NS4B, NS5A, and NS5B are responsible for regulating the life cycle of HCV.

The carboxy-terminal two-thirds of NS2 contain the catalytic triad of a cysteine protease (Lindenbach and Rice, 2005). The C-terminus of NS3 encodes a helicase which seems to function as a dimer (Serebrov and Pyle, 2004). NS5A interacts with cellular phosphorylases, generating different phosphoforms of this protein (Ide et al., 1997; Kim et al., 1999; Coito et al., 2004). An amino-terminal amphipathic alpha-helix mediates membrane association of the hepatitis C virus NS5A protein with cellular membranes (Brass et al., 2002).

NS5B encodes the RNA-dependent RNA polymerase and resembles the structure of a similar enzyme of bacteriophage φ6 (Butcher et al., 2001). For a detailed description of viral proteins and their functions, the reader is referred to the review by Lindenbach and Rice (2005).

During replication the mutation rate of HCV is high and amounts to 10^{-3} per nucleotide per generation (Levin et al., 2005). This results in an enormous accumulation of viral quasispecies in every persistently infected person, and also influences the immune response of the infected host.

Genome structure, translational properties and protein function classify HCV as a member of the Flavivirus family. It constitutes the sole representative of the genus hepacivirus (Robertson et al., 1998; Lauer and Walker, 2001). Thus far, it is the only member of the Flavivirus family to reveal oncogenic properties.

7.1.4
Infection, Transmission, and Viral DNA Persistence

Before the development of diagnostic tests for HCV, infection was transmitted through blood and blood-derived products, by hemodialysis, and by organ transplantation (Alter, 1997, 1999, 2002). Today, the majority of infections occurs in injecting drug users and their sexual partners (Alter, 1999). Sexual transmission appears to be of some importance, and inmates in correctional facilities frequently reveal a high degree of HCV positivity, whereas in the United States and many Western European countries approximately 2% of the general population is infected (Spaulding et al., 1999). Among HIV-infected individuals, up to 25% are coinfected with HCV (Choo et al., 1989). Besides transmission via blood products and sexual contacts, other – albeit less efficient – modes of transmission should exist, most likely via the digestive tract.

Approximately 10% of viremic mothers transmit HCV infections to their babies (Ohto et al., 1994), though the risk of transmission seems to be related to the extent of viremia in the mother. Mothers coinfected by HCV and HIV pose a much higher risk for HCV transmission to their newborns (Thaler et al., 1991; Novati et al., 1992).

In a typical infected person, about 10^{12} virus particles are produced each day, while chronically infected patients have viral loads in the range of 10^3 to 10^5 genomes per mL serum (Neumann et al., 1998; Lindenbach and Rice, 2005). As stated earlier, approximately 70% of infected persons become persistently infected, 20% of these will develop liver cirrhosis, and up to 2.5% will subsequently hepatocellular cancer (Bowen and Walker, 2005 a).

Since the acute infection is commonly mild, it remains frequently unrecognized. Prospective studies in humans at high risk for HCV exposure and experimental studies in chimpanzees revealed the control of acute primary viral replication by an expansion of antiviral CD4$^+$ and CD8$^+$ T cells (Bowen and Walker, 2005 b). Spontaneous resolution of HCV infection does not protect against later reinfections, but does reduce the risk for persistent infection upon re-exposure.

The studies on biological and molecular properties of HCV will be greatly facilitated by recent reports on the successful replication of this virus in tissue culture systems (Cai et al., 2005; Lindenbach et al., 2005; Zhong et al., 2005), with 10^5 infectious units per mL being produced within 48 h. The replication occurs in human hepatocyte-derived cells which had already previously been reported to permit low-efficiency replication of HCV (Kato et al., 2002, 2003). Replicon systems had been developed even earlier, though these neither allowed efficient replication nor produced infectious virus (Blight et al., 2000; Lohmann et al., 2001).

Recently, modulation of HCV RNA abundance by liver-specific microRNA has been described (Jopling et al., 2005). MicroRNA 122 is specifically expressed and abundant in human liver cells. This microRNA seems to facilitate the replication of viral RNA and may provide a clue for the hepatotropism of HCV infections.

A recent report on the association of HCV envelope proteins with exosomes and the association of CD81-carrying exosomes with viral RNA (Masciopinto et al., 2004) may point to a completely new mode of viral transmission, and may also explain some of the difficulties in finding HCV particles in infected tissues. Since similar reports appeared for specific retrovirus transmissions (see Chapter 8, Section 8.3), these observations, if confirmed, may also shed some light on the problems of immunologically clearing HCV infections.

7.1.5
Pathogenesis and Immune Interactions

7.1.5.1 Evasion of Host Defense Mechanisms

Infection with HCV triggers intracellular signaling which results in the production of interferons α and β (reviewed in Gale and Foy, 2005) via Toll-like receptors (Cook et al., 2004; Iwasaki and Medzhitov, 2004). The main components of this signaling are interferon (IFN) regulatory factor (IRF)-3 and nuclear factor κB (NF-κB) (Au et al., 1995; Lin et al., 1999; Richmond, 2002), which form an enhanceosome complex on the IFN-β promoter (Sen, 2001). NF-κB is also involved in the expression of chemokines and inflammatory cytokines (Tai et al., 2000). A large number of interferon-β-stimulated genes mediate the host response to virus infections (Der et al.,

1998). These result in the disruption of viral RNA translation and inhibition of viral RNA synthesis (Guo et al., 2001; Shimazaki et al., 2002; Gale and Foy, 2005).

Interferon-α is one of the induced genes which contribute to the maturation of immune effector cells and potentiates the synthesis of pro-inflammatory proteins (*Sen*, 2001). The expression levels of interferon-stimulated genes vary substantially in patients with chronic hepatitis C infection and cirrhosis (Smith et al., 2003). This shows that HCV infection is able to modify the host response and to evade a host cell-mediated control of this virus infection.

One of the cellular receptors binding double stranded (ds) RNA, and also of HCV, is the RNA helicase RIG-1 which signals the downstream activation of IRF-3 and NF-κB (Sumpter et al., 2005). Toll-like receptor (TLR) 3 is also activated by dsRNA and directs the activation of IRF-3 and NF-κB via a different pathway (for a review, see Gale and Foy, 2005).

Hepatitis C virus is able to interfere with these host cell control mechanisms and to evade them effectively. The NS3/4A protease functions counteract the IRF-3 activation and inhibit the interferon-β expression by blocking RIG-1 signaling and by cleaving the adaptor protein for TLR-3, TRIF, and thus impairing the function of TLR-3 (Foy et al., 2005; Li et al., 2005 a; Ferreon et al., 2005). The other function of NS3/A4 protease is the cleavage of nonstructural proteins from the HCV polyprotein during virus replication (De Francesco et al., 2000). A schematic outline of HCV pathogenesis is depicted in Figure 7.3.

Thus, HCV is using its protease activity, functioning as an essential component for viral replication, also to evade host cell control mechanisms by disrupting RIG-1 and TLR-3 signaling. This diminishes the function of two major pathways in interferon production (Li et al., 2005 b; Breiman et al., 2005). Overexpression of IKKε bypasses the HCV-mediated inhibition, restores transactivation of the IFN-β promoter, and impairs positive and negative replicative strands of the HCV replicon (Breiman et al., 2005).

Besides NS3/4A, NS5A antagonizes IFN-α functions (MacDonald and Harris, 2004; Zhang et al., 2005). This seems to be due to NS5A-mediated induction of IL-8

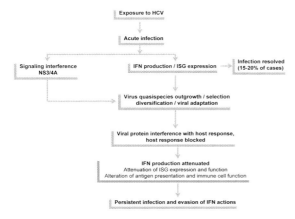

Fig. 7.3 Schematic outline of HCV pathogenesis. IFN: interferon; ISG: interferon-stimulated genes. (Modified from Gale and Foy, 2005.)

expression, a pro-inflammatory cytokine, which interferes with interferons (Khabar et al., 1997). In addition, HS5A and E2 proteins inhibit protein kinase R (PKR), apparently permitting evasion from the translation-suppressing functions of IFN and a PKR-mediated increased host response to infection (Gale et al., 1998; Taylor et al., 1999; Noguchi et al., 2001; Katze et al., 2002).

One other defense mechanism against host control results from the absence of a proofreading function of viral RNA-dependent RNA polymerase. This results in error-prone virus replication and creates closely related, but genetically different, quasispecies variants. It also influences the responsiveness to interferon therapy (Farci, 2001). Genetic variants occur at higher frequency during chronic infection and cirrhosis (Farci et al., 2000, 2002). A hotspot for genetic modifications appears to be a 40-residue interferon sensitivity-determining region of NS5A (Enomoto et al., 1996; Pascu et al., 2004; Schinkel et al., 2004).

7.1.5.2 Host Immune Responses

T cells play a central role in HCV control and clearance (for a review, see Bowen and Walker, 2005 a). The immunological memory does not protect against re-infection, although it does reduce the risk for viral persistence (Bowen and Walker, 2005 b).

Virus-specific antibodies commonly appear 7–8 weeks after infection (Pawlotzky, 1999). A major target to the antibody response is the hypervariable-1 region of the E2 envelope glycoprotein. Sequence variations in this region, occurring simultaneously with antibody seroconversion, determine the outcome of the infection in humans (Farci et al., 2000). The role of antibodies in resolving HCV infections is not entirely clear, since in some patients resolution may occur without detectable antibody response (Logvinoff et al., 2004; Meunier et al., 2005). HCV RNA genomes are detectable only a few days after infection, and reach the highest level 6–10 weeks later, irrespective of the outcome of infection (Abe et al., 1992; Beach et al., 1992; Alter et al., 1995).

Expansion of virus-specific CD8[+] T cells coincides with the immunopathological changes, monitored by elevated levels of transaminases in the serum (Cooper et al., 1999; Lechner et al., 2000; Thimme et al., 2002, 2003; Shoukry et al., 2003). Although higher concentrations of cytotoxic T-lymphocytes (CTLs) are found in chronically infected livers, they are not generally correlated with severity of disease (Nelson et al., 1997; He et al., 1999; Freeman et al., 2003). In chronic HCV infection, CTLs commonly target only a few epitopes (Koziel et al., 1992; Wedemeyer et al., 2002; Lauer et al., 2004). Occasionally, however, a broader spectrum is recognized during several years of persistent infection (Erickson et al., 2001; Kimura et al., 2005).

In chronically HCV-infected patients CD4[+] T-cell responses are low or not detectable (Diepolder et al., 1995; Takaki et al., 2000; Rosen et al., 2002). In resolved hepatitis C infection a broad specificity of virus-specific CD4[+] T-helper cell responses has been observed (Day et al., 2002). Antibody-mediated depletion of CD4[+] cells in immune chimpanzees, re-challenged with the same HCV strain, resulted in persistent infection Grakoui et al., 2003). These data point to the important role of CD4[+]

T cells in the control of HCV infections. It seems that the interaction between the HCV core and the complement receptor gC1qR induces dysfunction of T lymphocytes via induction of the suppressor of cytokine signaling (SOCS) family members SOCS1 and SOCS3 through inhibition of the Jak/STAT pathway (Yao et al., 2005).

The production of the immune-suppressive cytokine interleukin 10 (IL-10) by a subset of CD8[+] T-cell lines derived from the liver of persistently infected patients provided a first hint for MHC class-I-restricted antigen-specific regulatory activity with the potential to suppress antiviral T cells (Koziel et al., 1995; Bowen and Walker, 2005 a). The observation that intrahepatic CD8[+] cells from persistently infected patients suppressed HCV-specific and IL-10-dependent in-vitro proliferation of liver-derived lymphocytes, lends further support to the virus antigen-specific suppression (Accapezzato et al., 2004).

By summarizing these studies, failure of CD4[+] T-cell responses predicts HCV persistence (Bowen and Walker, 2005 a). The HCV interference with innate immune mechanisms (see Section 7.1.5.1) may be linked with the defect in CD4[+] T-cell help. The role of CD8[+] T cells in resolving the HCV infection seems to depend on the effectiveness of viral interference with innate immunity. Yet, successes in the early therapy of HCV infection seem to be independent of broad CD8[+] T-cell responses (Lauer et al., 2005). Clearly, the present picture of host/virus immunological interactions is still incomplete and requires further investigation.

7.1.6
Role in Hepatocellular Carcinoma

7.1.6.1 Experimental Evidence for a Role of HCV in Liver Cancer

7.1.6.1.1 Evidence from Tissue Culture Studies and Transgenic Mice
The mechanism of HCV involvement in HCC is still not fully understood, although some progress has been made recently. The absence of integrated viral nucleotide sequences, or even of intranuclear episomal genomes, points more to an indirect involvement of this virus infection in the development of liver cancer. It seems, however, that – at least in the majority of HCV-linked HCCs – viral genomes persist within the cancer cells (Tang et al., 1995). Attempts to inhibit a specific gene function of the NS3 gene by recombinant intracellular antibodies also resulted in an inhibition of cell proliferation and loss of the transformed phenotype of NS3-transformed cells (Zemel et al., 2004). These last two results would be more compatible with a direct role of HCV infection in liver carcinogenesis.

Two approaches have attempted to contribute to the analysis of this question: first, measurements of the biological effects of transfection of individual viral genes of HCV into various tissue culture systems; and second, the implantation of these genes into transgenic mice. Carcinogenic effects have been reported for three individual HCV genes, but only two of these have repeatedly been shown to result in cell transformation and tumorigenicity of tissue culture cells and in transgenic animals.

Several reports claim malignant transformation of tissue culture cells by the HCV NS3 protein. NIH 3T3 cells transfected with the 5'-half cDNA of the NS3 serine protease sequence proliferated rapidly, lost contact inhibition, grew anchorage-independently in soft agar, and formed tumors in nude mice (Sakamuro et al., 1995). The transformed cells continued to harbor this viral DNA. These data were confirmed in another study in the human liver cell line QSG7701 (He et al., 2003). Sequence comparisons of NS3 clones isolated from hepatocellular carcinomas revealed unique changes at the vicinity of catalytic sites of this region. These were the insertion of a charged amino acid, or the substitution of a polar by a hydrophobic amino acid, or the substitution of a charged with a polar amino acid (Zemel et al., 2000). NS3 also transformed nontumorigenic rat fibroblasts to rapid and serum-independent growth, loss of contact inhibition, anchorage independence, and tumorigenicity for nude mice (Zemel et al., 2001). A mutation at the catalytic site (serine 139 to alanine) showed no transforming activity.

Studies on a potential oncogenic activity of other nonstructural proteins of HCV were less convincing: one report analyzed the cooperation of NS4B with Ha-ras and claimed a positive interaction (Park et al., 2000). The NS5A sequence has also been implicated in oncogenesis (Gosh et al., 1999; Lan et al., 2002), possibly acting by an inhibition of protein kinase R (Giminez-Barcons et al., 2005). NS5A-transgenic mice, however, exhibited no major histological change within the liver up to 24 months of age (Majumder et al., 2003). Thus, the involvement of these genes in liver carcinogenesis remains an open question.

Data on increased cell proliferation and transformation are more convincing for the HCV core protein. Two independent lines of core gene-transgenic mice developed hepatic steatosis early in life as a histological feature characteristic for chronic HCV infection. After 16 months, initially liver adenomas developed and subsequently also HCCs (Moriya et al., 1998). Additional reports support this observation (Naas et al., 2005). One report revealed malignant transformation of human Chang-liver cells (Shan et al., 2005), while the other showed that the HCV core protein aberrantly sequesters a nuclear transcription protein, designated as LZIP, in the cytoplasm, inactivates its function and potentiates cellular transformation (Jin et al., 2000). LZIP was suggested to serve as a cellular tumor suppressor factor targeted by the HCV core protein. In NIH 3T3 cells, the HCV core protein interacts directly with and activates STAT3 through phosphorylation of a tyrosine residue (Yoshida et al., 2002). This resulted in rapid proliferation, up-regulation of Bcl-XL and cyclin D1, anchorage-independent growth, and tumorigenesis. One other group reported the development of liver adenomas and malignant lymphomas in a line of transgenic mice at ages over 20 months (Ishikawa et al., 2003). In HCV transgenic mice treated with diethylnitrosamine, tumor progression was accelerated by the core protein-mediated suppression of apoptosis (Kamegaya et al., 2005). A cooperative interaction in the transformation of NIH 3T3 mouse fibroblasts and HCV core protein and hepatitis B X protein has also been noted (Jung et al., 2003). Hepatitis C virus replication in stably transfected HepG2 cells, where primarily core and NS5B proteins were detectable, resulted in growth in soft agar, and accelerated tumor growth in nude mice (Sun et al., 2004).

HCV core sequences isolated from liver tumors, but not from adjacent nontumor tissue, significantly reduce transforming growth factor (TGF)-β activity (Pavio et al., 2005). This appears to block the growth-inhibitory function of TGF-β. The effect is mediated by direct binding of the core protein to Smad3, preventing binding of the latter to DNA.

NF-κB is considered as a tumor promoter in inflammation-associated cancers (Pikarsky et al., 2004). Its activation is commonly triggered by tumor necrosis factor-α (TNF-α). HCV core protein, and also NS5A, activate NF-κB-dependent signaling and suppress TNF-α-mediated apoptosis in human cells (Marusawa et al., 1999; Miyasaka et al., 2003; Waris et al., 2003). The core protein associates with the TNF-R1-TRADD-TRAF2 signaling complex and synergistically activates the TNF-α induction of NF-κB (Chung et al., 2001; Yoshida et al., 2001). The core protein also associates with the TNF receptor-related lymphotoxin-β receptor and modulates the cytolytic activity of this receptor – ligand complex (You et al., 1999). Interestingly, HCV core protein also *trans*-activates the inducible nitric oxide synthase promoter via NF-κB activation (de Lucas et al., 2003). NF-κB also mediates the activation of cyclooxygenase-2 (Cox-2) and the product of Cox-2 activity prostaglandin E_2 (Waris and Siddiqui, 2005). This activation was sensitive to antioxidant and calpain inhibitors, underlining the role of HCV core protein in inducing oxidative stress. In contrast to hepatic cells, in macrophages HCV core protein suppresses NF-κB activation and Cox-2 expression by directly interacting with IκB kinase β (Joo et al., 2005). In macrophages, the core protein suppresses IL-12 and nitric oxide production that is critical for the induction of Th1 and innate immunity (Lee et al., 2001). Thus, these apparently opposing effects in hepatic cells and in macrophages seem to aid the virus in establishing its persistence. This interpretation is supported by the immune suppression and liver damage observed in HCV core protein transgenic mice (Soguero et al., 2002).

In NS5A-induced NF-κB activation, tyrosine phosphorylation of IκBα at tyrosine residues 42 and 305 induces the activation process (Waris et al., 2003). NS5A expression reduced the function of caspases 8, 9, and 3. Apparently, the inhibition of caspase 8 activation is the reason for the anti-apoptotic effect of NS5A protein (Miyasaka et al., 2003).

7.1.6.1.2 Potential Oncogenic Functions of HCV Proteins

The HCV core protein, which interacts with several cellular regulatory functions (Varaklioti et al., 2002; Yamanaka et al., 2002; Anzola, 2004), occurs in both an innate form (nucleotides 1–191) and in a processed mature form (nucleotides 1–173). The innate form is retained in the cytoplasm and enhances $p21^{WAF1}$ expression by activating p53, whereas the mature form persists in the nucleus and suppresses $p21^{WAF1}$ by a p53-independent pathway. The HCV core protein also interacts with p73 (Alisi et al., 2003; Benard et al., 2003). The interaction with p73α, but not with p73β, prevents growth arrest by the former. By interacting with these proteins, the HCV core protein can influence cell proliferation and apoptosis.

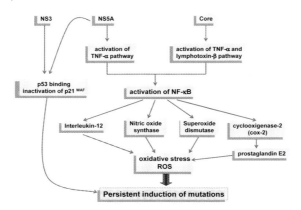

Fig. 7.4 Tentative scheme of potentially oncogenic functions of hepatitis C virus proteins.

NS3 protein is thought to form a complex with wild-type p53, and also may influence its functions (Ishido and Hotta, 1998). An additional report described inhibition of the promoter of p21^{WAF1} by NS3 (Muramatso et al., 1997). The repression of this promoter seems to be due to the modulation of p53 activity. NS3 acts synergistically with the HCV core protein in mediating these functions. NS3 is stabilized by co-expression of NS4A, and the complex is directed to the endoplasmic reticulum (Wölk et al., 2000).

NS5A binds directly to p53 and co-localizes p53 in the perinuclear region (Lan et al., 2002). Intramolecular cleavage of NS5A around amino acid 150 may target one of the truncated proteins to the nucleus (Song et al., 2000). These post-translationally modified truncated forms of NS5A may act as transcriptional activators, although the individual functions are still poorly defined (Khabar and Polyak, 2002; Reyes, 2002). A tentative scheme of potentially oncogenic functions of HCV is illustrated in Figure 7.4.

7.1.6.1.3 Alcohol as a Cofactor in HCV-Mediated Carcinogenesis

Besides immunosuppression by HIV or co-infection with hepatitis B virus, alcohol consumption emerges as the most important cofactor for HCV-linked carcinogenesis. It has been stated that chronic alcohol consumption of more than 80 g per day for more than 10 years increases the risk for liver cancer approximately five-fold (Morgan et al., 2004). In decompensated alcohol-induced cirrhosis, the risk for HCC approaches 1 % per year. Infection of the same individuals by HCV doubles the risk for liver cancer (Morgan et al., 2004). The prevalence of HCV infections is seven- to 10-fold higher in alcoholics in comparison to the general population, and up to 60 % of HCV patients have a past history of alcohol abuse (Jamal and Morgan, 2003). In addition, alcohol abuse causes decreased response to interferon treatment of HCV patients and accelerates progression to liver fibrosis, cirrhosis and liver cancer (Safdar and Schiff, 2004). In HCV replicon-containing cells, alcohol increased HCV replicon expression in a concentration-dependent manner (Zhang et al., 2003). One function of alcohol seems to be activation of the NF-κB promoter. A specific inhibitor of NF-κB, caffeic acid phenethyl ester, abolished alcohol-induced HCV RNA expression (Zhang et al., 2003). An additive activation of hepatic NF-κB by ethanol and HCV core protein has been described (Kim et al., 2001).

Thus, alcohol abuse emerges as the most important co-factor for liver cancer development in HCV-infected persons.

7.1.6.1.4 HCV – A Direct or Indirect Carcinogen: Does this Virus Fulfill Mediator Functions for Other Oncogenic Agents?

As highlighted previously, HCV exerts some functions which would be compatible with a more direct role in hepatocarcinogenesis. These include the frequent persistence of viral infection in carcinomatous tissue, and the use of recombinant antibodies in NS3-transformed cells which selectively inhibits proliferation of these cells. The significance of these observations appears questionable, however. Virus persistence is a poor indicator for a direct oncogenic role, and the sole description of a proliferation-inhibiting effect of recombinant antibodies requires further confirmation by other specific inhibitors of NS3.

The most persuasive evidence points to an indirect role of HCV infection in hepatocarcinogenesis. Tissue culture studies failed to demonstrate a direct growth-stimulating or immortalizing effect of specific HCV genes or complete viral genomes for primary human cells. Although murine and rat cells appear to be susceptible to transformation by HCV, these cells are also relatively susceptible to chemical and physical carcinogens (mutagens), and respond frequently with enhanced proliferation and transformation (Kuroki and Huh, 1993). Human cells transfected with HCV DNA or individual genes responding with increased carcinogenicity represent already immortalized lines or cells directly derived from liver tumors.

Combined with the studies in transgenic mice, the experimental evidence (even ignoring the vast body of epidemiologic studies) for a carcinogenic role of specific viral gene products emerges as increasingly compelling. It is particularly impressive for the HCV core protein expression, for the serine protease NS3 and, to a more limited degree, for NS5A. The described interaction of these proteins with p53, $p21^{WAF1}$ and p73 points to disturbances in mitotic checkpoint control and DNA repair. These observations found further support by an initial analysis for reactive oxygen species (ROS) and lipid and protein oxidation in HCV-positive patients (de Maria et al., 1996). Additional results show that superoxide dismutase is induced by HCV infection (Larrea et al., 1998), that mitochondrial injury, oxidative stress and antioxidant gene expression occur as the direct result of HCV core protein expression (Okuda et al., 2002; Korenaga et al., 2005), and that a differential contribution of NS5A and core protein results in oxidative and nitrosative stress generation (Garcia-Mediavilla et al., 2005). HCV infection activates the type II isoform of nitric oxide synthase, and thereby enhances DNA damage and mutations of cellular genes (Machida et al., 2004 a). Interestingly, ROS suppress HCV RNA replication, at least under tissue culture conditions (Choi et al., 2004). This may explain the relative paucity of HCV genomes observed in HCCs (Tang et al., 1995).

By summarizing these findings, it becomes increasingly likely that chronic DNA damage as a function of persisting HCV infections emerges as the main factor in HCV-mediated carcinogenicity. Nevertheless, it is clearly inappropriate to consider this interaction as a "hit and run" mechanism (Machida et al., 2004 b) since, at least in the majority of cancers, viral RNA continues to persist within the neoplastic cells.

These data do not exclude a mediator role of HCV for other carcinogenic agents. although to date no evidence has been produced to imply such function.

7.1.7
Role in Lymphoproliferative Diseases

7.1.7.1   Mixed Cryoglobulinemia

One of the most common lymphoproliferative extrahepatic manifestations of HCV infection is represented by cryoglobulinemia (reviewed in Sène et al., 2004). This condition is defined by circulating immunoglobulins that precipitate at cold temperatures and resolubilize when warmed. Mixed cryoglobulinemias with mono-clonal components (type II), but also with only polyclonal immunoglobulins (type III) are frequently found in HCV patients (Pascual et al., 1990; Casato et al., 1991; Disdier et al., 1991; Ferri et al., 1991; Galli, 1991; Agnello et al., 1992). Cryoglobulin-emia represents a clonal or polyclonal B cell proliferation accompanied by a small vessel vasculitis with vascular enluminal deposition of cryoprecipitates (Sène et al., 2004). Replication of HCV in B lymphocytes and neutrophils has been reported (Lerat et al., 1998; Crovatto et al., 2000; Fornasieri et al., 2000). HCV interacts with B cells via the CD81 receptor (Pileri et al., 1998). Lymphoproliferative conditions in HCV-infected patients are associated with lower expression of the CD81 receptor in peripheral B cells (Cacoub et al., 2003). It is likely that the expansion of clonal B-cell populations is enhanced by translocations of the Bcl-2, resulting in overexpression of this anti-apoptotic gene, as frequently observed in HCV-positive patients (Kitay-Cohen et al., 2000; Zignego et al., 2000, 2002). The core protein of HCV appears to be a constitutive component of cryoprecipitable immune complexes in type II mixed cryoglobulinemia (Sansonno et al., 2003).

Elevated serum levels of osteopontin are found in mixed cryoglobulinemia, and also in HCV-linked non-Hodgkin's lymphomas and in HCV-linked autoimmune disorders (Libra et al., 2005).

7.1.7.2   Splenic Lymphoma with Villous Lymphocytes

A second rare lymphoproliferation linked to HCV infections is splenic lymphoma with villous lymphocytes (for a review, see Sène et al., 2004). This condition is characterized by splenomegaly, pancytopenia, and clonal expansion of B cells with villous projections in the peripheral blood. The disease is closely related to im-munocytoma and splenic marginal-zone non-Hodgkin's lymphoma (NHL). A mul-ticentric French study pointed to the association between HCV infection and this condition (Hermine et al., 2002). Patients who were successfully treated with interferon-α and ribavirin and remained negative for HCV RNA for up to 27 months, also revealed a complete hematological response. A relapse of the lymphoproliferative condition was accompanied by the reappearance of HCV RNA.

7.1.7.3 Non-Hodgkin's Lymphoma

The third clearly malignant condition, NHL, remains controversial in its links to HCV infections. Initial suspicions for a link arose from serological studies conducted in Italy, where between 9% and 42% of NHL patients were HCV antibody-positive in contrast to 1–9% of control groups (Ferri et al., 1994; Cavanna et al., 1995; Luppi et al., 1996; Mazzaro et al., 1996; Silvestri et al., 1997; Zignego et al., 1997). Similar data were reported from Japan, with 8% to 17% antibody-positive NHL patients in comparison to 1–7% of the control groups (Izumi et al., 1997; Mizorogi et al., 2000; Kuniyoshi et al., 2001). The majority of studies in non-Italian European countries and in North America, with one notable exception (Zuckerman et al., 1997), failed to confirm this result (Brind et al., 1996; McColl et al., 1997; King et al., 1998; Bauduer et al., 1999; Hausfater et al., 2001; Rabkin et al., 2002).

One meta-analysis considers HCV infections as risk factors for NHL with an estimated odds ratio (OR) of 10.8 (Gisbert et al., 2003). It is clear, however, that the overall risk for NHL is not high in HCV-infected patients, ranging between 0.2% and 2.49% (Ohsawa et al., 1999; Hausfater et al., 2000; El-Serag et al., 2002). HCV-associated lymphomas are, in the majority of cases, low-grade B-cell immunocytomas or follicular lymphomas (Sène et al., 2004).

Besides lymphomas, several other extrahepatic manifestations of HCV infection have been reported. Approximately one-third of patients with chronic HCV infections develop type 2 diabetes mellitus (Bahtiyar et al., 2004). The rate is particularly high in HCV-positive cirrhotic patients receiving liver transplants. Complications of mixed cryoglobulinemia, such as renal disease, neuropathy, Sjögren's syndrome, noncryoglobulinemic systemic vasculitis, porphyria cutanea tarda, and autoantibody production, among others, represent further manifestations (for reviews, see Mayo, 2003; Sène et al., 2004; Soule et al., 2005).

In attempting to summarize the role of HCV infections in lymphoproliferative disorders, it seems evident that persistent HCV infections result in specific lymphoproliferative diseases such as mixed cryoglobulinemia. The data relating to splenic lymphoma with villous lymphocytes also seem to be persuasive. The role of HCV in NHL is clearly not settled. The likely function of HCV as an indirect carcinogen, however, could argue in favor of its role in neoplastic changes induced in persistently infected B lymphocytes.

7.1.8
Prevention and Control

7.1.8.1   **Vaccines**

To date, an effective vaccine against HCV infection has not been developed, though some hope arises from observations in convalescent humans and chimpanzees who, in the majority of cases, are protected against reinfection by the same virus (Bassett et al., 2001; Weiner et al., 2001; Mehta et al., 2002; Lanford et al., 2004). It is difficult to prime $CD8^+$ CTLs with polypeptide subunit vaccines, though some responses have been obtained (Polakos et al., 2001; Pearse and Drane, 2005). The use of recombinant HCV envelope glycoproteins gpE1 and gpE2 as vaccine antigens appears to be somewhat more promising (Ralston et al., 1993; Houghton and Abrignani, 2005). In studies on chimpanzees, the highest responding animals were completely protected against HCV infection (Choo et al., 1994). One of the important questions to be resolved concerns the crossprotection against heterologous HCV strains. Vaccinated chimpanzees infected with heterologous HCV acquired acute infections but did not develop virus persistence, whereas in control animals the infection became chronic (Houghton and Abrignani, 2005). In contrast to these results, ISCOMATRIX adjuvanted NS3–4-5 core polyprotein failed to prevent chronic infection, although it elicited broad $CD4^+$ and $CD8^+$ T-cell responses in the absence of measurable antibodies to envelope glycoproteins (Polakos et al., 2001; Pearse and Drane, 2005).

Other approaches have used adenoviral, avipox, alphaviral and vaccinia viral vectors that are in part presently explored in various animals, including chimpanzees (Brinster et al., 2002; Perri et al., 2003; Pancholi et al., 2003; Abraham et al., 2004; Catalucci et al., 2005). However, the high mutation rate of HCV genomes poses a substantial problem, and may require different approaches for successful vaccination.

Similar to preventive vaccines, therapeutic vaccines have thus far not been successfully applied. A number of candidate vaccines are presently undergoing preclinical and clinical testing (for a review, see Houghton and Abrignani, 2005), but their efficacy remains to be established.

7.1.8.2   **Therapy**

The first beneficial effects in the therapy of HCV infections were seen with IFN-α (Hoofnagle et al., 1986). This led to a reduction of HCV RNA in the serum and, in some instances, also to a resolution of chronic infection (Lau et al., 1998). After 12 months of treatment sustained response was only obtained in 16–20% of cases (Di Bisceglie and Hoofnagle, 2002). Additional improvements have been achieved with concomitant treatment with ribavirin, which doubled the response to 35–40% (McHutchison and Poynard, 1999), and also with pegylated IFN-α, which provides a longer half-life and improved antiviral activity (Glue et al., 2000; Heathcote et al., 2000; Zeuzem et al., 2000; Lindsay et al., 2001).

The application of HCV-targeted drugs suffers from the rapid development of resistance of the virus under selective pressure. Resistance develops quickly against HCV enzyme inhibitors, and also against small interfering RNA (siRNA) (Tomei et al., 2005). The NS3–4 serine protease, a heterodimeric protease containing the amino-terminal domain of NS3 protein and the small NS4A cofactor, and the NS5B RNA polymerase emerge as the most suitable targets (De Francesco and Migliaccio, 2005). Some protease inhibitors are presently undergoing clinical tests and show promising results (for a review, see De Francesco and Migliaccio, 2005). Inhibitors of NS5B polymerase include several nucleoside analogues which induce premature termination of RNA synthesis, though only one of these has demonstrated antiviral activity in clinical trials (De Francesco and Migliaccio, 2005). Some non-nucleoside inhibitors of the viral polymerase have also entered clinical trials, but the chemical details of these have not been disclosed by the respective companies.

A very different approach is represented by the use of nucleic acid-based antiviral drugs, which target the IRES at the 5' end of the viral genome. This is conserved among all HCV genotypes. A ribozyme and an anti-sense oligonucleotide were submitted for initial clinical studies, but showed either adverse effects or limited efficacy (Foster, 2004; De Francesco and Migliaccio, 2005). RNA interference (RNAi) is also currently being investigated for antiviral activity, but clinical data are not yet available (Kapadia et al., 2003; Randall et al., 2003; Wilson et al., 2003; Yokota et al., 2003).

Immunomodulatory agents stimulating Toll-like receptors are also undergoing analysis for anti-HCV activity, and agonists for Toll-like receptors 9 and 7 have revealed some promising properties. The stimulation of dendritic cells with short synthetic oligonucleotides containing unmethylated CpG motifs flanked by specific sequences leads to the production of TNF-α, IL-12, and high levels of IFN-α (Schetter and Vollmer, 2004). In addition, B-cell proliferation and antibody secretion are stimulated. A 7-thia-8-oxoguanosine represents an agonist for Toll-like receptor 7 (Lee et al., 2003). This leads to the release of inflammatory cytokines and of high levels of IFN-α. To date, clinical trials with these compounds have appeared to provide encouraging results (De Francesco and Migliaccio, 2005).

Although the prospects for a targeted chemotherapy of HCV infection are good, at present the possible interference with this infection – particularly during chronic state – is still very limited. Hopefully, some of the clinical trials which are presently being conducted will change this therapeutic outlook.

References

Abe, K., Inchauspe, G., Shikata, T., and Prince, A.M. Three different patterns of hepatitis C virus infection in chimpanzees. *Hepatology* 15: 690–695, **1992**.

Abraham, J.D., Himoudi, N., Kien, F., Berland, J.L., Codran, A., Bartosch, B., Baumert, T., Paranhos-Baccala, G.,

Schuster, C., Inchauspe, G., and Kieny, M.P. Comparative immunogenicity analysis of modified vaccinia Ankara vectors expressing native or modified forms of hepatitis C virus E1 and E2 glycoproteins. *Vaccine* 22: 3917–3928, **2004**.

Accapezzato, D., Francavilla, V., Paroli, M., Casciaro, M., Chircu, L.V., Cividini, A., Abrignani, S., Mondelli, M.U., and Barnaba, V. Hepatic expansion of a virus-specific regulatory CD8⁺ T cell population in chronic hepatitis C virus infection. *J. Clin. Invest.* 113: 963–972, **2004**.

Agnello, V., Chung, R.T., and Kaplan, L.M. A role for hepatitis C virus infection in type II cryoglobulinemia. *N. Engl. J. Med.* 327: 1490–1495, **1992**.

Alisi, A., Giambartolomei, S., Cupelli, F., Merlo, P., Fontemaggi, G., Spaziani, A., and Balsano, C. Physical and functional interaction between HCV core protein and the different p73 isoforms. *Oncogene* 22: 2573–2780, **2003**.

Alter, M.J. Epidemiology of hepatitis C. *Eur. J. Gastroenterol. Hepatol.* 8: 319–323, **1996**.

Alter, M.J. Epidemiology of hepatitis C. *Hepatology* 26: 62s–65s, **1997**.

Alter, M.J. Hepatitis C virus infection in the United States. *J. Hepatol.* 31 (Suppl. 1): 88–91, **1999**.

Alter, M.J. Prevention of spread of hepatitis C. Review. *Hepatology* 36 (Suppl.1): S93–S98, **2002**.

Alter, H.J. and Seeff, L.B. Recovery, persistence, and sequelae in hepatitis C virus infection: a perspective on long-term outcome. *Semin. Liver Dis.* 20: 17–35, **2000**.

Alter, H.J., Sanchez-Pescador, R., Urdea, M.S., Wilber, J.C., Lagier, R.J., Di Bisceglie, A.M., Shih, J.W., and Neuwald, P.D. Evaluation of branched DNA signal amplification for the detection of hepatitis C virus RNA. *J. Viral Hepatol.* 2: 121–132, **1995**.

Anzola, M., Hepatocellular carcinoma: role of hepatitis B and hepatitis C viruses proteins in hepatocarcinogenesis. *J. Viral Hepatol.* 11: 383–393, **2004**.

Au, W.C., Moore, P.A., Lowther, W., Juang, Y.T., and Pitha, P.M. Identification of a member of the interferon regulatory factor family that binds to the interferon-stimulated response element and activates expression of interferon-induced genes. *Proc. Natl. Acad. Sci. USA.* 92: 11657–11661, **1995**.

Bahtiyar, G., Shin, J.J., Aytaman, A., Sowers, J.R., and McFarlane, S. I. Association of diabetes and hepatitis C infection: epidemiologic evidence and pathophysiologic insights. *Curr. Diab. Rep.* 4: 194–198, **2004**.

Bassett, S. E., Guerra, B., Brasky, K., Miskovsky, E., Houghton, M., Klimpel, G.R., and Lanford, R.E. Protective immune response to hepatitis C virus in chimpanzees rechallenged following clearance of primary infection. *Hepatology* 33: 1479–1487, **2001**.

Bauduer, P., Katsahian, S., Blanchard, Y., Oui, B., Capdupuy, C., and Renoux, M. Descriptive epidemiology of non-Hodgkin lymphomas in a southwestern French hematology center: absence of significant relationship with hepatitis C virus infection. *Hematol. Cell. Ther.* 41: 191–193, **1999**.

Beach, M.J., Meeks, E.L., Mimms, L.T., Vallari, D., DuCharme, L., Spelbring, J., Taskar, S., Schleicher, J.B., Krawczynski, K., and Bradley, D.W. Temporal relationships of hepatitis C virus RNA and antibody responses following experimental infection of chimpanzees. *J. Med. Virol.* 36: 226–237, **1992**.

Benard, J., Douc-Rasy, S., and Ahomadegbe, J.C. TP53 family members and human cancers. *Hum. Mutat.* 21: 182–191, **2003**.

Blight, K.J., Kolykhalov, A.A., and Rice, C.M. Efficient initiation of HCV RNA replication in cell culture. *Science* 290: 1972–1974, **2000**.

Bowen, D.G. and Walker, C.M. The origin of quasispecies: cause or consequence of chronic hepatitis C viral infection? *J. Hepatol.* 42: 408–417, **2005 a**.

Bowen, D.G. and Walker, C.M. Adaptive immune responses in acute and chronic hepatitis C virus infection. *Nature* 436: 946–952, **2005 b**.

Brass, V., Bieck, E., Montserret, R., Wolk, B., Hellings, J.A., Blum, H.E., Penin, F., and Moradpour, D . An amino-terminal amphipathic alpha-helix mediates membrane association of the hepatitis C virus nonstructural protein 5A. *J. Biol. Chem.* 277: 8130–8139, **2002**.

Breiman, A., Grandvaux, N., Lin, R., Ottone, C., Akira, S., Yoneyama, M., Fujita, T., Hiscott, J., and Meurs, E.F. Inhibition of RIG-I-dependent signaling to the interferon pathway during hepatitis C virus expression and restoration of signaling by IKKå. *J. Virol.* 79: 3969–3978, **2005**.

Brind, A.M., Watson, J.P., Burt, A., Kestevan, P., Wallis, J., Proctor, S. J., and Bassendine, M.F. Non-Hodgkin's lymphoma and hepatitis C virus infection. *Leuk. Lymphoma* 21: 127–130, **1996**.

Brinster, C., Chen, M., Boucreux, D., Paran-hos-Baccala, G., Liljestrom, P., Lemmonier, F., and Inchauspe, G. Hepatitis C virus non-structural protein 3-specific cellular immune responses following single or combined immunization with DNA or recombinant Semliki Forest virus particles. *J. Gen. Virol.* 83: 369–81, **2002**.

Brown, R.S., Jr. Hepatitis C and liver transplantation. *Nature* 436: 973–978, **2005**.

Bukh, J., Miller, R.H., and Purcell, R.H. Genetic heterogeneity of hepatitis C virus: quasispecies and genotypes. *Semin. Liver Dis.* 15: 41–63, **1995**.

Butcher, S. J., Grimes, J.M., Makeyev, E.V., Bamford, D.H., and Stuart, D.I. A mechanism for initiating RNA-dependent RNA polymerization. *Nature* 410: 235–240, **2001**.

Cacoub, P., Bourliere, M., Hausfater, P., Charlotte, F., Khiri, H., Toci, S., Piette, J.C., Poynard, T., and Halfon, P. Lower expression of CD81 B-cell receptor in lymphoproliferative diseases associated with hepatitis C virus infection. *J. Viral Hepatol.* 10: 10–15, **2003**.

Cai, Z., Zhang, C., Chang, K.-S., Jiang, J., Ahn, B.-C., Wakita, T., Liang, T.J., and Luo, G. Robust production of infectious hepatitis C virus (HCV) from stably HCV cDNA-transfected human hepatoma cells. *J. Virol.* 79: 13 963–13 973, **2005**.

Casato, M., Taliani, G., Pucillo, L.P., Goffredo, F., Lagana, B., and Bonomo, L. Cryoglobulinaemia and hepatitis C virus. *Lancet* 337: 1047–1048, **1991**.

Catalucci, D., Sporeno, E., Cirillo, A., Ciliberto, G., Nicosia, A., and Colloca, S. An adenovirus type 5 (Ad5) amplicon-based packaging cell line for production of high-capacity helper-independent deltaE1-E2-E3-E4 Ad5 vectors. *J. Virol.* 79: 6400–6409, **2005**.

Cavanna, L., Sbolli, G., Tanzi, E., Romano, L., Civardi, G., Buscarini, E., Vallisa, D., Berte, R., and Rossi, A. High prevalence of antibodies to hepatitis C virus in patients with lymphoproliferative disorders. *Haematologica* 80: 486–487, **1995**.

Chisari, F.V. Unscrambling hepatitis C virus-host interactions. *Nature* 436: 930–932, **2005**.

Choi, J., Lee, K.J., Zheng, Y., Yamaga, A.K., Lai, M.M., and Ou, J.H. Reactive oxygen species suppress hepatitis C virus RNA replication in human hepatoma cells. *Hepatology.* 39: 81–89, **2004**.

Choo, Q.-L., Kuo, G., Weiner, A.J., Overby, L.R., Bradley, D.W., and Houghton, M. Isolation of a cDNA clone derived from a blood-borne non-A, non-B viral hepatitis genome. *Science* 244: 359–362, **1989**.

Choo, Q.-L., Kuo, G., Ralston, R., Weiner, A., Chien, D., Van Nest, G., Han, J., Berger, K., Thudium, K., Kuo, C., et al. Vaccination of chimpanzees against infection by the hepatitis C virus. *Proc. Natl. Acad. Sci. USA* 91: 1294–1298, **1994**.

Chung, Y.M., Park, K.J., Choi, S,Y., Hwang, S. B., and Lee, S. Y. Hepatitis C virus core protein potentiates TNF-α induced NF-κB activation through TRAF2-IKKβ-dependent pathway. *Biochem. Biophys. Res. Commun.* 284: 15–19, **2001**.

Coito, C., Diamond, D.L., Neddermann, P., Korth, M.J., and Katze, M.G. High-throughput screening of the yeast kinome: identification of human serine/threonine protein kinases that phosphorylate the hepatitis C virus NS5A protein. *J. Virol.* 78: 3502–3513, **2004**.

Cook, D.N., Pisetsky, D.S., and Schwartz, D.A. Toll-like receptors in the pathogenesis of human disease. *Nat. Immunol.* 5: 975–979, **2004**.

Cooper, S., Erickson, A.L., Adams, E.J., Kansopon, J., Weiner, A.J., Chien, D.Y., Houghton, M., Parham, P., and Walker, C.M. Analysis of a successful immune response against hepatitis C virus. *Immunity* 10: 439–449, **1999**.

Crovatto, M., Pozzato, G., Zorat, F., Pussini, E., Nascimben, F., Baracetti, S., Grando. M.G., Mazzarro, C., Reitano, M., Modolo, M.L., Martelli, P., Spada, A., and Santini, G. Peripheral blood neutrophils from hepatitis C virus-infected patients are replication sites of the virus. *Haematologica* 85: 356–361, **2000**.

Day, C.L., Lauer, G.M., Robbins, G.K., McGovern, B., Wurcel, A.G., Gandhi, R.T., Chung, R.T., and Walker, B.D. Broad specificity of virus-specific CD4+ T-helper-cell responses in resolved hepatitis C virus infection. *J. Virol.* 76: 12 584–12 595, **2002**.

De Francesco, R. and Migliaccio, G. Challenges and successes in developing new therapies for hepatitis C. *Nature* 436: 953–960, **2005**.

de Lucas, S., Bartolome, J., Amaro, M.J., and Carreno, V. Hepatitis C virus core protein transactivates the inducible nitric oxide synthase promoter via NF-κB activation. *Antiviral Res.* 60: 117–124, **2003**.

De Maria, N., Colantoni, A., Fagiuoli, S., Liu, G.J., Rogers, B.K., Farinati, F., Van Thiel, D.H., and Floyd, R.A. Association between reactive oxygen species and disease activity in chronic hepatitis C. *Free Radic. Biol. Med.* 21: 291–295, **1996**.

Der, S. D., Zhou, A., Williams, B.R.G., and Silverman, R.H. Identification of genes differentially regulated by interferons α, β, or γ using oligonucleotide arrays. *Proc. Natl. Acad. Sci. USA.* 95: 15 623–15 628, **1998**.

Di Bisceglie, A.M. and Hoofnagle, J.H. Optimal therapy of hepatitis C. *Hepatology* 36: S121–S127, **2002**.

Diepolder, H.M., Zachoval, R., Hoffmann, R.M., Wierenga, E.A., Santantonio, T., Jung, M.C., Eichenlaub, D., and Pape, G.R. Possible mechanism involving T-lymphocyte response to non-structural protein 3 in viral clearance in acute hepatitis C virus infection. *Lancet* 346: 1006–1007, **1995**.

Disdier, P., Harle, J.R., and Weiller, P.J. Cryoglobulinaemia and hepatitis C infection. *Lancet* 338: 1151–1152, **1991**.

El-Serag, H.B. Epidemiology of hepatocellular carcinoma. *Clin. Liver Dis.* 5: 87–107, **2001**.

El-Serag, H.B. and Mason, A.C. Rising incidence of hepatocellular carcinoma in the United States. *N. Engl. J. Med.* 340: 745–750, **1999**.

El-Serag, H.B., Hampel, H., Yeh, C., and Rabeneck, L. Extrahepatic manifestations of hepatitis C among United States male veterans. *Hepatology* 36: 1439–1445, **2002**.

Enomoto, N., Sakuma, I., Asahina, Y., Kurosaki, M., Murakami, T., Yamamoto, C., Ogura, Y., Izumi, N., Marumo, F., and Sato, C. Mutations in the non-structural protein 5A gene and response to interferon in patients with chronic hepatitis C virus 1 b infection. *N. Engl. J. Med.* 334: 77–81, **1996**.

Erickson, A.L., Kimura, Y., Igarashi, S., Eichelberger, J., Houghton, M., Sidney, J., McKinney, D., Sette, A., Hughes, A.L., and Walker, C.M. The outcome of hepatitis C virus infection is predicted by escape mutations in epitopes targeted by cytotoxic T lymphocytes. *Immunity* 15: 883–895, **2001**.

Farci, P. Hepatitis C virus. The importance of viral heterogeneity. *Clin. Liver Dis.* 5: 895–916, **2001**.

Farci, P., Shimoda, A., Coiana, A., Diaz, G., Peddis, G., Melpolder, J.C., Strazzera, A., Chien, D.Y., Munoz, S. J., Balestrieri, A., Purcell, R.H., and Alter, H.J. The outcome of acute hepatitis C predicted by the evolution of the viral quasispecies. *Science* 288: 339–344, **2000**.

Farci, P., Strazzera, R., Alter, H.J., Farci, S., Degioannis, D., Coiana, A., Peddis, G., Usai, F., Serra, G., Chessa, L., Diaz, G., Balestrieri, A., and Purcell, R.H. Early changes in hepatitis C viral quasispecies during interferon therapy predict the therapeutic outcome. *Proc. Natl. Acad. Sci. USA* 99: 3081–3086, **2002**.

Feinstone, S. M., Kapikian, A.Z., Purcell, R.H., Alter, H.J., and Holland, P.V. Transfusion-associated hepatitis not due to hepatitis type A or B. *N. Engl. J. Med.* 292: 767–770, **1975**.

Feld, J.J. and Hoofnagle, J.H. Mechanism of action of interferon and ribavirin in treatment of hepatitis C. *Nature* 436: 967–972, **2005**.

Ferreon, J.C., Ferreon, A.C., Li, K., and Lemon, S. M. Molecular determinants of TRIF proteolysis mediated by the hepatitis C virus NS3/4A protease. *J. Biol. Chem.* 280: 20 483–20 492, **2005**.

Ferri, C., Greco, F., Longombardo, G., Palla, P., Moretti, A., Marzo, E., Mazzoni, A., Pasero, G., Bombardieri, S., Highfield, P., and Corbishley, T. Association between hepatitis C virus and mixed cryoglobulinemia. *Clin. Exp. Rheumatol.* 9: 621–624, **1991**.

Ferri, C., Caracciolo, F., Zignego, A.L., La Civita, L., Monti, M., Longombardo, G., Lombardini, F., Greco, F., Capochiani, E., Mazzoni, A., Mazzaro, C., and Pasero, G. Hepatitis C virus infection in patients with non-Hodgkin's lymphoma. *Br. J. Haematol.* 88: 392–394, **1994**.

Fornasieri, A., Bernasconi, P., Ribero, M.L., Sinico, R.A., Fasola, M., Zhou, J., Portera, G., Tagger, A., Gibelli, A., and D'Amico, G. Hepatitis C virus (HCV) in lymphocyte subsets and in B lymphocytes expressing rheumatoid factor cross-reacting ideotype in type II mixed cryoglobulinaemia. *Clin. Exp. Immunol.* 122: 400–403, **2000**.

Foster, G.R. Past, present, and future hepatitis C treatments. *Semin. Liver Dis.* 24 (Suppl. 2): 97–104, **2004**.

Foy, E., Li, K., Sumpter, R., Jr., Loo, Y.M., Johnson, C.L., Wang, C., Fish, P.M., Yoneyama, M., Fujita, T., Lemon, S. M., and Gale. M., Jr. Control of antiviral defenses through hepatitis C virus disruption of retinoic acid-inducible gene-I signaling. *Proc. Natl. Acad. Sci. USA* 102: 2986–2991, **2005**.

Freeman, A.J., Pan, Y., Harvey, C.E., Post, J.J., Law, M.G., White, P.A., Rawlinson, W.D., Lloyd, A.R., Marinos, G., and Ffrench, R.A. The presence of an intrahepatic cytotoxic T lymphocyte response is associated with low viral load in patients with chronic hepatitis C virus infection. *J. Hepatol.* 38: 349–356, **2003**.

Gale, M., Jr. and Foy, E.M. Evasion of intracellular host defence by hepatitis C virus. *Nature* 436: 939–945, **2005**.

Gale, M., Jr., Blakely, C.M., Kwieciszewski, B., Tan, S. L., Dossett, M., Tang, N.M., Korth, M.J., Polyak, S. J., Gretch, D.R., and Katze, M.G. Control of PKR protein kinase by hepatitis C virus nonstructural 5A protein: molecular mechanisms of kinase regulation. *Mol. Cell. Biol.* 18: 5208–5218, **1998**.

Galli, M. Cryoglobulinaemia and serological markers of hepatitis viruses. *Lancet* 338: 758–759, **1991**.

Garcia-Mediavilla, M.V., Sanchez-Campos, S., Gonzalez-Perez, P., Gomez-Gonzalo, M., Majano, P.L., Lopez-Cabrera, M., Clemente, G., Garcia-Monzon, C., and Gonzalez-Gallego, J. Differential contribution of hepatitis C virus NS5A and core proteins to the induction of oxidative and nitrosative stress in human hepatocyte-derived cells. *J. Hepatol.* 43: 606–613, **2005**.

Gimenez-Barcons, M., Wang, C., Chen, M., Sanchez-Tapias, J.M., Saiz, J.C., and Gale, M., Jr. The oncogenic potential of hepatitis C virus NS5A sequence variants is associated with PKR regulation. *Interferon Cytokine Res.* 25: 152–164, **2005**.

Gisbert, J.P., Garcia-Buey, L., Pajares, J.M., and Moreno-Otero, R. Prevalence of hepatitis C virus infection in B-cell non-Hodgkin's lymphoma: systematic review and meta-analysis. *Gastroenterology* 125: 1723–1732, **2003**.

Glue, P., Fang, J.W., Rouzier-Panis, R., Raffanel, C., Sabo, R., Gupta, S. K., Salfi, M., and Jacobs, S. Pegylated interferon-alpha2b: pharmacokinetics, pharmacodynamics, safety, and preliminary efficacy data. Hepatitis C Intervention Therapy Group. *Clin. Pharmacol. Ther.* 68: 556–567, **2000**.

Gosh, A.K., Steele, R., Meyer, K., Ray, R., and Ray, R.B. Hepatitis C virus NS5A protein modulates cell cycle regulatory genes and promotes cell growth. *J. Gen. Virol.* 80: 1179–1183, **1999**.

Grakoui, A., Shoukry, N.H., Woollard, D.J., Han, J.H., Hanson, H.L., Ghrayeb, J., Murthy, K.K., Rice, C.M., and Walker, C.M. HCV persistence and immune evasion in the absence of memory T cell help. *Science* 302: 659–662, **2003**.

Griffin, S. D., Beales, L.P., Clarke, D.S., Worsfold, O., Evans, S. D., Jaeger, J., Harris, M.P., and Rowlands, D.J. The p7 protein of hepatitis C virus forms an ion channel that is blocked by the antiviral drug, Amantadine. *FEBS Lett.* 535: 34–38, **2003**.

Guo, J.T., Bichko, V.V., and Seeger, C. Effect of alpha interferon on the hepatitis C virus replicon. *J. Virol.* 75: 8516–8523, **2001**.

Hausfater, P., Cacoub, P., Rosenthal, E., Bernard, N., Loustaud-Ratti, V., Le Lostec, Z., Laurichesse, H., Turpin, F., Ouzan, D., Grasset, D., Perrone, C., Cabrol, M.P., and Piette, J.C. Hepatitis C virus infections and lymphoproliferative diseases in France: a national study. The GERMIVIC group. *Am. J. Hematol.* 64: 107–111, **2000**.

Hausfater, P., Cacoub, P., Sterkers, Y., Thibault, V., Amoura, Z., Nguyen, L., Ghillani, P., Leblond, V., and Piette, J.C. Hepatitis C virus infection and lymphoproliferative disease: prospective study on 1,576 patients in France. *Am. J. Hematol.* 67: 168–171, **2001**.

He, Q.Q., Cheng, R.X., Sun, Y., Feng, D.Y., Chen, Z.C., and Zheng, H. Hepatocyte transformation and tumor development induced by hepatitis C virus NS3 C-terminal deleted protein. *World J. Gastroenterol.* 9: 474–478, **2003**.

He, X.S., Rehermann, B., Lopez-Labrador, F.X., Boisvert, J., Cheung, R., Mumm, J., Wedemeyer, H., Berenguer, M., Wright, T.L., Davis, M.M., and Greenberg, H.B. Quantitative analysis of hepatitis C virus-specific CD8(+) T cells in peripheral blood and liver using peptide-MHC tetramers. *Proc. Natl. Acad. Sci. USA* 96: 5692–5697, **1999**.

Heathcote, E.J., Shiffman, M.L., Cooksley, W.G., Dusheiko, G.M., Lee, S. S., Balart, L., Reindollar, R., Reddy, R.K., Wright, T.L., Lin, A., Hoffman, J., and De Pamphilis, J. Peginterferon alfa-2 a in patients with chronic hepatitis C and cirrhosis. *N. Engl. J. Med.* 343: 1673–1680, **2000**.

Hermine, O., Lefrere, F., Bronowicki, J.P., Mariette, X., Jondeau, K., Eclache-Saudreau, V., Delmas, B., Valensi, F., Cacoub, P., Brechot, C., Varet, B., and Troussard, X. Regression of splenic lymphoma with villous lymphocytes after treatment of hepatitis C virus infection. *N. Engl. J. Med.* 347: 89–94, **2002**.

Hibbs, R.G., Corwin, A.L., Hassan, N.F., Kamel, M., Darwish, M., Edelman, R., Constantine, N.T., Rao, M.R., Khalifa, A.S., Mokhtar, S., et al. The epidemiology of antibody to hepatitis C in Egypt. *J. Infect. Dis.* 168: 789–790, **1993**.

Hoofnagle, J.H. Course and outcome of hepatitis C. *Hepatology* 36: S21–S29, **2002**.

Hoofnagle J.H., Mullen, K.D., Jones, D.B., Rustgi, V., Di Bisceglie, A., Peters, M., Waggoner, J.G., Park, Y., and Jones, E.A. Treatment of chronic non-A, non-B hepatitis with recombinant human alpha interferon. A preliminary report. *N. Engl. J. Med.* 315: 1575–1578, **1986**.

Houghton, M. and Abrignani, S. Prospects for a vaccine against the hepatitis C virus. *Nature* 436: 961–966, **2005**.

Ide, Y., Tanimoto, A., Sasaguri, Y. and Padmanabhan, R. Hepatitis C virus NS5A protein is phosphorylated in vitro by a stably bound protein kinase from HeLa cells and by cAMP-dependent protein kinase A-alpha catalytic subunit. Gene 201: 151–158, **1997**.

Ishido, S. and Hotta, H. Complex formation of the nonstructural protein 3 of hepatitis C virus with the p53 tumor suppressor. *FEBS Lett.* 438: 258–262, **1998**.

Ishikawa, T., Shibuya, K., Yasui, K., Mitamura, K., and Ueda, S. Expression of hepatitis C virus core protein associated with malignant lymphoma in transgenic mice. *Comp. Immunol. Microbiol. Infect. Dis.* 26: 115–124, **2003**.

Iwasaki, A. and Medzhitov, R. Toll-like receptor control of the adaptive immune responses. *Nat. Immunol.* 5: 987–995, **2004**.

Izumi, T., Sasaki, R., Tsunoda, S., Akutsu, M., Okamoto, H., and Miura, Y. B cell malignancy and hepatitis C virus infection. Leukemia 11 (Suppl. 3): 516–518, **1997**.

Jamal, M.M. and Morgan, T.R. Liver disease in alcohol and hepatitis C. *Best Pract. Res. Clin. Gastroenterol.* 17: 649–662, **2003**.

Ji, H., Fraser, C.S., Yu, Y., Leary, J., and Doudna, J.A. Coordinated assembly of human translation initiation complexes by the hepatitis C virus internal ribosome entry site RNA. *Proc. Natl. Acad. Sci. USA* 101: 16990–16995, **2004**.

Jin, D.Y., Wang, H.L., Zhou, Y., Chun, A.C., Kibler, K.V., Hou, Y.D., Kung, H., and Jeang, K.T. Hepatitis C virus core protein-induced loss of LZIP function correlates with cellular transformation. *EMBO J.* 19: 729–740, **2000**.

Joo, M., Hahn, Y.S., Kwon, M., Sadikot, R.T., Blackwell, T.S., and Christman, J.W. Hepatitis C virus core protein suppresses NF-κB activation and cyclooxygenase-2 expression by direct interaction with IκB kinase β. *J. Virol.* 79: 7648–7657, **2005**.

Jopling, C.L., Yi, M., Lancaster, A.M., Lemon, S. M., and Sarnow, P. Modulation of hepatitis C virus RNA abundance by a liver-specific microRNA. *Science* 309: 1577–1581, **2005**.

Jung, E.Y., Kang, H.K., Chang, J., Yu, D.Y., and Jang, K.L. Cooperative transformation of murine fibroblast NIH3T3 cells by hepatitis C virus core protein and hepatitis B virus X protein. *Virus Res.* 94: 79–84, **2003**.

Kamegaya, Y., Hiasa, Y., Zukerberg, L., Fowler, N., Blackard, J.T., Lin, W., Choe, W.H., Schmidt, E.V., and Chung, R.T. Hepatitis C virus acts as a tumor accelerator by blocking apoptosis in a mouse model of hepatocarcinogenesis. *Hepatology* 41: 660–667, **2005**.

Kao, J.H. and Chen, D.S. Transmission of hepatitis C virus in Asia: past and present perspectives. *J. Gastroenterol. Hepatol.* 15: Suppl. E91–E96, **2000**.

Kapadia, S. B., Brideau-Andersen, A., and Chisari, F.V. Interference of hepatitis C virus RNA replication by short interfering

RNAs. *Proc. Natl. Acad. Sci. USA* 100: 2014–2018, **2003**.

Kato, T., Furusaka, A., Miyamoto, M., Date, T., Yasui, K., Hiramoto, J., Nagayama, K., Tanaka, T., and Wakita, T. Sequence analysis of hepatitis C virus isolated from a fulminant hepatitis patient. *J. Med. Virol.* 64: 334–339, **2001** .

Kato, T., Date, T., Miyamoto, M., Furusaka, A., Tokushige, K., Mizokami, M., and Wakita, T. Efficient replication of the genotype 2a hepatitis C virus subgenomic replicon. Gastroenterology 125: 1808–1817, **2003**.

Katze, M.G., He, Y., and Gale, M., Jr. Viruses and interferon: a fight for supremacy. *Nat. Rev. Immunol.* 2: 675–687, **2002**.

Khabar, K.S. and Polyak, S. J. Hepatitis C virus-host interactions: the NS5A protein and the interferon/chemokine systems. *J. Interferon Cytokine Res.* 22: 1005–1012, **2002**.

Khabar, K.S., Al-Zoghaibi, F., Al-Ahdal, M.N., Murayama, T., Dhalla, M., Mukaida, N., Taha, M., Al-Sedairy, S. T., Siddiqui, Y., Kessie, G., and Matsushima, K. The α-chemokine, interleukin 8, inhibits the antiviral action of interferon α. *J. Exp. Med.* 186: 1077–1085, **1997**.

Kim, J., Lee, D., and Choe, J. Hepatitis C virus NS5A protein is phosphorylated by casein kinase II. *Biochem. Biophys. Res. Commun.* 257: 777–781, **1999**.

Kim, W.H., Hong, F., Jaruga, B., Hu, Z., Fan, S., Liang, T.J., and Gao, B. Additive activation of hepatic NF-kappaB by ethanol and hepatitis B protein X (HBX) or HCV core protein: involvement of TNF-alpha receptor 1-independent and -dependent mechanisms. *FASEB J.* 15: 2551–2553, **2001**.

Kimura, Y., Gushima, T., Rawale, S., Kaumaya, P., and Walker, C.M. Escape mutations alter proteasome processing of major histocompatibility complex class I-restricted epitopes in persistent hepatitis C virus infections. *J. Virol.* 79: 4870–4876, **2005**.

King, P.D., Wilkes, J.D., and Diaz-Arias, A.A. Hepatitis C virus infection in non-Hodgkin's lymphoma. *Clin. Lab. Haematol.* 20: 107–110, **1998**.

Kitay-Cohen, Y., Amiel, A., Hilzenrat, N., Buskila, D., Ashur, Y., Fejgin, M., Gaber, E., Safadi, R., Tur-Kaspa, R., and Lishner, M. Bcl-2 rearrangement in patients with chronic hepatitis C associated with essential mixed cryoglobulinemia type II. *Blood* 96: 2910–2912, **2000**.

Kiyosawa, K., Sodeyama, T., Tanaka, E., Gibo, Y., Yoshizawa, K., Nakano, Y., Furuta, S., Akahane, Y., Nishioka, K., Purcell, R.H., et al. Interrelationship of blood transfusion, non-A, non-B hepatitis and hepatocellular carcinoma: analysis by detection of antibody to hepatitis C virus. *Hepatology* 12: 671–675, **1990**.

Korenaga, M., Wang, T., Li, Y., Showalter, L.A., Chan, T., Sun, J., and Weinman, S. A. Hepatitis C virus core protein inhibits mitochondrial electron transport and increases reactive oxygen species (ROS) production. *J. Biol. Chem.* 280: 37481–37488, **2005**.

Koziel, M.J., Dudley, D., Wong, J.T., Dienstag, J., Houghton, M., Ralston, R., and Walker, B.D. Intrahepatic cytotoxic T lymphocytes specific for hepatitis C virus in persons with chronic hepatitis. *J. Immunol.* 149: 3339–3344, **1992** .

Koziel, M.J., Dudley, D., Afdhal, N., Choo, Q.-L., Houghton, M., Ralston, R., and Walker, B.D. Hepatitis C virus (HCV)-specific cytotoxic T lymphocytes recognize epitopes in the core and envelope proteins of HCV. *J. Virol.* 67: 7522–7532, **1993**.

Koziel, M.J., Dudley, D., Afdhal, N., Grakoui, A., Rice, C.M., Choo, Q.-L., Houghton, M., and Walker, B.D. HLA class I-restricted cytotoxic T lymphocytes specific for hepatitis C virus. Identification of multiple epitopes and characterization of patterns of cytokine release. *J. Clin. Invest.* 96: 2311–2321, **1995**.

Kuniyoshi, M., Nakamuta, M., Sakai, H., Enjoji, M., Kinukawa, N., Kotoh, K., Fukutomi, M., Yokota, M., Nishi, H., Iwamoto, H., Uike, N., Nishimura, J., Inaba, S., Maeda, Y., Nawata, H., and Muta, K. Prevalence of hepatitis B or C virus infections in patients with non-Hodgkin's lymphoma. *J. Gastroenterol. Hepatol.* 16: 215–219, **2001**.

Kuroki, T. and Huh, N.H. Why are human cells resistant to malignant cell transformation in vitro? *Jpn. J. Cancer Res.* 84: 1091–1100, **1993**.

Lan, K.H., Sheu, M.L., Hwang, S. J., Yen, S. H., Chen, S. Y., Wu, J.C., Wang, Y.J., Kato, N., Omata, M., Chang, F.Y., and Lee, S. D.

HCV NS5A interacts with p53 and inhibits p53-mediated apoptosis. *Oncogene* 21: 4801–4811, **2002** .

Lanford, R.E., Guerra, B., Chavez, D., Bigger, C., Brasky, K.M., Wang, X.H., Ray, S. C., and Thomas, D.L. Cross-genotype immunity to hepatitis C virus. *J. Virol.* 78: 1575–1581, **2004**.

Larrea, E., Beloqui, O., Munoz-Navas, M.A., Civeira, M.P., and Prieto, J. Superoxide dismutase in patients with chronic hepatitis C virus infection. *Free Radic. Biol. Med.* 24: 1235–1241, **1998**.

Lau, D.T., Kleiner, D.E., Ghany, M.G., Park, Y., Schmid, P., and Hoofnagle, J.H. 10-Year follow-up after interferon-alpha therapy for chronic hepatitis C. *Hepatology* 28: 1121–1127, **1998**.

Lauer, G.M. and Walker, B.D. Hepatitis C virus infection. *N. Engl. J. Med.* 345: 41–52, **2001**.

Lauer, G.M., Barnes, E., Lucas, M., Timm, J., Ouchi, K., Kim, A.Y., Day, C.L., Robbins, G.K., Casson, D.R., Reiser, M., Dusheiko, G., Allen, T.M., Chung, R.T., Walker, B.D., and Klenerman, P. High resolution analysis of cellular immune responses in resolved and persistent hepatitis C virus infection. *Gastroenterology* 127: 924–936, **2004**.

Lauer, G.M., Lucas, M., Timm, J., Ouchi, K., Kim, A.Y., Day, C.L., Schulze zur Wiesch, J.S., Paranhos-Baccala, G., Sheridan, I., Casson, D.R., Reiser, M., Gandhi, R.T., Li, B., Allen, T.M., Chung, R.T., Klenerman, P., and Walker, B.D. Full-breadth analysis of CD8⁺ T-cell responses in acute hepatitis C virus infection and early therapy. *J. Virol.* 79: 12 979–12 988, **2005**.

Lechner, F., Gruener, N.H., Urbani, S., Uggeri, J., Santantonio, T., Kammer, A.R., Cerny, A., Phillips, R., Ferrari, C., Pape, G.R., and Klenerman, P. CD8+ T lymphocyte responses are induced during acute hepatitis C virus infection but are not sustained. *Eur. J. Immunol.* 30: 2479–2487, **2000**.

Lee, C.H., Choi, Y.H., Yang, S. H., Lee, C.W., Ha, S. J., and Sung, Y.C. Hepatitis C virus core protein inhibits interleukin 12 and nitric oxide production from activated macrophages. *Virology* 279: 271–279, **2001**.

Lee, J., Chuang, T.H., Redecke, V., She, L., Pitha, P.M., Carson, D.A., Raz, E., and Cot-

tam, H.B. Molecular basis for the immunostimulatory activity of guanine nucleoside analogs: activation of Toll-like receptor 7. *Proc. Natl. Acad. Sci. USA* 100: 6646–6651, **2003**.

Lerat, H., Rumin, S., Habersetzer, F., Berby, F., Trabaud, M.A., Trepo, C., and Inchauspe, G. In vivo tropism of hepatitis C virus genomic sequences in hematopoietic cells: influence of viral load, viral genotype, and cell phenotype. *Blood* 91: 3841–3949, **1998**.

Levin, M.K., Gurjar, M., and Patel, S. S. A Brownian motor mechanism of translocation and strand separation by hepatitis C virus helicase. *Nat. Struct. Mol. Biol.* 12: 429–435, **2005**.

Li, K., Foy, E., Ferreon, J.C., Nakamura, M., Ferreon, A.C., Ikeda, M., Ray, S. C., Gale, M., Jr., and Lemon, S. M. Immune evasion by hepatitis C virus NS3/4A protease-mediated cleavage of the Toll-like receptor 3 adaptor protein TRIF. *Proc. Natl. Acad. Sci. USA* 102: 2992–2997, **2005 a**.

Li, K., Chen, Z., Kato, N., Gale, M., Jr., and Lemon, S. M. Distinct poly (I-C) and virus-activated signaling pathways leading to interferon-β production in hepatocytes. *J. Biol. Chem.* 280: 16 739–16 747, **2005 b**.

Liang, T.J. and Heller, T. Pathogenesis of hepatitis C-associated hepatocellular carcinoma. *Gastroenterology* 127 (5 Suppl. 1): S62–S71, **2004**.

Libra, M., Indelicato, M., De Re, V., Zignego, A.L., Chiocchetti, A., Malaponte, G., Dianzani, U., Nicoletti, F., Stivala, F., McCubrey, J.A., and Mazzarino, M.C. Elevated serum levels of osteopontin in HCV-associated lymphoproliferative disorders. *Cancer Biol. Ther.* 4: 1192–1194, **2005**.

Lin, H.-H., Kao, J.H., Hsu, H.-Y., Ni, Y.H., Yeh, S. H., Hwang, L.H., Chang, M.H., Hwang, S. C., Chen, P.J., and Chen, D.S. Possible role of high-titer maternal viremia in perinatal transmission of hepatitis C virus. *J. Infect. Dis.* 169: 638–641, **1994**.

Lin, R., Heylbroeck, C., Genin, P., Pitha, P.M., and Hiscott, J. Essential role of interferon regulatory factor 3 in direct activation of RANTES chemokine transcription. *Mol. Cell. Biol.* 19: 959–966, **1999**.

Lindenbach, B.D. and Rice, C.M. Unravelling hepatitis C virus replication from genome to function. *Nature* 436: 933–938, **2005**.

Lindenbach, B.D., Evans, M.J., Syder, A.J., Wölk, B., Tellinghuisen, T.L., Liu, C.C., Maruyama, T., Hynes, R.O., Burton, D.R., McKeating, J.A., and Rice, C.M. Complete replication of hepatitis C virus in cell culture. *Science* 309: 623–626, **2005**.

Lindsay, K.L., Trepo, C., Heintges, T., Shiffman, M.L., Gordon, S. C., Hoefs, J.C., Schiff, E.R., Goodman, Z.D., Laughlin, M., Yao, R., Albrecht, J.K., Hepatitis Interventional Therapy Group. A randomized, double-blind trial comparing pegylated interferon alfa-2 b to interferon alfa-2 b as initial treatment for chronic hepatitis C. *Hepatology*. 34: 395–403, **2001**.

Logvinoff, C., Major, M.E., Oldach, D., Heyward, S., Talal, A., Balfe, P., Feinstone, S. M., Alter, H., Rice, C.M., and McKeating, J.A. Neutralizing antibody response during acute and chronic hepatitis C virus infection. *Proc. Natl. Acad. Sci. USA* 101: 10 149–10 154, **2004**.

Lohmann, V., Koch, J.O., and Bartenschlager, R. Processing pathways of the hepatitis C virus proteins. *J. Hepatol*. 24 (2 Suppl.): 11–19, **1996**.

Lohmann, V., Korner, F., Dobierzewska, A., and Bartenschlager, R. Mutations in hepatitis C virus RNAs conferring cell culture adaptation. *J. Virol*. 75: 1437–1449, **2001**.

Luppi, M., Grazia Ferrari, M., Bonaccorsi, G., Longo, G., Narni, F., Barozzi, P., Marasca, R., Mussini, C., and Torelli, G. Hepatitis C virus infection in subsets of neoplastic lymphoproliferations not associated with cryoglobulinemia. *Leukemia* 10: 351–355, **1996**.

MacDonald, A. and Harris, M. Hepatitis C virus NS5 A: tales of a promiscuous protein. *J. Gen. Virol*. 85: 2485–2502, **2004**.

Machida, K., Cheng, K.T., Sung, V.M., Lee, K.J., Levine, A.M., and Lai, M.M. Hepatitis C virus infection activates the immunologic (type II) isoform of nitric oxide synthase and thereby enhances DNA damage and mutations of cellular genes. *J. Virol*. 78: 8835–8843, **2004 a**.

Machida, K., Cheng, K.T., Sung, V.M., Shimodaira, S., Lindsay, K.L., Levine, A.M., Lai, M.Y., and Lai, M.M. Hepatitis C induces a mutator phenotype: enhanced mutations of immunoglobulin and protooncogenes. *Proc. Natl. Acad. Sci. USA* 101: 4262–4267, **2004 b**.

Majumder, M., Steele, R., Gosh, A.K., Zhou, X.Y., Thornburg, L., Ray, R., Phillips, N.J., and Ray, R.B. Expression of hepatitis C virus non-structural 5 A protein in the liver of transgenic mice. *FEBS Lett*. 555: 528–532, **2003** .

Marusawa, H., Hijikata, M., Chiba, T., and Shimotohno, K. Hepatitis C virus core protein inhibits Fas- and tumor necrosis factor α-mediated apoptosis via NF-κB activation. *J. Virol*. 73: 4713–4720, **1999**.

Masciopinto, F., Giovani, C., Campagnoli, S., Galli-Stampino, L., Colombatto, P., Brunetto, M., Yen, T.S., Houghton, M., Pileri, P., and Abrignani, S. Association of hepatitis C virus envelope proteins with exosomes. *Eur. J. Immunol*. 34: 2834–2842, **2004**.

Mayo, M.J. Extrahepatic manifestations of hepatitis C infection. *Am. J. Med. Sci*. 325: 135–148, **2003**.

Mazzaro, C., Zagonel, V., Monfardini, S., Tulissi, P., Pussini, E., Fanni, M., Sorio, R., Bortolus, R., Crovatto, M., Santini, G., Tiribelli, C., Sasso, F., Masutti, R., and Pozzato, G. Hepatitis C virus and non-Hodgkin's lymphomas. *Br. J. Haematol* . 94: 544–550, **1996**.

McColl, M.D., Singer, I.O., Tait, R.C., McNeil, I.R., Cumming, R.L., and Hogg, R.B. The role of hepatitis C virus in the aetiology of non-Hodgkin's lymphoma – a regional association? *Leuk. Lymphoma* 26: 127–130, **1997**.

McHutchison, J.G. and Poynard, T. Combination therapy with interferon plus ribavirin for the initial treatment of chronic hepatitis C. *Semin. Liver Dis*. 19: 57–65, **1999**.

Mehta, S. H., Cox, A., Hoover, D.R., Wang, X.H., Mao, Q., Ray, S., Strathdee, S. A., Vlahov, D., and Thomas, D.L. Protection against persistence of hepatitis C. *Lancet* 359: 1478–1483, **2002**.

Meunier, J.C., Engle, R.E., Faulk, K., Zhao, M., Bartosch, B., Alter, H., Emerson, S. U., Cosset, F.L., Purcell, R.H., and Bukh, J. Evidence for cross-genotype neutralization of hepatitis C virus pseudo-particles and enhancement of infectivity by apolipoprotein C1. *Proc. Natl. Acad. Sci. USA* 102: 4560–4565, **2005**.

Miyasaka, Y., Enomoto, N., Kurosaki, M., Sakamoto, N., Kanazawa, N., Kohashi, T.,

Ueda, E., Maekawa, S., Watanabe, H., Izumi, N., Sato, C., and Watanabe, M. Hepatitis C virus nonstructural protein 5 A inhibits tumor necrosis factor-α-mediated apoptosis in Huh7 cells. *J. Infect. Dis.* 188: 1537–1544, **2003**.

Mizorogi, F., Hiramoto, J., Nozato, A., Takekuma, Y., Nagayama, K., Tanaka, T., and Takagi, K. Hepatitis C virus infection in patients with B-cell non-Hodgkin's lymphoma. *Intern. Med.* 39: 112–117, **2000**.

Morgan, T.R., Mandayam, S., and Jamal, M.M. Alcohol and hepatocellular carcinoma. *Gastroenterology* 127 (5 Suppl. 1): S87–S96, **2004**.

Moriya, K., Fujie, H., Shintani, Y., Yotsuyanagi, H., Tsutsumi, T., Ishibashi, K., Matsuura, Y., Kimura, S., Miyamura, T., and Koike, K. The core protein of hepatitis C virus induces hepatocellular carcinoma in transgenic mice. *Nat. Med.* 4: 1065–1067, **1998**.

Muramatso, S., Ishido, S., Fujita, T., Itoh, M., and Hotta, H. Nuclear localization of the NS3 protein of hepatitis C virus and factors affecting the localization. *J. Virol.* 71: 4954–4961, **1997**.

Naas, T., Ghorbani, M., Alvarez-Maya, I., Lapner, M., Kothary, R., De Repentigny, Y., Gomes, S., Babiuk, L., Giulivi, A., Soare, C., Azizi, A., and Diaz-Mitoma, F. Characterization of liver histopathology in a transgenic mouse model expressing genotype 1 a hepatitis C virus core and envelope proteins 1 and 2. *J. Gen. Virol.* 86: 2185–2196, **2005**.

Ndjomou, J., Pybus, O.G., and Matz, B. Phylogenetic analysis of hepatitis C virus isolates indicates a unique pattern of endemic infection in Cameroon. *J. Gen. Virol.* 84: 2333–2341, **2003**.

Nelson, D.R., Marousis, C.G., Davis, G.L., Rice, C.M., Wong, J., Houghton, M., and Lau, J.Y. The role of hepatitis C virus-specific cytotoxic T lymphocytes in chronic hepatitis C. *J. Immunol.* 158: 1473–1481, **1997**.

Neumann, A.U., Lam, N.P., Dahari, H., Gretch, D.R., Wiley, T.E., Layden, T.J., and Perelson, A.S. Hepatitis C viral dynamics in vivo and the antiviral efficacy of interferon-alpha therapy. *Science* 282: 103–107, **1998**.

Noguchi, T., Satoh, S., Noshi, T., Hatada, E., Fukuda, R., Kawai, A., Ikeda, S., Hijikata, M., and Shimotohno, K. Effects of mutation in hepatitis C virus nonstructural protein 5 A on interferon resistance mediated by inhibition of PKR kinase activity in mammalian cells. *Microbiol. Immunol.* 45: 829–840, **2001**.

Novati, R., Thiers, V., Monforte, A.D., Maisonneuve, P., Principi, N., Conti, M., Lazzarin, A., and Brechot, C. Mother-to-child transmission of hepatitis C virus detected by nested polymerase chain reaction. *J. Infect. Dis.* 165: 720–723, **1992**.

Ohsawa, M., Shingu, N., Miwa, H., Yoshihara, A., Kubo, M., Tsukuma, H., Teshima, H., Hashimoto, M., and Aozasa, K. Risk of non-Hodgkin's lymphoma in patients with hepatitis C virus infection. *Int. J. Cancer* 80: 237–239, **1999**.

Ohto, H., Terazawa, S., Sasaki, N., Sasaki, N., Hino, K., Ishiwata, C., Kako, M., Ujiie, N., Endo, C., Matsui, A., et al. Transmission of hepatitis C virus from mothers to infants. The Vertical Transmission of hepatitis C Virus Collaborative Study Group. *N. Engl. J. Med.* 330: 744–750, **1994**.

Okuda, M., Li, K., Beard, M.R., Showalter, L.A., Scholle, F., Lemon, S. M., and Weinman, S. A. Mitochondrial injury, oxidative stress, and antioxidant gene expression are induced by hepatitis C virus core protein. *Gastroenterology.* 122: 366–375, **2002**.

Oliveira, M.L., Bastos, F.I., Sabino, R.R., Paetzold, U., Schreier, E., Pauli, G., and Yoshida, C.F. Distribution of HCV genotypes among different exposure categories in Brazil. *Braz. J. Med. Biol. Res.* 32: 279–282, **1999**.

Otto, G.A. and Puglisi, J.D. The pathway of HCV IRES-mediated translation initiation. *Cell* 119: 369–380, **2004**.

Pancholi, P., Perkus, M., Tricoche, N., Liu, Q., and Prince, A.M. DNA immunization with hepatitis C virus (HCV) polycistronic genes or immunization by HCV DNA priming-recombinant canarypox virus boosting induces immune responses and protection from recombinant HCV-vaccinia virus infection in HLA-A2.1-transgenic mice. *J. Virol.* 77: 382–390, **2003**.

Park, J.S., Yang, J.M., and Min, M.K. Hepatitis C virus nonstructural protein NS4 B transforms NIH3 T3 cells in cooperation with the Ha-ras oncogene. *Biochem. Biophys. Res. Commun.* 267: 581–587, **2000**.

Pascu, M., Martus, P., Höhne, M., Wiedenmann, B., Hopf, U., Schreier, E., and Berg, T. Sustained virological response in hepatitis C virus type 1b infected patients is predicted by the number of mutations within the NS5 A-ISDR: a meta-analysis focused on geographical differences. *Gut* 53: 1345–1351, **2004**.

Pascual, M., Perrin, L., Giostra, E., and Schifferli, J.A. Hepatitis C virus in patients with cryoglobulinemia type II. *J. Infect. Dis.* 162: 569–570, **1990**.

Pavio, N., Battaglia, S., Boucreux, D., Arnulf, B., Sobesky, R., Hermine, O., and Brechot, C. Hepatitis C virus core variants isolated from liver tumor but not from adjacent non-tumor tissue interact with Smad3 and inhibit the TGF-β pathway. *Oncogene* 24: 6119–6132, **2005**.

Pavlovic, D., Neville, D.C., Argaud, O., Blumberg, B., Dwek, R.A., Fischer, W.B., and Zitzmann, N. The hepatitis C virus p7 protein forms an ion channel that is inhibited by long-alkyl-chain iminosugar derivatives. *Proc. Natl. Acad. Sci. USA* 100: 6104–6108, **2003**.

Pawlotsky, J.M. Diagnostic tests for hepatitis C. *J. Hepatol.* 31 (Suppl. 1): 71–79, **1999**.

Pearse, M.J. and Drane, D. ISCOMATRIX adjuvant for antigen delivery. *Adv. Drug Deliv. Rev.* 57: 465–474, **2005**.

Penin, F., Dubuisson, J., Rey, F.A., Moradpour, D., and Pawlotsky, J.M. Structural biology of hepatitis C virus. *Hepatology* 39: 5–19, **2004**.

Perri, S., Greer, C.E., Thudium, K., Doe, B., Legg, H., Liu, H., Romero, R.E., Tang, Z., Bin, Q., Dubensky, T.W., Jr., Vajdy, M., Otten, G.R., and Polo, J.M. An alphavirus replicon particle chimera derived from Venezuelan equine encephalitis and sindbis viruses is a potent gene-based vaccine delivery vector. *J. Virol.* 77: 10 394–10 403, **2003**.

Pikarsky, E., Porat, R.M., Stein, I., Abramovitch, R., Amit, S., Kasem, S., Gutkovich-Pyest, E., Urieli-Shoval, S., Galun, E., and Ben-Neriah, Y. NF-κB functions as a tumour promoter in inflammation-associated cancer. *Nature* 431: 461–466, **2004**.

Pileri, P., Uematsu, Y., Campagnoli, S., Galli, G., Falugi, F., Petracca, R., Weiner, A.J., Houghton, M., Rosa, D., Grandi, G., and Abrignani, S. Binding of hepatitis C virus to CD81. *Science* 282: 938–941, **1998**.

Polakos, N.K., Drane, D., Cox, J., Ng, P., Selby, M.J., Chien, D., O'Hagan, D.T., Houghton, M., and Paliard, X. Characterization of hepatitis C virus core-specific immune responses primed in rhesus macaques by a nonclassical ISCOM vaccine. *J. Immunol.* 166: 3589–3598, **2001**.

Rabkin, C.S., Tess, B.H., Christianson, R.E., Wright, W.E., Waters, D.J., Alter, H.J., and Van Den Berg, B.J. Prospective study of hepatitis C viral infection as a risk factor for subsequent B-cell neoplasia. *Blood* 99: 4240–4242, **2002**.

Ralston, R., Thudium, K., Berger, K., Kuo, C., Gervase, B., Hall, J., Selby, M., Kuo, G., Houghton, M., and Choo, Q.-L. Characterization of hepatitis C virus envelope glycoprotein complexes expressed by recombinant vaccinia viruses. *J. Virol.* 67: 6753–6761, **1993**.

Randall, G., Grakoui, A., and Rice, C.M. Clearance of replicating hepatitis C virus replicon RNAs in cell culture by small interfering RNAs. *Proc. Natl. Acad. Sci. USA* 100: 235–240, **2003**.

Reyes, G.R. The nonstructural NS5 A protein of hepatitis C virus: an expanding, multifunctional role in enhancing hepatitis C virus pathogenesis. *J. Biomed. Sci.* 9: 187–197, **2002**.

Richmond, A. NF-κB, chemokine gene transcription and tumour growth. *Nature Rev. Immunol.* 2: 664–674, **2002**.

Robertson, B., Myers, G., Howard, C., Brettin, T., Bukh, J., Gaschen, B., Gojobori, T., Maertens, G., Mizokami, M., Nainan, O., Netesov, S., Nishioka, K., Shin-I, T., Simmonds, P., Smith, D., Stuyver, L., and Weiner, A. Classification, nomenclature, and database development for hepatitis C virus (HCV) and related viruses: proposals for standardization. International Committee on Virus Taxonomy. *Arch. Virol.* 143: 2493–2503, **1998**.

Rosen, H.R., Miner, C., Sasaki, A.W., Lewinsohn, D.M., Conrad, A.J., Bakke, A., Bouwer, H.G., and Hinrichs, D.J. Frequencies of HCV-specific effector CD4+ T cells by flow cytometry: correlation with clinical disease stages. *Hepatology* 35: 190–198, **2002**.

Saeed, A.A., al-Admawi, A.M., al-Rasheed, A., Fairclough, D., Bacchus, R., Ring, C, and Garson, J. Hepatitis C virus infection in Egyptian volunteer blood donors in Riyadh. *Lancet* 338: 459–460, **1991**.

Safdar, K. and Schiff, E.R. Alcohol and hepatitis C. Semin. Liver Dis. 24: 305–315, **2004**.

Sakamuro, D., Furukawa, T., and Takegami, T. Hepatitis C virus nonstructural protein NS3 transforms NIH 3 T3 cells. *J. Virol*. 69: 3893–3896, **1995**.

Sansonno, D., Lauletta, G., Nisi, L., Gatti, P., Pesola, F., Pansini, N., and Dammacco, F. Non-enveloped HCV core protein as constitutive antigen of cold precipitable immune complexes in type II mixed cryoglobulinaemia. *Clin. Exp. Immunol*. 133: 275–282, **2003**.

Sarnow, P. Viral internal ribosome entry site elements: novel ribosome-RNA complexes and roles in viral pathogenesis. *J. Virol*. 77: 2801–2806, **2003**.

Schetter, C. and Vollmer, J. Toll-like receptors involved in the response to microbial pathogens: development of agonists for toll-like receptor 9. *Curr. Opin. Drug Discov. Dev*. 7: 204–210, **2004**.

Schinkel, J., Spoon, W.J., and Kroes, A.C. Meta-analysis of mutations in the NS5 A gene and hepatitis C virus resistance to interferon therapy: uniting discordant conclusions. *Antiviral Ther*. 9: 275–286, **2004**.

Seeff, L.B. Natural history of chronic hepatitis C. *Hepatology* 36 (5 Suppl. 1) S35–S46, **2002**.

Sen, G.C. Viruses and interferons. *Annu. Rev. Microbiol*. 55: 255–281, **2001**.

Sène, D., Limal, N., and Cacoub, P. Hepatitis C virus-associated extrahepatic manifestations: a review. *Metab. Brain Dis*. 19: 357–381, **2004**.

Serebrov, V. and Pyle, A.M. Periodic cycles of RNA unwinding and pausing by hepatitis C virus NS3 helicase. *Nature* 430: 476–480, **2004**.

Shan, Y., Chen, X.G., Huang, B., Hu, A.B., Xiao, D., and Guo, Z.M. Malignant transformation of the cultured human hepatocytes induced by hepatitis C virus core protein. *Liver Int*. 25: 141–147, **2005**.

Shimazaki, T., Honda, M., Kaneko, S., and Kobayashi, K. Inhibition of internal ribosomal entry site-directed translation of HCV by recombinant IFN-á correlates with a reduced La protein. *Hepatology* 35: 199–208, **2002**.

Shoukry, N.H., Grakoui, A., Houghton, M., Chien, D.Y., Ghrayeb, J., Reimann, K.A., and Walker, C.M. Memory CD8 + T cells are required for protection from persistent hepatitis C virus infection. *J. Exp. Med*. 197: 1645–1655, **2003**.

Silvestri, F., Barillari, G., Fanin, R., Pipan, C., Falasca, E., Salmaso, F., Zaja, F., Infanti, L., Patriarca, F., Botta, G.A., and Baccarini, M. Hepatitis C virus infection among cryoglobulinemic and non-cryoglobulinemic B-cell non-Hodgkin's lymphomas. *Haematologica* 82: 314–317, **1997**.

Simmonds, P. Reconstructing the origins of human hepatitis viruses. *Philos. Trans. R. Soc. Lond. B Biol. Sci*. 356: 1013–1026, **2001**.

Simmonds, P. Genetic diversity and evolution of hepatitis C virus – 15 years on. *J. Gen. Virol*. 85: 3173–3188, **2004**.

Simmonds, P., Bukh, J., Combet, C., Deleage, G., Enomoto, N., Feinstone, S., Halfon, P., Inchauspe, G., Kuiken, C., Maertens, G., Mizokami, M., Murphy, D.G., Okamoto, H., Pawlotsky, J.M., Penin, F., Sablon, E., Shin-I, T., Stuyver, L.J., Thiel, H.J., Viazov, S., Weiner, A.J., and Widell, A. Consensus proposals for a unified system of nomenclature of hepatitis C virus genotypes. *Hepatology* 42: 962–973, **2005**.

Smith, M.W., Yue, Z.N., Korth, M.J., Do, H.A., Boix, L., Fausto, N., Bruix, J., Carithers, R.L., Jr., and Katze, M.G. Hepatitis C virus and liver disease: global transcriptional profiling and identification of potential markers. *Hepatology* 38: 1458–1467, **2003**.

Soguero, C., Joo, M., Chianese-Bullock, K.A., Nguyen, D.T., Tung, K., and Hahn, Y.S. Hepatitis C virus core protein leads to immune suppression and liver damage in a transgenic murine model. *J. Virol*. 76: 9345–9354, **2002**.

Song, J., Nagano-Fujii, M., Wang, F., Florese, R., Fujita, T., Ishido, S., and Hotta, H. Nuclear localization and intramolecular cleavage of N-terminally deleted NS5 A protein of hepatitis C virus. *Virus Res.* 69: 109–117, **2000** .

Soule, J.L., Olyaei, A.J., Boslaugh, T.A., Busch, A.M., Schwartz, J.M., Morehouse, S. H., Ham, J.M., and Orloff, S. L. Hepatitis C infection increases the risk of new-onset diabetes after transplantation in liver allograft recipients. *Am. J. Surg* . 189: 552–557, **2005**.

Spahn, C.M., Kieft, J.S., Grassucci, R.A., Penczek, P.A., Zhou, K., Doudna, J.A., and Frank, J. Hepatitis C virus IRES RNA-induced changes in the conformation of the 40 S ribosomal subunit. *Science* 291: 1959–1962, **2001**.

Spaulding, A., Greene, C., Davidson, K., Schneidermann, M., and Rich, J. Hepatitis C in state correctional facilities. *Prev. Med.* 28: 92–100, **1999**.

Sumpter, R., Jr., Loo, Y.M., Foy, E., Li, K., Yoneyama, M., Fujita, T., Lemon, S. M., and Gale, M., Jr. Regulating intracellular antiviral defense and permissiveness to hepatitis C virus RNA replication through a cellular RNA helicase, RIG-1. *J. Virol.* 79: 2689–2699, **2005**.

Sun, B.S., Pan, J., Clayton, M.M., Liu, J., Yan, X., Matskevich, A.A., Strayer, D.S., Gerber, M., and Feitelson, M.A. Hepatitis C virus replication in stably transfected HepG2 cells promotes hepatocellular growth and tumorigenesis. *J. Cell Physiol* . 201: 447–458, **2004**.

Tabor, E., Purcell, R.H., Gerety, R.J. Primate animal models and titered inocula for the study of human hepatitis A, hepatitis B, and non-A, non-B hepatitis. *J. Med. Primatol.* 12: 305–318, **1983**.

Tai, D.I., Tsai, S. L., Chen, Y.M., Chuang, Y.L., Peng, C.Y., Sheen, I.S., Yeh, C.T., Chang, K.S., Huang, S. N., Kuo, G.C., and Liaw, Y.F. Activation of nuclear factor κB in hepatitis C virus infection: implications for pathogenesis and hepatocarcinogenesis. *Hepatology* 31: 656–664, **2000**.

Takaki, A., Wiese, M., Maertens, G., Depla, E., Seifert, U., Liebetrau, A., Miller, J.L., Manns, M.P., and Rehermann, B. Cellular immune responses persist and humoral responses decrease two decades after recovery from a single-source outbreak of hepatitis C. *Nat. Med.* 6: 578–582, **2000**.

Tang, L., Tanaka, Y., Enomoto, N., Marumo, F., and Sato, C. Detection of hepatitis C virus RNA in hepatocellular carcinoma by in situ hybridization. *Cancer* 76: 2211–2216, **1995**.

Taylor, D.R., Shi, S. T., Romano, P.R., Barber, G.N., and Lai, M.M.C. Inhibition of the interferon-inducible protein kinase PKR by HCV E2 protein. *Science*, 285: 107–110, **1999**.

Thaler, M.M., Park, C.K., Landers, D.V., Wara, D.W., Houghton, M., Veereman-Wauters, G., Sweet, R.L., and Han, J.H. Vertical transmission of hepatitis C virus. *Lancet* 338: 17–18, **1991**.

Thimme, R., Bukh, J., Spangenberg, H.C., Wieland, S., Pemberton, J., Steiger, C., Govindarajan, S., Purcell, R.H., and Chisari, F.V. Viral and immunological determinants of hepatitis C virus clearance, persistence, and disease. *Proc. Natl. Acad. Sci. USA* 99: 15 661–15 668, **2002**.

Thimme, R., Wieland, S., Steiger, C., Ghrayeb, J., Reimann, K.A., Purcell, R.H., and Chisari, F.V. CD8(+) T cells mediate viral clearance and disease pathogenesis during acute hepatitis B virus infection. *J. Virol.* 77: 68–76, **2003** .

Tomei, L., Altamura, S., Paonessa, G., De Francesco, R., and Migliaccio, G. HCV antiviral resistance: The impact of in vitro studies on the development of antiviral agents targeting the viral NS5 B polymerase. *Antiviral Chem. Chemother* . 16: 225–245, **2005**.

van der Poel, C.L. Hepatitis C virus. Epidemiology, transmission and prevention. In: Reesink, H.W. (Ed.), *Hepatitis C virus.* Karger, Amsterdam, pp. 137–163, **1991**.

van der Poel, C.L. Hepatitis C virus. Epidemiology, transmission and prevention. *Curr. Stud. Hematol. Blood Transfus.*, 137–163, **1994**.

Varaklioti, A., Vassilaki, N., Georgopoulou, U., and Mavromara, P. Alternate translation occurs within the core coding region of the hepatitis C viral genome. *J. Biol. Chem.* 277: 17 713–17 721, **2002**.

Waris, G. and Siddiqui, A. Hepatitis C virus stimulates the expression of cyclooxygenase-2 via oxidative stress: role of prostaglandin E2 in RNA replication. *J. Virol.* 79: 9725–9734, **2005**.

Waris, G., Livolsi, A., Imbert, V., Peyron, J.F., and Siddiqui, A. Hepatitis C virus NS5 A and subgenomic replicon activate NF-κB via tyrosine phosphorylation of IκBα and its degradation by calpain protease. *J. Biol. Chem.* 278: 40778–40787, **2003**.

Wedemeyer, H., He, X.S., Nascimbeni, M., Davis, A.R., Greenberg, H.B., Hoofnagle, J.H., Liang, T.J., Alter, H., and Rehermann, B. Impaired effector function of hepatitis C virus-specific CD8 + T cells in chronic hepatitis C virus infection. *J. Immunol.* 169: 3447–3458, **2002**.

Weiner, A.J., Paliard, X., Selby, M.J., Medina-Selby, A., Coit, D., Nguyen, S., Kansopon, J., Arian, C.L., Ng, P., Tucker, J., Lee, C.T., Polakos, N.K., Han, J., Wong, S., Lu, H.H., Rosenberg, S., Brasky, K.M., Chien, D., Kuo, G., and Houghton, M. Intrahepatic genetic inoculation of hepatitis C virus RNA confers cross-protective immunity. *J. Virol.* 75: 7142–7148, **2001**.

Wilson, J.A., Jayasena, S., Khvorova, A., Sabatinos, S., Rodrigue-Gervais, I.G., Arya, S., Sarangi, F., Harris-Brandts, M., Beaulieu, S., and Richardson, C.D. RNA interference blocks gene expression and RNA synthesis from hepatitis C replicons propagated in human liver cells. *Proc. Natl. Acad. Sci. USA* 100: 2783–2788, **2003**.

Wölk, B., Sansonno, D., Kräusslich, H.G., Dammacco, F., Rice, C.M., Blum, H.E., and Moradpour, D. Subcellular localization, stability, and trans-cleavage competence of the hepatitis C virus NS3-NS4 A complex expressed in tetracycline-regulated cell lines. *J. Virol.* 74: 2293–2304, **2000**.

Yamanaka, T., Uchida, M., and Doi, T. Innate form of HCV core protein plays an important role in the localization and the function of the HCV core protein. *Biochem. Biophys. Res. Commun.* 294: 521–527, **2002**.

Yao, Z.Q., Waggoner, S. N., Cruise, M.W., Hall, C., Xie, X., Oldach, D.W., and Hahn, Y.S. SOCS1 and SOCS3 are targeted by hepatitis C virus core/gC1 qR ligation to inhibit T-cell function. *J. Virol.* 79: 15417–15429, **2005**.

Yokota, T., Sakamoto, N., Enomoto, N., Tanabe, Y., Miyagishi, M., Maekawa, S., Yi, L., Kurosaki, M., Taira, K., Watanabe, M., and Mizusawa, H. Inhibition of intracellular hepatitis C virus replication by synthetic and vector-derived small interfering RNAs. *EMBO Rep.* 4: 602–608, **2003**.

Yoshida, H., Kato, N., Shiratori, Y., Otsuka, M., Maeda, S., Kato, J., and Omata, M. Hepatitis C virus core protein activates nuclear factor κB-dependent signaling through tumor necrosis factor receptor-associated factor. *J. Biol. Chem* . 276: 16399–16405, **2001**.

Yoshida, T., Hanada, T., Tokuhisa, T., Kosai, K., Sata, M., Kohara, M., and Yoshimura, A. Activation of STAT3 by the hepatitis C virus core protein leads to cellular transformation. *J. Exp. Med.* 196: 641–653, **2002**.

You, L.R., Chen, C.M., and Lee, Y.H. Hepatitis C virus core protein enhances NF-κB signal pathway triggering by lymphotoxin-β receptor ligand and tumor necrosis factor α. *J. Virol.* 73: 1672–1681, **1999**.

Zemel, R., Kazatsker, A., Greif, F., Ben-Ari, Z., Greif, H., Almog, O., and Tur-Kaspa, R. Mutations at vicinity of catalytic sites of hepatitis C virus NS3 serine protease gene isolated from hepatocellular carcinoma tissue. *Dig. Dis. Sci.* 45: 2199–2202, **2000**.

Zemel, R., Gerechet, S., Greif, H., Bachmatove, L., Birk, Y., Golan-Goldhirsh, A., Kunin, M., Berdichevsky, Y., Benhar, I., and Tur-Kaspa, R. Cell transformation induced by hepatitis C virus NS3 serine protease. *J. Viral. Hepatol.* 8: 96–102, **2001**.

Zemel, R., Berdichevsky, Y., Bachmatov, L., Benhar, I., and Tur-Kaspa, R. Inhibition of hepatitis C virus NS3-mediated cell transformation by recombinant intracellular antibodies. *J. Hepatol.* 40: 1000–1007, **2004**.

Zeuzem, S., Feinman, S. V., Rasenack, J., Heathcote, E.J., Lai, M.Y., Gane, E., O'Grady, J., Reichen, J., Diago, M., Lin, A., Hoffman, J., and Brunda, M.J. Peginterferon α-2 a in patients with chronic hepatitis C. *N. Engl. J. Med.* 343: 1666–1672, **2000**.

Zhang, T., Li, Y., Lai, J.P., Douglas, S. D., Metzger, D.S., O'Brien, C.P., and Ho, W.Z. Alcohol potentiates hepatitis C virus replicon expression. *Hepatology* 38: 57–65, **2003**.

Zhang, T., Lin, R.T., Li, Y., Douglas, S. D., Maxcey, C., Ho, C., Lai, J.P., Wang, Y.J., Wan, Q., and Ho, W.Z. Hepatitis C virus inhibits intracellular interferon α expression in human hepatic cell lines. *Hepatology* 42: 819–827, **2005**.

Zhong, J., Gastaminza, P., Cheng, G., Kapadia, S., Kato, T., Burton, D.R., Wieland, S. F., Uprichard, S. L., Wakita, T., and Chisari, F.V. Robust hepatitis C virus infection in vitro. *Proc. Natl. Acad. Sci. USA* 102: 9294–9299, **2005**.

Zignego, A.L., Ferri, C., Giannini, C., La Civita, L., Careccia, G., Longombardo, G., Bellesi, G., Caracciolo, F., Thiers, V., and Gentilini, P. Hepatitis C virus infection in mixed cryoglobulinemia and B-cell non-Hodgkin's lymphoma: evidence for a pathogenetic role. *Arch. Virol.* 142: 545–555, **1997**.

Zignego, A.L., Giannelli, F., Marrocchi, M.E., Mazzocca, A., Ferri, C., Giannini, C., Monti, M., Caini, P., La Villa, G.L., Laffi, G., and Gentilini, P. t(14;18) translocation in chronic hepatitis C virus infection. *Hepatology* 31: 474–479, **2000**.

Zignego, A.L., Ferri, C., Giannelli, F., Giannini, C., Caini, P., Monti, M., Marrocchi, M.E., Di Pietro, E., La Villa, G.L., Laffi, G., and Gentilini, P. Prevalence of bcl-2 rearrangement in patients with hepatitis C virus-related mixed cryoglobulinemia with or without B cell lymphomas. *Ann. Intern. Med.* 137: 571–580, **2002**.

Zuckerman, E., Zuckerman, T., Levine, A.M., Douer, D., Gutekunst, K., Mizokami, M., Qian, D.G., Velankar, M., Nathwani, B.N., and Fong, T.L. Hepatitis C virus infection in patients with B-cell non-Hodgkin lymphoma. *Ann. Intern. Med.* 127: 423–428, **1997**.

8
Retrovirus Family

Retroviruses have long been suspected to play a role in human cancers. They were initially identified as the causative agents of chicken sarcomas, murine mammary tumors and murine leukemias and lymphomas (see Chapter 1). Some retroviruses are acutely transforming viruses that evolved by capturing cellular genes during the course of virus replication, a process which resulted in the discovery of oncogenes (Stehelin et al., 1975). Their process of reverse transcription by the viral enzyme reverse transcriptase (Baltimore, 1970; Temin and Mizutani, 1970), preceding integration into the host cell genome, coupled with the experimental use of this enzyme, permitted the analysis of complementary DNA (cDNA) and, along these lines, the accurate composition of spliced RNA sequences. Moreover, retroviruses served as models to study the early events in animal carcinogenesis, in particular in lympho-proliferative conditions.

Three types of retroviral infection have been identified in humans. The first type – infections with human immunodeficiency viruses, HIV-1 and HIV-2 – cause severe immunosuppression and contribute indirectly to carcinogenesis. These viruses are not described in this chapter, and the interested reader is referred to specific textbooks dealing with infectious diseases. The well-studied structure of HIV particles shows characteristics of most retroviruses, and is depicted in Figure 8.1.

The other two types of retroviral infections in humans are represented by the human T-cell leukemia retrovirus and by a heterogeneous group of viruses that entered the human germline, the endogenous retroviruses. These types of infections will be described here.

Presently, the retrovirus family contains seven to eight clades, and representatives of human retroviruses are found in the beta-, delta-, and gamma-retroviral clades. HIV belongs into the subfamily of lentiviruses. In addition, a human spumavirus has been described as human foamy virus (Epstein et al., 1974). This virus may, however, originate from nonhuman primates and be transmitted accidentally to humans, though no clear-cut evidence is presently available for human-interspecies transmission. The individual retrovirus clades with representative members are shown in Figure 8.2.

Infections Causing Human Cancer. Harald zur Hausen
Copyright © 2006 WILEY-VCH Verlag GmbH & Co. KGaA, Weinheim
ISBN: 3-527-31056-8

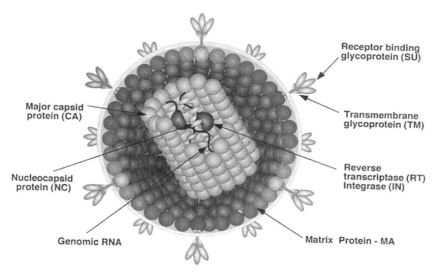

Fig. 8.1 The structural components of an HIV particle. (Reprinted from VIRUS TAXONOMY, Eighth Report of the International Committee on Taxonomy of Viruses, Vol 1, Fauquet, C.M., Mayo, M.A., Maniloff, J., Desselberger, U. and Ball, L.A. (Eds.), Part II – The DNA and RNA Reverse Transcribing Viruses, Retroviridae, 421. Copyright 2005, with permission from Elsevier.)

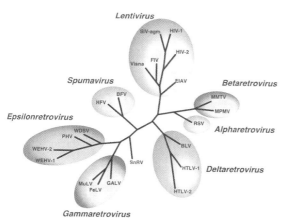

Fig. 8.2 The retrovirus family clades. (Reprinted from VIRUS TAXONOMY, Eighth Report of the International Committee on Taxonomy of Viruses, Vol 1, Fauquet, C.M., Mayo, M.A., Maniloff, J., Desselberger, U. and Ball, L.A. (Eds.), Part II – The DNA and RNA Reverse Transcribing Viruses, Retroviridae, 439. Copyright 2005, with permission from Elsevier.)

8.1
Human T-Lymphotropic Retrovirus (HTLV-1)

8.1.1
Historical Background

In 1979, a T-cell line was established by J. Minna, P. Bunn and A. Gazdar (quoted by Gallo, 2005) from a patient with a cutaneous T-cell lymphoma. From these cells a novel retrovirus, HTLV-1, has been identified (Poiesz et al., 1980). Prior to this discovery, in 1974 and 1977, Japanese researchers had described a specific T-cell leukemia in the coastal regions of Southern and Western Japan, with a remarkable clustering of cases in the Kyushu area (Yodoi et al., 1974; Uchiyama et al., 1977). The leukemic cells contained specific chromosomal markers and were cultivated *in vitro* (Miyoshi et al., 1979, 1980). The cells were found to contain a specific antigen which was detectable by indirect immunofluorescence tests with sera from adult T-cell leukemia (ATL) patients (Hinuma et al., 1981). Co-cultivation of these cells with normal lymphocytes resulted in immortalization of the latter (Miyoshi et al., 1981). In some of the cell lines a retrovirus was identified (Yoshida et al., 1982). The structure of the virus was determined by Seiki et al. (1983) and found to be identical with the Poiesz isolate.

8.1.2
Epidemiology and Transmission

Although HTLV-1 infections are most prevalent in the coastal regions of Southern Japan, virus carriers have also been noted in other regions of Asia, in the Caribbean, in South America, and in Africa (Blattner et al., 1982; Catovsky et al., 1982; Biggar et al., 1984; Merino et al., 1984; Saxinger et al., 1984). Besides Japan, focal areas of HTLV-1 infections occur in the South Pacific, in Iran, in Romania, in parts of West Africa, and in populations in the Western hemisphere, originating from endemic areas. ATL cases have also been observed in Italy (Manzari et al., 1985; Gradilone et al., 1986), New Guinea (Kazura et al., 1987), Israel (Ben-Ishai et al., 1985), the Arctic (Robert-Guroff et al., 1985), France, the United Kingdom (Taylor et al., 2005), and the United States (Blayney et al., 1983; Bunn et al., 1983). The number of HTLV-1 infected persons worldwide has been estimated at 10–20 million (de Thé and Bumford, 1993). In spite of a relative stability of the HTLV-1 genome during the course of evolution, strain differences among different geographical isolates (up to 9% of the nucleotide sequences) have been identified (Cassar et al., 2005). Phylogenetic studies permitted a classification in three well-defined subtypes: Cosmopolitan, Central African, and one found mainly in the Maroni Basin, French Guiana, and West Indies (Capdepont et al., 2005). A simian equivalent to HTLV-1 has been isolated from macaques and chimpanzees (Leendertz et al., 2004; for a review, see Franchini and Reitz, 1994).

Seroprevalence to HTLV-1 infections in endemic regions increases with greater age, and seropositivity is higher in females than in males (Blattner and Gallo, 1994).

Modes of transmission include the mother to infant route, and sexual as well as parenteral transmission. The breast milk of HTLV-1-positive mothers contains lymphocytes positive for HTLV-1 (Kinoshita et al., 1984). Thus, these infections occur mainly perinatally (Hino et al., 1985; Ando et al., 1987). Sexual transmission seems to occur more frequently from infected males to females with HTLV-1-infected lymphocytes in semen than from females to males (Brodine et al., 1992). Blood transfusions have also contributed in the past to HTLV-1 transmission (Sato and Okochi, 1986). Additional modes of transmission include needle sharing by intravenous drug users and male homosexual intercourse (Robert-Guroff et al., 1986; Bartholomew et al., 1987).

Only a small proportion of infected persons eventually develop ATL. After a latency period of several decades, approximately 6% of male and 2% of female carriers develop the disease (Taylor and Matsuoka, 2005). Risk factors for the development of ATL seem to include vertical or perinatal HTLV-1 transmission and increasing numbers of abnormal lymphocytes (Tajima, 1990; Hisada et al., 1998, 2001). The clinical picture of tropical spastic paraparesis, the HTLV-1-associated myelopathy (TSP/HAM) is mainly linked to infections at higher age, predominantly transmitted by sexual intercourse or blood products (Maloney and Blattner, 2003).

8.1.3
Viral Gene Organization and Gene Products

The HTLV-1 genome contains open reading frames (ORFs) typical for retroviruses, namely gag, pol, and env, and in addition a 3' region initially designated pX (Nicot et al., 2005). Several additional proteins are coded for by this region, among them two essential transcriptional and post-transcriptional regulators of viral gene expression, Tax and Rex proteins. A schematic outline of the genome organization and of virus-specific proteins transcribed from the genome is shown in Figure 8.3.

Following a short description of the structural proteins gag, pol, and env, and also of the virus-specific protease, the following sections will focus on proteins coded for by the X-region, which plays a clear role in HTLV-1-mediated oncogenesis and is profoundly engaged in regulatory processes of HTLV-1 and several cellular genes.

8.1.3.1   The gag Protein

The gag region is initially transcribed as a polyprotein precursor, and cleaved subsequently into the gag polypeptides, a 19-kDa matrix protein, the 24-kDa capsid protein, and a 15-kDa nucleocapsid protein (Copeland et al., 1983; Oroszlan et al., 1984). A post-transcriptional modification of p19 results in a covalently attached myristic acid tail at the amino terminus (Miwa et al., 1987). Myristoylation of the precursor 55-kDa gag protein emerges as a precondition for targeting it to the inner surface of the cell membrane (Hayakawa et al., 1992). Some immature precursors of the three major gag proteins are found in HTLV-1-infected cells (Cann and Chen, 1996).

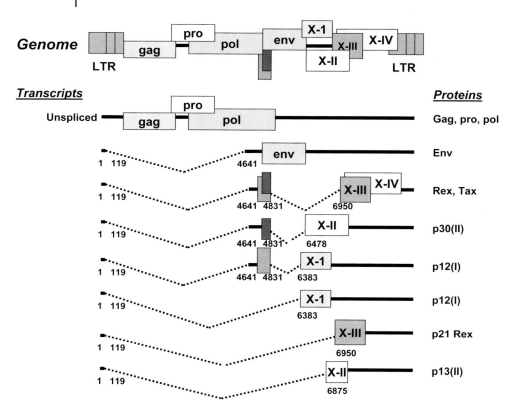

Fig. 8.3 Gene products of the HTLV-1 genome. (Modified from Nicot et al., 2005.)

8.1.3.2 HTLV Protease

The HTLV-1 protease is encoded by a region covering the 3' part of the gag and the 5' part of the pol ORFs. Ribosomal frameshifting as part of the gag polypeptide results in protease synthesis (Nam et al., 1988). This protease is responsible for processing of the mature gag products, and by autocatalyzation it generates the mature protease molecule (Kobayashi et al., 1991; Nam et al., 1993). The crystal structure of human T-cell leukemia virus protease has recently been unraveled (Li et al., 2005).

8.1.3.3 The Polymerase Protein

The pol region codes for an 896-amino acid product, including a ribosomal frame-shifting event, resulting eventually in an 864-amino acid peptide (Nam et al., 1988). The 5' end of the protein is responsible for the reverse transcriptase activity, while downstream sequences contain the information for the integrase and RNaseH functions. Divalent cations, most efficiently Mg^{2+}, are required for the reverse transcriptase function (Cann and Chen, 1996). The active HTLV-1 polymerase complex can exist as a p62/p49 heterodimer, formed by two cleaved products of the pol protein (Mitchell et al., 2006).

8.1.3.4 The env Protein

Depending on the cell line studied, the env glycoprotein is formed as a precursor protein of 61 to 69 kDa (Yamamoto et al., 1982; Lee et al., 1984; Schneider et al., 1984 a). The nonglycosylated precursor protein amounts to 54 kDa (Lee et al., 1984; Schneider et al., 1984 b). After cleavage of the precursor, a mature 46-kDa surface glycoprotein and a 21-kDa trans-membrane protein are formed, and Gp46 is shed from the surface of the cell. The conserved glycine-rich segment of the N-terminal fusion peptide of human T-cell leukemia virus type 1 transmembrane glycoprotein gp21 is a determinant of membrane fusion function and requires flexibility within the glycine-rich segment and hydrophobic contacts (Wilson et al., 2005).

8.1.3.5 The Tax Protein

The Tax proteins represent nonstructural regulatory proteins, occurring within the α-subgroup of retroviruses (for reviews, see Grassmann et al., 2005; Marriott and Semmes, 2005). These proteins are also required for viral replication, but stimulate at the same time proliferation of the infected host cells. In virus-producing cells, Tax acts as a transcriptional activator of the viral long terminal repeat (LTR). Tax does not bind directly to the promoter of the LTR but becomes linked with its N-terminus to the CREB protein which docks to the cyclic AMP-responsive motif of the LTR (Adya and Giam, 1995; Baranger et al., 1995). Tax represents a nuclear phosphoprotein, post-transcriptionally modified by ubiquitination (Chiari et al., 2004; Peloponese et al., 2004). Tax induces several cellular transcription factors, such as NF-κB, CREB, SRF and Ap-1 (Jeang, 2001; Azran et al., 2004), and also recruits transcriptional co-activators, such as CBP and p300 (Giebler et al., 1997; Bex et al., 1998; Harrod et al., 2000). The C-terminal activation domain of Tax attaches directly to the TATA-box-bound TBP protein (Caron et al., 1993), promoting the initiation of transcription and RNA polymerase elongation (Chung et al., 2003). Some of the early effects of Tax are shown schematically in Figure 8.4.

Tax expression profoundly modifies the cell cycle by accelerating the G_1-phase (Lemoine and Marriott, 2001). This seems to be due to transcriptional activation of cyclins E and D2. In addition, the levels of Cdk 4/6 and Cdk 2 are increased (Santiago et al., 1999; Huang et al., 2001). Tax binds directly to cyclins D3, D2, Cdk 4 and stabilizes cyclin D/Cdk4 complexes (Haller et al., 2002; Fraedrich et al., 2005). The additional binding to $p16^{INK4}$ prevents this cyclin-dependent kinase inhibitor from inactivating Cdk 4 and Cdk 6 (Low et al., 1997). As a result of binding to Cdk4, Tax promotes Rb phosphorylation and release of the transcription factor E2F, thus further

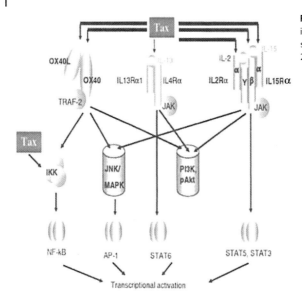

Fig. 8.4 Tax-induced pathways in stimulating cellular transcription. (Grassmann et al., 2005. With permission.)

facilitating cell-cycle progression (Lemasson et al., 1998; Ohtani et al., 2000). Moreover, Tax binds to the hypophosphorylated form of Rb and promotes its proteasome degradation (Kehn et al., 2005). Tax also constitutively activates NF-κB by forming a ternary complex of IKK/PP2A/Tax in which PP2A becomes inactivated (Carter et al., 2001; Fu et al., 2003).

Tax impairs the function of p53 (Mulloy et al., 1998; Pise-Masison et al., 1998). Tax-expressing cells fail to generate an appropriate p53-dependent response to DNA damage. Although Tax does not bind directly to p53, the effect seems to be due to a nuclear stabilization of transcriptionally inactive p53 (Cereseto et al., 1996; Tubakin-Fix et al., 2006), possibly due to a competitive binding of Tax and p53 to the ubiquitous co-activator CREB-binding protein CBP/p300, thus interfering with the p53 target gene activation (Suzuki et al., 1999a; Van et al., 2001). Tax activates the p21[WAF1] gene independent of p53 (de la Fuente et al., 2000). In contrast to regular p21 functions, Tax-induced expression is associated with resistance to apoptosis (Kawata et al., 2003).

Tax also binds and interferes with functions of the Drosophila discs large tumor suppressor protein, hDLG (Suzuki et al., 1999b), and in this function resembles the E6 protein of high-risk papillomaviruses (see Chapter 5). The repression of cyclin A by Tax may permit redundant DNA replication and contribute to aneuploidy (Kibler and Jeang, 2001).

Although Tax expression impairs the induction of human telomerase reverse transcriptase (hTERT), transduction of Tax into primary lymphocytes is sufficient to activate and maintain telomerase expression and telomere length when cultured in the absence of any exogenous stimulation (Sinha-Datta et al., 2004). Tax has a profound effect on a protein complex named shelterin, which includes the telomerase DNA-binding proteins TRF1, TRF2, and Pot1 (Escoffier et al., 2005). The down-regulation of hTERT transcription by Tax in HTLV-1 transformed or in Tax-expressing T lymphocytes is correlated with a significant increase of TRF2 and/or Pot1mRNAs. This interesting down-regulation of hTERT by a viral oncogene has been proposed also to contribute at an early phase of carcinogenesis to the intensive ploidy changes associated with the development of HTLV-1-associated malignancies (Escoffier et al., 2005).

De-novo expression of Tax causes accumulation of cells in G_2/M (Tyler et al., 2001; Liang et al., 2002; Haoudi and Semmes, 2003; Kino and Pavlakis, 2004). Tax forms a complex with Chk2 and Chk1, both of which are in the ATM/ATR signaling pathway and normally activate several downstream targets including p53 (Marriott and Semmes, 2005). The progression through mitosis by Tax seems to be delayed by its direct binding to, and premature activation of, APC^{clb2p}, which leads to improper cyclin B and securing degradation (Liu et al., 2003, 2005).

Tax suppresses nucleotide excision repair (Kao and Marriott, 1999). This inhibition correlates with the transcriptional activation of the proliferating cell nuclear antigen (PCNA) promoter (Ressler et al., 1997; Kao et al., 2000; Lemoine et al., 2000). Tax expression results in increased frequency of mutations within the cellular genome (Miyake et al., 1999), most likely as the result of a failing nuclear excision repair in response to environmental mutagens. Tax also suppresses the human DNA polymerase β promoter (Jeang et al., 1990); this enzyme is involved in base excision and mismatch DNA repair (Wilson et al., 1988). It has been shown directly that Tax expression specifically suppresses base excision repair of DNA (Philpott and Buehring, 1999). In addition, Tax also seems negatively to influence the repair of double-stranded DNA breaks (Ng et al., 2001). Apparently, the Ku80 protein plays an important role in the induction of micronuclei formation and Tax-mediated clastogenic activity, since Ku80-negative cells are protected from these aberrations (Majone et al., 2005). Thus, Tax expression is responsible for various forms of genetic instability.

8.1.3.6 The Rex Protein

Rex is a 27-kDA RNA binding protein that is essential for the splicing and transport of viral mRNA (Kashanchi and Brady, 2005). Although not required for cellular immortalization *in vitro*, Rex is indispensable for efficient viral replication, infection and spreading of the infection (Ye et al., 2003; Younis and Green, 2005). Rex influences the cytoplasmic levels of singly spliced and unspliced mRNA at the expense of doubly spliced mRNA (Hidaka et al., 1988). Rex expression leads to a reduction of splicing and to increased stability of mRNAs (Grone et al., 1996).

Rex proteins are found in multimers that are required for their function (Malim et al., 1990). A highly basic N-terminal RNA-binding domain, located within the first 19 amino acids, is essential for binding of Rex to the Rex-responsive element within the U and R regions of the 3' LTR (Seiki et al., 1988; Bogerd et al., 1991; Grassmann et al., 1991). The same domain serves as a nucleolus-targeting signal and mediates the transport of unspliced viral mRNA into the cytoplasm (Siomi et al., 1988; Nosaka et al., 1989; Bohnlein et al., 1991).

Another domain within residues 66–118 is important for the interaction with several cellular factors (Hope et al., 1991; Weichselbraun et al., 1992). It is also important for targeting Rex to the nuclear pore complex (Palmeri and Malim, 1996; Rehberger et al., 1997). Many of these cellular factors bind to the Rex-responsive elements in the 3′ LTR and interfere with Rex binding. This accounts for the heterogeneous nuclear ribonucleoprotein A1, the splicing factor SF2, the exportin protein, CRM1, and the nucleolar protein B-23 (Dodon et al., 2002). Rex functions as a multimer (Malim et al., 1990), the nucleotides 54–69 being critical for multimerization (Weichselbraun et al., 1992).

The available data indicate that Rex plays an important role as a post-transcriptional regulator of HTLV-1.

8.1.3.7 The p12(I) Protein

This protein is encoded by either singly or doubly spliced mRNA by splicing from nucleotide 119 from the LTR to the splice acceptor at position 6383 (Ciminale et al., 1992; Koralnik et al., 1992, 1993). The doubly spliced product should yield a Rex/p12(I) hybrid protein, but expression of this message in HeLa cells leads only to p12(I) (Koralnik et al., 1992). p12(I) is found in the cellular endomembranes, in the endoplasmic reticulum, and in the Golgi apparatus (Koralnik et al., 1993; Ding et al., 2001; Johnson et al., 2001). This protein is not required for in-vitro replication of HTLV-1 (Derse et al., 1997; Robek et al., 1998; Albrecht et al., 2000), but contributes to infectivity *in vivo*. CTLs and serum antibodies from HTLV-1-infected persons recognize peptides within this protein (Dekaban et al., 2000; Pique et al., 2000).

The p12(I) protein is highly hydrophobic and contains four proline-rich (PXXP) Src homology 3 (SH3) binding domains (Franchini, 1995). It is able to form dimers (Trovato et al., 1999). Interestingly, this protein shows a 50% amino acid identity with part of the bovine papillomavirus (BPV) E5 protein (Franchini et al., 1993). It also cooperates with BPV E5 in a focus formation assay. Similar to E5, p12(I) binds to the 16-kDa subunit of the vacuolar ATPase (Franchini et al., 1993; Koralnik et al., 1995). It also interacts with the IL-2 receptor β and γ_c chains and decreases their surface expression (Mulloy et al., 1996). As a consequence of this interaction, p12(I) induces an increase in DNA binding and in transcriptional activity of STAT5 (Nicot et al., 2001). By STAT5 activation, p12(I) induces synthesis of IL-2 and contributes to the proliferation of infected T cells (Nicot et al., 2005).

p12(I) also influences T-cell activation and permits T cells to enter S-phase, even under conditions of suboptimal antigen stimulation, and induces a linker of activated T- cell-independent increase in intracellular calcium levels (Lewis, 2001). It has been suggested that p12(I) interferes with MHC presentation of viral peptides, as it binds to MHC class I heavy chains encoded by HLA-A2, -B7, and -Cw4 alleles (Nicot et al., 2005). This results in a failure of these MHC class I heavy chains to associate with β_2-microglobulin, in retransportation to the cytosol, and in degradation by the proteasome complex.

8.1.3.8 The p30(II) Protein

p30(II) represents a nucleolar protein, and is encoded by a doubly spliced mRNA, placing the Tax AUG in frame with ORF II (Ciminale et al., 1992; Koralnik et al., 1992). A CTL immune response and antibodies against this protein are observed in HTLV-1-infected individuals (Pique et al., 2000). P30(II) is a negative regulator of viral gene expression (Nicot et al., 2004). The autologous down-regulation of HTLV-1 expression seems to permit viral persistence within an immunocompetent host. Freshly isolated lymphatic cells from HTLV-1-infected individuals express only low or almost undetectable levels of viral antigens (Kinoshita et al., 1989; Gessain et al., 1991; Berneman et al., 1992; Yoshida, 2005).

p30(II) selectively reduces the level of Tax/Rex mRNA, but does not substantially affect the levels of Gag-Pol, Env, and p21Rex spliced mRNA (Nicot et al., 1993, 2004; Younis et al., 2004). The reduction is accompanied by nuclear accumulation of Tax/Rex mRNA which is bound specifically to p30(II). The trapping of Tax/Rex mRNA results in a reduction of productive viral replication.

p30(II) expression also affects several cellular transcription factors. It interacts with the transcriptional cofactors p300/CREB-binding protein. Overexpression represses cellular CREB-driven reporter gene activity, independent of Tax expression, whereas lower concentrations enhance the HTLV-1 LTR-driven reported gene activity, again independent of Tax expression (Zhang et al., 2000, 2001). p30(II) co-localizes with p300 in cell nuclei and binds directly to CBP/p300 in cells (Zhang et al., 2001). Other cellular genes affected by p30(II) are integrins and cadherins. Their expression is repressed, whereas the expression of genes involved in T-cell activation and apoptosis is increased (Michael et al., 2004). p30(II) also interacts with Myc-containing transcription complexes and transactivates the human D2 promoter (Awasthi et al., 2005). Co-expression of this protein with Myc enhances Myc-dependent cellular transformation of immortalized human fibroblasts. Thus, p30(II) may contribute to HTLV-1-mediated cell transformation.

8.1.3.9 The p13(II) Protein

p13(II) mRNA was initially detected in HTLV-1-positive cell lines and in patients with ATL (Berneman et al., 1992; Koralnik et al., 1992; Cereseto et al., 1997). The protein corresponds to the 87 C-terminal amino acids of p30(II), and is expressed from a singly spliced mRNA (Ciminale et al., 1992; Koralnik et al., 1992). p13(II) targets primarily the inner part of the mitochondrial membrane and becomes an integral protein at this site (Ciminale et al., 1999; D'Agustino et al., 2002). It induces marked changes in the morphology of mitochondria, which seem to swell. p13(II) increases mitochondrial permeability to small monovalent cations, particularly to K^+ (D'Agustino et al., 2002). The protein also negatively influences cell proliferation at high density and tumor growth *in vivo* (Silic-Benussi et al., 2004). In addition, the protein increases sensitivity to ceramide-induced apoptosis in T cells, although p13(II) itself did not induce apoptosis (Silic-Benussi et al., 2004; D'Agostino et al., 2005; Hiraragi et al., 2005). The Fas ligand-induced apoptosis of T cells was also increased by p13(II).

8.1.4
Diseases Caused by HTLV-1 Infection

The most prominent disease that may develop as consequence of a persisting HTLV-1 infection is represented by ATL, which is discussed separately in the following sections. The other relatively prominent condition that may be caused by long-term persistence of this virus is HAM, or TSP. This condition was initially observed in the West Indies (Gessain et al., 1985), but occurs in all areas where HTLV-1 infections are endemic (Gessain et al., 1986; Osame et al., 1987; Rodgers-Johnson et al., 1988). The lifetime risk for the development of HAM/TSP in HTLV-1 infected persons has been estimated at < 1% (Kaplan et al., 1990).

Besides neurological symptoms, the cerebrospinal fluid of these patients contains antibodies to HTLV-1 and reveals lymphocytic pleocytosis. In the peripheral blood, the lymphocyte counts remain normal, but some lymphocytes reveal an atypical morphology (Osame et al., 1989; Furukawa et al., 1992).

Although a number of attempts have been made to link additional hematologic disorders to HTLV-1 infections, the reported data remain non-reproducible. One other rare complication of HTLV-1 infections is represented by chronic inflammatory arthropathy (Kitajima et al., 1991; Sato et al., 1991; Nishioka et al., 1993). Similar arthropathies have been observed in HTLV-1 transgenic mice (Iwakura et al., 1991). Uveitis has also been reported to be linked to HTLV-1 infections (Nakao et al., 1989; Mochizuki et al., 1992), and has also been observed in a rabbit infected with HTLV-1 (Taguchi et al., 1993).

ATL is also associated with an impairment of the cellular immune response (Hinuma et al., 1983; Capell et al., 1987; Taguchi and Miyoshi, 1989; Murai et al., 1990). This may cause problems with parasitic or other opportunistic infections (O'Doherty et al., 1984; Newton et al., 1992; Robinson et al., 1994).

8.1.5
Immune Response to HTLV-1 Infections

In contrast to the sequence variation, observed for example in HIV infections, and in spite of an error-prone reverse transcriptase, there is relatively little variation between different HTLV-1 isolates (Daenke et al., 1990; Kinoshita et al., 1991; Slattery et al., 1999). In HTLV-1-infected persons, more than 30% of peripheral mononuclear cells and more than 50% of CD4$^+$ cells represent proliferating provirus-containing cells (Cavrois et al., 1996; Etoh et al., 1997; Eiraku et al., 1998). In ATL patients the tumor cells are mostly of CD4$^+$ and CD25$^+$ mature T-lymphocyte phenotype (Uchiyama et al., 1977). HTLV-1 virions seem to be absent, and virus-specific mRNA or proteins are difficult to detect within those cells. Yet, an antibody response to HTLV-1, including IgM antibodies (Nagasato et al., 1991; Kira et al., 1992; Ishihara et al., 1994) and an activated CTL response, particularly to Tax (Jacobson et al.,

1990; Kannagi et al., 1991; Goon et al., 2004a), point to HTLV-1 antigen expression. Indeed, a low level of HTLV-1mRNA has been detected in non-cultivated tumor cells and in lymph nodes of ATL patients (Kinoshita et al., 1989; Oshima et al., 1996). The inoculation of uncultured formalin-treated ATL-cells into naïve rats also resulted in the induction of a HTLV-1-specific T-cell response (Kurihara et al., 2005).

If explanted into tissue culture under appropriate conditions, CD4$^+$ cells from about 50% of HTLV-1-infected persons begin to express viral antigens starting 12 h after explantation (Hinuma et al., 1982; Hanon et al., 2000). The addition of CD8$^+$ T cells reduces the viral antigen expression in a dose-dependent manner. Thus, CTLs present in the CD8$^+$ T-cell preparations seem able to suppress Tax and other viral antigen expression (Bangham, 2003; Bangham and Osame, 2005). *In vivo*, CTLs appear to play a very active role in eliminating Tax-expressing cells (Vine et al., 2004). Thus, a very low Tax expression may permit escape of HTLV-1 provirus-carrying cells from immune surveillance mechanisms. This leaves the question open as to how HTLV-1 infections are transmitted to other susceptible T cells. It has been suggested that this may occur through cell contact-triggered "virological synapses" formed due to virus-induced polarization of the cytoskeleton (Igakura et al., 2003). However, an alternative route may exist via cellular exosomes containing the whole viral genome and being fused to previously uninfected cells (Duelli et al., 2005).

ATL-cells from approximately half of the patients do not induce viral antigens upon *in-vitro* cultivation (Kannagi et al., 2005). The HTLV-1 genome appears to be irreversibly silenced. It has been suggested that this is due to deletions in the 5' LTR region or within the gag/pol genes (Konishi et al., 1984; Tamiya et al., 1996).

Interestingly, there seems to exist no correlation between proviral load and CTL activity (Kubota et al., 2000; Wodarz et al., 2001). A slightly positive correlation appears to exist in TSP patients, who usually reveal a higher frequency of HTLV-1-specific CTLs (Elovaara et al., 1993; Greten et al., 1998). In contrast to TSP patients, who commonly reveal highly activated CTL activity, HTLV-1-specific CTLs are only rarely induced in ATL patients (for a review, see Kannagi et al., 2005). They are apparently present, but expand insufficiently (Arnulf et al., 2004), a finding which points to some immune suppression or tolerance in these patients.

Genetic polymorphisms influence the efficacy of the immune response to HTLV-1 (Nagai et al., 1998; Jeffery et al., 1999, 2000; Vine et al., 2002). One strong genetic determinant is an HLA-class I genotype; indeed, genes HLA-A*02 and HLA-Cw*08 were associated with a lower proviral load and a lower risk of TSP. It has been suggested that these data point to a particularly efficient CTL response in persons with those genotypes (Bangham and Osame, 2005). Minor sequence variations within HLA-A*02 were associated with significant differences in the prevalence of TSP in Kagoshima, Japan (Furukawa et al., 2000). Another genotype increasing the risk for TSP development is HLA-DRB1*0101 (HLA-DR1) (Usuku et al., 1990; Nishimura et al., 1991; Kitze et al., 1998; Sabouri et al., 2005).

Much less is known about the effects of natural killer (NK) cells, although HTLV-1-associated inflammatory conditions reveal a lower frequency of NK cells (Fujihara et al., 1991; Yu et al., 1991; Saito et al., 2003). Similarly, the role of CD4$^+$ (helper) T cells is also poorly understood, although they seem to recognize most commonly the env protein, contrasting the preferential recognition of Tax by CD8[+] T cells (Goon et al., 2004 b).

8.1.6
Animal Studies

HTLV-1 effectively infects rabbits (Akagi et al., 1985; Lairmore et al., 1992), cynomolgus and squirrel monkeys (Nakamura et al., 1987; Murata et al., 1996; Kazanji, 2000) and, less efficiently, rats (Suga et al., 1991; Ibrahim et al., 1994).

Oral infection of rats results in virus persistence without measurable immune response (Kato et al., 1998), whereas intravenous routes of infection lead to strong antibody and T-cell responses (Kannagi et al., 2000). HTLV-1 infected rats appear to be a model for TSP, since immunosuppressed animals develop spastic paraparesis with degenerative spinal cord and peripheral nerve lesions several months following infection (Ishiguro et al., 1992; Kushida et al., 1993). HTLV-1 provirus was found in microglial cells and macrophages at lesional sites (Kasai et al., 1999). An ATL-like lymphoproliferative disease was established in adult nude rats after inoculation of HTLV-1 immortalized cell lines (Ohashi et al., 1999). Tax-specific small interfering RNA (siRNA) protected against this proliferative condition (Nomura et al., 2004).

Rabbits turned out to be suitable animal models to study HTLV-1 infection, although these animals rarely, if ever, show clinical symptoms (Lairmore et al., 2005). Rabbits can transfer the virus via blood, semen, or milk (Kotani et al., 1986; Uemura et al., 1987; Hirose et al., 1988; Iwahara et al., 1990). Rabbits also served as convenient models to study the development of antibodies against HTLV-1 (Cockerell et al., 1990), and to analyze env epitopes for protective immunization studies (Tanaka et al., 1994). Furthermore, they permitted an evaluation of the role of accessory proteins of the pX region for in-vivo infections (Collins et al., 1998; Bartoe et al., 2000; Silverman et al., 2004).

Experimental infection of nonhuman primates can be achieved by the inoculation of HTLV-1-transformed cell lines. Some of these animals may develop malignant lymphomas (Homma et al., 1984; Kanki et al., 1985), although the majority of the infections remain asymptomatic. Most experimental studies were conducted in squirrel monkeys and macaques. These animals also served for testing potential HTLV-1 vaccines (Nakamura et al., 1987) and hyperimmune globulin treatment (Murata et al., 1996; Akari et al., 1997).

ATL cells grow successfully in severe combined immunodeficiency (SCID) mice (Ishihara et al., 1992; Feuer et al., 1993), which succumb to lymphomas. Non-leukemic HTLV-1-infected cells only grow in these mice when their NK cell activity has been suppressed (Feuer et al., 1995). Transgenic mouse models have been used successfully to study the role of targeted tax gene expression and the respective host response. By using the HTLV-1 LTR promoter, the development of neurofibromas was observed (Hinrichs et al., 1987), while in other analogous experiments lymphocyte-mediated arthropathy developed (Iwakura et al., 1991; Yamamoto et al., 1993; Fujisawa et al., 1996). Tax expression under the control of the CD3-ε promoter-enhancer led to salivary and mammary adenomas (Hall et al., 1998). These experiments underlined the oncogene function of the *Tax* gene.

By targeting the mature T-cell compartment with the GzmB promoter, large granular lymphocytic tumors developed (Grossman et al., 1995). Cell lines derived from such tumors exhibited high levels of NF-κB expression and a wide variety of NF-κB target genes (Grossman and Ratner, 1997; Portis et al., 2001). The significance of these models is somewhat questionable in view of the different tumor type induced under these conditions in comparison to ATL.

Animal models are certainly useful in analyzing specific functions of viral genes. However, they have their limitations in cases where the mode of persistence or the induced clinical symptoms do not parallel the clinical situation in humans.

8.1.7
Mechanism of Cell Transformation by HTLV-1

The X-region of the HTLV genome carrying genes for the regulatory Tax proteins is unique among α-retroviruses. These proteins are required for productive viral infection, as well as for growth stimulation of infected lymphatic cells. Even in non-leukemic HTLV-1 positive patients, the infected cells expand clonally and persist for prolonged periods of time (Etoh et al., 1997; Gabet et al., 2000).

The virus enters CD4 cells via their GLUT1 (glucose transporter) receptor (for a review, see Manel et al., 2005). Other cell types can also be infected in patients, specifically CD8$^+$ lymphocytes, monocytes, and B lymphocytes (Koyanagi et al., 1993; Eiraku et al., 1998; Nagai et al., 2001; Grant et al., 2002). *In vitro* even non-lymphatic cells may become infected, such as primary human endothelial cells (Ho et al., 1984; Hoxie et al., 1984), microglial cells (Hoffman et al., 1992), and basal mammary epithelial cells (LeVasseur et al., 1998).

The primary factor for the stimulation of cell growth is the transcriptional activator Tax. This protein can be considered as a viral oncogene since it is able, in cooperation with Ras, to immortalize primary rodent cells which produce tumors when inoculated into nude mice (Pozzatti et al., 1990). In NIH 3T3 and Rat 1 cells, Tax antagonizes contact inhibition, and induces anchorage-independent growth in soft agar and nude mouse tumorigenicity (Tanaka et al., 1990). Tax-transformed cells also reveal an elevated resistance to apoptosis (Fujita and Shiku, 1995). Tax is also able to immortalize human T cells *in vitro*: if expressed from rhabdoviral (Grassmann et al., 1989, 1992) or retroviral vectors (Akagi and Shimotohno, 1993), T cells become immortalized, but depend on IL-2 for growth (Akagi et al., 1995; Rosin et al., 1998; Schmitt et al., 1998).

The analysis of Tax mutants permitted analyses of cellular factors required for immortalization. Interestingly, Tax mutants deficient for either interfering with CREB- or NF-κB pathways were still able to transform rodent fibroblasts (Smith and Greene, 1991; Yamaoka et al., 1996; Matsumoto et al., 1997). On the other hand, the serum responsive factor (SRF) was found to play a major role in the transformation of primary rat fibroblasts by Tax (Matsumoto et al., 1997). For immortalization of human lymphocytes, the CREB and/or SPF pathways had to be activated to clonally expand CD4$^+$ and CD8$^+$ T cells (Akagi et al., 1997; Rosin et al., 1998).

In Tax-immortalized cells, and also in ATL cells, Tax induces a multitude of changes in cellular gene expression and signaling cascades. The α-chain of the IL-2 receptor is up-regulated (Ballard et al., 1988; Ruben et al., 1988) which, jointly with β- and the γ-chain, forms the high-affinity IL-2 receptor (IL-2R) (Grassmann et al., 2005). In addition, the IL-2 gene is also activated by Tax (Hoyos et al., 1989; McGuire et al., 1993; Good et al., 1996). The hypothesis that Tax causes T-cell proliferation by an autocrine IL-2/IL-2R loop is weakened by Tax-immortalized cells, which still require the exogenous addition of IL-2 for proliferation. Besides IL-2, IL-15mRNA expression and its receptor, IL-15Rα is also elevated by Tax (Azimi et al., 1998; Mariner et al., 2001). In HTLV-1-transformed cells IL-13 is also up-regulated (Chung et al., 2003; Wäldele et al., 2004). Increased levels of IL-13 are also noted in Hodgkin's lymphoma cells. In addition to interleukins, the expression of one member of the tumor necrosis factor (TNF) family, OX40, is also increased (Pankow et al., 2000) and constitutively expressed in HTLV-1-producing cells, but not in resting T cells.

Several signaling cascades are influenced by the Tax activity. The phosphorylated signal transducers of activated T cells (STAT5 a and STAT5 b) are highly activated in HTLV-1-immortalized T-cell lines and in lymphocytes from ATL patients (Migone et al., 1995). The expression of TGF-β is also stimulated by Tax (Kim et al., 1990), but its signaling activity is negatively influenced by a Tax-mediated repression of the DNA-binding activity of transcription factors Smad3 and Smad4 (Mori et al., 2001; Arnulf et al., 2002; Lee et al., 2002). Another enzyme involved in signaling events influenced by Tax is the phosphoinositide 3-kinase (P13K) (Liu et al., 2001). One of this enzyme's downstream targets is Akt (Kelly-Welch et al., 2003), the pathway responsible for growth stimulation and anti-apoptotic activity.

The stimulation of various phases of the cell cycle by Tax and the interaction of Tax with p53 and Rb has been discussed previously. Overexpression of Tax, similar to other growth-promoting genes such as Myc, E2F, E7 and E1A, triggers apoptosis. At the same time, Tax possesses an anti-apoptotic effect which seems to be mediated by the transactivation of cellular regulators of apoptosis, such as Bcl-Xl and Bcl-2A1 (Tsukahara et al., 1999; Nicot et al., 2000; de la Fuente et al., 2003). Clearly, there is a fine balance between apoptotic and anti-apoptotic effects (as is also noted for other viral oncogenes), and this plays an important role in cell transformation by Tax. The long latency periods for ATL development indicate, in addition, that specific host cell modifications must take place prior to malignant conversion (see chapter on cellular interfering factors). The previously reported effects of Tax on DNA damage and genetic and chromosomal instability further underline the importance of host cell modifications prior to the onset of malignant transformation.

The available data provide sufficient evidence that HTLV-1 infection via Tax induction acts as a direct carcinogen for humans. In line with other human tumorvirus infections, viral oncogene expression *per se* is not sufficient for tumor induction. The latter requires changes in specific host cell genes which counteract the oncogenic function of the infectious agent.

8.1.8
Prevention and Therapy

The most effective mode of preventing HTLV-1 infections is the avoidance of breast-feeding in case of virus-carrying mothers. Although some attempts have been made in animals to develop vaccines against this infection, it is presently difficult to foresee their clinical application (for a review, see Lairmore et al., 2005). The comparatively low rate of mutations of this virus in relation to other retroviruses should render it a suitable candidate for vaccine development. The low number of infected persons globally, however, will be a restrictive factor for the interests of pharmaceutical companies engaged in vaccine production.

Although combination chemotherapy protocols have been developed for the treatment of ATL, the median survival time does not exceed 13 months (Yamada et al., 2001). Some ATL patients respond to anti-CD25 monoclonal antibody treatment (Waldmann et al., 1993), and a higher response rate has been achieved with the combination of azidothymidine and interferon-α, without however preventing a relapse (Gill et al., 1995; Hermine et al., 1995). A limited hope is presently based on allogenic human stem cell transplantation therapies leading to a longlasting complete remission in some ATL patients (Tsukasaki et al., 1999; Utsunomiya et al., 2001).

References

Adya, N. and Giam CZ. Distinct regions in human T-cell lymphotropic virus type I tax mediate interactions with activator protein CREB and basal transcription factors. *J. Virol.* 69: 1834–1841, **1995**.

Akagi, T. and Shimotohno, K. Proliferative response of Tax1-transduced primary human T cells to anti-CD3 antibody stimulation by an interleukin-2-independent pathway. *J. Virol.* 67: 1211–1217, **1993**.

Akagi, T., Takeda, I., Oka, T., Ohtsuki, Y., Yano, S., and Miyoshi, I. Experimental infection of rabbits with human T-cell leukemia virus type I. *Jpn. J. Cancer Res.* 76: 86–94, **1985**.

Akagi, T., Ono, H., and Shimotohno, K. Characterization of T cells immortalized by Tax1 of human T-cell leukemia virus type 1. *Blood* 86: 4243–4249, **1995**.

Akagi, T., Ono, H., Nyunoya, H., and Shimotohno, K. Characterization of peripheral blood T-lymphocytes transduced with HTLV-I Tax mutants with different trans-activating phenotypes. *Oncogene* 14: 2071–2078, **1997**.

Akari, H., Suzuki, T., Ikeda, K., Hoshino, H., Tomono, T., Murotsuka, T., Terao, K., Ito, H., and Yoshikawa, Y. Prophylaxis of experimental HTLV-I infection in cynomolgus monkeys by passive immunization. *Vaccine* 15: 1391–1395, **1997**.

Albrecht, B., Collins, N.D., Burniston, M.T., Nisbet, J.W., Ratner, L., Green, P.L., and Lairmore, M.D. Human T-lymphotropic virus type 1 open reading frame I p12(I) is required for efficient viral infectivity in primary lymphocytes. *J. Virol.* 74: 9828–9835, **2000**.

Ando, Y., Nakano, S., Saito, K., Shimamoto, I., Ichijo, M., Toyama, T., and Hinuma, Y. Transmission of adult T-cell leukemia retrovirus (HTLV-I) from mother to child: comparison of bottle- with breast-fed babies. *Jpn. J. Cancer Res.* 78: 322–324, **1987**.

Arnulf, B., Villemain, A., Nicot, C., Mordelet, E., Charneau, P., Kersual, J., Zermati, Y., Mauviel, A., Bazarbachi, A., and Hermine, O. Human T-cell lymphotropic virus oncoprotein Tax represses TGF-beta 1 signaling in human T cells via c-Jun activation: a potential mechanism of HTLV-I leukemogenesis. *Blood* 100: 4129–4138, **2002**.

Arnulf, B., Thorel, M., Poirot, Y., Tamouza, R., Boulanger, E., Jaccard, A., Oksenhendler, E., Hermine, O., and Pique, C. Loss of the ex vivo but not the reinducible CD8+ T-cell response to Tax in human T-cell leukemia virus type 1-infected patients with adult T-cell leukemia/lymphoma. *Leukemia* 18: 126–132, **2004**.

Awasthi, S., Sharma, A., Wong, K., Zhang, J., Matlock, E.F., Rogers, L., Motloch, P., Takemoto, S., Taguchi, H., Cole, M.D., Lüscher, B., Dittrich, O., Tagami, H., Nakatani, Y., McGee, M., Girard, A.M., Gaughan, L., Robson, C.N., Monnat, R.J., Jr., and Harrod, R. A human T-cell lymphotropic virus type 1 enhancer of Myc transforming potential stabilizes Myc-TIP60 transcriptional interactions. *Mol. Cell. Biol.* 25: 6178–6198, **2005**.

Azimi, N., Brown, K., Bamford, R.N., Tagaya, Y., Siebenlist, U., Waldmann, T.A. Human T cell lymphotropic virus type I Tax protein trans-activates interleukin 15 gene transcription through an NF-kappaB site. *Proc. Natl. Acad. Sci. USA* 95: 2452–2457, **1998**.

Azran, I., Schavinsky-Khrapunsky, Y., and Aboud, M. Role of Tax protein in human T-cell leukemia virus type-I leukemogenicity. *Retrovirology* 1: 20, **2004**.

Ballard, D.W., Bohnlein, E., Lowenthal, J.W., Wano, Y., Franza, B.R., Greene, W.C. HTLV-I tax induces cellular proteins that activate the kappa B element in the IL-2 receptor alpha gene. *Science* 241: 1652–1655, **1988**.

Baltimore, D. RNA-dependent DNA polymerase in virions of RNA tumour viruses. *Nature* 226: 1209–1211, **1970**.

Bangham, C.R. Human T-lymphotropic virus type 1 (HTLV-1): persistence and immune control. *Int. J. Hematol.* 78: 297–303, **2003**.

Bangham, C.R. and Osame, M. Cellular immune response to HTLV-1. *Oncogene* 24: 6035–6046, **2005**.

Baranger, A.M., Palmer, C.R., Hamm, M.K., Giebler, H.A., Brauweiler, A., Nyborg, J.K., and Schepartz, A. Mechanism of DNA-binding enhancement by the human T-cell leukaemia virus transactivator Tax. *Nature* 376: 606–608, **1995**.

Bartholomew, C., Saxinger, W.C., Clark, J.W., Gail, M., Dudgeon, A., Mahabir, B., Hull-Drysdale, B., Cleghorn, F., Gallo, R.C., and Blattner, W.A. Transmission of HTLV-I and HIV among homosexual men in Trinidad. *JAMA* 257: 2604–2608, **1987**.

Bartoe, J.T., Albrecht, B., Collins, N.D., Robek, M.D., Ratner, L., Green, P.L., and Lairmore, M.D. Functional role of pX open reading frame II of human T-lymphotropic virus type 1 in maintenance of viral loads in vivo. *J. Virol.* 74: 1094–1100, **2000**.

Ben-Ishai, Z., Haas, M., Triglia, D., Lee, V., Nahmias, J., Bar-Shany, S., Jensen, F.C. Human T-cell lymphotropic virus type-I antibodies in Falashas and other ethnic groups in Israel. *Nature* 315: 665–666, **1985**.

Berneman, Z.N., Gartenhaus, R.B., Reitz, M.S., Jr., Blattner, W.A., Manns, A., Hanchard, B., Ikehara, O., Gallo, R.C., and Klotman, M.E. Expression of alternatively spliced human T-lymphotropic virus type I pX mRNA in infected cell lines and in primary uncultured cells from patients with adult T-cell leukemia/lymphoma and healthy carriers. *Proc. Natl. Acad. Sci. USA* 89: 3005–3009, **1992**.

Bex, F., Yin, M.J., Burny, A., Gaynor, R.B. Differential transcriptional activation by human T-cell leukemia virus type 1 Tax mutants is mediated by distinct interactions with CREB binding protein and p300. *Mol. Cell Biol.* 18: 2392–2405, **1998**.

Biggar, R.J., Saxinger, C., Gardiner, C., Collins, W.E., Levine, P.H., Clark, J.W., Nkrumah, F.K., and Blattner, W.A. Type-I HTLV antibody in urban and rural Ghana, West Africa. *Int. J. Cancer.* 34: 215–219, **1984**.

Blattner, W.A. and Gallo, R.C. Epidemiology of HTLV-I and HTLV-II infection. In: Takatsuki, K. (Ed.), *Adult T-Cell Leukaemia.* Oxford University Press, pp. 45–90, **1994**.

Blattner, W.A., Kalyanaraman, V.S., Robert-Guroff, M., Lister, T.A., Galton, D.A., Sarin, P.S., Crawford, M.H., Catovsky, D., Greaves, M., and Gallo, R.C. The human type-C retrovirus, HTLV, in Blacks from the Caribbean region, and relationship to adult T-cell leukemia/lymphoma. *Int. J. Cancer* 30(3): 257–264, **1982**.

Blayney, D.W., Jaffe, E.S., Blattner, W.A., Cossman, J., Robert-Guroff, M., Longo, D.L., Bunn, P.A., Jr., and Gallo, R.C. The human T-cell leukemia/lymphoma virus associated with American adult T-cell leukemia/lymphoma. *Blood* 62: 401–405, **1983**.

Bogerd, H.P., Huckaby, G.L., Ahmed, Y.F., Hanly, S. M., and Greene, W.C. The type I human T-cell leukemia virus (HTLV-I) Rex trans-activator binds directly to the HTLV-I Rex and the type 1 human immunodeficiency virus Rev RNA response elements. *Proc. Natl. Acad. Sci. USA* 88: 5704–5708, **1991**.

Bohnlein, S., Pirker, F.P., Hofer, L., Zimmermann, K., Bachmayer, H., Bohnlein, E., and Hauber, J. Transdominant repressors for human T-cell leukemia virus type I rex and human immunodeficiency virus type 1 rev function. *J. Virol.* 65: 81–88, **1991**.

Brodine, S. K., Oldfield, E.C., III, Corwin, A.L., Thomas, R.J., Ryan, A.B., Holmberg, J., Molgaard, C.A., Golbeck, A.L., Ryden, L.A., Benenson, A.S., et al. HTLV-I among U.S. Marines stationed in a hyperendemic area: evidence for female-to-male sexual transmission. *J. Acquir. Immune Defic. Syndr.* 5: 158–162, **1992**.

Bunn, P.A., Jr., Schechter, G.P., Jaffe, E., Blayney, D., Young, R.C., Matthews, M.J., Blattner, W., Broder, S., Robert-Guroff, M., and Gallo, R.C. Clinical course of retrovirus-associated adult T-cell lymphoma in the United States. *N. Engl. J. Med.* 309: 257–264, **1983**.

Cann, A.J. and Chen, I.S. Y. Human T-cell leukemia viruses types I and II. In: Fields, B.N., Knipe, D.M., and Howley, P.M. (Eds.), *Fields Virology*. Lippincott-Raven, Philadelphia, New York, pp. 1849–1880, **1996**.

Capdepont, S., Londos-Gagliardi, D., Joubert, M., Correze, P., Lafon, M.E., Guillemain, B., and Fleury, H.J. New insights in HTLV-I phylogeny by sequencing and analyzing the entire envelope gene. *AIDS Res. Hum. Retroviruses* 21: 28–42, **2005**.

Cappell, M.S. and Chow, J. HTLV-I-associated lymphoma involving the entire alimentary tract and presenting with an acquired immune deficiency. *Am. J. Med.* 82: 649–654, **1987**.

Caron, C., Rousset, R., Beraud, C., Moncollin, V., Egly, J.M., and Jalinot, P. Functional and biochemical interaction of the HTLV-I Tax1 transactivator with TBP. *EMBO J.* 12: 4269–4278, **1993**.

Carter, R.S., Geyer, B.C., Xie, M., Acevedo-Suarez, C.A., and Ballard, D.W. Persistent activation of NF-κB by the tax transforming protein involves chronic phosphorylation of IκB kinase subunits IKKβ and IKKγ. *J. Biol. Chem.* 276: 24445–24448, **2001**.

Cassar, O., Capuano, C., Meertens, L., Chungue, E., and Gessain, A. Human T-cell leukemia virus type 1 molecular variants, Vanuatu, Melanesia. *Emerg. Infect. Dis.* 11: 706–710, **2005**.

Catovsky, D., Greaves, M.F., Rose, M., Galton, D.A., Goolden, A.W., McCluskey, D.R., White, J.M., Lampert, I., Bourikas, G., Ireland, R., Brownell, A.I., Bridges, J.M., Blattner, W.A., and Gallo, R.C. Adult T-cell lymphoma-leukaemia in Blacks from the West Indies. *Lancet* 1: 639–643, **1982**.

Cavrois, M., Gessain, A., Wain-Hobson, S., and Wattel, E. Proliferation of HTLV-1 infected circulating cells in vivo in all asymptomatic carriers and patients with TSP/HAM. *Oncogene* 12: 2419–2423, **1996**.

Cereseto, A., Diella, F., Mulloy, J.C., Cara, A., Michieli, P., Grassmann, R., Franchini, G., and Klotman, M.E. p53 functional impairment and high p21waf1/cip1 expression in human T-cell lymphotropic/leukemia virus type I-transformed T cells. *Blood* 88: 1551–1560, **1996**.

Cereseto, A., Berneman, Z.N., Koralnik, I.J., Vaughn, J., Franchini, G., and Klotman, M.E. Differential expression of alternatively spliced pX mRNAs in HTLV-I-infected cell lines. *Leukemia* 11: 866–870, **1997**.

Chiari, E., Lamsoul, I., Lodewick, J., Chopin, C., Bex, F., and Pique, C. Stable ubiquitination of human T-cell leukemia virus type 1 tax is required for proteasome binding. *J. Virol.* 78: 11823–11832, **2004**.

Chung, H.K., Young, H.A., Goon, P.K., Heidecker, G., Princler, G.L., Shimozato, O., Taylor, G.P., Bangham, C.R., and Derse, D. Activation of interleukin-13 expression in T cells from HTLV-1-infected individuals and in chronically infected cell lines. *Blood* 102: 4130–4136, **2003**.

Ciminale, V., Pavlakis, G.N., Derse, D., Cunningham, C.P., and Felber, B.K. Complex splicing in the human T-cell leukemia virus (HTLV) family of retroviruses: novel mRNAs and proteins produced by HTLV type I. *J. Virol.* 66: 1737–1745, **1992**.

Ciminale, V., Zotti, L., D'Agostino, D.M., Ferro, T., Casareto, L., Franchini, G., Bernardi, P., and Chieco-Bianchi, L. Mitochondrial targeting of the p13II protein coded by the x-II ORF of human T-cell leukemia/lymphotropic virus type I (HTLV-I). *Oncogene* 18: 4505–4514, **1999**.

Cockerell, G.L., Lairmore, M., De, B., Rovnak, J., Hartley, T.M., and Miyoshi, I. Persistent infection of rabbits with HTLV-I: patterns of anti-viral antibody reactivity and detection of virus by gene amplification. *Int. J. Cancer* 45: 127–130, **1990**.

Collins, N.D., Newbound, G.C., Albrecht, B., Beard, J.L., Ratner, L., and Lairmore, M.D. Selective ablation of human T-cell lymphotropic virus type 1 p12I reduces viral infectivity in vivo. *Blood* 91: 4701–4707, **1998**.

Copeland, T.D., Oroszlan, S., Kalyanaraman, V.S., Sarngadharan, M.G., and Gallo, R.C. Complete amino acid sequence of human T-cell leukemia virus structural protein p15. *FEBS Lett.* 162: 390–395, **1983**.

Daenke, S., Nightingale, S., Cruickshank, J.K., and Bangham, C.R. Sequence variants of human T-cell lymphotropic virus type I from patients with tropical spastic paraparesis and adult T-cell leukemia do not distinguish neurological from leukemic isolates. *J. Virol.* 64: 1278–1282, **1990**.

D'Agostino, D.M., Ranzato, L., Arrigoni, G., Cavallari, I., Belleudi, F., Torrisi, M.R., Silic-Benussi, M., Ferro, T., Petronilli, V., Marin, O., Chieco-Bianchi, L., Bernardi, P., and Ciminale, V. Mitochondrial alterations induced by the p13II protein of human T-cell leukemia virus type 1. Critical role of arginine residues. *J. Biol. Chem.* 277: 34424–34433, **2002**.

D'Agostino, D.M., Silic-Benussi, M., Hiraragi, H., Lairmore, M.D., and Ciminale, V. The human T-cell leukemia virus type 1 p13II protein: effects on mitochondrial function and cell growth. *Cell Death Differ.* 12 (Suppl 1): 905–915, **2005**.

Dekaban, G.A., Peters, A.A., Mulloy, J.C., Johnson, J.M., Trovato, R., Rivadeneira, E., and Franchini, G. The HTLV-I orfI protein is recognized by serum antibodies from naturally infected humans and experimentally infected rabbits. *Virology.* 274: 86–93, **2000**.

de la Fuente, C., Santiago, F., Chong, S. Y., Deng, L., Mayhood, T., Fu, P., Stein, D., Denny, T., Coffman, F., Azimi, N., Mahieux, R., and Kashanchi, F. Overexpression of p21(waf1) in human T-cell lymphotropic virus type 1-infected cells and its association with cyclin A/cdk2. *J. Virol.* 74: 7270–7283, **2000**.

de la Fuente, C., Wang, L., Wang, D., Deng, L., Wu, K., Li, H., Stein, L.D., Denny, T., Coffman, F., Kehn, K., Baylor, S., Maddukuri, A., Pumfery, A., and Kashanchi, F. Paradoxical effects of a stress signal on pro- and anti-apoptotic machinery in HTLV-1 Tax expressing cells. *Mol. Cell. Biochem.* 245: 99–113, **2003**.

Derse, D., Mikovits, J., and Ruscetti, F. X-I and X-II open reading frames of HTLV-I are not required for virus replication or for immortalization of primary T-cells in vitro. *Virology* 237: 123–128, **1997**.

Ding, W., Albrecht, B., Luo, R., Zhang, W., Stanley, J.R., Newbound, G.C., and Lairmore, M.D. Endoplasmic reticulum and cis-Golgi localization of human T-lymphotropic virus type 1 p12(I): association with calreticulin and calnexin. *J. Virol.* 75: 7672–7682, **2001**.

de Thé, G. and Bumford, R. An HTLV-1 vaccine: why, how, for whom? *AIDS Res. Hum. Retroviruses* 9: 381–386, **1993**.

Dodon, M.D., Hamaia, S., Martin, J., and Gazzolo, L. Heterogeneous nuclear ribonucleoprotein A1 interferes with the binding of the human T cell leukemia virus type 1 rex regulatory protein to its response element. *J. Biol. Chem.* 277: 18744–18752, **2002**.

Duelli, D.M., Hearn, S., Myers, M.P., and Lazebnik, Y. A primate virus generates transformed human cells by fusion. *J. Cell Biol.* 171: 493–503, **2005**.

Eiraku, N., Hingorani, R., Ijichi, S., Machigashira, K., Gregersen, P.K., Monteiro, J., Usuku, K., Yashiki, S., Sonoda, S., Osame, M., and Hall, W.W. Clonal expansion within CD4+ and CD8+ T cell subsets in human T lymphotropic virus type I-infected individuals. *J. Immunol.* 161: 6674–6680, **1998**.

Elovaara, I., Koenig, S., Brewah, A.Y., Woods, R.M., Lehky, T., and Jacobson, S. High human T cell lymphotropic virus type 1 (HTLV-1)-specific precursor cytotoxic T lymphocyte frequencies in patients with HTLV-1-associated neurological disease. *J. Exp. Med.* 177: 1567–1573, **1993**.

Epstein, M.A., Achong, B.G., Ball, G. Further observations on a human syncytial virus from a nasopharyngeal carcinoma. *J. Natl. Cancer Inst.* 53: 681–688, **1974**.

Escoffier, E., Rezza, A., Roborel de Climens, A., Belleville, A., Gazzolo, L., Gilson, E., and Duc Dodon, M. A balanced transcription between telomerase and the telomeric DNA-binding proteins TRF1, TRF2 and Pot1 in resting, activated, HTLV-1 transformed and Tax-expressing human T lymphocytes. *Retrovirology* 2: 77, **2005**.

Etoh, K., Tamiya, S., Yamaguchi, K., Okayama, A., Tsubouchi, H., Ideta, T., Mueller, N., Takatsuki, K., and Matsuoka, M. Persistent clonal proliferation of human T-lymphotropic virus type I-infected cells in vivo. *Cancer Res.* 57: 4862–4867, **1997**.

Feuer, G., Zack, J.A., Harrington, W.J., Jr., Valderama, R., Rosenblatt, J.D., Wachsman, W., Baird, S. M., and Chen, I.S. Establishment of human T-cell leukemia virus type I T-cell lymphomas in severe combined immunodeficient mice. *Blood* 82: 722–731, **1993**.

Feuer, G., Stewart. S. A., Baird, S. M., Lee, F., Feuer, R., and Chen, I.S. Potential role of natural killer cells in controlling tumorigenesis by human T-cell leukemia viruses. *J. Virol.* 69: 1328–1333, **1995**.

Fraedrich, K., Müller, B., and Grassmann, R. The HTLV-1 Tax protein binding domain of cyclin-dependent kinase 4 (CDK4) includes the regulatory PSTAIRE helix. *Retrovirology* 2: 54, **2005**.

Franchini, G. Molecular mechanisms of human T-cell leukemia/lymphotropic virus type I infection. *Blood* 86: 3619–3639, **1995**.

Franchini, G. and Reitz, M.S., Jr. Phylogenesis and genetic complexity of the non-human primate retroviridae. *AIDS Res. Hum. Retroviruses* 10: 1047–1060, **1994**.

Franchini, G., Mulloy, J.C., Koralnik, I.J., Lo Monico, A., Sparkowski, J.J., Andresson, T., Goldstein, D.J., and Schlegel, R. The human T-cell leukemia/lymphotropic virus type I p12I protein cooperates with the E5 oncoprotein of bovine papillomavirus in cell transformation and binds the 16-kilodalton subunit of the vacuolar H+ ATPase. *J. Virol.* 67: 7701–7704, **1993**.

Fu, D.X., Kuo, Y.L., Liu, B.Y., Jeang, K.T., and Giam, C.Z. Human T-lymphotropic virus type 1 tax inactivates I-κB kinase by inhibiting I-κB kinase-associated serine/threonine protein phosphatase 2 A. *J. Biol. Chem.* 278: 1487–1493, **2003**.

Fujihara, K., Itoyama, Y., Yu, F., Kubo, C., and Goto, I. Cellular immune surveillance against HTLV-I infected T lymphocytes in HTLV-I associated myelopathy/tropical spastic paraparesis (HAM/TSP). *J. Neurol. Sci.* 105: 99–107, **1991** .

Fujisawa, K., Asahara, H., Okamoto, K., Aono, H., Hasunuma, T., Kobata, T., Iwakura, Y., Yonehara, S., Sumida, T., and Nishioka, K. Therapeutic effect of the anti-Fas antibody on arthritis in HTLV-1 tax transgenic mice. *J. Clin. Invest.* 98: 271–278, **1996**.

Fujita, M. and Shiku, H. Differences in sensitivity to induction of apoptosis among rat fibroblast cells transformed by HTLV-I tax gene or cellular nuclear oncogenes. *Oncogene* 11: 15–20, **1995**.

Furukawa, Y., Fujisawa, J., Osame, M., Toita, M., Sonoda, S., Kubota, R., Ijichi, S., and Yoshida, M. Frequent clonal proliferation of human T-cell leukemia virus type 1 (HTLV-1)-infected T cells in HTLV-1-associated myelopathy (HAM-TSP). *Blood* 80: 1012–1016, **1992**.

Furukawa, Y., Yamashita, M., Usuku, K., Izumo, S., Nakagawa, M., and Osame, M. Phylogenetic subgroups of human T cell lymphotropic virus (HTLV) type I in the tax gene and their association with different risks for HTLV-I-associated myelopathy/tropical spastic paraparesis. *J. Infect. Dis.* 182: 1343–1349, **2000**.

Gabet, A.S., Mortreux, F., Talarmin, A., Plumelle, Y., Leclercq, I., Leroy, A., Gessain, A., Clity, E., Joubert, M., and Wattel, E. High circulating proviral load with oligoclonal expansion of HTLV-1 bearing T cells in HTLV-1 carriers with strongyloidiasis. *Oncogene* 19: 4954–4960, **2000**.

Gallo, R.C. History of the discoveries of the first human retroviruses: HTLV-1 and HTLV-2. *Oncogene* 24: 5926–5930, **2005**.

Gessain, A., Barin, F., Vernant, J.C., Gout, O., Maurs, L., Calender, A., de Thé, G. Antibodies to human T-lymphotropic virus type-I in patients with tropical spastic paraparesis. *Lancet* 2: 407–410, **1985**.

Gessain, A., Francis, H., Sonan, T., Giordano, C., Akani, F., Piquemal, M., Caudie, C., Malone, G., Essex, M., and de Thé, G. HTLV-I and tropical spastic paraparesis in Africa. *Lancet* 2: 698, **1986**.

Gessain, A., Louie, A., Gout, O., Gallo, R.C., and Franchini, G. Human T-cell leukemia-lymphoma virus type I (HTLV-I) expression in fresh peripheral blood mononuclear cells from patients with tropical spastic paraparesis/HTLV-I-associated myelopathy. *J. Virol.* 65: 1628–1633, **1991**.

Giebler, H.A., Loring, J.E., van Orden, K., Colgin, M.A., Garrus, J.E., Escudero, K.W., Brauweiler, A., and Nyborg, J.K. Anchoring of CREB binding protein to the human T-cell leukemia virus type 1 promoter: a molecular mechanism of Tax transactivation. *Mol. Cell. Biol.* 17: 5156–5164, **1997**.

Gill, P.S., Harrington, W., Jr., Kaplan, M.H., Ribeiro, R.C., Bennett, J.M., Liebman, H.A., Bernstein-Singer, M., Espina, B.M., Cabral, L., Allen, S., et al. Treatment of adult T-cell leukemia-lymphoma with a combination of interferon alfa and zidovudine. *N. Engl. J. Med.* 332: 1744–1748, **1995**.

Good, L., Maggirwar, S. B., and Sun, S. C. Activation of the IL-2 gene promoter by HTLV-I tax involves induction of NF-AT complexes bound to the CD28-responsive element. *EMBO J.* 15: 3744–3750, **1996**.

Goon, P.K., Biancardi, A., Fast, N., Igakura, T., Hanon, E., Mosley, A.J., Asquith, B., Gould, K.G., Marshall, S., Taylor, G.P., and Bangham, C.R. Human T cell lymphotropic virus (HTLV) type-1-specific CD8+ T cells: frequency and immunodominance hierarchy. *J. Infect. Dis.* 189: 2294–2298, **2004 a**.

Goon, P.K., Igakura, T., Hanon, E., Mosley, A.J., Barfield, A., Barnard, A.L., Kaftantzi, L., Tanaka, Y., Taylor, G.P., Weber, J.N., and Bangham, C.R. Human T cell lymphotropic virus type I (HTLV-I)-specific CD4+ T cells: immunodominance hierarchy and preferential infection with HTLV-I. *J. Immunol.* 172: 1735–1743, **2004 b**.

Gradilone, A., Zani, M., Barillari, G., Modesti, M., Agliano, A.M., Maiorano, G., Ortona, L., Frati, L., and Manzari, V. HTLV-I and HIV infection in drug addicts in Italy. *Lancet* 2: 753–754, 1986.

Grant, C., Barmak, K., Alefantis, T., Yao, J., Jacobson, S., and Wigdahl, B. Human T cell leukemia virus type I and neurologic disease: events in bone marrow, peripheral blood, and central nervous system during normal immune surveillance and neuroinflammation. *J. Cell Physiol.* 190: 133–159, **2002**.

Grassmann, R., Dengler, C., Müller-Fleckenstein, I., Fleckenstein, B., McGuire, K., Dokhelar, M.C., Sodroski, J.G., and Haseltine, W.A. Transformation to continuous growth of primary human T lymphocytes by human T-cell leukemia virus type I X-region genes transduced by a Herpesvirus saimiri vector. *Proc. Natl. Acad. Sci. USA* 86: 3351–3355, **1989**.

Grassmann, R., Berchtold, S., Aepinus, C., Ballaun, C., Boehnlein, E., and Fleckenstein, B. In vitro binding of human T-cell leukemia virus rex proteins to the rex-response element of viral transcripts. *J. Virol.* 65: 3721–3727, **1991** .

Grassmann, R., Berchtold, S., Radant, I., Alt, M., Fleckenstein, B., Sodroski, J.G., Haseltine, W.A., and Ramstedt, U. Role of human T-cell leukemia virus type 1X region proteins in immortalization of primary human lymphocytes in culture. *J. Virol.* 66: 4570–4575, **1992**.

Grassmann, R., Aboud, M., and Jeang, K.-T. Molecular mechanisms of cellular transformation by HTLV-1 Tax. *Oncogene* 24: 5976–5985, **2005**.

Greten, T.F., Slansky, J.E., Kubota, R., Soldan, S. S., Jaffee, E.M., Leist, T.P., Pardoll, D.M., Jacobson, S., and Schneck, J.P. Direct visualization of antigen-specific T cells: HTLV-1 Tax11–19- specific CD8(+) T cells are activated in peripheral blood and accumulate in cerebrospinal fluid from HAM/TSP patients. *Proc. Natl. Acad. Sci. USA* 95: 7568–7573, **1998**.

Grone, M., Koch, C., and Grassmann, R. The HTLV-1 Rex protein induces nuclear accumulation of unspliced viral RNA by avoiding intron excision and degradation. *Virology* 218: 316–325, **1996**.

Grossman, W.J. and Ratner, L. Cytokine expression and tumorigenicity of large granular lymphocytic leukemia cells from mice transgenic for the tax gene of human T-cell leukemia virus type I. *Blood* 90: 783–794, **1997**.

Grossman, W.J., Kimata, J.T., Wong, F.H., Zutter, M., Ley, T.J., and Ratner, L. Development of leukemia in mice transgenic for the tax gene of human T-cell leukemia virus type I. *Proc. Natl. Acad. Sci. USA* 92: 1057–1061, **1995**.

Hall, A.P., Irvine, J., Blyth, K., Cameron, E.R., Onions, D.E., and Campbell, M.E. Tumours derived from HTLV-I tax transgenic mice are characterized by enhanced levels of apoptosis and oncogene expression. *J. Pathol.* 186: 209–214, **1998**.

Haller, K., Wu, Y., Derow, E., Schmitt, I., Jeang, K.T., and Grassmann, R. Physical interaction of human T-cell leukemia virus type 1 Tax with cyclin-dependent kinase 4 stimulates the phosphorylation of retinoblastoma. *Mol. Cell. Biol.* 22: 3327–3338, **2002**.

Hanon, E., Hall, S., Taylor, G.P., Saito, M., Davis, R., Tanaka, Y., Usuku, K., Osame, M., Weber, J.N., and Bangham, C.R. Abundant tax protein expression in CD4+ T cells infected with human T-cell lymphotropic virus type I (HTLV-I) is prevented by cytotoxic T lymphocytes. *Blood* 95: 1386–1392, **2000**.

Haoudi, A. and Semmes, O.J. The HTLV-1 tax oncoprotein attenuates DNA damage induced G1 arrest and enhances apoptosis in p53 null cells. *Virology* 305: 229–239, **2003**.

Harrod, R., Kuo, Y.L., Tang, Y., Yao, Y., Vassilev, A., Nakatani, Y., and Giam, C.Z. p300 and p300/cAMP-responsive element-binding protein associated factor interact with human T-cell lymphotropic virus type-1 Tax in a multi-histone acetyltransferase/activator-enhancer complex. *J. Biol. Chem.* 275: 11852–11857, **2000**.

Hayakawa, T., Miyazaki, T., Misumi, Y., Kobayashi, M., and Fujisawa, Y. Myristoylation-dependent membrane targeting and release of the HTLV-I Gag precursor, Pr53 gag, in yeast. *Gene* 119: 273–277, **1992**.

Hermine, O., Bouscary, D., Gessain, A., Turlure, P., Leblond, V., Franck, N., Buzyn-Veil, A., Rio, B., Macintyre, E., Dreyfus, F., et al. Brief report: treatment of adult T-cell leukemia-lymphoma with zidovudine and interferon alfa. *N. Engl. J. Med.* 332: 1749–1751, **1995**.

Hidaka, M., Inoue, J., Yoshida, M., and Seiki, M. Post-transcriptional regulator (rex) of HTLV-1 initiates expression of viral structural proteins but suppresses expression of regulatory proteins. *EMBO J.* 7: 519–523, **1988**.

Hino, S., Yamaguchi, K., Katamine, S., Sugiyama, H., Amagasaki, T., Kinoshita, K., Yoshida, Y., Doi, H., Tsuji, Y., and Miyamoto, T. Mother-to-child transmission of human T-cell leukemia virus type-I. *Jpn. J. Cancer Res.* 76: 474–480, **1985**.

Hinrichs, S. H., Nerenberg, M., Reynolds, R.K., Khoury, G., and Jay, G. A transgenic mouse model for human neurofibromatosis. *Science* 237: 1340–1343, **1987**.

Hinuma, Y., Nagata, K., Hanaoka, M., Nakai, M., Matsumoto, T., Kinoshita, K.I., Shirakawa, S., and Miyoshi, I. Adult T-cell leukemia: antigen in an ATL cell line and detection of antibodies to the antigen in human sera. *Proc. Natl. Acad. Sci. USA* 78: 6476–6480, **1981**.

Hinuma, Y., Gotoh, Y., Sugamura, K., Nagata, K., Goto, T., Nakai, M., Kamada, N., Matsumoto, T., and Kinoshita, K. A retrovirus associated with human adult T-cell leukemia: in vitro activation. *GANN* 73: 341–344, **1982**.

Hinuma, Y., Chosa, T., Komoda, H., Mori, I., Suzuki, M., Tajima, K., Pan, I.H., and Lee, M. Sporadic retrovirus (ATLV)-seropositive individuals outside Japan. *Lancet* 1: 824–825, **1983**.

Hiraragi, H., Michael, B., Nair, A., Silic-Benussi, M., Ciminale, V., and Lairmore, M. Human T-lymphotropic virus type 1 mitochondrion-localizing protein p13II sensitizes Jurkat T cells to Ras-mediated apoptosis. *J. Virol.* 79: 9449–9457, **2005**.

Hirose, S., Kotani, S., Uemura, Y., Fujishita, M., Taguchi, H., Ohtsuki, Y., and Miyoshi, I. Milk-borne transmission of human T-cell leukemia virus type I in rabbits. *Virology* 162: 487–489, **1988**.

Hisada, M., Okayama, A., Tachibana, N., Stuver, S. O., Spiegelman, D.L., Tsubouchi, H., and Mueller, N.E. Predictors of level of circulating abnormal lymphocytes among human T-lymphotropic virus type I carriers in Japan. *Int. J. Cancer* 77: 188–192, **1998**.

Hisada, M., Okayama, A., Spiegelman, D., Mueller, N.E., and Stuver, S. O. Sex-specific mortality from adult T-cell leukemia among carriers of human T-lymphotropic virus type I. *Int. J. Cancer* 91: 497–499, **2001**.

Ho, D.D., Rota, T.R., and Hirsch, M.S. Infection of human endothelial cells by human T-lymphotropic virus type I. *Proc. Natl. Acad. Sci. USA* 81: 7588–7590, **1984**.

Hoffman, P.M., Dhib-Jalbut, S., Mikovits, J.A., Robbins, D.S., Wolf, A.L., Bergey, G.K., Lohrey, N.C., Weislow, O.S., and Ruscetti, F.W. Human T-cell leukemia virus type I infection of monocytes and microglial cells in primary human cultures. *Proc. Natl. Acad. Sci. USA* 89: 11 784–11 788, **1992**.

Homma, T., Kanki, P.J., King, N.W., Jr., Hunt, R.D., O'Connell, M.J., Letvin, N.L., Daniel, M.D., Desrosiers, R.C., Yang, C.S., and Essex, M. Lymphoma in macaques: association with virus of human T lymphotrophic family. *Science* 225: 716–718, **1984**.

Hope, T.J., Bond, B.L., McDonald, D., Klein, N.P., and Parslow, T.G. Effector domains of human immunodeficiency virus type 1 Rev and human T-cell leukemia virus type I Rex are functionally interchangeable and share an essential peptide motif. *J. Virol.* 65: 6001–6007, **1991**.

Hoxie, J.A., Matthews, D.M., and Cines, D.B. Infection of human endothelial cells by human T-cell leukemia virus type I. *Proc. Natl. Acad. Sci. USA* 81: 7591–7595, **1984**.

Hoyos, B., Ballard, D.W., Bohnlein, E., Siekevitz, M., and Greene, W.C. Kappa B-specific DNA binding proteins: role in the regulation of human interleukin-2 gene expression. *Science* 244: 457–460, **1989**.

Huang, Y., Ohtani, K., Iwanaga, R., Matsumura, Y., and Nakamura, M. Direct trans-activation of the human cyclin D2 gene by the oncogene product Tax of human T-cell leukemia virus type I. *Oncogene* 20: 1094–1102, **2001**.

Ibrahim, F., Fiette, L., Gessain, A., Buisson, N., de Thé, G., and Bomford, R. Infection of rats with human T-cell leukemia virus type-I: susceptibility of inbred strains, antibody response and provirus location. *Int. J. Cancer* 58: 446–451, **1994**.

Igakura, T., Stinchcombe, J.C., Goon, P.K., Taylor, G.P., Weber, J.N., Griffiths, G.M., Tanaka, Y., Osame, M., and Bangham, C.R. Spread of HTLV-I between lymphocytes by

virus-induced polarization of the cytoskeleton. *Science* 299: 1713–1716, **2003**.

Ishiguro, N., Abe, M., Seto, K., Sakurai, H., Ikeda, H., Wakisaka, A., Togashi, T., Tateno, M., and Yoshiki, T. A rat model of human T lymphocyte virus type I (HTLV-I) infection. 1. Humoral antibody response, provirus integration, and HTLV-I-associated myelopathy/tropical spastic paraparesis-like myelopathy in seronegative HTLV-I carrier rats. *J. Exp. Med.* 176: 981–989, **1992**.

Ishihara, S., Tachibana, N., Okayama, A., Murai, K., Tsuda, K., and Mueller, N. Successful graft of HTLV-I-transformed human T-cells (MT-2) in severe combined immunodeficiency mice treated with anti-asialo GM-1 antibody. *Jpn. J. Cancer Res.* 83: 320–323, **1992**.

Ishihara, S., Okayama, A., Stuver, S., Horinouchi, H., Shioiri, S., Murai, K., Kubota, T., Yamashita, R., Tachibana, N., Tsubouchi, H., et al. Association of HTLV-I antibody profile of asymptomatic carriers with proviral DNA levels of peripheral blood mononuclear cells. *J. Acquir. Immune Defic. Syndr.* 7: 199–203, **1994**.

Iwahara, Y., Takehara, N., Kataoka, R., Sawada, T., Ohtsuki, Y., Nakachi, H., Maehama, T., Okayama, T., and Miyoshi, I. Transmission of HTLV-I to rabbits via semen and breast milk from seropositive healthy persons. *Int. J. Cancer* 45: 980–983, **1990**.

Iwakura, Y., Tosu, M., Yoshida, E., Takiguchi, M., Sato, K., Kitajima, I., Nishioka, K., Yamamoto, K., Takeda, T., Hatanaka, M., et al. Induction of inflammatory arthropathy resembling rheumatoid arthritis in mice transgenic for HTLV-I. *Science* 253: 1026–1028, **1991**.

Jacobson, S., Shida, H., McFarlin, D.E., Fauci, A.S., and Koenig, S. Circulating CD8+ cytotoxic T lymphocytes specific for HTLV-I pX in patients with HTLV-I associated neurological disease. *Nature* 348: 245–248, **1990**.

Jeang, K.T. Functional activities of the human T-cell leukemia virus type I Tax oncoprotein: cellular signaling through NF-kappa B. *Cytokine Growth Factor Rev.* 12: 207–217, **2001**.

Jeang, K.T., Widen, S. G., Semmes, O.J., IV, and Wilson, S. H. HTLV-I trans-activator protein, tax, is a trans-repressor of the human beta-polymerase gene. *Science* 247: 1082–1084, **1990**.

Jeffery, K.J., Usuku, K., Hall, S. E., Matsumoto, W., Taylor, G.P., Procter, J., Bunce, M., Ogg, G.S., Welsh, K.I., Weber, J.N., Lloyd, A.L., Nowak, M.A., Nagai, M., Kodama, D., Izumo, S., Osame, M., and Bangham, C.R. HLA alleles determine human T-lymphotropic virus-I (HTLV-I) proviral load and the risk of HTLV-I-associated myelopathy. *Proc. Natl. Acad. Sci. USA* 96: 3848–3853, **1999**.

Jeffery, K.J., Siddiqui, A.A., Bunce, M., Lloyd, A.L., Vine, A.M., Witkover, A.D., Izumo, S., Usuku, K., Welsh, K.I., Osame, M., and Bangham, C.R. The influence of HLA class I alleles and heterozygosity on the outcome of human T cell lymphotropic virus type I infection. *J. Immunol.* 165: 7278–7284, **2000**.

Johnson, J.M., Nicot, C., Fullen, J., Ciminale, V., Casareto, L., Mulloy, J.C., Jacobson, S., and Franchini, G. Free major histocompatibility complex class I heavy chain is preferentially targeted for degradation by human T-cell leukemia/lymphotropic virus type 1 p12(I) protein. *J. Virol.* 75: 6086–6094, **2001**.

Kanki, P.J., Homma, T., Lee, T.H., King, N.W., Jr., Hunt, R.D., and Essex, M. Antibodies to human T-cell leukemia virus-membrane antigens in macaques with malignant lymphoma. *Haematol Blood Transfus.* 29: 345–349, **1985**.

Kannagi, M., Harada, S., Maruyama, I., Inoko, H., Igarashi, H., Kuwashima, G., Sato, S., Morita, M., Kidokoro, M., Sugimoto, M., et al. Predominant recognition of human T cell leukemia virus type I (HTLV-I) pX gene products by human CD8+ cytotoxic T cells directed against HTLV-I-infected cells. *Int. Immunol.* 3: 761–767, **1991**.

Kannagi, M., Ohashi, T., Hanabuchi, S., Kato, H., Koya, Y., Hasegawa, A., Masuda, T., and Yoshiki, T. Immunological aspects of rat models of HTLV type 1-infected T lymphoproliferative disease. *AIDS Res. Hum. Retroviruses* 16: 1737–1740, **2000**.

Kannagi, M., Harashima, N., Kurihara, K., Ohashi, T., Utsunomiya, A., Tanosaki, R., Masuda, M., Tomonaga, M., and Okamura, J. Tumor immunity against adult T-cell leukemia. *Cancer Sci.* 96: 249–255, **2005**.

Kao, S. Y. and Marriott, S. J. Disruption of nucleotide excision repair by the human T-cell leukemia virus type 1 Tax protein. *J. Virol.* 73: 4299–4304, **1999**.

Kao, S. Y., Lemoine, F.J., and Marriott, S. J. Suppression of DNA repair by human T cell leukemia virus type 1 Tax is rescued by a functional p53 signaling pathway. *J. Biol. Chem.* 275: 35926–35931, **2000**.

Kaplan, J.E., Osame, M., Kubota, H., Igata, A., Nishitani, H., Maeda, Y., Khabbaz, R.F., and Janssen, R.S. The risk of development of HTLV-I-associated myelopathy/tropical spastic paraparesis among persons infected with HTLV-I. *J. Acquir. Immune Defic. Syndr.* 3: 1096–1101, **1990**.

Kasai, T., Ikeda, H., Tomaru, U., Yamashita, I., Ohya, O., Morita, K., Wakisaka, A., Matsuoka, E., Moritoyo, T., Hashimoto, K., Higuchi, I., Izumo, S., Osame, M., and Yoshiki, T. A rat model of human T lymphocyte virus type I (HTLV-I) infection: in situ detection of HTLV-I provirus DNA in microglia/macrophages in affected spinal cords of rats with HTLV-I-induced chronic progressive myeloneuropathy. *Acta Neuropathol. (Berl.)* 97: 107–112, **1999**.

Kashanchi, F. and Brady, J.N. Transcriptional and post-transcriptional gene regulation of HTLV-1. *Oncogene* 24: 5938–5951, **2005**.

Kato, H., Koya, Y., Ohashi, T., Hanabuchi, S., Takemura, F., Fujii, M., Tsujimoto, H., Hasegawa, A., and Kannagi, M. Oral administration of human T-cell leukemia virus type 1 induces immune unresponsiveness with persistent infection in adult rats. *J. Virol.* 72: 7289–7293, **1998**.

Kawata, S., Ariumi, Y., and Shimotohno, K. p21(Waf1/Cip1/Sdi1) prevents apoptosis as well as stimulates growth in cells transformed or immortalized by human T-cell leukemia virus type 1-encoded tax. *J. Virol.* 77: 7291–7299, **2003**.

Kazanji, M. HTLV type 1 infection in squirrel monkeys (*Saimiri sciureus*): a promising animal model for HTLV type 1 human infection. *AIDS Res. Hum. Retroviruses* 16: 1741–1746, **2000**.

Kazura, J.W., Saxinger, W.C., Wenger, J., Forsyth, K., Lederman, M.M., Gillespie, J.A., Carpenter, C.C., and Alpers, M.A. Epidemiology of human T cell leukemia virus type I infection in East Sepik Province, Papua New Guinea. *J. Infect. Dis.* 155: 1100–1107, **1987**.

Kehn, K., de la Fuente, C. L., Strouss, K., Berro, R., Jiang, H., Brady, J., Mahieux, R., Pumfery, A., Bottazzi, M.E., and Kashanchi, F. The HTLV-I Tax oncoprotein targets the retinoblastoma protein for proteasomal degradation. *Oncogene*24: 525–540, **2005**.

Kelly-Welch, A.E., Hanson, E.M., Boothby, M.R., and Keegan, A.D. Interleukin-4 and interleukin-13 signaling connections maps. *Science* 300: 1527–1528, **2003**.

Kibler, K.V. and Jeang, K.T. CREB/ATF-dependent repression of cyclin a by human T-cell leukemia virus type 1 Tax protein. *J. Virol.* 75: 2161–2173, **2001**.

Kim, S. J., Kehrl, J.H., Burton, J., Tendler, C.L., Jeang, K.T., Danielpour, D., Thevenin, C., Kim, K.Y., Sporn, M.B., and Roberts, A.B. Transactivation of the transforming growth factor beta 1 (TGF-beta 1) gene by human T lymphotropic virus type 1 tax: a potential mechanism for the increased production of TGF-beta 1 in adult T cell leukemia. *J. Exp. Med.* 172: 121–129, **1990**.

Kino, T. and Pavlakis, G.N. Partner molecules of accessory protein Vpr of the human immunodeficiency virus type 1 DNA. *Cell Biol.* 23: 193–205, **2004**.

Kinoshita, K. Hino, S., Amagasaki, T., Ikeda, S., Yamada, Y., Suzuyama, J., Momita, S., Toriya, K., Kamihira, S., and Ichimaru, M. Demonstration of adult T-cell leukemia virus antigen in milk from three sero-positive mothers. *GANN* 75: 103–105, **1984**.

Kinoshita, T., Shimoyama, M., Tobinai, K., Ito, M., Ito, S., Ikeda, S., Tajima, K., Shimotohno, K., and Sugimura, T. Detection of mRNA for the tax1/rex1 gene of human T-cell leukemia virus type I in fresh peripheral blood mononuclear cells of adult T-cell leukemia patients and viral carriers by using the polymerase chain reaction. *Proc. Natl. Acad. Sci. USA* 86: 5620–5624, **1989**.

Kinoshita, T., Tsujimoto, A., and Shimotohno, K. Sequence variations in LTR and env regions of HTLV-I do not discriminate between the virus from patients with HTLV-I-associated myelopathy and adult T-cell leukemia. *Int. J. Cancer.* 47: 491–495, **1991**.

Kira, J., Nakamura, M., Sawada, T., Koyanagi, Y., Ohori, N., Itoyama, Y., Yamamoto, N., Sakaki, Y., and Goto, I. Antibody titers to HTLV-I-p40 tax protein and gag-env hybrid protein in HTLV-I-associated myelopathy/ tropical spastic paraparesis: correlation with increased HTLV-I proviral DNA load. *J. Neurol. Sci.* 107: 98–104, **1992**.

Kitajima, I., Yamamoto, K., Sato, K., Nakajima, Y., Nakajima, T., Maruyama, I., Osame, M., and Nishioka, K. Detection of human T cell lymphotropic virus type I proviral DNA and its gene expression in synovial cells in chronic inflammatory arthropathy. *J. Clin. Invest.* 88: 1315–1322, **1991**.

Kitze, B., Usuku, K., Yamano, Y., Yashiki, S., Nakamura, M., Fujiyoshi, T., Izumo, S., Osame, M., and Sonoda, S. Human CD4+ T lymphocytes recognize a highly conserved epitope of human T lymphotropic virus type 1 (HTLV-1) env gp21 restricted by HLA DRB1*0101. *Clin. Exp. Immunol.* 111: 278–285, **1998**.

Kobayashi, M., Ohi, Y., Asano, T., Hayakawa, T., Kato, K., Kakinuma, A., and Hatanaka, M. Purification and characterization of human T-cell leukemia virus type I protease produced in *Escherichia coli. FEBS Lett.* 293: 106–110, **1991**.

Konishi, H., Kobayashi, N. and Hatanaka, M. Defective human T-cell leukemia virus in adult T-cell leukemia patients. *Mol. Biol. Med.* 2: 273–283, **1984**.

Koralnik, I.J., Gessain, A., Klotman, M.E., Lo Monico, A., Berneman, Z.N., and Franchini, G. Protein isoforms encoded by the pX region of human T-cell leukemia/ lymphotropic virus type I. *Proc. Natl. Acad. Sci. USA* 89: 8813–8817, **1992** .

Koralnik, I.J., Fullen, J., and Franchini, G. The p12I, p13II, and p30II proteins encoded by human T-cell leukemia/lymphotropic virus type I open reading frames I and II are localized in three different cellular compartments. *J. Virol.* 67: 2360–2366, **1993**.

Koralnik, I.J., Mulloy, J.C., Andersson, T., Fullen, J., and Franchini, G. Mapping of the intermolecular association of human T cell leukaemia/lymphotropic virus type I p12I and the vacuolar H+-ATPase 16kDa subunit protein. *J. Gen. Virol.* 76: 1909–1916, **1995**.

Kotani, S., Yoshimoto, S., Yamato, K., Fujishita, M., Yamashita, M., Ohtsuki, Y., Taguchi, H., and Miyoshi, I. Serial transmission of human T-cell leukemia virus type I by blood transfusion in rabbits and its prevention by use of X-irradiated stored blood. *Int. J. Cancer* 37: 843–847, **1986**.

Koyanagi, Y., Itoyama, Y., Nakamura, N., Takamatsu, K., Kira, J., Iwamasa, T., Goto, I., and Yamamoto, N. In vivo infection of human T-cell leukemia virus type I in non-T cells. *Virology* 196: 25–33, **1993**.

Kubota, R., Nagai, M., Kawanishi, T., Osame, M., and Jacobson, S. Increased HTLV type 1 tax specific CD8+ cells in HTLV type 1-associated myelopathy/tropical spastic paraparesis: correlation with HTLV type 1 proviral load. *AIDS Res. Hum. Retroviruses* 16: 1705–1709, **2000**.

Kurihara, K., Harashima, N., Hanabuchi, S., Masuda, M., Utsunomiya, A., Tanosaki, R., Tomonaga, M., Ohashi, T., Hasegawa, A., Masuda, T., Okamura, J., Tanaka, Y., and Kannagi, M. Potential immunogenicity of adult T cell leukemia cells in vivo. *Int. J. Cancer* 114: 257–267, **2005**.

Kushida, S., Matsumura, M., Tanaka, H., Ami, Y., Hori, M., Kobayashi, M., Uchida, K., Yagami, K., Kameyama, T., Yoshizawa, T., et al. HTLV-1-associated myelopathy/tropical spastic paraparesis-like rats by intravenous injection of HTLV-1-producing rabbit or human T-cell line into adult WKA rats. *Jpn. J. Cancer Res.* 84: 831–833, **1993**.

Lairmore, M.D., Roberts, B., Frank, D., Rovnak, J., Weiser, M.G., and Cockerell, G.L. Comparative biological responses of rabbits infected with human T-lymphotropic virus type I isolates from patients with lymphoproliferative and neurodegenerative disease. *Int. J. Cancer* 50: 124–130, **1992**.

Lairmore, M.D., Silverman, L., and Ratner, L. Animal models for human T-lymphotropic virus type 1 (HTLV-1) infection and transformation. *Oncogene* 24: 6005–6015, **2005**.

Lee, D.K., Kim, B.C., Brady, J.N., Jeang, K.T., and Kim, S. J. Human T-cell lymphotropic virus type 1 tax inhibits transforming growth factor-beta signaling by blocking the association of Smad proteins with Smad-binding element. *J. Biol. Chem.* 277: 33 766–33 775, **2002**.

Lee, T.H., Coligan, J.E., Homma, T., McLane, M.F., Tachibana, N., and Essex, M. Human T-cell leukemia virus-associated membrane antigens: identity of the major antigens recognized after virus infection. *Proc. Natl. Acad. Sci. USA* 81: 3856–3860, **1984**.

Leendertz, F.H., Junglen, S., Boesch, C., Formenty, P., Couacy-Hymann, E., Courgnaud, V., Pauli, G., and Ellerbrok, H. High variety of different simian T-cell leukemia virus type 1 strains in chimpanzees (*Pan troglodytes verus*) of the Taï National Park, Côte d'Ivoire. *J. Virol.* 78: 4352–4356, **2004**.

Lemasson, I., Thebault, S., Sardet, C., Devaux, C., and Mesnard, J.M. Activation of E2F-mediated transcription by human T-cell leukemia virus type I Tax protein in a p16(INK4A)-negative T-cell line. *J. Biol. Chem.* 273: 23 598–23 604, **1998**.

Lemoine, F.J. and Marriott, S. J. Accelerated G(1) phase progression induced by the human T cell leukemia virus type I (HTLV-I) Tax oncoprotein. *J. Biol. Chem.* 276: 31 851–31 857, **2001**.

Lemoine, F.J., Kao, S. Y., and Marriott, S. J. Suppression of DNA repair by HTLV type 1 Tax correlates with Tax trans-activation of proliferating cell nuclear antigen gene expression. *AIDS Res. Hum. Retroviruses* 16: 1623–1627, **2000** .

LeVasseur, R.J., Southern, S. O., and Southern, P.J. Mammary epithelial cells support and transfer productive human T-cell lymphotropic virus infections. *J. Hum. Virol.* 1: 214–223, **1998**.

Lewis, R.S. Calcium signaling mechanisms in T lymphocytes. *Annu. Rev. Immunol.* 19: 497–521, **2001**.

Li, M., Laco, G.S., Jaskolski, M., Rozycki, J., Alexandratos, J., Wlodawer, A., and Gustchina, A. Crystal structure of human T cell leukemia virus protease, a novel target for anticancer drug design. *Proc. Natl. Acad. Sci. USA* 102: 18 332–18 337, **2005**.

Liang, M.H., Geisbert, T., Yao, Y., Hinrichs, S. H., and Giam, C.Z. Human T-lymphotropic virus type 1 oncoprotein tax promotes S-phase entry but blocks mitosis. *J. Virol.* 76: 4022–4033, **2002**.

Liu, B., Liang, M.H., Kuo, Y.L., Liao, W., Boros, I., Kleinberger, T., Blancato, J., and Giam, C.Z. Human T-lymphotropic virus type 1 oncoprotein tax promotes unscheduled degradation of Pds1p/securin and Clb2p/cyclin B1 and causes chromosomal instability. *Mol. Cell. Biol.* 23: 5269–5281, **2003**.

Liu, B., Hong, S., Tang, Z., Yu, H., and Giam, C.Z. HTLV-I Tax directly binds the Cdc20-associated anaphase-promoting complex and activates it ahead of schedule. *Proc. Natl. Acad. Sci. USA* 102: 63–68, **2005**.

Liu, Y., Wang, Y., Yamakuchi, M., Masuda, S., Tokioka, T., Yamaoka, S., Maruyama, I., and Kitajima, I. Phosphoinositide-3 kinase-PKB/Akt pathway activation is involved in fibroblast Rat-1 transformation by human T-cell leukemia virus type I tax. *Oncogene* 20: 2514–2526, **2001**.

Low, K.G., Dorner, L.F., Fernando, D.B., Grossman, J., Jeang, K.T., and Comb, M.J. Human T-cell leukemia virus type 1 Tax releases cell cycle arrest induced by p16INK4a. *J. Virol.* 71: 1956–1962, **1997**.

Majone, F., Luisetto, R., Zamboni, D., Iwanaga, Y., and Jeang, K.-T. Ku protein as a potential human T-cell leukaemia virus type 1 (HTLV-1) Tax target in clastogenic chromosomal instability of mammalian cells. *Retrovirology* 2: 45, **2005**.

Malim, M.H., Tiley, L.S., McCarn, D.F., Rusche, J.R., Hauber, J., and Cullen, B.R. HIV-1 structural gene expression requires binding of the Rev trans-activator to its RNA target sequence. *Cell* 60: 675–683, **1990**.

Maloney, E.M. and Blattner, W.A. HTLV-I worldwide patterns and disease associations. In: Sugamura, K. (Ed.), Two decades of adult T-cell leukemia and HTLV-I research. GANN Monograph *Cancer Res.* No. 50, Karger, Basel and Japan Scientific Soc. Press, Tokyo, pp. 339–361, **2003**.

Manel, N., Battini, J.L., Taylor, N., and Sitbon, M. HTLV-1 tropism and envelope receptor. *Oncogene* 24: 6016–6025, **2005**.

Manzari, V., Gradilone, A., Barillari, G., Zani, M., Collalti, E., Pandolfi, F., De Rossi, G., Liso, V., Babbo, P., Robert-Guroff, M., et al. HTLV-I is endemic in southern Italy: detection of the first infectious cluster in a white population. *Int. J. Cancer* 36: 557–559, **1985**.

Mariner, J.M., Lantz, V., Waldmann, T.A., and Azimi, N. Human T cell lymphotropic virus type I Tax activates IL-15R alpha gene expression through an NF-kappa B site. *J. Immunol.* 166: 2602–2609, **2001**.

Marriott, S. J. and Semmes, O.J. Impact of HTLV-I Tax on cell cycle progression and the cellular DNA damage repair response. *Oncogene* 24: 5986–5995, **2005**.

Matsumoto, K., Shibata, H., Fujisawa, J.I., Inoue, H., Hakura, A., Tsukahara, T., and

Fujii, M. Human T-cell leukemia virus type 1 Tax protein transforms rat fibroblasts via two distinct pathways. *J. Virol.* 71: 4445–4451, **1997**.

McGuire, K.L., Curtiss, V.E., Larson, E.L., and Haseltine, W.A. Influence of human T-cell leukemia virus type I tax and rex on interleukin-2 gene expression. *J. Virol.* 67: 1590–1599, **1993**.

Merino, F., Robert-Guroff, M., Clark, J., Biondo-Bracho, M., Blattner, W.A., and Gallo, R.C. Natural antibodies to human T-cell leukemia/lymphoma virus in healthy Venezuelan populations. *Int. J. Cancer* 34: 501–506, **1984**.

Michael, B., Nair, A.M., Hiraragi, H., Shen, L., Feuer, G., Boris-Lawrie, K., and Lairmore, M.D. Human T lymphotropic virus type-1 p30II alters cellular gene expression to selectively enhance signaling pathways that activate T lymphocytes. *Retrovirology* 1: 39, **2004**.

Migone, T.S., Lin, J.X., Cereseto, A., Mulloy, J.C., O'Shea, J.J., Franchini, G., and Leonard, W.J. Constitutively activated Jak-STAT pathway in T cells transformed with HTLV-I. *Science* 269: 79–81, **1995**.

Mitchell, M.S., Tozser, J., Princler, G., Lloyd, P.A., Ashleigh, A., and David, D. Synthesis, processing and composition of the virion-associated HTLV-1 reverse transcriptase. *J. Biol. Chem.* 281: 3964–3971, **2006**.

Miyake, H., Suzuki, T., Hirai, H., and Yoshida, M. Trans-activator Tax of human T-cell leukemia virus type 1 enhances mutation frequency of the cellular genome. *Virology* 253: 155–161, **1999**.

Miyoshi, I., Sumita, M., Sano, K., Nishihara, R., Miyamoto, K., Kimura, I., and Sato, J. Marker chromosome 14q+ in adult T-cell leukemia. *N. Engl. J. Med.* 300: 921, **1979**.

Miyoshi, I., Kubonishi, I., Sumida, M., Hiraki, S., Tsubota, T., Kimura, I., Miyamoto, K., and Sato, J. A novel T-cell line derived from adult T-cell leukemia. *GANN* 71: 155–156, **1980**.

Miyoshi, I., Kubonishi, I., Yoshimoto, S., Akagi, T., Ohtsuki, Y., Shiraishi, Y., Nagata, K., and Hinuma, Y. Type C virus particles in a cord T-cell line derived by co-cultivating normal human cord leukocytes and human leukaemic T cells. *Nature* 294: 770–771, **1981**.

Miwa, M., Shimotohno, K., Kitamura, T., Shima, H., Shimizu, N., Ootsuyama, Y., Tsujimoto, A., Watanabe, S., Shimoyama, M., and Sugimura, T. HTLV and ATL. In: Gallo, R.C., Haseltine, W., Klein, G., and zur Hausen, H. (Eds.), *Viruses and Human Cancer*. Alan R. Liss, Inc., New York, pp. 131–140, **1987**.

Mochizuki, M., Watanabe, T., Yamaguchi, K., Yoshimura, K., Nakashima, S., Shirao, M., Araki, S., Takatsuki, K., Mori, S., and Miyata, N. Uveitis associated with human T-cell lymphotropic virus type I. *Am. J. Ophthalmol*. 114: 123–129, **1992**.

Mori, N., Morishita, M., Tsukazaki, T., Giam, C.Z., Kumatori, A., Tanaka, Y., and Yamamoto, N. Human T-cell leukemia virus type I oncoprotein Tax represses Smad-dependent transforming growth factor beta signaling through interaction with CREB-binding protein/p300. *Blood* 97: 2137–2144, **2001**.

Mulloy, J.C., Crownley, R.W., Fullen, J., Leonard, W.J., and Franchini, G. The human T-cell leukemia/lymphotropic virus type 1 p12I proteins bind the interleukin-2 receptor beta and gamma chains and affects their expression on the cell surface. *J. Virol*. 70: 3599–3605, **1996**.

Mulloy, J.C., Kislyakova, T., Cereseto, A., Casareto, L., Lo Monico, A., Fullen, J., Lorenzi, M.V., Cara, A., Nicot, C., Giam, C., and Franchini, G. Human T-cell lymphotropic/leukemia virus type 1 Tax abrogates p53-induced cell cycle arrest and apoptosis through its CREB/ATF functional domain. *J. Virol*. 72: 8852–8860, **1998**.

Murai, K., Tachibana, N., Shioiri, S., Shishime, E., Okayama, A., Ishizaki, J., Tsuda, K., and Mueller, N. Suppression of delayed-type hypersensitivity to PPD and PHA in elderly HTLV-I carriers. *J. Acquir. Immune Defic. Syndr*. 3: 1006–1009, **1990**.

Murata, N., Hakoda, E., Machida, H., Ikezoe, T., Sawada, T., Hoshino, H., and Miyoshi, I. Prevention of human T cell lymphotropic virus type I infection in Japanese macaques by passive immunization. *Leukemia* 10: 1971–1974, **1996**.

Nagai, M., Usuku, K., Matsumoto, W., Kodama, D., Takenouchi, N., Moritoyo, T., Hashiguchi, S., Ichinose, M., Bangham, C.R., Izumo, S., and Osame, M. Analysis of HTLV-I proviral load in 202 HAM/TSP patients and 243 asymptomatic HTLV-I carriers: high proviral load strongly predisposes to HAM/TSP. *J. Neurovirol*. 4: 586–593, **1998**.

Nagai, M., Brennan, M.B., Sakai, J.A., Mora, C.A., and Jacobson, S. CD8(+) T cells are an in vivo reservoir for human T-cell lymphotropic virus type I. *Blood* 98: 1858–1861, **2001**.

Nagasato, K., Nakamura, T., Ohishi, K., Shibayama, K., Motomura, M., Ichinose, K., Tsujihata, M., and Nagataki, S. Active production of anti-human T-lymphotropic virus type I (HTLV-I) IgM antibody in HTLV-I-associated myelopathy. *J. Neuroimmunol* . 32: 105–109, **1991**.

Nakamura, H., Hayami, M., Ohta, Y., Ishikawa, K., Tsujimoto, H., Kiyokawa, T., Yoshida, M., Sasagawa, A., and Honjo, S. Protection of cynomolgus monkeys against infection by human T-cell leukemia virus type-I by immunization with viral env gene products produced in Escherichia coli. *Int. J. Cancer* 40: 403–407, **1987**.

Nakao, K., Ohba, N., and Matsumoto, M. Noninfectious anterior uveitis in patients infected with human T-lymphotropic virus type I. *Jpn. J. Ophthalmol*. 33: 472–481, **1989**.

Nam, S. H., Kidokoro, M., Shida, H., and Hatanaka, M. Processing of gag precursor polyprotein of human T-cell leukemia virus type I by virus-encoded protease. *J. Virol*. 62: 3718–3728, **1988**.

Nam, S. H., Copeland, T.D., Hatanaka, M., and Oroszlan, S. Characterization of ribosomal frameshifting for expression of pol gene products of human T-cell leukemia virus type I. *J. Virol*. 67: 196–203, **1993**.

Newton, R.C., Limpuangthip, P., Greenberg, S., Gam, A., and Neva, F.A. *Strongyloides stercoralis* hyperinfection in a carrier of HTLV-I virus with evidence of selective immunosuppression. *Am. J. Med*. 92: 202–208, **1992** .

Ng, P.W., Iha, H., Iwanaga, Y., Bittner, M., Chen, Y., Jiang, Y., Gooden, G., Trent, J.M., Meltzer, P., Jeang, K.T., and Zeichner, S. L. Genome-wide expression changes induced by HTLV-1 Tax: evidence for MLK-3 mixed lineage kinase involvement in Tax-mediated NF-kappaB activation. *Oncogene* 20: 4484–4496, **2001**.

Nicot, C., Astier-Gin, T., Edouard, E., Legrand, E., Moynet, D., Vital, A., Londos-Gagliardi, D., Moreau, J.P., and Guillemain, B. Establishment of HTLV-I-infected cell lines from French, Guianese and West Indian patients and isolation of a proviral clone producing viral particles. *Virus Res.* 30: 317–334, **1993**.

Nicot, C., Mahieux, R., Takemoto, S., and Franchini, G. Bcl-X(L) is up-regulated by HTLV-I and HTLV-II in vitro and in ex vivo ATL samples. *Blood* 96: 275–281, **2000**.

Nicot, C., Mulloy, J.C., Ferrari, M.G., Johnson, J.M., Fu, K., Fukumoto, R., Trovato, R., Fullen, J., Leonard, W.J., and Franchini, G. HTLV-1 p12(I) protein enhances STAT5 activation and decreases the interleukin-2 requirement for proliferation of primary human peripheral blood mononuclear cells. *Blood* 98: 823–829, **2001**

Nicot, C., Dundr, M., Johnson, J.M., Fullen, J.R., Alonzo, N., Fukumoto, R., Princler, G.L., Derse, D., Misteli, T., and Franchini, G. HTLV-1-encoded p30II is a post-transcriptional negative regulator of viral replication. *Nat. Med.* 10: 197–201, **2004**.

Nicot, C., Harrod, R.L., Ciminale, V., and Franchini, G. Human T-cell leukemia/lymphoma virus type 1 nonstructural genes and their functions. *Oncogene* 24: 6026–6034, **2005**.

Nishimura, Y., Okubo, R., Minato, S., Itoyama, Y., Goto, I., Mori, M., Hirayama, K., and Sasazuki, T. A possible association between HLA and HTLV-I-associated myelopathy (HAM) in Japanese. *Tissue Antigens* 37: 230–231, **1991**.

Nishioka, K., Nakajima, T., Hasunuma, T., and Sato, K. Rheumatic manifestation of human leukemia virus infection. *Rheum. Dis. Clin. North Am.* 19: 489–503, **1993**.

Nomura, M., Ohashi, T., Nishikawa, K., Nishitsuji, H., Kurihara, K., Hasegawa, A., Furuta, R.A., Fujisawa, J., Tanaka, Y., Hanabuchi, S., Harashima, N., Masuda, T., and Kannagi, M. Repression of tax expression is associated both with resistance of human T-cell leukemia virus type 1-infected T cells to killing by tax-specific cytotoxic T lymphocytes and with impaired tumorigenicity in a rat model. *J. Virol.* 78: 3827–3836, **2004**.

Nosaka, T., Siomi, H., Adachi, Y., Ishibashi, M., Kubota, S., Maki, M., and Hatanaka, M. Nucleolar targeting signal of human T-cell leukemia virus type I rex-encoded protein is essential for cytoplasmic accumulation of unspliced viral mRNA. *Proc. Natl. Acad. Sci. USA* 86: 9798–9802, **1989**.

O'Doherty, M.J., Van de Pette, J.E., Nunan, T.O., and Croft, D.N. Recurrent *Strongyloides stercoralis* infection in a patient with T-cell lymphoma-leukaemia. *Lancet* 1: 858, **1984**.

Ohashi, T., Hanabuchi, S., Kato, H., Koya, Y., Takemura, F., Hirokawa, K., Yoshiki, T., Tanaka, Y., Fujii, M., and Kannagi, M. Induction of adult T-cell leukemia-like lymphoproliferative disease and its inhibition by adoptive immunotherapy in T-cell-deficient nude rats inoculated with syngeneic human T-cell leukemia virus type 1-immortalized cells. *J. Virol.* 73: 6031–6040, **1999**.

Ohtani, K., Iwanaga, R., Arai, M., Huang, Y., Matsumura, Y., and Nakamura, M. Cell type-specific E2F activation and cell cycle progression induced by the oncogene product Tax of human T-cell leukemia virus type I. *J. Biol. Chem.*275: 11 154–11 163, **2000**.

Oroszlan, S., Copeland, T.D., Rice, N.R., Smythers, G.W., Tsai, W.P., Yoshinaka, Y., and Shimotohno, K. Structural and antigenic characterization of the proteins of human T-cell leukemia viruses and their relationships to the gene products of other retroviruses. *Princess Takamatsu Symp.* 15: 147–157, **1984**.

Osame, M., Matsumoto, M., Usuku, K., Izumo, S., Ijichi, N., Amitani, H., Tara, M., and Igata, A. Chronic progressive myelopathy associated with elevated antibodies to human T-lymphotropic virus type I and adult T-cell leukemia-like cells. *Ann. Neurol.* 21: 117–122, **1987**.

Osame, M., Igata, A., Matsumoto, M., Kohka, M., Usuku, K., and Izumo, S. HTLV-1-associated myelopathy (HAM) treatment trials, retrospective survey and clinical and laboratory findings. *Hematol. Res. Commun.* 3: 271–284, **1989**.

Ohshima, K., Suzumiya, J., Izumo, S., Mukai, Y., Tashiro, K., and Kikuchi, M. Detection of human T-lymphotropic virus type-I DNA and mRNA in the lymph nodes; using polymerase chain reaction in situ hybridization (PCR/ISH) and reverse transcription (RT-PCR/ISH). *Int. J. Cancer* 66: 18–23, **1996**.

Palmeri, D. and Malim, M.H. The human T-cell leukemia virus type 1 posttranscriptional trans-activator Rex contains a nuclear export signal. *J. Virol.* 70: 6442–6445, **1996**.

Pankow, R., Durkop, H., Latza, U., Krause, H., Kunzendorf, U., Pohl, T., and Bulfone-Paus, S. The HTLV-I tax protein transcriptionally modulates OX40 antigen expression. *J. Immunol.* 165: 263–270, **2000**.

Peloponese, J.M., Jr., Iha, H., Yedavalli, V.R., Miyazato, A., Li, Y., Haller, K., Benkirane, M., and Jeang, K.T. Ubiquitination of human T-cell leukemia virus type 1 tax modulates its activity. *J. Virol.* 78: 11 686–11 695, **2004**.

Philpott, S. M. and Buehring, G.C. Defective DNA repair in cells with human T-cell leukemia/bovine leukemia viruses: role of tax gene. *J. Natl. Cancer Inst.* 91: 933–942, **1999**.

Pique, C., Ureta-Vidal, A., Gessain, A., Chancerel, B., Gout, O., Tamouza, R., Agis, F., and Dokhelar, M.C. Evidence for the chronic in vivo production of human T cell leukemia virus type I Rof and Tof proteins from cytotoxic T lymphocytes directed against viral peptides. *J. Exp. Med.* 191: 567–572, **2000**.

Pise-Masison, C.A., Radonovich, M., Sakaguchi, K., Appella, E., and Brady, J.N. Phosphorylation of p53: a novel pathway for p53 inactivation in human T-cell lymphotropic virus type 1-transformed cells. *J. Virol.* 72: 6348–6355, **1998** .

Poiesz, B.J., Ruscetti, F.W., Gazdar, A.F., Bunn, P.A., Minna, J.D., and Gallo, R.C. Detection and isolation of type C retrovirus particles from fresh and cultured lymphocytes of a patient with cutaneous T-cell lymphoma. *Proc. Natl. Acad. Sci. USA* 77: 7415–7419, **1980**.

Portis, T., Harding, J.C., and Ratner, L. The contribution of NF-kappa B activity to spontaneous proliferation and resistance to apoptosis in human T-cell leukemia virus type 1 Tax-induced tumors. *Blood* 98: 1200–1208, **2001**.

Pozzatti, R., Vogel, J., and Jay, G. The human T-lymphotropic virus type I tax gene can cooperate with the ras oncogene to induce neoplastic transformation of cells. *Mol. Cell. Biol.* 10: 413–417, **1990**.

Rehberger, S., Gounari, F., DucDodon, M., Chlichlia, K., Gazzolo, L., Schirrmacher, V., and Khazaie, K. The activation domain of a hormone inducible HTLV-1 Rex protein determines colocalization with the nuclear pore. *Exp. Cell Res.* 233: 363–371, **1997**.

Ressler, S., Morris, G.F., and Marriott, S. J. Human T-cell leukemia virus type 1 Tax transactivates the human proliferating cell nuclear antigen promoter. *J. Virol.* 71: 1181–1190, **1997**.

Robek, M.D., Wong, F.H., and Ratner, L. Human T-cell leukemia virus type 1pX-I and pX-II open reading frames are dispensable for the immortalization of primary lymphocytes. *J. Virol.* 72: 4458–4462, **1998**.

Robert-Guroff, M., Clark, J., Lanier, A.P., Beckman, G., Melbye, M., Ebbesen, P., Blattner, W.A., and Gallo, R.C. Prevalence of HTLV-I in Arctic regions. *Int. J. Cancer* 36: 651–655, **1985**.

Robert-Guroff, M., Weiss, S. H., Giron, J.A., Jennings, A.M., Ginzburg, H.M., Margolis, I.B., Blattner, W.A., and Gallo, R.C. Prevalence of antibodies to HTLV-I, -II, and -III in intravenous drug abusers from an AIDS endemic region. *JAMA.* 255: 3133–3137, **1986**.

Robinson, R.D., Lindo, J.F., Neva, F.A., Gam, A.A., Vogel, P., Terry, S. I., and Cooper, E.S. Immunoepidemiologic studies of *Strongyloides stercoralis* and human T lymphotropic virus type I infections in Jamaica. *J. Infect. Dis.* 169: 692–696, **1994**.

Rodgers-Johnson, P., Morgan, O.S., Mora, C., Sarin, P., Ceroni, M., Piccardo, P., Garruto, R.M., Gibbs, C.J., Jr., and Gajdusek, D.C. The role of HTLV-I in tropical spastic paraparesis in Jamaica. *Ann Neurol.* 23 (Suppl): S121–S126, **1988**.

Rosin, O., Koch, C., Schmitt, I., Semmes, O.J., Jeang, K.T., and Grassmann, R. A human T-cell leukemia virus Tax variant incapable of activating NF-kappaB retains its immortalization potential for primary T-lymphocytes. *J. Biol. Chem.* 273: 6698–6703, **1998**.

Ruben, S., Poteat, H., Tan, H., Kawakami, K., Roeder, R., Haseltine, W., and Rosen, C.A. Cellular transcription factors and regulation of IL-2 receptor gene expression by

HTLV-I tax gene product. *Science* 241: 89–92, **1988**.

Sabouri, A.H., Saito, M., Usuku, K., Bajestan, S. N., Mahmoudi, M., Forughipour, M., Sabouri, Z., Abbaspour, Z., Goharjoo, M.E., Khayami, E., Hasani, A., Izumo, S., Arimura, K., Farid, R., and Osame, M. Differences in viral and host genetic risk factors for development of human T-cell lymphotropic virus type 1 (HTLV-1)-associated myelopathy/tropical spastic paraparesis between Iranian and Japanese HTLV-1-infected individuals. *J. Gen. Virol.* 86: 773–781, **2005**.

Saito, M., Braud, V.M., Goon, P., Hanon, E., Taylor, G.P., Saito, A., Eiraku, N., Tanaka, Y., Usuku, K., Weber, J.N., Osame, M., and Bangham, C.R. Low frequency of CD94/NKG2A+ T lymphocytes in patients with HTLV-1-associated myelopathy/tropical spastic paraparesis, but not in asymptomatic carriers. *Blood* 102: 577–584, **2003**.

Santiago, F., Clark, E., Chong, S., Molina, C., Mozafari, F., Mahieux, R., Fujii, M., Azimi, N., and Kashanchi, F. Transcriptional up-regulation of the cyclin D2 gene and acquisition of new cyclin-dependent kinase partners in human T-cell leukemia virus type 1-infected cells. *J. Virol.* 73: 9917–9927, **1999**.

Sato, H. and Okochi, K. Transmission of human T-cell leukemia virus (HTLV-I) by blood transfusion: demonstration of proviral DNA in recipients' blood lymphocytes. *Int. J. Cancer.* 37: 395–400, **1986**.

Sato, K., Maruyama, I., Maruyama, Y., Kitajima, I., Nakajima, Y., Higaki, M., Yamamoto, K., Miyasaka, N., Osame, M., and Nishioka, K. Arthritis in patients infected with human T lymphotropic virus type I. Clinical and immunopathologic features. *Arthritis Rheum.* 34: 714–721, **1991**.

Saxinger, W., Blattner, W.A., Levine, P.H., Clark, J., Biggar, R., Hoh, M., Moghissi, J., Jacobs, P., Wilson, L., Jacobson, R., et al. Human T-cell leukemia virus (HTLV-I) antibodies in Africa. *Science* 225: 1473–1476, **1984**.

Schmitt, I., Rosin, O., Rohwer, P., Gossen, M., and Grassmann, R. Stimulation of cyclin-dependent kinase activity and G1- to S-phase transition in human lymphocytes by the human T-cell leukemia/lymphotropic virus type 1 Tax protein. *J. Virol.* 72: 633–640, **1998**.

Seiki, M., Hattori, S., Hirayama, Y., and Yoshida, M. Human adult T-cell leukemia virus: complete nucleotide sequence of the provirus genome integrated in leukemia cell DNA. *Proc. Natl. Acad. Sci. USA* 80: 3618–3622, **1983**.

Seiki, M., Inoue, J., Hidaka, M., and Yoshida, M. Two cis-acting elements responsible for posttranscriptional trans-regulation of gene expression of human T-cell leukemia virus I. *Proc. Natl. Acad. Sci. USA* 85: 7124–7128, **1988** .

Schneider, J., Yamamoto, N., Hinuma, Y., and Hunsmann, G. Precursor polypeptides of adult T-cell leukaemia virus: detection with antisera against isolated polypeptides gp68, p24 and p19. *J. Gen. Virol.* 65: 2249–2258, **1984 a**.

Schneider, J., Yamamoto, N., Hinuma, Y., and Hunsmann, G. Sera from adult T-cell leukemia patients react with envelope and core polypeptides of adult T-cell leukemia virus. *Virology* 132: 1–11, **1984 b**.

Silic-Benussi, M., Cavallari, I., Zorzan, T., Rossi, E., Hiraragi, H., Rosato, A., Horie, K., Saggioro, D., Lairmore, M.D., Willems, L., Chieco-Bianchi, L., D'Agostino, D.M., and Ciminale, V. Suppression of tumor growth and cell proliferation by p13 II, a mitochondrial protein of human T cell leukemia virus type 1. *Proc. Natl. Acad. Sci. USA* 101: 6629–6634, **2004**.

Silverman, L.R., Phipps, A.J., Montgomery, A., Ratner, L., and Lairmore, M.D. Human T-cell lymphotropic virus type 1 open reading frame II-encoded p30II is required for in vivo replication: evidence of in vivo reversion. *J. Virol.* 78: 3837–3845, **2004**.

Sinha-Datta, U., Horikawa, I., Michishita, E., Datta, A., Sigler-Nicot, J.C., Brown, M., Kazanji, M., Barrett, J.C., and Nicot, C. Transcriptional activation of hTERT through NK-kappaB pathway in HTLV-I-transformed cells. *Blood* 104: 2523–2531, **2004**.

Siomi, H., Shida, H., Nam, S. H., Nosaka, T., Maki, M., and Hatanaka, M. Sequence requirements for nucleolar localization of human T cell leukemia virus type I pX protein, which regulates viral RNA processing. *Cell* 55: 197–209, **1988** .

Slattery, J.P., Franchini, G., and Gessain, A. Genomic evolution, patterns of global dissemination, and interspecies transmission of human and simian T-cell leukemia/lymphotropic viruses. *Genome Res.* 9: 525–540, **1999**.

Smith, M.R. and Greene, W.C. Type I human T cell leukemia virus tax protein transforms rat fibroblasts through the cyclic adenosine monophosphate response element binding protein/activating transcription factor pathway. *J. Clin. Invest.* 88: 1038–1042, **1991**.

Stehelin, D., Varmus, H.E., and Bishop, J.M. Detection of nucleotide sequences associated with transformation by avian sarcoma viruses. *Bibl. Haematol.* 43: 539–541, **1975**.

Suga, T., Kameyama, T., Kinoshita, T., Shimotohno, K., Matsumura, M., Tanaka, H., Kushida, S., Ami, Y., Uchida, M., Uchida, K., et al. Infection of rats with HTLV-1: a small-animal model for HTLV-1 carriers. *Int. J. Cancer* 49: 764–769, **1991**.

Suzuki, T., Uchida-Toita, M., and Yoshida M. Tax protein of HTLV-1 inhibits CBP/p300-mediated transcription by interfering with recruitment of CBP/p300 onto DNA element of E-box or p53 binding site. *Oncogene* 18: 4137–4143, **1999 a**.

Suzuki, T., Ohsugi, Y., Uchida-Toita, M., Akiyama, T., and Yoshida, M. Tax oncoprotein of HTLV-1 binds to the human homologue of *Drosophila* discs large tumor suppressor protein, hDLG, and perturbs its function in cell growth control. *Oncogene* 18: 5967–5972, **1999 b**.

Taguchi, H. and Miyoshi, I. Immune suppression in HTLV-I carriers: a predictive sign of adult T-cell leukemia. *Acta Med. Okayama* 43: 317–321, **1989**.

Taguchi, H., Sawada, T., Fukushima, A., Iwata, J., Ohtsuki, Y., Ueno, H., and Miyoshi, I. Bilateral uveitis in a rabbit experimentally infected with human T-lymphotropic virus type I. *Lab. Invest.* 69: 336–339, **1993**.

Tajima, K. The 4th nation-wide study of adult T-cell leukemia/lymphoma (ATL) in Japan: estimates of risk of ATL and its geographical and clinical features. The T- and B-cell Malignancy Study Group. *Int. J. Cancer* 45: 237–243, **1990** .

Tamiya, S., Matsuoka, M., Etoh, K., Watanabe, T., Kamihira, S., Yamaguchi, K., and Takatsuki, K. Two types of defective human T-lymphotropic virus type I provirus in adult T-cell leukemia. *Blood* 88: 3065–3073, **1996**.

Tanaka, A., Takahashi, C., Yamaoka, S., Nosaka, T., Maki, M., and Hatanaka, M. Oncogenic transformation by the tax gene of human T-cell leukemia virus type I in vitro. *Proc. Natl. Acad. Sci. USA* 87: 1071–1075, **1990**.

Tanaka, Y., Tanaka, R., Terada, E., Koyanagi, Y., Miyano-Kurosaki, N., Yamamoto, N., Baba, E., Nakamura, M., and Shida, H. Induction of antibody responses that neutralize human T-cell leukemia virus type I infection in vitro and in vivo by peptide immunization. *J. Virol.* 68: 6323–6331, **1994**.

Taylor, G.P. and Matsuoka, M. Natural history of adult T-cell leukemia/lymphoma and approaches to therapy. *Oncogene* 24: 6047–6057, **2005**.

Taylor, G.P., Bodéus, M., Courtois, F., Pauli, G., Del Mistro, A., Machuca, A., Padua, E., Andersson, S., Goubau, P., Chieco-Bianchi, L., Soriano, V., Coste, J., Ades, A.E., and Weber, J.N. The seroepidemiology of human T-lymphotropic viruses: types I and II in Europe: a prospective study of pregnant women. *J. Acquir. Immune Defic. Syndr.* 38: 104–109, **2005**.

Temin, H. and Mizutani, S. A RNA-dependent DNA polymerase and a DNA endonuclease in virions of Rous sarcoma virus. *Nature* 228: 424–427, **1970**.

Trovato, R., Mulloy, J.C., Johnson, J.M., Takemoto, S., de Oliveira, M.P., and Franchini, G. A lysine-to-arginine change found in natural alleles of the human T-cell lymphotropic/leukemia virus type 1 p12(I) protein greatly influences its stability. *J. Virol.* 73: 6460–6467, **1999**.

Tsukahara, T., Kannagi, M., Ohashi, T., Kato, H., Arai, M., Nunez, G., Iwanaga, Y., Yamamoto, N., Ohtani, K., Nakamura, M., and Fujii, M. Induction of Bcl-x(L) expression by human T-cell leukemia virus type 1 Tax through NF-kappaB in apoptosis-resistant T-cell transfectants with Tax. *J. Virol.* 73: 7981–7987, **1999**.

Tsukasaki, K., Maeda, T., Arimura, K., Taguchi, J., Fukushima, T., Miyazaki, Y., Moriuchi, Y., Kuriyama, K., Yamada, Y., and Tomonaga, M. Poor outcome of autologous stem cell transplantation for adult T cell leukemia/lymphoma: a case report and review of the literature. *Bone Marrow Transplant* 23: 87–89, **1999**.

Tubakin-Fix, Y., Azran, I., Schavinsky-Khrapunsky, Y., Levy, O., and Aboud, M. Functional inactivation of p53 by human T-cell leukaemia virus type 1 Tax protein: mechanisms and clinical implications. *Carcinogenesis* 27: 673–681, **2006** .

Tyler, K.L., Clarke, P., DeBiasi, R.L., Kominsky, D., and Poggioli, G.J. Retroviruses and the host cell. *Trends Microbiol.* 9: 560–564, **2001**.

Uchiyama, T., Yodoi, J., Sagawa, K., Takatsuki, K., and Uchino, H. Adult T-cell leukemia: clinical and hematologic features of 16 cases. *Blood* 50: 481–492, **1977**.

Uemura, Y., Kotani, S., Yoshimoto, S., Fujishita, M., Yamashita, M., Ohtsuki, Y., Taguchi, H., and Miyoshi, I. Mother-to-offspring transmission of human T cell leukemia virus type I in rabbits. *Blood* 69: 1255–1258, **1987**.

Usuku, K., Nishizawa, M., Matsuki, K., Tokunaga, K., Takahashi, K., Eiraku, N., Suehara, M., Juji, T., Osame, M., and Tabira, T. Association of a particular amino acid sequence of the HLA-DR beta 1 chain with HTLV-I-associated myelopathy. *Eur. J. Immunol.* 20: 1603–1606, **1990**.

Utsunomiya, A., Miyazaki, Y., Takatsuka, Y., Hanada, S., Uozumi, K., Yashiki, S., Tara, M., Kawano, F., Saburi, Y., Kikuchi, H., Hara, M., Sao, H., Morishima, Y., Kodera, Y., Sonoda, S., and Tomonaga, M. Improved outcome of adult T cell leukemia/lymphoma with allogeneic hematopoietic stem cell transplantation. *Bone Marrow Transplant.* 27: 15–20, **2001**.

Van, P.L., Yim, K.W., Jin, D.Y., Dapolito, G., Kurimasa, A., Jeang, K.T. Genetic evidence of a role for ATM in functional interaction between human T-cell leukemia virus type 1 Tax and p53. *J. Virol.* 75: 396–407, **2001**.

Vine, A.M., Witkover, A.D., Lloyd, A.L., Jeffery, K.J., Siddiqui, A., Marshall, S. E., Bunce, M., Eiraku, N., Izumo, S., Usuku, K., Osame, M., and Bangham, CR. Polygenic control of human T lymphotropic virus type I (HTLV-I) provirus load and the risk of HTLV-I-associated myelopathy/tropical spastic paraparesis. *J. Infect. Dis.* 186: 932–939, **2002**.

Vine, A.M., Heaps, A.G., Kaftantzi, L., Mosley, A., Asquith, B., Witkover, A., Thompson, G., Saito, M., Goon, P.K., Carr, L., Martinez-Murillo, F., Taylor, G.P., and Bangham, C.R. The role of CTLs in persistent viral infection: cytolytic gene expression in CD8+ lymphocytes distinguishes between individuals with a high or low proviral load of human T cell lymphotropic virus type 1. *J. Immunol.* 173: 5121–5129, **2004**.

Wäldele, K., Schneider, G., Ruckes, T., and Grassmann, R. Interleukin-13 overexpression by tax transactivation: a potential autocrine stimulus in human T-cell leukemia virus-infected lymphocytes. *J. Virol.* 78: 6081–6090, **2004**.

Waldmann, T.A., White, J.D., Goldman, C.K., Top, L., Grant, A., Bamford, R., Roessler, E., Horak, I.D., Zaknoen, S., Kasten-Sportes, C., et al. The interleukin-2 receptor: a target for monoclonal antibody treatment of human T-cell lymphotrophic virus I-induced adult T-cell leukemia. *Blood* 82: 1701–1712, **1993**.

Weichselbraun, I., Farrington, G.K., Rusche, J.R., Bohnlein, E., and Hauber, J. Definition of the human immunodeficiency virus type 1 Rev and human T-cell leukemia virus type I Rex protein activation domain by functional exchange. *J. Virol.* 66: 2583–2587, **1992**.

Wilson, K.A., Bar, S., Maerz, A.L., Alizon, M., and Poumbourios, P. The conserved glycine-rich segment linking the N-terminal fusion peptide to the coiled coil of human T-cell leukemia virus type 1 transmembrane glycoprotein gp21 is a determinant of membrane fusion function. *J. Virol.* 79: 4533–4539, **2005**.

Wilson, S., Abbotts, J., and Widen, S. Progress toward molecular biology of DNA polymerase beta. *Biochim. Biophys. Acta* 949: 149–157, **1988**.

Wodarz, D., Hall, S. E., Usuku, K., Osame, M., Ogg, G.S., McMichael, A.J., Nowak, M.A., and Bangham, C.R. Cytotoxic T-cell abundance and virus load in human immunodeficiency virus type 1 and human T-cell leukaemia virus type 1. *Proc. Biol. Sci.* 268: 1215–1221, **2001**.

Yamada, Y., Tomonaga, M., Fukuda, H., Hanada, S., Utsunomiya, A., Tara, M., Sano, M., Ikeda, S., Takatsuki, K., Kozuru, M., Araki, K., Kawano, F., Niimi, M., Tobinai, K., Hotta, T., and Shimoyama, M. A new G-CSF-supported combination chemotheraphy, LSG15, for adult T-cell leukaemia-lymphoma: Japan Clinical Oncology Group Study 9303. *Br. J. Haematol.* 113: 375–382, **2001**.

Yamamoto, H., Sekiguchi, T., Itagaki, K., Saijo, S., and Iwakura, Y. Inflammatory polyarthritis in mice transgenic for human T cell leukemia virus type I. *Arthritis Rheum.* 36: 1612–1620, **1993**.

Yamamoto, N., Schneider, J., Hinuma, Y., and Hunsmann, G. Adult T-cell leukemia-associated antigen (ATLA): detection of a glycoprotein in cell- and virus-free supernatant. *Z. Naturforsch [C]* 37: 731–732, **1982**.

Yamaoka, S., Inoue, H., Sakurai, M., Sugiyama, T., Hazama, M., Yamada, T., and Hatanaka, M. Constitutive activation of NF-kappa B is essential for transformation of rat fibroblasts by the human T-cell leukemia virus type I Tax protein. *EMBO J.* 15: 873–887, **1996**.

Ye, J., Silverman, L., Lairmore, M.D., and Green, P.L. HTLV-1 Rex is required for viral spread and persistence in vivo but is dispensable for cellular immortalization in vitro. *Blood* 102: 3963–3969, **2003**.

Yodoi, J., Takatsuki, K., and Masuda, T. Two cases of T-cell chronic lymphocytic leukemia in Japan. *N. Engl. J. Med.* 290: 572–573, **1974**.

Yoshida, M. Discovery of HTLV-1, the first human retrovirus, its unique regulatory mechanisms, and insights into pathogenesis. *Oncogene* 24: 5931–5937, **2005**.

Yoshida, M., Miyoshi, I., and Hinuma, Y. Isolation and characterization of retrovirus from cell lines of human adult T-cell leukemia and its implication in the disease. *Proc. Natl. Acad. Sci. USA* 79: 2031–2035, **1982**.

Younis, I. and Green, P.L. The human T-cell leukemia virus Rex protein. *Front. Biosci.* 10: 431–445, **2005**.

Younis, I., Khair, L., Dundr, M., Lairmore, M.D., Franchini, G., and Green, P.L. Repression of human T-cell leukemia virus type 1 and type 2 replication by a viral mRNA-encoded posttranscriptional regulator. *J. Virol.* 78: 11077–11 083, **2004**.

Yu, F., Itoyama, Y., Fujihara, K., and Goto, I. Natural killer (NK) cells in HTLV-I-associated myelopathy/tropical spastic paraparesis-decrease in NK cell subset populations and activity in HTLV-I seropositive individuals. *J. Neuroimmunol.* 33: 121–128, **1991**.

Zhang, W., Nisbet, J.W., Bartoe, J.T., Ding, W., and Lairmore, M.D. Human T-lymphotropic virus type 1 p30(II) functions as a transcription factor and differentially modulates CREB-responsive promoters. *J. Virol.* 74: 11 270–11 277, **2000**.

Zhang, W., Nisbet, J.W., Albrecht, B., Ding, W., Kashanchi, F., Bartoe, J.T., and Lairmore, M.D. Human T-lymphotropic virus type 1 p30(II) regulates gene transcription by binding CREB binding protein/p300. *J. Virol.* 75: 9885–9895, **2001**.

8.2
Human T-Lymphotropic Retrovirus-2 (HTLV-2)

HTLV-2 was isolated from a T-cell line of a patient with hairy cell T-cell leukemia (Kalyanaraman et al., 1982). The line had been established four years earlier (Saxon et al., 1978). Epidemiological studies showed this infection to occur frequently in Central and West Africa (Gessain et al., 1993; Goubau et al., 1993), and to occur at a higher rate in native American populations throughout the continent (Hjelle et al., 1990, 1991; Lairmore et al., 1990; Heneine et al., 1991). Serological analysis revealed that this retrovirus is related to – but different from – HTLV-1, and it was therefore designated as HTLV-2. A second isolate was obtained four years later, again from a T-cell lymphocytosis (Rosenblatt et al., 1986). A few more isolates have been obtained subsequently.

Serological assays distinguishing between HTLV-1 and -2 infections revealed HTLV-2-positive sera among intravenous drug abusers in Great Britain (Tedder et al., 1984), and New York (Robert-Guroff et al., 1986). Within the same risk group, high incidences of HTLV-2 infections were noted in New Orleans (Lee et al., 1989; Rosenblatt et al., 1990). In several of these patients, the CD8+ T-cell counts were elevated, although the patients remained asymptomatic. Occasional observations noted spontaneous lymphocyte proliferation (Wiktor et al., 1991), mucosis fungoides (Zucker-Franklin et al., 1992), large granular lymphocyte leukemia (Loughran et al., 1992; Martin et al., 1993), and neurological complications corresponding to TSP (Harrington et al., 1993; Jacobson et al., 1993) in an occasional HTLV-2-infected person.

HTLV-2 shares approximately 70% of its nucleotides with HLTV-1, and encodes similar regulatory and accessory genes from pX regions ORFs (Feuer and Green, 2005). The availability of an infectious HTLV-2 clone (Chen et al., 1983 a) permitted earlier studies on HTLV gene structure and function than for HTLV-1 (Kimata et al., 1994; Derse et al., 1995).

HTLV-2 infections occur preferentially in CD8$^+$ cells (Miyamoto et al., 1991; Ijichi et al., 1992; Lal et al., 1993; Wang et al., 2000), although CD4$^+$ cells also become infected. In contrast to HTLV-1-immortalized lines, HTLV-2-transformed cells do not reveal an activated Jak/STAT signaling pathway (Lal et al., 1992; Mulloy et al., 1998).

HTLV-2 also immortalizes human peripheral blood T cells *in vitro* (Chen et al., 1983 b). As observed in HTLV-1 infections, Tax plays a decisive role in this process (Ross et al., 1996). The Tax activation of NF-κB and CREB/ATF is required for IL-1-independent T-cell proliferation (Ross et al., 1996).

The HTLV-1-encoded Tax (Tax-1) and the HTLV-2 Tax (Tax-2) share approximately 78% of amino acids, and both display characteristics of viral oncogenes (Feuer and Green, 2005). Similar to Tax-1, Tax-2 protects cells from Fas-mediated apoptosis (Zehender et al., 2001). Yet, both proteins differ in their transforming activities. They show differences in inducing cellular gene transcription (Ejima et al., 1993; Lal et al., 1993; Mori and Prager, 1996), and Tax-1 more effectively transactivates the viral LTR (Ye et al., 2003). The reduced transforming activity of Tax-2 seems to be due to the missing carboxy terminus of Tax-1 (Feuer and Green, 2005). Tax-2 also inhibits p53 function to a lesser extent than Tax-1 (Mahieux et al., 2000), and it is less efficient in transforming rat embryo fibroblasts *in vitro* (Endo et al., 2002). The tumorigenic potential of Tax-2-transformed lymphoid cell lines is also reduced in comparison to Tax-1-transformed cells (Feuer et al., 1995). There exists also a difference in intracellular localization between Tax-1 and Tax-2, the latter being found predominantly in the cytoplasm (Meertens et al., 2004).

The available data suggest that differences in the C-terminal part of Tax determine the higher pathogenicity of HTLV-1 in comparison to HTLV-2. Thus, the inconclusive evidence linking HTLV-2 infections with ATL-like lymphoproliferations seems to be determined by the C-terminal fragment of Tax. Interestingly, this part in Tax-1 contains the PDZ binding motif (Hall and Fujii, 2005). PDZ binding proteins play a key role in cell signaling and cell communication (Fanning and Anderson, 1999; Harris and Lim, 2001). Chimeric Tax-2, encoding the last 53 amino acids of Tax-1, regained increasing transforming potential for rat fibroblasts (Hirata et al., 2004).

References

Chen, I.S., McLaughlin, J., Gasson, J.C., Clark, S. C., and Golde, D.W. Molecular characterization of genome of a novel human T-cell leukaemia virus. *Nature* 305: 502–505, **1983a**.

Chen, I.S., Quan, S. G., and Golde, D.W. Human T-cell leukemia virus type II transforms normal human lymphocytes. *Proc. Natl. Acad. Sci. USA* 80: 7006–7009, **1983b**.

Derse, D., Mikovits, J., Polianova, M., Felber, B.K., and Ruscetti, F. Virions released from cells transfected with a molecular clone of human T-cell leukemia virus type I give rise to primary and secondary infections of T cells. *J. Virol.* 69: 1907–1912, **1995**.

Ejima, E., Rosenblatt, J.D., Massari, M., Quan, E., Stephens, D., Rosen, C.A., and Prager, D. Cell-type-specific transactivation of the parathyroid hormone-related protein gene promoter by the human T-cell leukemia virus type I (HTLV-I) tax and HTLV-II tax proteins. *Blood* 81: 1017–1024, **1993**.

Endo, K., Hirata, A., Iwai, K., Sakurai, M., Fukushi, M., Oie, M., Higuchi, M., Hall, W.W., Gejyo, F., and Fujii, M. Human T-cell leukemia virus type 2 (HTLV-2) Tax protein transforms a rat fibroblast cell line but less efficiently than HTLV-1 Tax. *J. Virol.* 76: 2648–2653, **2002**.

Fanning, A.S. and Anderson, J.M. PDZ domains: fundamental building blocks in the organization of protein complexes at the plasma membrane. *J. Clin. Invest.* 103: 767–727, **1999**.

Feuer, G. and Green, P.L. Comparative biology of human T-cell lymphotropic virus type 1 (HTLV-1) and HTLV-2. *Oncogene* 24: 5996–6004, **2005**.

Feuer, G., Stewart, S. A., Baird, S. M., Lee, F., Feuer, R., and Chen, I.S. Potential role of natural killer cells in controlling tumorigenesis by human T-cell leukemia viruses. *J. Virol.* 69: 1328–1333, **1995**.

Gessain, A., Fretz, C., Koulibaly, M., Boudret, M.L., Bah, A., Raphael, M., de Thé, G., and Fournel, J.J. Evidence of HTLV-II infection in Guinea, West Africa. *J. Acquir. Immune Defic. Syndr.* 6: 324–325, **1993**.

Goubau, P., Desmyter, J., Swanson, P., Reynders, M., Shih, J., Surmont, I., Kazadi, K., and Lee, H. Detection of HTLV-I and HTLV-II infection in Africans using type-specific envelope peptides. *J. Med. Virol.* 39: 28–32, **1993**.

Hall, W.W. and Fujii, M. Deregulation of cell-signaling pathways in HTLV-1 infection. *Oncogene* 24: 5965–5975, **2005**.

Harrington, W.J., Jr., Sheremata, W., Hjelle, B., Dube, D.K., Bradshaw, P., Foung, S. K., Snodgrass, S., Toedter, G., Cabral, L., and Poiesz, B. Spastic ataxia associated with human T-cell lymphotropic virus type II infection. *Ann. Neurol.* 33: 411–414, **1993**.

Harris, B.Z. and Lim, W.A. Mechanism and role of PDZ domains in signaling complex assembly. *J. Cell Sci.* 114: 3219–3231, **2001**.

Heneine, W., Kaplan, J.E., Gracia, F., Lal, R., Roberts, B., Levine, P.H., and Reeves, W.C. HTLV-II endemicity among Guaymi Indians in Panama. *N. Engl. J. Med.* 324: 565, **1991**.

Hirata, A., Higuchi, M., Niinuma, A., Ohashi, M., Fukushi, M., Oie, M., Akiyama, T., Tanaka, Y., Gejyo, F., and Fujii, M. PDZ domain-binding motif of human T-cell leukemia virus type 1 Tax oncoprotein augments the transforming activity in a rat fibroblast cell line. *Virology* 318: 327–336, **2004**.

Hjelle, B., Scalf, R., and Swenson S. High frequency of human T-cell leukemia-lymphoma virus type II infection in New Mexico blood donors: determination by sequence-specific oligonucleotide hybridization. *Blood* 76: 450–454, **1990**.

Hjelle, B., Cyrus, S., Swenson, S., and Mills, R. Serologic distinction between human T-lymphotropic virus (HTLV) type I and HTLV type II. *Transfusion* 31: 731–736, **1991**.

Ijichi, S., Ramundo, M.B., Takahashi, H., and Hall, W.W. In vivo cellular tropism of human T cell leukemia virus type II (HTLV-II). *J. Exp. Med.* 176: 293–296, **1992**.

Jacobson, S., Lehky, T., Nishimura, M., Robinson, S., McFarlin, D.E., and Dhib-Jalbut, S. Isolation of HTLV-II from a patient with chronic, progressive neurological disease clinically indistinguishable from HTLV-I-associated myelopathy/tropical spastic paraparesis. *Ann. Neurol.* 33: 392–396, **1993**.

Kalyanaraman, V.S., Sarngadharan, M.G., Robert-Guroff, M., Miyoshi, I., Golde, D., and Gallo, R.C. A new subtype of human T-cell leukemia virus (HTLV-II) associated with a T-cell variant of hairy cell leukemia. *Science* 218: 571–573, **1982**.

Kimata, J.T., Wong, F.H., Wang, J.J., and Ratner, L. Construction and characterization of infectious human T-cell leukemia virus type 1 molecular clones. *Virology*. 204: 656–664, **1994**.

Lairmore, M.D., Jacobson, S., Gracia, F., De, B.K., Castillo, L., Larreategui, M., Roberts, B.D., Levine, P.H., Blattner, W.A., and Kaplan, J.E. Isolation of human T-cell lymphotropic virus type 2 from Guaymi Indians in Panama. *Proc. Natl. Acad. Sci. USA* 87: 8840–8844, **1990**.

Lal, R.B., Hjelle, B., and Rudolph, D.L. Spontaneous proliferation of HTLV-II-infected peripheral blood lymphocytes: HLA-DR-driven, IL-2-dependent response. *Microbiol. Immunol.* 36: 865–872, **1992**.

Lal, R.B., Rudolph, D.L., Folks, T.M., and Hooper, W.C. Over expression of insulin-like growth factor receptor type-I in T-cell lines infected with human T-lymphotropic virus types-I and -II. *Leuk. Res.* 17: 31–35, **1993**.

Lee, H., Swanson, P., Shorty, V.S., Zack, J.A., Rosenblatt, J.D., and Chen, I.S. High rate of HTLV-II infection in seropositive i.v. drug abusers in New Orleans. *Science* 244: 471–475, **1989**.

Loughran, T.P., Jr., Coyle, T., Sherman, M.P., Starkebaum, G., Ehrlich, G.D., Ruscetti, F.W., and Poiesz, B.J. Detection of human T-cell leukemia/lymphoma virus, type II, in a patient with large granular lymphocyte leukemia. *Blood* 80: 1116–1169, **1992**.

Mahieux, R., Pise-Masison, C.A., Nicot, C., Green, P., Hall, W.W., and Brady, J.N. Inactivation of p53 by HTLV type 1 and HTLV type 2 Tax trans-activators. *AIDS Res. Hum. Retroviruses* 16: 1677–1681, **2000**.

Martin, M.P., Biggar, R.J., Hamlin-Green, G., Staal, S., and Mann, D. Large granular lymphocytosis in a patient infected with HTLV-II. *AIDS Res. Hum. Retroviruses* 9:715–719, **1993**.

Meertens, L., Chevalier, S., Weil, R., Gessain, A., and Mahieux, R. A 10-amino acid

domain within human T-cell leukemia virus type 1 and type 2 tax protein sequences is responsible for their divergent subcellular distribution. *J. Biol. Chem.* 279: 43 307–43 320, **2004**.

Miyamoto, K., Kamiya, T., Minowada, J., Tomita, N., and Kitajima, K. Transformation of CD8+ T-cells producing a strong cytopathic effect on CD4+ T-cells through syncytium formation by HTLV-II. *Jpn. J. Cancer Res.* 82: 1178–1183, **1991**.

Mori, N. and Prager, D. Transactivation of the interleukin-1 alpha promoter by human T-cell leukemia virus type I and type II Tax proteins. *Blood.* 87: 3410–3417, **1996**.

Mulloy, J.C., Migone, T.S., Ross, T.M., Ton, N., Green, P.L., Leonard, W.J., and Franchini, G. Human and simian T-cell leukemia viruses type 2 (HTLV-2 and STLV-2(pan-p)) transform T cells independently of Jak/STAT activation. *J. Virol.*72: 4408–4412, **1998**.

Robert-Guroff, M., Weiss, S. H., Giron, J.A., Jennings, A.M., Ginzburg, H.M., Margolis, I.B., Blattner, W.A., and Gallo, R.C. Prevalence of antibodies to HTLV-I, -II, and -III in intravenous drug abusers from an AIDS endemic region. *JAMA* 255: 3133–3137, **1986**.

Rosenblatt, J.D., Golde, D.W., Wachsman, W., Giorgi, J.V., Jacobs, A., Schmidt, G.M., Quan, S., Gasson, J.C., and Chen, I.S. A second isolate of HTLV-II associated with atypical hairy-cell leukemia. *N. Engl. J. Med.* 315: 372–377, **1986** .

Rosenblatt, J.D., Plaeger-Marshall, S., Giorgi, J.V., Swanson, P., Chen, I.S., Chin, E., Wang, H.J., Canavaggio, M., Hausner, M.A., and Black, A.C. A clinical, hematologic, and immunologic analysis of 21 HTLV-II-infected intravenous drug users. *Blood* 76: 409–417, **1990**.

Ross, T.M., Pettiford, S. M., and Green, P.L. The tax gene of human T-cell leukemia virus type 2 is essential for transformation of human T lymphocytes. *J. Virol.* 70: 5194–5202, **1996**.

Saxon, A., Stevens, R.H., Quan, S. G., and Golde, D.W. Immunologic characterization of hairy cell leukemias in continuous culture. *J. Immunol.* 120: 777–782, **1978**.

Tedder, R.S., Shanson, D.C., Jeffries, D.J., Cheingsong-Popov, R., Clapham, P., Dalgleish, A., Nagy, K., and Weiss, R.A. Low prevalence in the UK of HTLV-I and HTLV-II infection in subjects with AIDS, with extended lymphadenopathy, and at risk of AIDS. *Lancet* 2: 125–128, **1984**.

Wang, T.G., Ye, J., Lairmore, M.D., and Green, P.L. In vitro cellular tropism of human T cell leukemia virus type 2. *AIDS Res. Hum. Retroviruses* 16: 1661–1668, **2000**.

Wiktor, S. Z., Jacobson, S., Weiss, S. H., Shaw, G.M., Reuben, J.S., Shorty, V.J., McFarlin, D.E., and Blattner, W.A. Spontaneous lymphocyte proliferation in HTLV-II infection. *Lancet* 337: 327–328, **1991**.

Ye, J., Xie, L., and Green, P.L. Tax and overlapping rex sequences do not confer the distinct transformation tropisms of human

T-cell leukemia virus types 1 and 2. *J. Virol.* 77: 7728–7735, **2003**.

Zehender, G., Varchetta, S., De Maddalena, C., Colasante, C., Riva, A., Meroni, L., Moroni, M., and Galli, M. Resistance to Fas-mediated apoptosis of human T-cell lines expressing human T-lymphotropic virus type-2 (HTLV-2) Tax protein. *Virology* 281: 43–50, **2001**.

Zucker-Franklin, D., Hooper, W.C., and Evatt, B.L. Human lymphotropic retroviruses associated with mycosis fungoides: evidence that human T-cell lymphotropic virus type II (HTLV-II) as well as HTLV-I may play a role in the disease. *Blood* 80: 1537–1545, **1992**.

8.3
Human Endogenous Retroviruses

A large proportion of mammalian (including human) genomes originated from ancient transposable elements. DNA transposon-like structures and retroelements cover between 3% and 43% of the human genome (Deininger and Batzer, 2002; van de Lagemaat et al., 2003; Bannert and Kurth, 2004). DNA transposons are amplified without an RNA intermediate, while retroelements are transcribed into RNA and retrotranscribed by reverse transcriptase before they may re-enter the mammalian genome.

The retroelements can be subdivided into two major groups. One group, which is most abundant, carries no LTR, and the elements are usually 90 to 300 bp in length. These short interspersed elements (SINEs) are non-autonomous and seem to depend on long interspersed elements (LINEs) for their amplification (Weiner et al., 1986; Okada and Hamada, 1997). SINEs and LINEs will not be discussed here, but they are most likely derived from various tRNA genes (Daniels and Deininger, 1985; Deininger and Daniels, 1986) or the 7SL RNA gene (Ullu and Tschudi, 1984).

In this chapter, attention will be focused on a second group of human endogenous retroviruses (HERVs) which entered the human host by infecting germline cells. Most of these proviruses have acquired extensive mutations and deletions, and some have retained the coding capacity for functional proteins. The estimated percentage of such elements in the human genome amounts to slightly more than 8% (Bannert and Kurth, 2004).

The taxonomy of HERVs is based on the amino acid specificity of tRNA hybridizing to the primer binding site. The name is defined by adding its one-letter code as a suffix to the acronym HERV (Larsson et al., 1989; Bannert and Kurth, 2004). This approach leads to some confusion, as even distantly related HERVs may use the same tRNA. Clearly, there is a need for a detailed re-classification of these proviruses, preferentially on the basis of nucleotide comparisons.

Table 8.1 Classification of human endogenous retroviruses

Class	Related to	Human HERVs	Presence in nonhuman primates
Class I	γ-retroviruses (murine leukemia virus)	HERV-W HERV-H	Old and New World primates
Class II	β-retroviruses (mouse mammary tumor virus)	HERV-K	Only humans and chimpanzees (HERV-K-HML2 only in humans)
Class III	distantly related to spumaviruses	HERV-L HERV-S	Old and New World primates

Based on genome organization and sequence similarities, HERVs have been grouped into three classes (Griffiths, 2001):

- Class I HERVs are related to γ-retroviruses such as murine leukemia virus, and includes HERV-W and HERV-H.
- Class II HERVs are related to β-retroviruses which also harbor the mouse mammary tumor virus and several types of HERV-K.
- Class III HERVs are distantly related to spumaviruses, and include HERV-L and HERV-S.

Class I and class III HERVs have been discovered throughout the primate lineage, whereas many loci containing class II HERV-K proviruses are restricted to chimpanzees and humans. A summary of some characteristics of HERVs is shown in Table 8.1.

8.3.1
The Discovery of HERVs

The discovery of human endogenous proviruses relied initially on the detection of genome sequences related to animal retroviral elements (Repaske et al., 1983; Ono et al., 1987). Degenerate primers and chance observations made during the analysis of specific gene loci and chromosomal regions further contributed to a growing number of HERV-like sequences (Maeda, 1985; Harada et al., 1987). The availability of human databases has greatly facilitated the detection of HERV-sequences during recent years. The three major ORFs of retroviruses (gag, pol, and env) were maintained in only a small fraction of identified HERV sequences (Mayer et al., 1999; Griffiths, 2001; Turner et al., 2001).

Initially, typical retroviral structures were identified electronmicroscopically in the syncytial layer of full-term human placentas (Kalter et al., 1973; Vernon et al., 1974). Complete retroviral particles as well as specific antigens were also detected in human teratocarcinoma cell lines (Fig. 8.5) and in testicular tumors (Bronson et al., 1979; Boller et al., 1993, 1997). The latter particles were identified in teratocarci-

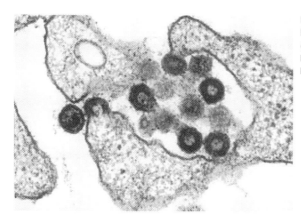

Fig. 8.5 HERV particles from a human teratocarcinoma line. (Illustration courtesy of K. Boller, Paul-Ehrlich-Institut, Langen.)

noma cells as HERV-K (Kurth et al., 1980). Cloning was first performed in 1981 (Martin et al.), since then endogenous retroviral particles belonging to the HERV-H and HERV-W families have also been identified (Perron et al., 2001; Christensen et al., 2003). Today, research in this field is actively growing, and is especially motivated by a possible role for reactivated HERVs in chronic inflammatory conditions, auto-immune diseases, and cancer.

8.3.2
Genome Organization and Transcription

8.3.2.1 **HERV-K**

HERV-K exists in a larger number of copies within the human genome (Bannert and Kurth, 2004). One subgroup (HERV-K HLM-2) is entirely human-specific (Medstrand and Mager, 1998; Buzdin et al., 2003). Approximately 113 elements of this DNA are present in the human genome, and eight to eleven of these are insertionally polymorphic (Belshaw et al., 2005). Fifteen of the HERV-K HLM-2 elements represent full-length genomes, while 98 are solely LTRs. It appears that the majority of the full-length elements were inserted relatively recently into the human genome, since their LTRs reveal a low level of mutational divergence (Turner et al., 2001; Belshaw et al., 2005). The HERV-K113 provirus is located on chromosome 19p13.11, and is also not completely fixed in the human population. It contains ORFs for all retroviral genes and remains an excellent candidate for a still active provirus in humans (Turner et al., 2001).

The structure of the HERV-K genome is outlined in Figure 8.6. Two types of HERV-K proviruses have been detected, differing by the presence or absence of a 292-bp sequence at the pol-env boundary (Löwer et al., 1993). Almost completely intact HERV-K proviruses were identified in human chromosome 7, and also reported as an allelic variant in the human population (Barbulescu et al., 1999; Mayer et al., 1999; Tönjes et al., 1999; Turner et al., 2001; Belshaw et al., 2005).

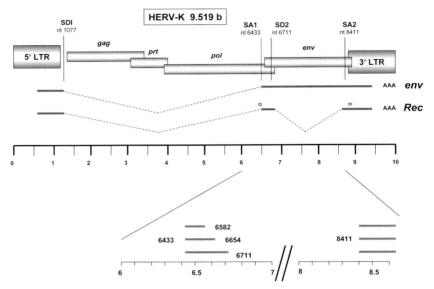

Fig. 8.6 Genomic organization of the HERV-K genome. (Modified from Mayer et al., 2004.)

A strong expression of HERV-K transcripts was noted in germ cell tumors which expressed all classical retroviral genes also as proteins (Sauter et al., 1995, 1996). In addition to these transcripts, within the *env* gene a 14kDa protein is expressed that shares 87 amino acids with the env protein and reveals additional 18 amino acids upstream from the 3' LTR in an ORF that differs from *env* (Löwer et al., 1995). Two additional smaller variants of this transcript have been also identified (Mayer et al., 2004); their structure is shown in Figure 8.6.

In addition, a 9-kDA protein, designated NP9, is produced is produced exclusively by HERV-K proviruses that contain the 292 bp deletion. Np9 shares the first 15 amino acids with the Rec and env proteins, while the C-terminal 59 amino acids are derived from the third (non-env, non-Rec) ORF. Np9 is expressed in various tumor tissues and transformed cell lines, but not in normal, nontransformed cells (Armbruester et al., 2002) (Fig. 8.7). Np9 interacts with the ligand of the Numb protein X (LNX) and can affect the subcellular localization of LNX. LNX has been reported to target the cell fate determinant and Notch antagonist Numb for proteasome-dependent degradation, thereby causing an increase in the transactivational activity of Notch. Np9 is unstable and is degraded via the proteasome pathway, whereas ectopic Numb can stabilize recombinant Np9. This may point to the possibility that Np9 is engaged in tumorigenesis through the LNX/Numb/Notch pathway (Armbruester et al., 2004).

The 14-kDa protein was termed Rec or K-Rev, and is only produced by those proviruses that do not contain the 292-bp deletion. The Rec protein appears to be functionally similar to HIV_{Rev} which exports unspliced HIV transcripts from the nucleus (Yang et al., 1999). It possesses an arginine-rich nuclear localization signal

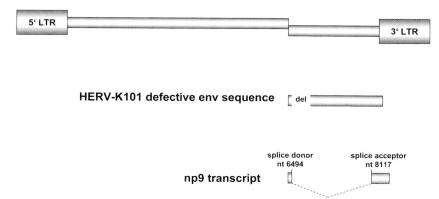

Fig. 8.7 Transcript of the *np9* gene in HERV-K 101. (Modified from Armbruester, V., et al., 2002.)

(Magin et al., 2000), and interacts with a cellular nuclear export factor (Crm1) and with the promyelocytic leukemia zinc finger protein (Boese et al., 2000).

Recent data indicate that HERV-K (HLM2) insertions result from reinfection rather than retrotransposition within germline cells (Belshaw et al., 2004), and that members of this family are likely to be infectious as well as insertionally active.

8.3.2.2 HERV-H

HERV-H is estimated to exist in about 1000 copies in the human genome (Wilkinson et al., 1994). These entered the human genome prior to the split of Old and New World monkeys (~30 million years ago), and expanded particularly in Old World primates (Anderssen et al., 1997; Mager and Freeman, 1995). The basic structure of the HERV-H genome corresponds to that of HERV-K. Most HERV-Hs are defective in one or several regions of their genome. HERV-H was defined based on histidine primer binding site (Mager and Henthorn, 1984). Based on the analysis of the pol region (~2800 bp), there are also variants that use phenylalanine tRNA as primer (Jern et al., 2004). Subsequently, Southern blots and LTR similarity also confirmed this classification (Anderssen et al., 1997; Wilkinson et al., 1994).

In teratocarcinoma cells producing retroviral particles, both HERV-K and HERV-H sequences are expressed (Löwer et al., 1993). Whereas the majority of HERV-H elements within the human genome reveals large deletions in pol and most of the *env* gene, 5–10% of them are full-length elements (Hirose et al., 1993; Wilkinson et al., 1993; Jern et al., 2002) and possess an almost complete env gene coding for transcripts that have been found in T-cell leukemia cell lines and lymphocytes from healthy blood donors (Lindeskog and Blomberg, 1997). Whereas gag and pol products are translated from full-length mRNA, env-encoded surface and transmembrane proteins are regulatory proteins and translated from spliced subgenomic mRNAs (Lindeskog and Blomberg, 1997). A rec/rev-like sequence, as detected in

HERV-K genomes, has also been described for HERV-H (Jern et al., 2004). A hybrid structure between the ORFs of HERV-H protease and HERV-E integrase and the HERV-E envelope surface glycoprotein was identified in six different human chromosomes, existing also in multiple copies in chimpanzees and gorillas, but not in orangutans or Old World monkeys (Lindeskog et al., 1998). This results in a relatively large part of HERV-E elements under the transcriptional control of HERV-H LTRs.

The most abundant subclass of HERV-H transcripts originates from a partially deleted subclass of these elements of 5.8 kb which is transcribed as ~5.6-kb unit length RNA and a ~3.7-kb spliced derivative (Goodchild et al., 1995; Kelleher et al., 1996).

8.3.2.3 HERV-W

The presence of extracellular particles with reverse transcriptase activity in leptomeningeal cells and monocyte cultures from patients with multiple sclerosis (Perron et al., 1989, 1991) resulted in intensive studies analyzing endogenous retroviruses possibly linked to the etiology of multiple sclerosis (MS). Retroviral sequences were partially cloned from the cerebrospinal fluid, plasma or cell culture supernatants of MS patients (Dolei, 2005), and expression of these sequences was demonstrated in both MS and normal brain tissues and in normal full-term placentas (Lefebvre et al., 1995; Blond et al., 1999). The isolated sequences belong to a multicopy endogenous retrovirus family now named HERV-W (Blond et al., 1999). The complete endogenous genome appears to be in a 10.4-kb genome sequence. Most – if not all – HERV-W sequences are defective for replication-containing mutations in one or more of the ORFs. Particle formation may thus result from *trans*-complementation events, supported by other HERV types.

Transcripts were obtained from placental tissue, consisting of three bands at 8, 3.1, and 1.3 kb. Probes from either gag, prt, pol and env recognized the 8-kb transcript, whereas the 3.1-kb transcript hybridized exclusively with the *env* probe (Blond et al., 1999). The protein coded for by *env* is highly conserved (Mallet et al., 2004), and deserves specific interest: it seems to serve an important function in the human host. The protein, syncytin, induces the formation of giant syncytia and seems to mediate placental cytotrophoblast fusion in placental morphogenesis (Mi et al., 2000). It can be considered as a specific marker of the human trophoblast (Malassine et al., 2005). Syncytin is synthesized as a glycosylated gPR73 precursor, which is cleaved into two mature proteins, a gp50 surface subunit and a gp24 transmembrane subunit. The intracytoplasmic tail is critical for the fusogenic phenotype (Cheynet et al., 2005). The crystal structure of the central fragment of syncytin-2 permitted a remarkable superposition with the structures of corresponding domains of present-day infectious retroviruses, in spite of a more than 60% divergent sequence (Renard et al., 2005).

8.3.2.4 Other Endogenous Human Retrovirus Genomes

Some additional sequences have been analyzed and assigned to HERV-A (Sugino et al., 1992), HERV-E (Medstrand et al., 1992), HERV-I (Maeda and Kim, 1990; Martin et al., 1997), HERV-L (Cordonnier et al., 1995; Benit et al., 1999), HERV-R (Kato et al., 1987, 1990; Andersson et al., 2002), HERV-S (Yi et al., 2004), and HERV-FRD (Blaise et al., 2004). All of these proviruses entered the human germline far back in our evolutionary history and, except for HERV-E, I, and L, they have been less intensively studied than the previously discussed members of these elements.

8.3.3
HERV Proteins and the Immune Response

Thus far, at least 16 ORFs coding for the env protein (six of them HERV-K) are apparently able to code for functional proteins (de Parseval et al., 2003). One of the env functions in forming syncytin in trophoblasts of the human placenta is discussed in Section 8.2.2.3 as a specific property of HERV-W env. Its fusogenic property is also shared by some other members of the HERV group (Blaise et al., 2003). Env may confer resistance to reinfection by the same or closely related agents by blocking the receptor for these events (Melder et al., 2003; Ponferrada et al., 2003). Endogenous Jaagsiekte sheep retrovirus blocks the entry of exogenous Jaagsiekte virus (Spencer et al., 2003). A similar effect could be attributed to gag functions, as the expression of a gag sequence of an endogenous murine retrovirus blocks infection by several murine leukemia viruses soon after entering the respective cell (Best et al., 1996).

The first report on antibody responses to proteins of endogenous retroviruses appeared in 1975 (Charman et al.), and was subsequently confirmed in animals and humans (Toth et al., 1985; Denner et al., 1996). Clearly, under certain conditions the anticipated immune tolerance of "self-antigens" breaks down. Antibodies to multiple epitopes of HERV-K env protein were even demonstrated in about one-third of healthy individuals and in approximately two-thirds of patients suffering from seminoma (Boller et al., 1997; Herve et al., 2002). Pregnant women also reveal elevated antibody titers twice as often as nonpregnant controls (Simpson et al., 1996; Boller et al., 1997) Inflammatory conditions seem to contribute to antibody development against HERVs, as for example identified in Sjögren's syndrome, multiple sclerosis (Clerici et al., 1999; Christensen et al., 2003), psoriasis (Moles et al., 2005), lupus erythematosus (Bengtsson et al., 1996), and rheumatoid arthritis (Hishikawa et al., 1997; Nakagawa et al., 1997).

Two other properties of specific HERV proteins deserve attention, namely immunosuppression and the potential function as superantigens. Cleavage of the env protein results in two components: the surface protein (gp70), and a transmembrane protein (gp15E) containing an immunosuppressive region (Larsson and Andersson, 1998). The immunosuppressive sequence from the Moloney murine leukemia virus LQNRRGLDLLFLKEGGLC is remarkably similar to the HERV-H19 sequence LQNRRGLDLLTAEKGGLC, and to similar sequences in HERV-R and HERV-E (Nelson et al., 2003). An experimental demonstration of immunosuppressive properties of the HERV-H env was published by Mangeney et al. (2001). The immunosuppressive functions are advantageous not only for the virus, but also for the host as they should protect viral protein-expressing cells from an immune attack. At the same time, its expression in syncytiotrophoblasts of the placenta should protect the developing fetus from maternal immune responses (Venables et al., 1995; Swerdlow, 2000).

Superantigens elicit a strong primary T-cell response and are presented to T cells by major histocompatibility complex (MHC) class II complex on antigen-presenting cells (for reviews, see Herman et al., 1991; Huber et al., 1996). The superantigens bind solely to the Vβ portion of the T-cell receptor, bridging the T cell with the antigen-presenting cell (Jardetzky et al., 1994). This induces T cells to secrete cytokines that activate further T cells, resulting in a strong primary T-cell activation. Besides Rhabdoviridae and Herpesviridae, a retrovirus, mouse mammary tumor virus (MMTV), encodes a superantigen in its infective and its endogenous form (Dyson et al., 1991; Frankel et al., 1991; Marrack et al., 1991; Woodland et al., 1991). Since the HERV-K family is closely related to type B retroviruses, superantigen activity was analyzed and reported for the *env* gene of HERV-K18 (IDDMK$_{1,2}$22), located on chromosome 1 (Conrad et al., 1994, 1997; Stauffer et al., 2001; Sutkowski et al., 2001). ORFs, however, expressed from the putative superantigen region did not provide evidence for stimulation of human or murine T cells in a Vβ-specific pattern (Lapatschek et al., 2000). A few additional observations recently provided additional support for superantigen activity of HERV-K18: a superantigen activity previously described for Epstein–Barr virus (EBV) (Sutkowski et al., 1996) turned out to be due to the transactivation of HERV-K18 by EBV (Sutkowski et al., 2001). Subsequently, it was shown that the EBV latent membrane protein LMP2 A is sufficient for this transactivation and induction of HERV-K18 superantigen activity (Sutkowski et al., 2004). Although these data require further confirmation, such observations may contribute to novel insights into the potential pathogenesis of endogenous retrovirus reactivation. According to Meylan et al. (2005), negative thymocyte selection for HERV K18 superantigens constitutes a first checkpoint controlling peripheral tolerance compared with superantigen reactivity.

Interferons α and β are also able to strongly induce HERV-R and HERV-K18 expression in human vascular endothelial cells and in peripheral blood cells (Katsumata et al., 1999; Stauffer et al., 2001). This may have interesting implications in chronic inflammatory diseases, as discussed in the following section.

8.3.4
HERV: The Role in Human Tumors and Autoimmune Diseases

The difficulties in establishing a potential role of endogenous viral genomes for cancer development are substantial. The presence of retrovirus-like sequences comprising approximately 8% of the human genome renders it exceptionally difficult to pinpoint a transformation event to one of these sequences, especially, if insertional mutagenesis somewhat distant from the target gene results in transcriptional activation of the latter. A more direct proof could originate from specific infection or transfection experiments resulting in proliferative modification of the respective target cells. In the absence of specific integration patterns, transformation by insertional mutagenesis must be an extremely rare event. The situation would be different, however, if specific viral proteins were to exert oncogenic functions.

The risk of insertional mutagenesis became evident in leukemia development of children receiving mouse leukemia virus vector-driven gene therapy for severe combined immunodeficiency (Hacein-Bey-Abina et al., 2003; Baum et al., 2004). In these patients, vector integration occurred in the proximity of the LMO2 gene and initiated enhanced cell proliferation. Oncogenesis also follows the high copy delivery of nonprimate lentiviral gene therapy to fetal and neonatal mice (Themis et al., 2005). It can almost be predicted that the transposition of endogenous retroviral genomes or infection after induction of retroviruses could lead to the same consequence.

A large number of reports have described an enhanced expression of proteins of endogenous retroviruses in human tumors. An insertional polymorphism of endogenous HERV-K113 and HERV-K115 retroviruses was reported in breast cancer patients that however, did not differ significantly from that in age-matched controls (Burmeister et al., 2004). The expression of spliced env and rec was found in 45% of metastatic melanoma biopsies and 44% of melanoma cell lines (Büscher et al., 2005). Neonatal melanocytes expressed only spliced rec, but no env.

Two endogenous retroviruses, SERPINB5 and a not fully characterized HERV-H, showed a high expression in colon adenomas and colon cancers, without significant expression in corresponding normal tissue (Wentzensen et al., 2004). Similarly, HERV-H was the only family expressed in cancers of the intestine, bone marrow, bladder, and cervix, and was highly expressed in cancers of the stomach, colon, and prostate (Stauffer et al., 2004) and in various cancer-derived cell lines (Yi et al., 2006). Expression of HERV-E in prostate cancer biopsies was suggested to serve as a novel marker for the early diagnosis of patients with prostate carcinomas (Wang-Johanning et al., 2003). The pol gene of the HERV-S family was reported to be more active in cancer cells than in other human tissues (Yi et al., 2004). Increased expression of HERV-K env transcripts was found in ovarian carcinomas, kidney cancer, and testicular carcinomas (de Parseval et al., 2003). Several studies analyzed the expression of endogenous retroviruses in leukemias and lymphomas and in cell lines obtained from these malignancies. A novel human endogenous retrovirus, HERV-H/F, was found in some B-cell lines of leukemic origin and in myeloid lines (Patzke et al., 2002). A HERV-K10-like *gag* gene was found to be overexpressed in six of eight leukemia samples (Depil et al., 2002). In megakaryocytes from patients with essential thrombocythemia, even HERV-K particles have been detected (Morgan and Brodsky, 2004). A less-characterized sequence highly homologous to human endogenous retroviruses was overexpressed in childhood acute lymphoblastic leukemia (Iwabuchi et al., 2004).

It remains an open question in virtually all of these studies as to whether the expression of proteins of endogenous retroviruses is a consequence of the malignant proliferation or contributed to the process of cell transformation. Similarly, increased seroreactivity against endogenous retroviral antigens, as observed for example in seminoma and germ cell tumor patients (Löwer et al., 1995; Herbst et al., 1996; Sauter et al., 1996; Magin et al., 1999; Yang et al., 1999), suffer from the same difficulties in interpreting this as cause or effect of malignant growth.

Only one study has attempted to address the biological activity of a specific viral gene experimentally. Galli et al. (2005) showed that the *rec*-gene of HERV-K (related to the HIV *rev*-gene) in transgenic mice disturbed germ cell development and, at 19 months of age, induced changes reminiscent of a carcinoma *in situ*, as a precursor lesion of seminoma. If confirmed, this represents the first report of an organ-specific tumorigenesis by a human endogenous retrovirus gene in a transgenic mouse model.

Endogenous retroviral genomes in mice and man are readily induced by specific herpes infections. In murine systems, the first observations were published as early as the late 1970s by infecting or transfecting cells with partially UV-inactivated herpes simplex virus type 2 (Hampar et al., 1976; Boyd et al., 1978, 1980). This activation of murine type C viruses is not limited to transformed murine cells, but occurs also in nontransformed cells (Hampar et al., 1977). Herpes simplex virus infection also activates endogenous HERV-K and HERV-W retrovirus LTRs in human cells (Kwun et al., 2002; Lee et al., 2003). There are no reports on endogenous retrovirus activation by human herpesvirus type 6, yet, this agent – similar to herpes simplex virus infections – is able to up-regulate expression of an exogenous retrovirus infection, HIV-1, by inducing the LTR activity of that virus (Ensoli et al., 1989; Campbell et al., 1991; Garzino-Demo et al., 1996). The previously described activation of HERV-K expression by LMP-2 A of EBV (Sutkowski et al., 2004) reveals that herpesvirus infections are probably, to a large extent, able to activate endogenous retroviruses. A herpesvirus infection of chicken with Marek's disease virus seems to underline this statement: Marek virus DNA contains two integrated copies of avian leukosis virus, subgroup J (Isfort et al., 1992; Davidson et al., 2002). When activation of endogenous retroviruses plays a role in human carcinogenesis, herpesvirus infections may act as indirect carcinogens by activating those agents.

It is probably easier to analyze the role of endogenous retrovirus activation in the induction of autoimmune diseases. Although this will not be covered here in detail, the organ-specific strictly localized autoimmune disorders, such as MS (Christensen et al., 2000; Firouzi et al., 2003; Brudek et al., 2004), diabetes mellitus (Suenaga and Yoon, 1988; Badenhoop et al., 1996; Conrad et al., 1997; Marguerat et al., 2004), thyroiditis (Shiroma et al., 2001), and others such as Sjögren's syndrome and rheumatoid arthritis (Talal et al., 1990; Gaudin et al., 2000; Bessis et al., 2004) have been suspected to be linked to endogenous retrovirus activity. In MS, the haplotypes of human endogenous retrovirus HRES-1 LTR sequences differ from those of non-MS control groups (Clausen, 2003). Yet, none of the available data are presently conclusive.

8.3.5
The Trojan Exosome Hypothesis

In 2003 an interesting hypothesis was put forward by Gould et al., the Trojan exosome hypothesis. Basically, this hypothesis states that retroviruses may exploit a cell-encoded pathway of intercellular vesicle traffic, the exosomes, for biogenesis of retroviral particles and a low-efficiency but mechanistically important mode of infection. The hypothesis predicts that retroviral particles and exosomes contain a similar array of host cell lipids and proteins in the absence of retroviral env proteins. The theory was mainly derived from observations in HIV systems: HIV buds into endosomes in macrophages and dendritic cells (Blom et al., 1993; Raposo et al., 2002; Greene Nguyen et al., 2003). HIV strains, defective for the gene Vpu, bud into endosomes even in T cells (Klimkait et al., 1990; Gottlinger et al., 1993; Li et al., 1995). One other type of observation supports this hypothesis for HIV: env-independent infections have been well documented in different systems (Chalvet et al., 1999; Pang et al., 2000; Chow et al., 2002).

This model could explain a failure of adaptive immunity in controlling retrovirus infections and, since exosomes carry MHC/peptide complexes (Raposo et al., 1996; Escola et al., 1998; Clayton et al., 2001; Denzer et al., 2000; Wolfers et al., 2001), they may specifically target T cells. In this respect it may be interesting to note that the human CD46 lymphocyte surface antigen shares crossreacting antigenic epitopes with the envelope gp70 glycoproteins of gibbon ape leukemia viruses and Mason-Pfizer monkey virus primate retroviruses (Purcell et al., 1989), but is also a constituent of human immunodeficiency viruses (Montefiori et al., 1994). These authors speculate that a human endogenous retroviral sequence may partially or completely encode the CD49 antigen.

Exosomes have been discovered which carry the genetic information of hepatitis C virus (Masciopinto et al., 2004). Thus, it may also transpire that this novel mode of transporting even partially defective genomes to previously uninfected cells plays a very important role in the transmission of viral genomes which are unable to form infectious viral particles. This might represent a remarkably effective way of bypassing the immune surveillance system of the host. Recently, a very interesting example of Mason-Pfizer retrovirus transmission via exosomes was described where infectious viral RNA-containing exosomes infect human cells by cell fusion (Duelli et al., 2005). It is clear that this mechanism deserves further attention for its possible role in permitting the transmission of endogenous human viruses to different cell compartments and cell types.

References

Anderssen, S., Sjøttem, E., Svineng, G., and Johansen, T. Comparative analyses of LTRs of the ERV-H family of primate-specific retrovirus-like elements isolated from marmoset, African green monkey, and man. *Virology* 234: 14–30, **1997** .

Andersson, A.C., Venables, P.J., Tönjes, R.R., Scherer, J., Eriksson, L., and Larsson, E.

Developmental expression of HERV-R (ERV3) and HERV-K in human tissue. *Virology* 297: 220–225, **2002**.

Armbruester, V., Sauter, M., Krautkraemer, E., Meese, E., Kleiman, A., Best, B., Roemer, K., and Müller-Lantzsch, N. A novel gene from the human endogenous retrovirus K expressed in transformed cells. *Clin. Cancer Res.* 8: 1800–1807, **2002**.

Armbruester, V., Sauter, M., Roemer, K., Best, B., Hahn, S., Nty, A., Schmid, A., Philipp, S., Mueller, A., and Müller-Lantzsch, N. Np9 protein of human endogenous retrovirus K interacts with ligand of numb protein X. *J. Virol.* 78: 10 310–10 319, **2004**.

Badenhoop, K., Tönjes, R.R., Rau, H., Donner, H., Rieker, W., Braun, J., Herwig, J., Mytilineos, J., Kurth, R., and Usadel, K.H. Endogenous retroviral long terminal repeats of the HLA-DQ region are associated with susceptibility to insulin-dependent diabetes mellitus. *Hum. Immunol.* 50: 103–110, **1996**.

Bannert, N. and Kurth, R. Retroelements and the human genome: new perspectives on an old relation. *Proc. Natl. Acad. Sci. USA* 101: 14 572–14 579, **2004**.

Barbulescu, M., Turner, G., Seaman, M.I., Deinard, A.S., Kidd, K.K., and Lenz, J. Many human endogenous retrovirus K (HERV-K) proviruses are unique in humans. *Curr. Biol.* 9: 861–868, **1999**.

Baum, C., von Kalle, C., Staal, F.J.T., Li, Z., Fehse, B., Schmidt, M., Weerkamp, F., Karlsson, S., Wagemaker, G., and Williams, D.A. Chance or necessity? Insertional mutagenesis in gene therapy and its consequences. *Mol. Therapy* 9: 5–13, **2004**.

Belshaw, R., Pereira, A., Katzourakis, G., Talbot, J., Paèes, J., Burt, A., and Tristem, M. Long-term reinfection of the human genome by endogenous retroviruses. *Proc. Natl. Acad. Sci. USA* 101: 4894–4899, **2004**.

Belshaw, R., Dawson, A.L.A., Woolven-Allen, J., Redding, J., Burt, A., and Tristem, M. Genome-wide screening reveals high levels of insertional polymorphism in the human endogenous retrovirus family HERV-K(HLM2): implications for present day activity. *J. Virol.* 79: 12 507–12 514, **2005**.

Bengtsson, A., Blomberg, J., Nived, O., Pipkorn, R., Toth, L., and Sturfelt, G. Selective antibody reactivity with peptides from human endogenous retroviruses and non-viral poly(amino acids) in patients with systemic lupus erythematosus. *Arthritis Rheum.* 39: 1654–1663, **1996**.

Benit, L., Lallemand, J.B., Casella, J.F., Philippe, H., and Heidmann, T. ERV-L elements: a family of endogenous retrovirus-like elements active throughout the evolution of mammals. *J. Virol.* 73: 3301–3308, **1999**.

Bessis, D., Moles, J.P., Basset-Seguin, N., Tesniere, A., Arpin, C., and Guilhou, J.J. Differential expression of human endogenous retrovirus E transmembrane envelope glycoprotein in normal, psoriatic and atopic dermatitis human skin. *Br. J. Dermatol.* 151: 737–745, **2004**.

Best, S., Le Tissier, P., Towers, G., and Stoye, J.P. Positional cloning of the mouse retrovirus restriction gene Fv1. *Nature.* 382: 826–829, **1996**.

Blaise, S., de Parseval, N., Benit, L., and Heidmann, T. Genomewide screening for fusogenic human endogenous retrovirus envelopes identifies syncytin 2, a gene conserved on primate evolution. *Proc. Natl. Acad. Sci. USA.* 100: 13 013–13 018, **2003**.

Blaise, S., Ruggieri, A., Dewannieux, M., Cosset, F.L., and Heidmann, T. Identification of an envelope protein from the FRD family of human endogenous retroviruses (HERV-FRD) conferring infectivity and functional conservation among simians. *J. Virol.* 78: 1050–1054, **2004**.

Blom, J., Nielsen, C., and Rhodes, J.M. An ultrastructural study of HIV-infected human dendritic cells and monocytes/macrophages. *APMIS* 101: 672–680, **1993**.

Blond, J.-L., Besème, F., Duret, L., Bouton, O., Bedin, F., Perron, H., Mandrand, B., and Mallet, F. Molecular characterization and placental expression of HERV-W, a new human endogenous retrovirus family. *J. Virol.* 73: 1175–1185, **1999**.

Boese, A., Sauter, M., Galli, U., Best, B., Herbst, H., Mayer, J., Kremmer, E., Roemer, K., and Mueller-Lantzsch, N. Human endogenous retrovirus protein cORF supports cell transformation and associates with the promyelocytic leukemia zinc finger protein. *Oncogene* 19: 4328–4336, **2000**.

Boller, K., König. H., Sauter, M., Mueller-Lantzsch, N., Löwer, R., Löwer, J., and

Kurth, R. Evidence that HERV-K is the endogenous retrovirus sequence that codes for the human teratocarcinoma-derived retrovirus HTDV. *Virology* 196: 349–353, **1993**.

Boller, K., Janssen, O., Schuldes, H., Tönjes, R.R., and Kurth, R. Characterization of the antibody response specific for the human endogenous retrovirus HTDV/HERV-K. *J. Virol.* 71: 4581–4588, **1997**.

Boyd, A.L., Derge, J.G., and Hampar, B. Activation of endogenous type C virus in BALB/c mouse cells by herpesvirus DNA. *Proc. Natl. Acad. Sci. USA* 75: 4558–4562, **1978**.

Boyd, A.L., Enquist, L., Vande Woude, G.F., and Hampar, B. Activation of mouse retrovirus by herpes simplex virus type 1 cloned DNA fragments. *Virology* 103: 228–231, **1980**.

Bronson, D.L., Fraley, E.E., Fogh, J., and Kalter, S. S. Induction of retrovirus particles in human testicular tumor (Tera-1) cell cultures: an electron microscopic study. *J. Natl. Cancer Inst.* 63: 337–339, **1979**.

Brudek, T. Christensen, T., Hansen, H.J., Bobecka, J., and Moller-Larsen, A. Simultaneous presence of endogenous retrovirus and herpes virus antigens has profound effect on cell-mediated immune responses: implications for multiple sclerosis. *AIDS. Res. Hum. Retroviruses* 20: 415–423, **2004**.

Buzdin, A., Ustyugova, S., Khodosevich, K., Mamedow, L., Lebedev, Y., Hunsmann, G., and Sverdlov, E. Human-specific subfamilies of HERV-K (HML-2) long terminal repeats: three master genes were active simultaneously during branching of hominoid lineages. *Genomics* 81: 149–156, **2003**.

Burmeister, T., Ebert, A.D., Pritze, W., Loddenkemper, C., Schwartz, S., and Thiel, E. Insertional polymorphisms of endogenous HERV-K113 and HERV-K115 retroviruses in breast cancer patients and age-matched controls. *AIDS Res. Hum. Retroviruses* 20: 1223–1229, **2004**.

Büscher, K., Trefzer, U., Hofmann, M., Sterry, W., Kurth, R., and Denner, J. Expression of human endogenous retrovirus K in melanomas and melanoma cell lines. *Cancer Res.* 65: 4172–4180, **2005**.

Campbell, M.E., McCorkindale, S., Everett, R.D., and Onions, D.E. Activation of gene expression by human herpesvirus 6 is reported gene-dependent. *J. Gen. Virol.* 72: 1123–1130, **1991**.

Chalvet, F., Teysset, L., Terzian, C., Prud'homme, N., Santamaria, P., Bucheton, A., and Pelisson, A. Proviral amplification of the Gypsy endogenous retrovirus of *Drosophila melanogaster* involves env-independent invasion of the female germline. *EMBO J.* 18: 2659–2669, **1999**.

Charman, H.P., Kim, N., White, M., Marquardt, H., Gilden, R.V., and Kawakami, T. Natural and experimentally induced antibodies to defined mammalian type-C virus proteins in primates. *J. Natl. Cancer Inst.* 55: 1419–1424, **1975**.

Cheynet, V., Ruggieri, A., Oriol, G., Blond, J.L., Boson, B., Vachot, L., Verrier, B., Cosset, F.L., and Mallet, F. Synthesis, assembly, and processing of the env ERV-WE1/syncytin human endogenous retroviral envelope. *J. Virol.* 79: 5585–5593, **2005**.

Chow, Y.H., Yu, D., Zhang, J.Y., Xie, Y., Wei, O.L., Chiu, C., Foroohar, M., Yang, O.O., Park, N.H., Chen, I.S. Pang, S. gp120-Independent infection of CD4(-) epithelial cells and CD4(+) T-cells by HIV-1. *J. Acquir. Immune Defic. Syndr.* 30: 1–8, **2002**.

Christensen, T., Dissing Sørensen, P., Riemann; H., Hansen, H.J., Munch, M., Haahr, S., and Møller-Larsen, A. Molecular characterization of HERV-H variants associated with multiple sclerosis. *Acta Neurol. Scand.* 101: 229–238, **2000**.

Christensen, T., Sørensen, P.D., Hansen, H.J., and Møller-Larsen, A. Antibodies against a human endogenous retrovirus and the preponderance of env splice variants in multiple sclerosis patients. *Mult. Scler.* 9: 6–15, **2003**.

Clausen, J. Endogenous retroviruses and MS: using ERVs as disease markers. *Int. MS J.* 10: 22–28, **2003**.

Clayton, A., Court, J., Navabi, H., Adams, M., Mason, M.D., Hobot, J.A., Newman, G.R., and Jasani, B. Analysis of antigen presenting cell derived exosomes, based on immuno-magnetic isolation and flow cytometry. *J. Immunol. Methods* 247: 163–174, **2001**.

Clerici, M., Fusi, M.L., Caputo, D., Guerini, F.R., Trabattoni, D., Salvaggio, A., Cazzullo, C.L., Arienti, D., Villa, M.L. Urnovitz, H.B., and Ferrante P. Immune responses to antigens of human endogenous retroviruses in patients with acute or stable multiple sclerosis. *J. Neuroimmunol.* 99: 173–182, **1999**.

Conrad, B., Weidmann, E., Trucco, G., Rudert, N.A., Behboo, R., Ricordi, C., Rodriguez-Rilo, H., Finegold, D., and Trucco, M. Evidence for superantigen involvement in insulin-dependent diabetes mellitus aetiology. *Nature* 371: 351–355, **1994**.

Conrad, B., Weissmahr, R.N., Boni, J., Arcari, R., Schupbach, J., and Mach, B. A human endogenous retroviral superantigen as candidate autoimmune gene in type I diabetes. *Cell* 90: 303–313, **1997**.

Cordonnier, A., Casella, J.F., and Heidmann, T. Isolation of novel human endogenous retrovirus-like elements with foamy virus-related pol sequence. *J. Virol.* 69: 5890–5897, **1995**.

Daniels, G.R. and Deininger, P.L. Repeat sequence families derived from mammalian tRNA genes. *Nature* 317: 819–822, **1985**.

Davidson, I., Borenshtain, R., Kung, H.J., and Witter, R.L. Molecular indications for in vivo integration of the avian leukosis virus, subgroup J-long terminal repeat into the Marek's disease virus in experimentally dually-infected chickens. *Virus Genes* 24: 173–180, **2002**.

Deininger, P.L. and Daniels, G.R. The recent evolution of mammalian repetitive DNA elements. *Trends Genet.* 2: 76–80, **1986**.

Deininger, P.L. and Batzer, M.A. Mammalian retroelements. *Genome Res.* 12: 1455–1465, **2002**.

Denner, J., Persin, C., Vogel, T., Haustein, D., Norley, S., and Kurth, R.J. The immunosuppressive peptide of HIV-1 inhibits T and B lymphocyte stimulation. *J. Acquir. Immune Defic. Syndr. Hum. Retrovirol.* 12: 442–450, **1996**.

Denzer, K., van Eijk, M., Kleijmeer, M.J., Jakobson, E., de Groot, C., and Geuze, H.J. Follicular dendritic cells carry MHC class II-expressing microvesicles at their surface. *J. Immunol.* 165: 1259–1265, **2000**.

de Parseval, N., Lazar, V., Casella, J.F., Benit, L., and Heidmann, T. Survey of human genes of retroviral origin: identification and transcriptome of the genes with coding capacity for complete envelope proteins. *J. Virol.* 77: 10414–10422, **2003**.

Depil, S., Roche, C., Dussart, P., and Prin, L. Expression of a human endogenous retrovirus, HERV-K, in the blood cells of leukemia patients. *Leukemia* 16: 254–259, **2002**.

Dolei, A. MSRV/HERV-W/syncytin and its linkage to multiple sclerosis: the usability and the hazard of a human endogenous retrovirus. *J. Neurovirol.* 11: 232–235, **2005**.

Duelli, D.M., Hearn, S., Myers, M.P., and Lazebnik, Y. A primate virus generates transformed human cells by fusion. *J. Cell Biol.* 171: 493–503, **2005**.

Dyson, P.J., Knight, A.M., Fairchild, S., Simpson, E., and Tomonari, K. Genes encoding ligands for deletion of Vβ11T cells cosegregate with mammary tumour virus genomes. *Nature* 349: 531–532, **1991**.

Ensoli, B., Lusso, P., Schachter, F., Josephs, S. F., Rappaport, J., Negro, F., Gallo, R.C., and Wong-Staal, F. Human herpes virus-6 increases HIV-1 expression in co-infected T cells via nuclear factors binding to the HIV-1 enhancer. *EMBO J.* 8: 3019–3027, **1989**.

Escola, J.M., Kleijmeer, M.J., Stoorvogel, W., Griffith, J.M., Yoshie, O., and Geuze, H.J. Selective enrichment of tetraspan proteins on the internal vesicles of multivesicular endosomes and on exosomes secreted by human B-lymphocytes. *J. Biol. Chem.* 273: 20121–20127, **1998**.

Firouzi, R., Rolland, A., Michel, M., Jouvin-Marche, E., Hauw, J.J., Malcus-Vocanson, C., Lazarini, F., Gebuhrer, L., Seigneurin, J.M., Touraine, J.L., Sanhadji, K., Marche, P.N., and Perron, H. Multiple sclerosis-associated retrovirus particles cause T lymphocyte-dependent death with brain hemorrhage in humanized SCID mice model. *J. Neurovirol.* 9: 79–93, **2003**.

Frankel, W.N., Rudy, C., Coffin, J.M., and Huber, B.T. Linkage of Mls genes to endogenous mammary tumour viruses of inbred mice. *Nature* 349: 526–528, **1991**.

Galli, U.M., Sauter, M., Lecher, B., Maurer, S., Herbst, H., Roemer, K., and Mueller-Lantzsch, N. Human endogenous retrovirus rec interferes with germ cell development in mice and may cause carcinoma in situ, the predecessor lesion of germ cell tumors. *Oncogene* 24: 3223–3228, **2005**.

Garzino-Demo, A., Chen, M., Lusso, P., Berneman, Z., and DiPaolo, J.A. Enhancement of TAT-induced transactivation of the HIV-1 LTR by two genomic fragments of HIV-6. *J. Med. Virol.* 50: 20–24, **1996**.

Gaudin, P., Ijaz, S., Tuke, P.W., Marcel, F., Paraz, A., Seigneurin, J.M., Mandrand, B., Perron, H., and Garson, J.A. Infrequency of detection of particle-associated MSRV/HERV-W RNA in the synovial fluid of patients with rheumatoid arthritis. *Rheumatology (Oxford)* 39: 950–954, **2000**.

Goodchild, N.L., Freeman, J.D., and Mager, D.L. Spliced HERV-H endogenous retroviral sequences in human genomic DNA: evidence for amplification via retrotransposition. *Virology* 206: 164–173, **1995**.

Gottlinger, H.G., Dorfman, T., Cohen, E.A., and Haseltine, W.A. Vpu protein of human immunodeficiency virus type 1 enhances the release of capsids produced by gag gene constructs of widely divergent retroviruses. *Proc. Natl. Acad. Sci. USA* 90: 7381–7385, **1993**.

Gould, S. J., Booth, A.M., and Hildreth, J.E.K. The Trojan exosome hypothesis. *Proc. Natl. Acad. Sci. USA* 100: 10 592–10 597, **2003**.

Greene Nguyen, D., Booth, A., Gould, S. J., and Hildreth, J.E.K. Evidence that HIV budding in primary macrophages occurs through the exosome release pathway. *J. Biol. Chem.* 278: 52 347–52 354, **2003**.

Griffiths, D.J. Endogenous retroviruses in the human genome sequence. *Genome Biol.* 2: 1017.1–1017.5, **2001**.

Hacein-Bey-Abina, S., von Kalle, C., Schmidt, M., McCormack, M.P., Wulffraat, N., Leboulch, P., Lim, A., Osborne, C.S., Pawliuk, R., Morillon, E., Sorensen, R., Forster, A., Fraser, P., Cohen, J.I., de Saint Basile, G., Alexander, I., Wintergerst, U., Frebourg, T., Aurias, A., Stoppa-Lyonnet, D., Romana, S., Radford-Weiss, I., Gross, F., Valensi, F., Delabesse, E., Macintyre, E., Sigaux, F., Soulier, J., Leiva, L.E., Wissler, M., Prinz, C., Rabbitts, T.H., Le Deist, F., Fischer, A., and Cavazzana-Calvo, M. LMO2-associated clonal T cell proliferation in two patients after gene therapy for SCID-X1. *Science* 302, 415–419, **2003**.

Hampar, B., Aaronson, S. A., Derge, J.G., Chakrabarty, M., Showalter, S. D., and Dunn, C.Y. Activation of an endogenous mouse type C virus by ultraviolet-irradiated herpes simplex virus types 1 and 2. *Proc. Natl. Acad. Sci. USA.* 73: 646–650, **1976**.

Hampar, B., Hatanaka, M., Aulakh, G., Derge, J.G., Lee, L., and Showalter, S. Type C virus activation in "nontransformed" mouse cells by UV-irradiated herpes simplex virus. *Virology* 76: 876–881, **1977**.

Harada, F., Tsukada, N., and Kato, N. Isolation of three kinds of human endogenous retrovirus-like sequences using tRNA(Pro) as a probe. *Nucleic Acids Res.* 15: 9153–9162, **1987**.

Herman, A., Kappler, J.W., Marrack, P., and Pullen, A.M. Superantigens: mechanism of T cell stimulation and role in immune responses. *Annu. Rev. Immunol.* 9: 745–772, **1991**.

Herbst, H., Sauter, M., and Mueller-Lantzsch, N. Expression of human endogenous retrovirus K elements in germ cell and trophoblastic tumors. *Am. J. Pathol.* 149: 1727–1735, **1996**.

Herve, C.A., Lugli, E.B., Brand, A., Griffiths, D.J., and Venables, P.J. Autoantibodies to human endogenous retrovirus-K are frequently detected in health and disease and react with multiple epitopes. *Clin. Exp. Immunol.* 128: 75–82, **2002**.

Hirose, Y., Takamatsu, M., and Harada, F. Presence of env genes in members of the RTVL-H family of human endogenous retrovirus-like elements. *Virology* 192: 52–61, **1993**.

Hishikawa, T., Ogasawara, H., Kaneko, H., Shirasawa, T., Matsuura, Y., Sekigawa, I., Takasaki, Y., Hashimoto, H., Hirose, S., Handa, S., Nagasawa, R., and Maruyama, N. Detection of antibodies to a recombinant gag protein derived from human endogenous retrovirus clone 4–1 in autoimmune diseases. *Viral Immunol.* 10: 137–147, **1997**.

Huber, B.T., Hsu, P.N., and Sutkowski, N. Virus-encoded superantigens. *Microbiol. Rev.* 60: 473–482, **1996**.

Isfort, R., Jones, D., Kost, R., Witter, R., and Kung, H.J. Retrovirus insertion into herpesvirus in vitro and in vivo. *Proc. Natl. Acad. Sci. USA* 89: 991–995, **1992**.

Iwabuchi, H., Kakihara, T., Kobayashi, T., Imai, C., Tanaka, A., Uchiyama, M., and Fukuda, T. A gene homologous to human endogenous retrovirus overexpressed in childhood acute lymphoblastic leukaemia. *Leuk. Lymphoma* 45: 2303–2306, **2004**.

Jardetzky, T.S., Brown, J.H., Gorga,. J.C., Stern, L.J., Urban, R.G., Chi, Y., Stauffacher, C., Strominger, J.L., and Wiley, D.C. Three dimensional structure of human class II histocompatibility molecule complexed with superantigen. *Nature* 368: 711–718, **1994**.

Jern, P., Lindeskog, M., Karlsson, D., and Blomberg, J. Full-length HERV-H elements with env SU open reading frames in the human genome. *AIDS Res. Hum. Retroviruses* 18: 671–676, **2002**.

Jern, P., Sperber, G.O., and Blomberg, J. Definition and variation of human endogenous retrovirus H. *Virology* 327: 93–110, **2004**.

Kalter, S. S., Helmke, R.J., Heberling, R.L., Panigel, M., Fowler, A.K., Strickland, J.E., and Hellman, A. C-type particles in normal human placentas. *J. Natl. Cancer Inst.* 50: 1081–1084, **1973**.

Kato, N., Pfeifer-Ohlsson, S., Kato, M., Larsson, E., Rydnert, J., Ohlsson, R., and Cohen, M. Tissue-specific expression of human provirus ERV3 mRNA in human placenta: two of the three ERV3 mRNAs contain human cellular sequences. *J. Virol.* 61: 2182–2191, **1987**.

Kato, N., Shimotohno, K., VanLeeuwen, D., and Cohen, M. Human proviral mRNAs down regulated in choriocarcinoma encode a zinc finger protein related to Krüppel. *Mol. Cell. Biol.* 10: 4401–4405, **1990**.

Katsumata, K., Ikeda, H., Sato. M., Ishuzu, A., Kawarada, Y., Kato, H., Wakisaka, A., Koike, T., and Yoshiki, T. Cytokine regulation of env gene expression of human endogenous retrovirus-R in human vascular endothelial cells. *Clin. Immunol.* 93: 75–80, **1999**.

Kelleher, C.A., Wilkinson, A., Freeman, J.D., Mager, D.L., and Gelfand, E.W. Expression of novel-transposon-containing mRNAs in human T cells. *J. Gen. Virol.* 77: 1101–1110, **1996**.

Klimkait, T., Strebel, K., Hoggan, M.D., Martin, M.A., and Orenstein, J.M. The human immunodeficiency virus type 1-specific protein vpu is required for efficient virus maturation and release. *J. Virol.* 64: 621–629, **1990**.

Kurth, R., Löwer, R., Löwer, J., Harzmann, R., Pfeiffer, R., Schmidt, C.G., Fogh, J., and Frank, H. Oncornavirus synthesis in human teratocarcinomas cultures and an increased antiviral immune reactivity in corresponding patients. In: Todaro, G., Essex, M., and zur Hausen, H. (Eds.), *Viruses in Naturally Occurring Cancers.* Cold Spring Harbor Laboratory Press, pp. 835–846, **1980**.

Kwun, H.J., Han, H.J., Lee, W.J., Kim, H.S., and Jang, K.L. Transactivation of the human endogenous retrovirus K long terminal repeat by herpes simplex virus type 1 immediate early protein 0. *Virus Res.* 86: 93–100, **2002**.

Lapatschek, M., Dürr, S., Löwer, R., Magin, C., Wagner, H., and Miethke, T. Functional analysis of the env open reading frame in human endogenous retrovirus IDDMK$_{1,2}$22 encoding superantigen activity. *J. Virol.* 74: 6386–6393, **2000**.

Larsson, E. and Andersson, G. Beneficial role of human endogenous retroviruses: facts and hypotheses. *Scand. J. Immunol.* 48: 329–338, **1998**.

Larsson, E., Kato, N., and Cohen, M. Human endogenous proviruses. *Curr. Top. Microbiol. Immunol.* 148: 115–132, **1989**.

Lee, W.J., Kwun, H.J., Kim, H.S., and Jang, K.L. Activation of human endogenous retrovirus W long terminal repeat by herpes simplex virus type 1 immediate early protein 1. *Mol. Cells* 15: 75–80, **2003**.

Lefebvre, S., Hubert, B., Tekaia, F., Brahic, M., and Bureau, J.F. Isolation from human brain of six previously unreported cDNAs related to the reverse transcriptase of human endogenous retroviruses. *AIDS Res. Hum. Retroviruses* 11: 231–237, **1995**.

Li, Q.G., Zhang, Y.J., Liang, Y., Feng, C.Q., Li, Y.Z., Sjoberg, R., Jiang, Y., Wang, N.F., and Wadell, G. The morphogenesis of a Chinese strain of HIV-1 forming inclusion bodies in Jurkat-tat III cells. *J. Acquir. Immune Defic. Syndr. Hum. Retrovirol.* 9: 103–113, **1995**.

Lindeskog, M. and Blomberg, J. Spliced human endogenous retroviral HERV-H env transcripts in T-cell leukaemia cell lines and normal leukocytes: alternative splicing pattern of HERV-H transcripts. *J. Gen. Virol.* 78: 2575–2585, **1997** .

Lindeskog, M., Medstrand, P., Cunningham, A.A., and Blomberg, J. Coamplification and dispersion of adjacent human endogenous retroviral HERV-H and HERV-E elements; presence of spliced hybrid transcripts in normal leukocytes. *Virology* 244: 219–229, **1998**.

Löwer, R., Boller, K., Hasenmaier, B., Korbmacher, C., Müller-Lantzsch, N., Löwer, J., and Kurth, R. Identification of human endogenous retroviruses with complex mRNA expression and particle formation. *Proc. Natl. Acad. Sci. USA* 90: 4480–4484, **1993**.

Löwer, R., Tönjes, R.R., Korbmacher, C., Kurth, R., and Löwer, J. Identification of Rev-related protein by analysis of spliced transcripts of the human endogenous retroviruses HTVDV/HERV-K. *J. Virol.* 69: 141–149, **1995**.

Maeda, N. Nucleotide sequence of the haptoglobin and haptoglobin-related gene pair. The haptoglobin-related gene contains a retrovirus-like element. *J. Biol. Chem.* 260: 6698–6709, **1985**.

Maeda, N. and Kim, H.S. Three independent insertions of retrovirus-like sequences in the haptoglobin gene cluster of primates. *Genomics* 8: 671–683, **1990**.

Mager, D.L. and Henthorn, P.S. Identification of a retrovirus-like repetitive element in human DNA. *Proc. Natl. Acad. Sci. USA* 81: 7510–7514, **1984**.

Mager, D.L. and Freeman, J.D. HERV-H endogenous retroviruses: presence in the New World branch but amplification in the Old World primate lineage. *Virology* 213: 395–404, **1995**.

Magin, C., Löwer, R., and Löwer, J. cORF and RcRE, the Rev/Rex and RRE/RxRE homologues of the human endogenous retrovirus family HTDV/HERV-K. *J. Virol.* 73: 9496–9507, **1999**.

Magin, C., Hesse, J., Löwer, J., and Löwer, R. Corf, the Rev/Rex homologue of HTDV/ HERV-K, encodes an arginine-rich nuclear localization signal that exerts a trans-dominant phenotype when mutated. *Virology* 274: 11–16, **2000**.

Malassine, A., Handschuh, K., Tsatsaris, V., Gerbaud, P., Cheynet, V., Oriol, G., Mallet, F., and Evain-Brion, D. Expression of HERV-W env glycoprotein (syncytin) in the extravillous trophoblast of first trimester human placenta. *Placenta* 26: 556–562, **2005**.

Mallet, F., Bouton, U., Prudhomme, S., Cheynet, V., Oriol, G., Bonnaud, B., Lucotte, G., Duret, L., and Mandrand, B. The endoge-

nous retroviral locus ERVWE1 is a bona fide gene involved in hominoid placental physiology. *Proc. Natl. Acad. Sci. USA* 101: 1731–1736, **2004**.

Mangeney, M., de Parseval, N., Thomas, G., and Heidmann, T. The full-length envelope of an HERV-H human endogenous retrovirus has immunosuppressive properties. *J. Gen. Virol.* 82: 2515–2518, **2001**.

Marguerat, S., Wang, W.Y., Todd, J.A., and Conrad, B. Association of human endogenous retrovirus K-18 polymorphisms with type 1 diabetes. *Diabetes* 53: 852–854, **2004**.

Marrack, P., Kushnir, E., and Kappler, J. A maternally inherited superantigen encoded by mammary tumour virus. *Nature* 349: 524–526, **1991**.

Martin, J., Herniou, E., Cook, J., Waugh O'Neill, R., and Tristem, M. Human endogenous retrovirus type I-related viruses have an apparently widespread distribution within vertebrates. *J. Virol.* 71: 437–443, **1997**.

Martin, M.A., Bryan, T., Rasheed, S., and Khan, A.S. Identification and cloning of endogenous retroviral sequences present in human DNA. *Proc. Natl. Acad. Sci. USA* 78: 4892–4896, **1981**.

Masciopinto, F., Giovani, C., Campagnoli, S., Galli-Stampino, L., Colombatto, P., Brunetto, M., Yen, T.S., Houghton, M., Pileri, P., and Abrignani, S. Association of hepatitis C virus envelope proteins with exosomes. *Eur. J. Immunol.* 34: 2834–2842, **2004**.

Mayer, J., Sauter, M., Racz, A., Scherer, D., Mueller-Lantzsch, N., and Meese, E. An almost-intact human endogenous retrovirus K on human chromosome 7. *Nat. Genet.* 21: 257–258, **1999**.

Mayer, J., Ehlhardt, S., Seifert, M., Sauter, M., Müller-Lantzsch, N., Mehraein, Y., Zang, K.-D., and Meese, E. Human endogenous retrovirus HERV-K(HLM-2) proviruses with Rec protein coding capacity and transcriptional activity. *Virology* 322: 190–198, **2004**.

Medstrand, P. and Mager, D.L. Human-specific integrations of the HERV-K endogenous retrovirus family. *J. Virol.* 72: 9782–9787, **1998**.

Medstrand, P., Lindeskog, M., and Blomberg, J. Expression of human endogenous retroviral sequences in peripheral blood mononuclear cells of healthy individuals. *J. Gen. Virol.* 73: 2463–2466, **1992**.

Melder, D.C., Pankratz, V.S., and Federspiel, M.J. Evolutionary pressure of a receptor competitor selects different subgroup a avian leukosis virus escape variants with altered receptor interactions. *J. Virol.* 77: 10 504–10 514, **2003**.

Meylan, F., De Smedt, M., Leclercq, G., Plum, J., Leupin, O., Marguerat, S., and Conrad, B. Negative thymocyte selection to HERV-K18 superantigens in humans. *Blood* 105: 4377–4382, **2005**.

Mi, S., Lee, X., Li, X., Veldman, G.M., Finnerty, H., Racie, L., LaVallie, E., Tang, X.Y., Edouard, P., Howes, S., Keith, J.C., Jr., and McCoy, J.M. Syncytin is a captive retroviral envelope protein involved in human placental morphogenesis. *Nature* 403: 785–789, **2000**.

Moles, J.P., Tesniere, A., and Gilhou, J.J. A new endogenous retroviral sequence is expressed in skin of patients with psoriasis. *Br. J. Dermatol.* 153: 83–89, **2005**.

Montefiori, D.C., Cornell, R.J., Zhou, J.Y., Zhou, J.T., Hirsch, V.M., and Johnson, P.R. Complement control proteins, CD46, CD55, and CD59, as common surface constituents of human and simian immunodeficiency viruses and possible targets for vaccine protection. *Virology* 205: 82–92, **1994**.

Morgan, D. and Brodsky, I. Human endogenous retrovirus (HERV-K) particles in megakaryocytes cultured from essential thrombocythemia peripheral blood stem cells. *Exp. Hematol.* 32: 520–525, **2004**.

Nakagawa, K., Brusic, V., McColl, G., and Harrison, L.C. Direct evidence for the expression of multiple endogenous retroviruses in the synovial compartment in rheumatoid arthritis. *Arthritis Rheum.* 40: 627–638, **1997**.

Nelson, P.N., Carnegie, P.R., Martin, J., Davari Ejtehadi, H., Hooley, P., Roden, D., Rowland-Jones, S., Warren, P., Astley, J., and Murray, P.G. Demystified. Human endogenous retroviruses. *Mol. Pathol.* 56: 11–18, **2003**.

Okada, N. and Hamada, M. The 3' ends of tRNA-derived SINEs originated from the 3' ends of LINEs: a new example from the bovine genome. *J. Mol. Evol. Suppl.* 1, 44: 52–56, **1997**.

Ono, M., Kawakami, M., and Ushikubo, H. Stimulation of expression of the human endogenous retrovirus genome by female steroid hormones in human breast cancer cell line T47D. *J. Virol.* 61: 2059–2062, **1987**.

Pang, S., Yu, D., An, D.S., Baldwin, G.C., Xie, Y., Poon, B., Chow, Y.H., Park, N.H., and Chen, I.S. Human immunodeficiency virus Env-independent infection of human CD4(-) cells. *J. Virol.* 74: 10 994–11 000, **2000**.

Patzke, S., Lindeskog, M., Munthe, E., and Aasheim, H.C. Characterization of a novel human endogenous retrovirus, HERV-H/F, expressed in human leukaemia cell lines. *Virology* 303: 164–173, **2002**.

Perron, H., Geny, C., Laurent, A.., Mouriquand, C., Pellat, J., Perret, J., and Seigneurin, J.M. Leptomeningeal cell line from multiple sclerosis with reverse transcriptase activity and viral particles. *Res. Virol.* 140: 551–561, **1989** .

Perron, H., Geny, C., Genoulaz, O., Pellat, J., Perret, J., and Seigneurin, J.M. Antibody to reverse transcriptase of human retroviruses in multiple sclerosis. *Acta Neurol. Scand.* 84: 507–513, **1991**.

Perron, H., Jouvin-Marche, E., Michel, M., Ounanian-Paraz, A., Camelo, S., Dumon, A., Jolivet-Reynaud, C., Marcel, F., Souillet, Y., Borel, E., Gebuhrer, L., Santoro, L., Marcel, S., Seigneurin, J.M., Marche, P.N., and Lafon, M. Multiple sclerosis retrovirus particles and recombinant envelope trigger an abnormal immune response in vitro, by inducing polyclonal Vâ16 T-lymphocyte activation. *Virology* 287: 321–332, **2001**.

Ponferrada, V.G., Mauck, B.S., and Wooley, D.P. The envelope glycoprotein of human endogenous retrovirus HERV-W induces cellular resistance to spleen necrosis virus. *Arch. Virol.* 148: 659–675, **2003**.

Purcell, D.F., Deacon, N.J., and McKenzie, I.F. The human non-lineage CD46 (HuLy-m5) and primate retroviral gp70 molecules share protein-defined antigenic determinants. *Immunol. Cell. Biol.* 67: 279–289, **1989**.

Raposo, G., Nijman, H.W., Stoorvogel, W., Liejendekker, R., Harding, C.V., Melief, C.J., and Geuze, H.W. B lymphocytes secrete antigen-presenting vesicles. *J. Exp. Med.* 183: 1161–1172, **1996**.

Raposo, G., Moore, M., Innes, D., Leijen-dekker, R., Leigh-Brown, A., Benaroch, P., and Geuze, H. Human macrophages accumulate HIV-1 particles in MHC II compartments. *Traffic* 3: 718–729, **2002**.

Renard, M., Varela, P.F., Letzelter, C., Duquerroy, S., Rey, F.A., and Heidmann, T. Crystal structure of a pivotal domain of human syncytin-2, a 40 million years old endogenous retrovirus fusogenic envelope gene captured by primates. *J. Mol. Biol .* 352: 1029–1034, **2005**.

Repaske, R., O'Neill, R.R., Steele, P.E., and Martin, M.A. Characterization and partial nucleotide sequence of endogenous type C retrovirus segments in human chromosomal DNA. *Proc. Natl. Acad. Sci. USA* 80: 678–682, **1983**.

Sauter, M., Schommer, S., Kremmer, E., Remberger, K., Dölken, G., Lemm, I., Buck, M., Best, B., Neumann-Haefelin, D., and Mueller-Lantzsch, N. Human endogenous retrovirus K10 expression of Gag protein and detection of antibodies in patients with seminomas. *Cancer Res. J. Virol.* 69: 414–421, **1995**.

Sauter, M., Roemer, K., Best, B., Afting, M., Schommer, S., Seitz, G., Hartmann, M., and Mueller-Lantzsch, N. Specificity of antibodies directed against Env protein of human endogenous retroviruses in patients with germ cell tumors. *Cancer Res.* 56: 4362–4365, **1996**.

Shiroma, T., Sugimoto, J., Oda, T., Jinno, Y., and Kanaya, F. Search for active endogenous retroviruses: identification and characterization of a HERV-E gene that is expressed in the pancreas and thyroid. *J. Hum. Genet.* 46: 619–625, **2001**.

Simpson, G.R., Patience, C., Löwer, R., Tönjes, R.R., Moore, H.D., Weiss, R.A., and Boyd, M.T. Endogenous D-type (HERV-K) related sequences are packaged into retroviral particles in the placenta and possess open reading frames for reverse transcriptase. *Virology* 222: 451–456, **1996**.

Spencer, T.E., Mura, M., Gray, C.A., Griebel, P.J., and Palmarini, M. Receptor usage and fetal expression of ovine endogenous betaretroviruses: implications for coevolution of endogenous and exogenous retroviruses. *J. Virol.* 77: 749–753, **2003**.

Stauffer, Y., Marguerat, S., Meylan, F., Ucla, C., Sutkowski, N., Huber, B., Pelet, T., and Conrad, B. Interferon-α-induced endogenous superantigen. A model linking environment and autoimmunity. *Immunity* 15: 591–601, **2001**.

Stauffer, Y., Theiler, G., Sperisen, P., Lebedev, Y., and Jongeneel, C.V. Digital expression profiles of human endogenous retroviral families in normal and cancerous tissues. *Cancer Immun.* 4: 2, **2004**.

Suenaga, K. and Yoon, J.W. Association of β-cell-specific expression of endogenous retrovirus with development of insulitis and diabetes in NOD mice. *Diabetes* 37: 1722–1726, **1988**.

Sugino, H., Oshimura, M., and Matsubara, K. Banding profiles of LTR of human endogenous retrovirus HERV-A in 24 chromosomes in somatic cell hybrids. *Genomics* 13: 461–464, **1992**.

Sutkowski, N., Palkama, T., Ciurli, C., Sekaly, R.P., Thorley Lawson, D.A., and Huber, B.T. An Epstein-Barr virus-associated superantigen. *J. Exp. Med.* 184: 971–980, **1996**.

Sutkowski, N., Conrad, B., Thorley-Lawson, D.A., and Huber, B.T. Epstein-Barr virus transactivates the human endogenous retrovirus HERV-K18 that encodes a superantigen. *Immunity* 15: 579–589, **2001**.

Sutkowski, N., Chen, G., Calderon, G., and Huber, B.T. Epstein-Barr virus latent membrane protein LMP-2A is sufficient for transactivation of the human endogenous retrovirus HERV-K18 superantigen. *J. Virol.* 78: 7852–7860, **2004**.

Swerdlow, E.D. Retroviruses and primate evolution. *BioEssays* 22: 161–171, **2000**.

Talal, N., Dauphinee, M.J., Dang, H., Alexander, S. S., Hart, D.J., and Garry, R.F. Detection of serum antibodies to retroviral proteins in patients with primary Sjogren's syndrome (autoimmune exocrinopathy). *Arthritis Rheum.* 33: 774–781, **1990**.

Themis, M., Waddington, S. M., Schmidt, M., von Kalle, C., Wang, Y., Al-Allaf, F., Gregory, L.G., Nivsarkar, M., Themis, M., Holderr, M.V., Buckley, S. M., Dighe, N., Ruthe, A.T., Mistry, A., Bigger, B., Rahim, A., Nguyen, T.H., Trono, D., Thraasher, A.J., and Coutelle, C. Oncogenesis following delivery of nonprimate lentiviral gene therapy vector to fetal and neonatal mice. *Mol. Ther.* 12: 763–771, **2005**.

Tönjes, R.R., Czauderna, F., and Kurth, R. Genome-wide screening, cloning, chromosomal assignment, and expression of full-length human endogenous retrovirus type K. *J. Virol.* 73: 9187–9195, **1999**.

Toth, F.D., Vaczi, L., Szabo, B., Kiss, J., Rethy, A., Kiss, A., Telek, B., Kovacs, I., Kiss, C., and Rak, K. Detection of main core proteins of simian C-type viruses and human retrovirus HTLV and antibodies to them in patients with lymphoid malignancies. *Acta Microbiol. Hung.* 32: 267–273, **1985**.

Turner, G., Barbulescu, M., Su, M., Jensen-Seaman, M.I., Kidd, K.K., and Lenz, J. Insertional polymorphisms of full-length endogenous retroviruses in humans. *Curr. Biol.* 11: 1531–1535, **2001**.

Ullu, E. and Tschudi, C. Alu sequences are processed 7SL RNA genes. *Nature* 312: 171–172, **1984**.

van de Lagemaat, L.N., Landry, J.R., Mager, D.L., and Medstrand, OP. Transposable elements in mammals promote regulatory variation and diversification of genes with specialized functions. *Trends Genet.* 19: 530–536, **2003**.

Venables, P.J.W., Brookes, S. M., Griffiths, D., Weiss, R.A., and Boyd, M.T. Abundance of an endogenous retroviral envelope protein in placental trophoblasts suggests a biological function. *Virology* 211: 589–592, **1995**.

Vernon, M.L., McMahon, J.M., and Hackett, J.J. Additional evidence of type-C particles in human placentas. *J. Natl. Cancer Inst.* 52: 987–989, **1974**.

Wang-Johanning, F., Frost, A.R., Jian, B., Azerou, R., Lu, D.W., Chen, D.T., and Johanning, G.L. Detecting the expression of human endogenous retrovirus E envelope transcripts in human prostate adenocarcinoma. *Cancer* 98: 187–197, **2003** .

Weiner, A.M., Deininger, P.L., Efstratiadis, A. Nonviral retroposons: genes, pseudogenes and transposable elements generated by the reverse flow of genetic information. *Annu. Rev. Biochem.* 55: 631–661, **1986**.

Wentzensen, N., Wilz, B., Findeisen, P., Wagner, R., Dippold, W., von Knebel Doeberitz, M., and Gebert, J. Identification of differentially expressed genes in colorectal adenoma compared to normal tissue by suppression subtractive hybridization. *Int. J. Oncol.* 24: 987–994, **2004**.

Wilkinson, D.A., Goodchild, N.L., Saxton, T.M., Wood, S., and Mager, D.L. Evidence for a functional subclass of the RTVL-H family of human endogenous retrovirus-like sequences. *J. Virol.* 67: 2981–2989, **1993**.

Wilkinson, D.A., Mager, D.L., and Leong, J.C. Endogenous human retroviruses. In: Levy, J. (Ed.), *The Retroviridae*. Plenum Press New York, pp. 465–535, **1994**.

Wolfers, J., Lozier, A., Raposo, G., Regnault, A., Thery, C., Masurier, C., Flamant, C., Pouzieux, S., Faure, F., Tursz, T., Angevin, E., Amigorena, S., and Zitvogel, L. Tumor-derived exosomes are a source of shared tumor rejection antigens for CTL cross-priming. *Nat. Med.* 7: 297–303, **2001**.

Woodland, D.L., Lund, F.E., Happ, M.P., Blackman, M.A., Palmer, E., and Corley, R.B. Endogenous superantigen expression is controlled by mouse mammary tumor proviral loci. *J. Exp. Med.* 174: 1255–1258, **1991**.

Yang, J., Bogerd, H.P., Peng, S., Wiegand, H., Truant, R., and Cullen, B.R. An ancient family of human endogenous retroviruses encodes a functional homolog of the HIV-1 Rev protein. *Proc. Natl. Acad. Sci. USA* 96: 13404–13408, **1999**.

Yi, J.M., Kim, T.H., Huh, J.W., Park, K.S., Jang, S. B., Kim, H.M., and Kim, H.S. Human endogenous retroviral elements belonging to the HERV-S family from human tissues, cancer cells, and primates: expression, structure, phylogeny and evolution. *Gene* 342: 283–292, **2004**.

Yi, J.M., Kim, H.M., and Kim, H.S. Human endogenous retrovirus HERV-H family in human tissues and cancer cells: expression, identification, and phylogeny. *Cancer Lett.* 231: 228–239, **2006**.

8.4
Gibbon Ape Leukemia Virus and Simian Sarcoma Virus

Although several different types of retrovirus infections have been noted in non-human primates – among them simian T-lymphotropic virus (STLV), simian immunodeficiency virus (SIV), simian type D retrovirus (SRV), and simian foamy virus (for a review, see Lerche and Osborn, 2003) – gibbon ape leukemia virus (GALV) and simian sarcoma virus (SSV) deserve a specific discussion. Besides STLV, GALV and SSV were both isolated from malignant proliferations (leukemias and sarcomas) in their native hosts, the gibbon ape and the woolly monkey, respectively (De Paoli and Garner, 1968; Theilen et al., 1971; Kawakami et al., 1972; Snyder et al., 1973; Todaro and Gallo, 1973; Gallo et al., 1978). The second reason originates from recent observations of sequences relatively closely related to these agents within the human genome, in part retaining the complete set of retroviral genes (see below).

GALV and SSV belong to the genus α of the retrovirus family, and are thus related to murine leukemia viruses and human endogenous virus types HERV-W and HERV-H. Several strains of GALV have been identified (Krakower et al., 1978; Reitz et al., 1979): the GALV-SF from gibbon lymphosarcomas (Kawakami et al., 1972; Snyder et al., 1973), GALV-S from a gibbon granulocytic leukemia (Kawakami and Buckley, 1974), GALV-H from an acute lymphatic leukemia in gibbons (Gallo et al., 1978), and also from frozen brain tissues of non-leukemic gibbons (GALV-Br) (Todaro et al., 1973). The woolly monkey SSV is closely related to these isolates, and shares 78% of amino acid identity with GALV-S (Ting et al., 1998). A cell-derived oncogene was not discovered within the isolates obtained from malignant proliferations of gibbons (Gelmann et al., 1982). It has, however, been discovered within the SSV genome (Dalla-Favera et al., 1981). A structural relationship of this sequence (v-sis) was subsequently discovered with human platelet-derived growth factor (PDGF) (Waterfield et al., 1983; Doolittle et al., 1983). This sequence is expressed in SSV-transformed cells (Deuel et al., 1983). The cellular homologue to v-sis, c-sis, was identified as one chain of PDGF (Josephs et al., 1984).

The viruses are apparently transmitted from viremic animals to their offspring either prenatally or postnatally (Kawakami et al., 1978). In prenatal infections – in contrast to postnatal exposure – large quantities of proviral DNA are commonly observed.

Studies on the biological activity of these viruses are still rare. SSV was able to induce tumors in marmoset monkeys (Wolfe et al., 1971), while a SSV isolate, supposedly originating from human leukemic cells, was shown capable of inducing tumors in these monkeys (Bergholz et al., 1977). The infection of young gibbons with GALV resulted in the development of chronic granulocytic leukemia with multifocal bone lesions and metastases after latency periods of 5–11 months (Kawakami et al., 1980). Gibbons infected at the age of 14 months developed persisting neutralizing antibodies to the virus and remained free of hematopoietic disease. Infection of human blood cells with either GALV or SSV led to enhanced induction of growth of B lymphoblasts (Markham et al., 1979).

A number of reports described the identification of SSV and GALV or the detection of antibodies directed against their antigens in human tumors or sera. Most of these studies were published during the 1970s or the early 1980s. One series of reports attempted to characterize a virus isolated from acute myelogenous leukemia (Gallagher and Gallo, 1975; Gallagher et al., 1975; Teich et al., 1975). At that time, GALV or SSV-related p30 antigens were demonstrated in peripheral white blood cells of humans with acute leukemia (Sherr and Todaro, 1975). Another report described the characterization of an RNA-directed DNA polymerase from human leukemic blood cells corresponding to the GALV-enzyme and being inhibited by antisera to reverse transcriptase from SSV (Mondal et al., 1975). A virus isolate from an AIDS patient with C-type virus characteristics was identified as a lymphocytopathic agent (Levy et al., 1984) and, after sequencing, as a new subtype of GALV (Parent et al., 1998). The demonstration of cytotoxicity of lymphocytes or antibodies against autologous tumor cells in patients with myeloid leukemia or preleukemic disorders was reported to be blocked by the gp70 antigen of GALV, and also by the corresponding protein of baboon endogenous retrovirus (Szabo et al., 1983). The close relationship of the human leukemia isolates to GALV and SSV, as initially demonstrated by tryptic digest mapping of peptides, raised the suspicion that they may have been derived from inadvertent contamination of the respective materials with gibbon and woolly monkey viruses (Fuqua and Naso, 1982). Reports demonstrating the presence of natural antibodies in 74–78% of sera from healthy humans to antigens of GALV (Aoki et al., 1976 a,b) added to the difficulties in interpreting the results of this period (see also Chapter 1).

It is interesting to note that virtually all isolates of GALV and SSV from human leukemic materials date back to more than 20 years ago. The data do not exclude an obviously extremely rare horizontal transmission of these nonhuman primate retroviruses to humans. It became clear, however, that neither GALV nor SSV sequences persist as endogenous genomes within the human germline. This seems to exclude a reactivation of such endogenous DNA in the course of leukemogenesis.

More recent studies point to the existence of a novel subgenus of human endogenous retroviruses most closely related to GALV and SSV. This sequence was apparently obtained from a patient with chronic myelogenous leukemia, and at present is only available in the human genome data bank (Xu and Zheng, 2003 a,b). The sequence represents a full-length retrovirus genome with the typical ORFs not interrupted by stop codons. At the nucleotide level it shares at various genomic sites between 54 and 66% of homology with the sequenced GALV isolate, and the individual ORFs show the following homology at the amino acid level: within the polymerase sequence of 47% for 1183 amino acids, for the gag sequence 34% for 506 amino acids, and for the env sequence 33% for 231 amino acids. The genomic organization of HVML is shown in Figure 8.8.

Our own studies revealed that at least three complete copies of this agent exist within the human genome (E.-M. de Villiers, R. Schmidt, and H. zur Hausen, unpublished results). Partial sequences are found in various chromosomal sites (see Fig. 8.9).

HCML – V Genome Structure

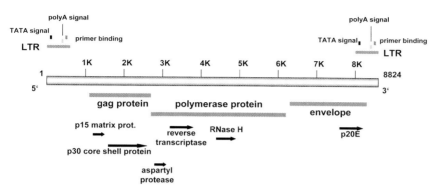

Fig. 8.8 HVML genome structure.

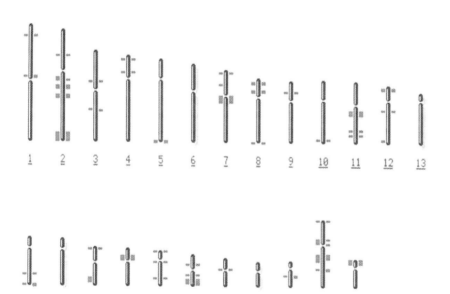

Fig. 8.9 Localization of HCML genomes in human chromosomes.

Besides HERV-K this seems to represent a second subgroup of human endogenous viruses which should be able to code for complete particles. The significance of
these observations is presently difficult to assess. The original observation of the
isolation of these GALV-related novel agents from a human chronic myelogenous
leukemia, a condition which in gibbons is clearly induced by such infections, should
create some interest in these or related agents.

References

Aoki, T., Liu, M., Walling, M.J., Bushar, G.S., Brandchaft, O.B., and Kawakami, T.G. Specificity of naturally occurring antibody in normal gibbon serum. *Science* 191: 1180–1183, **1976a**.

Aoki, T., Walling, M.J., Bushar, G.S., Liu, M., and Hsu, K.C. Natural antibodies in sera from healthy humans to antigens on surfaces of type C RNA viruses and cells from primates. *Proc. Natl. Acad. Sci. USA* 73: 2491–2495, **1976b**.

Bergholz, C.M., Wolfe, L.G., Deinhardt, F., Thakkar, B., and Marczynska, B. Oncogenicity in marmosets of HL-23V, a type C oncornavirus isolated from human leukemic cells, and comparison with simian sarcoma virus type 1 (SSV-1/SSAV-1). *J. Natl. Cancer Inst.* 58: 1041–1046, **1977**.

Dalla-Favera, R., Gelmann, E.P., Gallo, R.C., and Wong-Staal, F. A human onc gene homologous to the transforming gene (v-sis) of simian sarcoma virus. *Nature* 292: 31–35, **1981**.

De Paoli, A. and Garner, E.M. Acute lymphocytic leukaemia in a white-cheeked gibbon (*Hylobates concolor*). *Cancer Res.* 28: 2559–2561, **1968**.

Deuel, T.F., Huang, J.S., Huang, S. S., Stroobant, P., and Waterfield, M.D. Expression of a platelet-derived growth factor-like protein in simian sarcoma virus transformed cells. *Science* 221: 1348–1350, **1983**.

Doolittle, R.F., Hunkapiller, M.W., Hood, L.E., Devare, S. G., Robbins, K.C., Aaronson, S. A., and Antoniades, H.N. Simian sarcoma virus onc gene, v-sis, is derived from the gene (or genes) encoding a platelet-derived growth factor. *Science* 221: 275–277, **1983**.

Fuqua, S. A. and Naso, R.B. A comparison of the intracellular precursor polyproteins of simian sarcoma-associated virus [SiSV(SiAV)] and three human virus isolates: HL23V, HEL12V and A1476V. *J. Gen Virol.* 62: 49–63, **1982**.

Gallagher, R.E. and Gallo, R.C. Type C RNA tumor virus isolated from cultured human acute myelogenous leukemia cells. *Science* 187, 350–353, **1975**.

Gallagher, R.E., Salahuddin, S. Z., Hall, W.T., McCredie, K.B., and Gallo, R.C. Growth and differentiation in culture of leukemic leukocytes from a patient with acute myelogenous leukemia and re-identification of type-C virus. *Proc. Natl. Acad. Sci. USA* 72: 4137–4141, **1975**.

Gallo, R.C., Gallagher, R.E., Wong-Staal, F., Aoki, T., Markham, P.D., Schetters, H., Ruscetti, F., Valerio, M., Walling, M.J., O'Keefe, R.T., Saxinger, W.C., Smith, R.G., Gillespie, D.H., and Reitz, M.S., Jr. Isolation and tissue distribution of type-C virus and viral components from a gibbon ape (*Hylobates lar*) with lymphocytic leukemia. *Virology* 84: 359–373, **1978**.

Gelmann, E.P., Trainor, C.D., Wong-Staal, F., and Reitz, M.S. Molecular cloning of circular unintegrated DNA of two types of the SEATO-strain of gibbon ape leukemia virus. *J. Virol.* 44: 269–275, **1982**.

Josephs, S. F., Guo, C., Ratner, L., and Wong-Staal, F. Human-proto-oncogene nucleotide sequences corresponding to the transforming region of simian sarcoma virus. *Science* 223: 487–491, **1984**.

Kawakami, T.G., Huff, S. D., Buckley, P.M., Dungworth, D.L., Snyder, S. P., and Gilden, R.V. C-type virus associated with gibbon lymphosarcoma. *Nat. New Biol.* 235: 170–171, **1972**.

Kawakami, T. and Buckley, P.M. Antigenic studies in gibbon type C viruses. *Transplant. Proc.* 6: 193–196, **1974**.

Kawakami, T.G., Sun, L., and McDowell, T.S. Natural transmission of gibbon leukemia virus. *J. Natl. Cancer Inst.* 61: 1113–1115, **1978**.

Kawakami, T.G., Kollias, G.V., Jr., and Holmberg, C. Oncogenicity of gibbon type-C myelogenous leukemia virus. *Int. J. Cancer* 25: 641–646, **1980**.

Krakower, J.M., Tronick, S. R., Gallagher, R.E., Gallo, R.C., and Aaronson, S. A. Antigenic characterization of a new gibbon ape leukemia virus isolate: seroepidemiologic assessment of an outbreak of gibbon leukemia. *Int. J. Cancer* 22: 715–721, **1978**.

Lerche, N.W. and Osborn, K.G. Simian retrovirus infections: potential confounding variables in primate toxicology studies. *Toxicol. Pathol.* 31: 103–110, **2003**.

Levy, J.A., Hoffman, A.D., Kramer, S. M., Landis, J.A., Shimabukuro, J.M., and Oshiro, L.S. Isolation of lymphocytopathic retroviruses from San Francisco patients with AIDS. *Science* 225: 840–842, **1984**.

Markham, P.D., Ruscetti, F., Salahuddin, S. Z., Gallagher, R.E., and Gallo, R.C. Enhanced induction of growth of B lymphoblasts from fresh human blood by primate type-C retroviruses (gibbon ape leukemia virus and simian sarcoma virus). *Int. J. Cancer* 23: 148–156, **1979**.

Mondal, H., Gallagher, R.E., and Gallo, R.C. RNA-directed DNA polymerase from human leukemic blood cells and from primate type-C virus-producing cells: high and low-molecular-weight forms with variant biochemical and immunological properties. *Proc. Natl. Acad. Sci. USA* 72: 1194–1198, **1975**.

Parent, I., Qin, Y., Vandenbroucke, A.T., Walon, C., Delferriere, N., Godfroid, E., and Burtonboy, G. Characterization of a C-type retrovirus isolated from an HIV infected cell line: complete nucleotide sequence. *Arch. Virol.* 143: 1077–1092, **1998**.

Reitz, M.S., Jr., Wong-Staal, F., Haseltine, W.A., Kleid, D.G., Trainor, C.D., Gallagher, R.E., and Gallo, R.C. Gibbon ape leukemia virus-Hall's Island: new strain of gibbon ape leukemia virus. *J. Virol.* 29: 395–400, **1979**.

Sherr, C.J. and Todaro, G.J. Primate type C virus p30 antigen in cells from humans with acute leukemia. *Science* 187: 855–857, **1975**.

Snyder, S. P., Dungworth, D.L., Kawakami, T.G., Callaway, E., and Lau, D.T. Lymphosarcomas in two gibbons (*Hylobates lar*) with associated C-type virus. *J. Natl. Cancer Inst.* 51: 89–94, **1973**.

Szabo, B., Toth, F.D., Vaczi, L., Rethy, A., Kiss, A., and Rak, K. Cytotoxicity of lymphocytes and antibodies against autologous tumor cells in patients with myeloid leukemias and preleukemic disorders. I.

Blocking activity of gp70 antigens of primate type C viruses. *Neoplasma* 30: 129–135, **1983**.

Teich, N.M., Weiss, R.A., Salahuddin, S. Z., Gallagher, R.E., Gillespie, D.H., and Gallo, R.C. Infective transmission and characterisation of a C-type virus released by cultured human myeloid leukaemia cells. *Nature* 256: 551–555, **1975** .

Theilen, G.H., Gould, D., Fowler, M., and Dungworth, D.L. C-type virus in tumor tissue of a woolly monkey (*Lagothrix* spp.) with fibrosarcoma. *J. Natl. Cancer Inst.* 47: 881–889, **1971**.

Ting, Y.T., Wilson, C.A., Farrell, K.B., Chaudry, G.J., and Eiden, M.V. Simian sarcoma-associated virus fails to infect Chinese hamster cells despite the presence of functional gibbon ape leukemia virus receptors. *J. Virol.* 72: 9453–9458, **1998**.

Todaro, G.J. and Gallo, RC. Immunological relationship of DNA polymerase from human acute leukaemia cells and primate and mouse leukaemia virus reverse transcriptase. *Nature* 244: 206–209, **1973**.

Todaro, G.J., Lieber, M.M., Beneveniste, R.E., and Sherr, C.J. Infectious primate type C viruses: Three isolates belonging to a new subgroup from the brains of normal gibbons. *Virology* 67: 335–343, **1975**.

Waterfield, M.D., Scrace, G.T., Whittle, N., Stroobant, P., Johnsson, A., Wasteson, A., Westermark, B., Heldin, C.H., Huang, J.S., and Deuel, T.F. Platelet-derived growth factor is structurally related to the putative transforming protein p28sis of simian sarcoma virus. *Nature* 304: 35–39, **1983**.

Wolfe, L.G., Deinhardt, F., Theilen, G.H., Rabin, H., Kawakami, T., and Bustad, L.K. Induction of tumors in marmoset monkeys by simian sarcoma virus, type 1 (Lagothrix): a preliminary report. *J. Natl. Cancer Inst.* 47: 1115–1120, **1971**.

Xu, R.Z. and Zheng, S. Data Base Accession Number AF499232, unpublished **2003 a**.

Xu, R.Z. and Zheng, S. Data Base Accession Number AY2o8746, unpublished, **2003 b**.

9
Other Virus Infections Possibly Involved in Human Cancers

9.1
Polyomaviruses (JC, BK, and SV40)

Members of the polyomavirus family represent small (~40 nm) non-enveloped viruses (Fig. 9.1) containing a circular double-stranded (ds) DNA genome of about 5200 base pairs. Open reading frames (ORFs) for one of these viruses (SV40) are shown in Figure 9.2.

To date, two human polyoma-type viruses have been isolated, and both have received designations with the initials of the patient from whom they were isolated: the BK virus was isolated in 1971 (Gardner et al.), and the JC virus within the same year by Padgett et al. Both of these agents are widely spread among all human populations, and cause persistent infections that may be reactivated under conditions of severe immunosuppression. In the latter case, specifically JC virus may cause progressive multifocal leukencephalopathy.

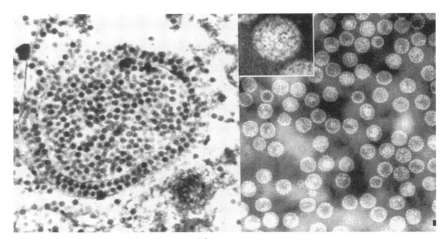

Fig. 9.1 Polyoma-type particles. (Reprinted from VIRUS TAXONOMY, Eighth Report of the International Committee on Taxonomy of Viruses, Vol 1, Fauquet, C.M., Mayo, M.A., Maniloff, J., Desselberger, U. and Ball, L.A. (Eds.), Part II – The Double Stranded DNA Viruses, Polyomaviridae, 232. Copyright 2005, with permission from Elsevier.)

Infections Causing Human Cancer. Harald zur Hausen
Copyright © 2006 WILEY-VCH Verlag GmbH & Co. KGaA, Weinheim
ISBN: 3-527-31056-8

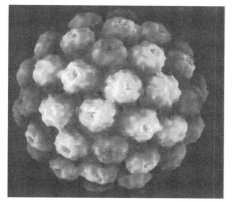
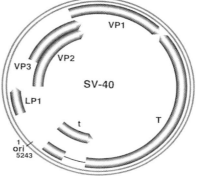

Fig. 9.2 Schematic representation of a polyoma virus particle and of the open reading frames within the SV40 genome. (Reprinted from VIRUS TAXONOMY, Eighth Report of the International Committee on Taxonomy of Viruses, Vol 1, Fauquet, C.M., Mayo, M.A., Maniloff, J., Desselberger, U. and Ball, L.A. (Eds.), Part II – The Double Stranded DNA Viruses, Polyomaviridae, 231. Copyright 2005, with permission from Elsevier.)

Several additional polyoma-type viruses have also been identified in nonhuman primates and other mammalian and avian species. Here, we will discuss only polyoma-type viruses in nonhuman primates. The first isolate in this group is the simian virus 40 (SV40), initially identified as a contamination of rhesus monkey kidney cells (Eddy et al., 1961, 1962). In addition to SV40, simian agent 12 is regularly found in baboons, while a novel polyoma virus was recently discovered in the feces of a chimpanzee (Johne et al., 2005). An additional polyoma-type virus was isolated from lymphoblastoid cell cultures of an African green monkey and labeled as B-lymphotropic polyomavirus (zur Hausen and Gissmann, 1979). A number of human sera contain antibodies neutralizing this virus, yet, attempts to isolate this or a related agent from human specimens thus far have been unsuccessful (Brade et al., 1981).

The majority of polyoma-type viruses are effective carcinogens. As a rule, with few exceptions, they do not induce tumors within their natural hosts but do this efficiently upon inoculation into newborn rodents. One of these viruses (JC) also induces gliomas upon intracerebral infection of adult owl monkeys (London et al., 1978).

It remains one of the most interesting – but poorly studied – questions as to how the natural host of these viruses inhibits the potential oncogenicity of these agents. Indeed, besides polyoma-type viruses a number of human adenovirus types have been identified which also represent effective carcinogens for newborn rodents, but have not been identified in any malignant human condition. The control for polyoma-type viruses can neither be solely immunological nor a question of permissiveness, since BK, JC, and SV40 viruses persist in their natural hosts despite a clearly measurable immune response. The suspicion that cells of the natural host succumb to lytic infections by these agents and thus cannot be transformed, must also be incorrect, since at least JC virus infects human cells in tissue culture abortively without lysing or transforming them. The life-long persistence of some of these agents also argues against this hypothesis.

The evidence for a tumorigenic function of primate polyomaviruses in their natural hosts is at best poor (see below), although most of these virus types induce effectively tumors in the nonpermissive heterologous hosts. This led to the question of whether a reciprocal situation might exist for some animal viruses potentially infecting humans (*zur Hausen*, 2001). In this case, the nonpermissive human cells, not being adapted to the respective infection, may have failed to develop the necessary cellular interfering factors to cope with these then potentially transforming infections. Careful studies along those lines have not yet been conducted.

During the past four decades, polyoma-type viruses have attracted intense attention, in particular the SV40 and murine polyomaviruses. This led to many early studies on the molecular biology of virus-induced oncogenesis, with the viruses serving as vector systems for gene technological experiments (Strayer et al., 2005), and last – but certainly not least – as potential human tumor viruses.

It is not the intention of this chapter to review the vast body of literature covering the molecular biology of these viruses and their transforming activities *in vitro* and *in vivo*. In this respect, the reader is referred to reviews by White and Khalili (2004), Ahuja et al. (2005), and Arroyo and Hahn (2005). This chapter will outline only those data related to human carcinogenesis and to the potential role of BK, JC, and SV40 viruses.

9.1.1
BK Virus

BK virus infections commonly occur early in childhood. In the vast majority of cases the primary infection is asymptomatic, but it may very occasionally lead to mild respiratory symptoms (Mantyjärvi et al., 1973; Goudsmit et al., 1982). Very rarely, the infection causes cystitis and kidney disease in children (Padgett and Walker, 1983; Saitoh et al., 1993). The virus persists apparently for the patient's lifetime, and may be reactivated during pregnancy, with slightly more than 3% of pregnant women excreting BK virus in the urine (Coleman et al., 1980). Under immunosuppression – for example in renal transplant patients or bone marrow transplant recipients – virus excretion occurs in 25–45% of cases (Hogan et al., 1980; Gardner et al., 1984; Andrews et al., 1988). Hemorrhagic cystitis is a common complication especially in allogeneic bone marrow recipients. This condition is regularly accompanied by – and probably caused by – the excretion of BK virus (Arthur et al., 1986; Apperley et al., 1987; Chapman et al., 1991).

9.1.1.1 Tumorigenicity of BK Virus in Experimental Animals

The immortalization of rabbit, rat, mouse, and monkey cells by BK virus infections was reported as early as the 1970s (Mason and Takemoto, 1977; Portolani and Borgatti, 1978; Seehafer et al., 1979). All immortalized cells produced the BK virus-specific T-antigen, commonly contained episomal virus DNA, and were not tumorigenic when heterografted into immunoincompetent hosts (nude mice).

The inoculation of BK virus into newborn rodents, however, resulted in tumors, with tumor development depending on the animal species, the site of inoculation, and on the amount of virus administered. Brain tumors were the most frequently observed, such as ependymomas in hamsters (Uchida et al., 1976; Corralini et al., 1977), choroid plexus papillomas (Greenlee et al., 1977), gliomas, neuroblastomas, insulinomas, neuroblastomas, nephroblastomas, osteosarcomas, fibrosarcomas, and lymphomas (Corralini et al., 1978, 1982; Yogo et al., 1980). It was noted at an early stage that histologically corresponding cancers in humans were devoid of detectable BK virus sequences and BK virus T-antigen (Grossi et al., 1981).

Transgenic mice containing the early BK virus regions developed liver and renal cell cancers at 8–10 months of age, and expressed viral mRNA within the tumor tissue (Small et al., 1986 a). Thymoproliferative disorders and lymphomas were induced in another set of experiments, besides renal adenocarcinomas (Dalrymple and Beemon, 1990). Transgenic mice carrying the HIV tat gene in addition to the BK early region developed skin leiomyosarcomas, squamous cell papillomas and carcinomas, adenocarcinomas of skin adnexa, glands, and B-cell lymphomas (Corallini et al., 1993).

9.1.1.2 Immortalization of Human Cells by BK Virus, and BK Virus in Human Cancers

Immortalization was also observed in BK virus-infected human kidney and human fetal brain cells, although the cells retained a semi-permissive state and continued to produce small quantities of infectious BK virus (Purchio and Fareed, 1979; Takemoto et al., 1979).

BK DNA has been reported in human neuroblastomas (Flaegstad et al., 1999), although neuroblastoma cell lines were negative for BK (Stolt et al., 2005). In addition, viral DNA was also reported in an occasional glioma (5/150) and in a single medulloblastoma (Huang et al., 1999). One report claimed the presence of episomal BK virus DNA in primary human brain tumors, in Kaposi's sarcoma and in cell lines from brain tumors, in Ewing sarcoma and in osteogenic sarcoma. Infectious BKV was rescued from several of these tumors and tumor cell lines by transfecting the total cellular DNA derived from such sources into human embryonic fibroblasts (Negrini et al., 1990). Since all these positive samples contained the DNA of one specific BK virus variant previously isolated from a tumor of the pancreatic islet by the same group, the risk of inadvertent contamination appears to be relatively high and, indeed, other groups were unable to confirm this finding (Weggen et al., 2000; Kim et al., 2002; Rollison et al., 2005 a). There was also no serological indication for elevated BK virus antibody levels in patients with brain tumors (Rollison et al., 2003).

Thus, the presently available data provide no hint that BK virus is involved in human cancer development.

9.1.2
JC Virus

JC virus, similar to BK virus, is widely spread among all human populations, apparently persisting within the central nervous system for the patient's lifetime. The primary infection is commonly asymptomatic, but under conditions of severe immunosuppression it may cause a subacute fatal demyelinating disease, progressive multifocal leukoencephalopathy (PML). Although during the past few decades PML has been mainly seen among elderly patients, the current AIDS epidemic has resulted in PML being identified in younger patients. Oligodendrocytes in PML lesions produce large quantities of the JC virus.

9.1.2.1 Tumorigenicity of JC Virus in Experimental Animals

An initial report described the transformation of primary hamster brain cells by JC virus or by viral DNA (Frisque et al., 1980). NIH 3T3 cells can be also transformed by JC, although at lower efficiency than with BK or SV40 DNA (Hayashi et al., 2001). In cell lines obtained from mice transgenic for the early region of JC virus, there was no T-Ag expression in mesenchymal fibroblasts. Instead, T-Ag-positive lines had characteristics consistent with a neural crest origin (Beggs et al., 1990). Primary brain cultures from the same animals contained many T-Ag-positive astrocytes, but no expression was detected in macrophages, epithelial cells, neuronal cells, or in oligodendrocytes. Thus, the strict tissue specificity of JCV T-antigen expression was maintained. This tissue specificity of early gene expression and function is determined by the JC virus promoter (Feigenbaum et al., 1992).

The virus effectively induces tumors upon inoculation into hamsters, mainly cerebellar medulloblastomas and plexus tumors (Nagashima et al., 1984). Intracranial injection of JC virus into newborn Sprague-Dawley rats resulted in brain tumors in the cerebrum, but not in the cerebellum. Most of the tumor cells were of an undifferentiated neuroectodermal nature (Ohsumi et al., 1986). One of the most interesting observations was the induction of brain tumors in owl monkeys at 18 and 25 months after intracerebral inoculation of JC virus (London et al., 1978). The first of these tumors represented one grade 3 to grade 4 astrocytoma, resembling a human glioblastoma multiforme; the second malignant tumor contained both, glial and neuronal cell types. A cell line established from one of the tumors continued to express the JC virus T-antigen (Major et al., 1984).

In mice, transgenic for the early region of JC virus, dysmyelination in the central nervous system was observed, but not in the peripheral nervous system (Small et al., 1986 b). Some of these animals also developed adrenal neuroblastomas (Small et al.,

1986 a). In another line of transgenic mice the development of massive, undifferentiated, solid mesenteric tumors of neural crest origin was noted, without obvious neurological symptoms (Franks et al., 1996; Krynska et al., 1997). Other animals developed tumors which closely resembled the human medulloblastoma/primitive neuroectodermal tumors (PNETs) in location, histologic appearance, and expression of marker proteins (Krynska et al., 1999 a). Approximately 50 % of the animals developed pituitary tumors by 1 year of age (Shollar et al., 2004), although a small subset developed solid masses arising from the soft tissues surrounding the salivary gland, the sciatic nerve, and along the extremities. Histologically, the tumors resembled malignant peripheral nerve sheath tumors, a rare type of neoplasm which occur in individuals with neurofibromatosis type 1 (NF1) (Shollar et al., 2004).

9.1.2.2 Immortalization of Human Cells by JC Virus, and JC Virus in Human Cancers

Primary human fetal glial cells can be transformed *in vitro* by JC virus infection and retain a partial permissivity for JC virus replication (Mandl et al., 1987). Few data exist on cell transformation in human systems, most likely due to the stringent cell tropism of the virus. Yet, transfection of BK virus DNA into human fibroblasts already infected with human cytomegalovirus results in pronounced replication of JC DNA (Heilbronn et al., 1993; Winklhofer et al., 2000).

In contrast to the paucity of reports on transformation of human cells by JC viruses, a larger number of publications claim a role for this virus in human carcinogenesis. Reports on the co-existence of cancerous lesions within PML foci raised the suspicion that JC virus may cause different types of brain tumor (Castaigne et al., 1974; Sima et al., 1983; Gullotta et al., 1992). In these studies, astrocytomas and gliomas were recorded, but unfortunately the tumors were not fully analyzed for JC virus DNA persistence or T-antigen expression, and no cell lines have been established from them. A few brain tumors, however, have been reported to be positive for JC virus DNA, RNA and T-antigen: one of these tumors was an oligoastrocytoma (Rencic et al., 1996). The tumor material consisted partly of an oligodendroglioma and partly of an astrocytoma, though the JCV T-antigen was only detected within the oligodendroglioma portion. In another observation, JCV DNA was identified in a pleomorphic xanthoastrocytoma of a nine-year-old child (Boldorini et al., 1998). A further report described JC virus DNA in 11 out of 23 childhood medulloblastomas (Krynska et al., 1999 b), with four of these tumors also expressing T-antigen in the nuclei of the cancer cells. One study suggested a role for the JC virus agnoprotein in the development of T-antigen-negative tumors (Del Valle et al., 2002); immunohistochemical analysis showed a cytoplasmic localization and widespread distribution of agnoprotein in the neoplastic cells in 11 of 20 samples (55 %). The JCV early gene product, T-antigen, was present in the nucleus of some – but not all – of the neoplastic cells. Other medulloblastoma samples that expressed agnoprotein had no sign of T-antigen expression. Among 32 medulloblastomas, 18 ependymomas, five choroid plexus papillomas, and seven pilocytic astrocytomas analyzed for the presence of JC virus DNA by Southern blot hybridization and direct sequencing, JC viral DNA sequence was detected in only five ependymomas and one choroid plexus papilloma (Okamoto et al., 2005). In this study, immunohistochemistry revealed nuclear expression of the large T-antigen in one choroid plexus papilloma, but none of the medulloblastomas or pilocytic astrocytomas contained JC virus DNA. In another study, JCV DNA was found in nine out of 22 brain tumors, including eight astrocyte-derived tumors (seven glioblastomas and one astrocytoma) and one oligodendroglioma, and in two of 15 cerebrospinal fluid specimens with positive tumor tissue (one glioblastoma and one astrocytoma) (Boldorini et al., 2003). By using gene amplification techniques, Del Valle et al. (2001) demonstrated the presence of JC viral early sequence in 49 of 71 samples (69%) (oligodendroglioma, astrocytoma, pilocytic astrocytoma, oligoastrocytoma, anaplastic astrocytoma, anaplastic oligodendroglioma, glioblastoma multiforme, gliomatosis cerebri, gliosarcoma, ependymoma, and subependymoma). In this series, an immunohistochemistry analysis revealed expression of the JCV T-antigen in the nuclei of tumor cells in 28 of 85 (32.9 %) tested samples.

This impressive list of positive data was contrasted by some studies unable to detect JC virus DNA in brain tumors. For example, Arthur et al. (1994) failed to detect JC sequences in 75 glial tumors and tumor-derived cell lines; likewise, Herbarth et al. (1998) could not find JC virus DNA in 52 gliomas or tumor-derived cell lines. Similarly, in eight cases of medulloblastoma, Hayashi et al. (2001) did not find any evidence of JC viral DNA or expression of T-antigens; neither was any JC virus DNA noted in 15 primary medulloblastomas and five supratentorial primitive neuroectodermal tumors (Kim et al., 2002). Another study conducted between two separate laboratories found only three out of 225 brain tumors to be positive for JC virus DNA (Rollison et al., 2005 a).

The major problem in interpreting all of these results stems from the strict neurotropism of JC virus. It is difficult to exclude a passenger role of JC virus in DNA samples of, or even T-antigen-positive brain tumors, although at least some of the data appear suggestive of an etiological role. In order to analyze the question of causality more stringently, experiments are required to demonstrate the need for viral gene transcription and/or protein expression for maintenance of the malignant phenotype. The induction of polyploidy was noted in JC virus-infected cells (Neel et al., 1996), as well as increased chromosomal abnormalities in lymphocytes of patients with high antibody titers to JC antigens (Lazutka et al., 1996). This may suggest an indirect contribution of JC virus infections to carcinogenesis, though obviously additional studies are required to clarify the situation.

Some groups have reported the presence of JC viral DNA and T-antigens in a high percentage of samples from colorectal cancer and from normal colon mucosa (Laghi et al., 1999; Casini et al., 2005; Theodoropoulos et al., 2005). Another group was unable to confirm this finding in an analysis of 233 colorectal tumor samples (Newcomb et al., 2004), even though they were able to detect JC virus DNA in 70% of urine samples of such patients. This group found no evidence to indicate that JCV is the cause of genetic instability in colorectal cancer. Thus, the possible role of JC virus in colorectal cancer remains controversial and also requires further studies.

9.1.3
SV40

Since its discovery during the early 1960s, SV40 has been the prototype of a DNA tumor virus, besides mouse polyoma virus. It easily transforms a wide variety of cells in tissue culture and efficiently induces tumors when inoculated into newborn rodents. SV40 is present as a latent infection in rhesus monkeys and, at least at the time of the discovery of this agent, there was no evidence for SV40 infections in humans. A well-documented exposure of humans to this virus, however, occurred between 1955 and 1963 as the consequence of immunization with SV40 virus-contaminated poliovirus vaccines (Shah and Nathanson, 1976; Strickler and Goedert, 1998). In Europe and the United States, it is likely that several million people were vaccinated with this contaminated vaccine.

Since that time there have been many discussions on whether this inadvertent infection of humans with an established tumor virus might have contributed to human carcinogenesis. In particular, human cancers were studied which correspond to SV40-induced tumors in animal systems, such as a variety of brain tumors, including choroids plexus papillomas, mesotheliomas, and lymphomas.

9.1.3.1   Tumorigenicity of SV40 in Experimental Animals

It is not the intention of this section to review the extensive literature on tumor induction of SV40 in animal systems. Rather, the reader is referred to reviews by Shah (1996) and Ahuja et al. (2005). These authors also refer to the transforming properties of SV40 early proteins and the signaling pathway affected by the expression of these proteins. The infection into newborn mice, hamsters, rats, and other rodents results in tumor formation several months later. A remarkable chromosomal instability is induced by these infections as a function of T-antigen expression (for a review, see Lavia et al., 2003).

9.1.3.2   Immortalization of Human Cells by SV40, and SV40 in Human Cancers

The detection of SV40 sequences in human cancers is rendered difficult due to three technical problems:
- SV40 sequences, spanning almost the complete genome, are present in the majority of commercially used gene vector systems (Völter et al., 1997, 1998; Lopez-Rios et al., 2004; Vera and Fortes, 2004; Strayer et al., 2005). An example of the commonly used vectors that contain SV40 sequences is shown in Figure 9.3. Only a short stretch of 286 bp of the SV40 genome, 3' of VP 2 and VP3 and 5' of VP1, is not represented in any of more than 200 vector sequences present in the databanks (Fig. 9.3) (C. Völter and E.-M. de Villiers, unpublished results). Clearly, the frequent presence of

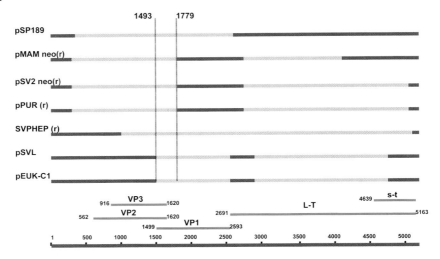

Fig. 9.3 SV40 sequences in some commonly used vector systems. The SV40 sequences are indicated in dark red. The corresponding open reading frames are colored light red. The scale at the bottom reveals the linearized SV40 DNA. (C. Völter and E.-M. de Villiers, unpublished results.)

SV40 sequences in vector DNA poses a substantial problem for possible contaminations (Lopez-Rios et al., 2004).

- A second problem stems from a high degree of homology between SV40 and JC viral DNA. This affects in particular the immunohistochemical detection of viral T antigens. Even a monoclonal antibody to SV40 large T-antigen labels a nuclear antigen in JC virus-transformed cells and in PML brain infected with JC virus (Stoner et al., 1988). Crossreactivity between these polyoma-type viral antigens seems difficult to avoid.

- A third problem is posed by the existence of an extensive homology between part of the SV40 T-antigen and human cellular DNA (Martini et al., 2002; zur Hausen, 2003). This is particularly problematic when polymerase chain reaction primers are used covering a region from nucleotides 4476–4104 (373 bp at the amino terminus) and from nucleotides 2774–2630 (145 bp at the carboxy terminus). These regions show a 97% homology with human genomic sequences in the telomeric regions of chromosomes 10 (191 of 195 bp) and 11 (340 of 348 bp) (Martini et al., 2002).

These considerations must be borne in mind during any analysis of the multiple positive findings of SV40 DNA in human tumors.

Initial observations of SV40 DNA sequences were made in brain tumors, including ependymomas and choroid plexus papillomas (Bergsagel et al., 1992), in five meningeomas, in one astrocytoma, one oligodendroglioma, and one medulloblastoma (Krieg et al., 1981). A number of additional reports claimed the presence of SV40 DNA in brain tumors: Woloschak et al. (1995) found SV40 DNA in one human brain tumor and sequenced the viral genome. Several other groups reported a number of different brain tumors positive for SV40 DNA (Huang et al., 1999; Zhen et al., 1999; Kouhata et al., 2001; Malkin et al., 2001). The T-antigen region of SV40 was amplified from four ependymomas and three gliomas (Suzuki et al., 1997). Sequence analysis of two brain and one osteosarcoma SV40 sequences did not provide evidence for a "human-specific" SV40 sequence (Stewart et al., 1998). Two human glioblastoma cell lines were reported to contain both, BK virus and SV40 T-antigens (Martini et al., 1996).

Early and contemporary reports were unable to confirm these findings: Greenlee et al. (1978) failed to find SV40 T-antigen in human cerebral tumors. Even in northern India, where rhesus monkeys – the natural host of SV40 – are abundant, human brain tumors were found to be negative for SV40 DNA (Engels et al., 2002).

In addition to brain tumors, primarily methotheliomas, as well as osteosarcomas, renal cancer, thyroid carcinomas, lymphomas and Hodgkin's disease materials were reported to contain SV40 DNA. Human osteosarcomas were found to be positive for SV40 DNA sequences by several groups (Lednicky et al., 1997; Butel et al., 1998; Mendoza et al., 1998; Heinsohn et al., 2000; Yamamoto et al., 2000).

The first reports on SV40 DNA in human mesotheliomas appeared during the mid-1990s (Carbone et al., 1994, 1996), and several other positive reports followed shortly thereafter (Pepper et al., 1996; Galateau-Salle et al., 1998; Testa et al., 1998; Mayall et al., 1999; Shivapurkar et al., 1999; McLaren et al., 2000). SV40 genome-positive mesotheliomas were reported to have a poor prognosis (Procopio et al., 2000). One report described geographical differences for SV40-positive mesotheliomas that were found in the United States, but not in Turkey (De Rienzo et al., 2002). Another report noted that SV40-specific cytotoxic T cells had been generated from the peripheral blood of malignant pleural mesothelioma patients (Bright et al., 2002). One report from Japan indicated that SV40-positive mesotheliomas had occurred among a population which was unlikely to have been exposed to SV40-contaminated poliovirus vaccine (Jin et al., 2004). Furthermore, SV40 was reported to enhance the risk of malignant mesothelioma among people exposed to asbestos (Cristaudo et al., 2005). It should be noted that the listing provided here omits a larger number of reviews published on this topic.

Although at first glance impressive, an equally long list of negative findings contrast these reports: a number of epidemiological studies failed to find any increased incidence of mesotheliomas or other cancer in those populations exposed to SV40-contaminated poliovirus vaccines (Olin and Gieseke, 1998; Strickler et al., 1998, 2003; Engels et al., 2003; Rollison et al., 2004, 2005a; Engels, 2005). Similarly, seroepidemiological studies analyzing populations previously exposed to contaminated vaccines for SV40 antibodies failed to detect evidence for persistent SV40 infections (Carter et al., 2003; Shah et al., 2004). Failure to detect SV40 T-antigens in mesotheliomas was published repeatedly (Pilatte et al., 2000; Simsir et al., 2001). In addition, a larger number of reports failed to confirm the presence of SV40 DNA in mesotheliomas obtained from various regions of the world (Krainer et al., 1995; Strickler et al., 1996, 2001; Hirvonen et al., 1999; Mulatero et al., 1999; Emri et al., 2000; Hubner and Van Marck, 2002; Leithner et al., 2002; Manfredi et al., 2005). A critical discussion of positive data pointed to the problems linked to the finding of SV40 DNA in human tumors (Griffiths et al., 1998; Lopez-Rios et al., 2004).

An initial report showing the presence of SV40 DNA in human lymphomas, in Hodgkin's disease and in lymphadenopathies was published in 1998 (Martini et al., 1998). The same group had previously found SV40 sequences in the peripheral blood (Martini et al., 1996). These data were supported by other reports which also claimed SV40 sequences in a substantial percentage of blood cells from healthy donors (David et al., 2001). A surprisingly high percentage of SV40-positive non-Hodgkin lymphomas (NHL) and Hodgkin lymphomas was reported by Vilchez et al. (2002 a,b, 2005) and Shivapurkar et al. (2002, 2004). Several positive tumors were also found in Japan (Nakatsuka et al., 2003).

Initial data not fully compatible with these observations were published in 2003 (de Sanjose et al.). These authors failed to find serologic evidence for SV40 infections in lymphoma patients. In addition, epidemiological surveys provided no evidence for an increased risk of previously SV40-exposed persons for NHL (Engels et al., 2003, 2004; Rollison et al., 2005 b; Schuler et al., 2005; Thu et al., 2006). A large series of NHL (n = 152) from the United Kingdom turned out to be negative for SV40 DNA (MacKenzie et al., 2003). Other reports also failed to find SV40 DNA in human lymphomas (Montesinos-Rongen et al., 2004; Sui et al., 2005). An immunohistological search provided no evidence for the presence of SV40 T-antigen in a large series of NHL and Hodgkin's lymphomas (Brousset et al., 2004).

Sporadic reports of SV40 sequences in a larger number of additional tumors have been published, but remain as yet unconfirmed. Tests in cell lines obtained from bladder carcinomas, Hodgkin lymphomas, and Kaposi's sarcoma, as well as DNA from meningiomas and Kaposi's tumors were negative for any known polyoma virus DNA (Völter et al., 1997).

9.1.3.3 Does SV40 Represent a Human Carcinogen?

In comparison to other viral carcinogens discussed in this book, the data published on the role of SV40 in human cancers are at least disturbing. A large number of conflicting reports cover the three tumor localizations or major tumor types reported to be linked to this infection, namely brain tumors, mesotheliomas, and NHL. Neither does epidemiology support an increased cancer risk for the SV40-exposed population; nor does seroepidemiology point to an increased risk of the low number of SV40-seroreactive probands for cancers.

Given the limitations of the test systems discussed in the first section of this chapter, it becomes increasingly questionable as to whether this virus does indeed cause any proliferative disease in the human host. Possible pitfalls in SV40 DNA analysis have been pointed out succinctly by Lopez-Rios et al. (2004), but clearly these do not explain all the positive claims made until today. Moreover, the present author is not convinced that the allocation of further funds into this problem will be of any help in this respect.

What remains therefore is one of the most intriguing questions: why human polyomaviruses and SV40 – all of which are equipped with potent oncogenes (with the possibility of rare exceptions) – do not represent tumorviruses for their natural hosts.

References

Ahuja, D., Saenz-Robles, M.T., and Pipas, J.M. SV40 large T antigen targets multiple cellular pathways to elicit cellular transformation. *Oncogene* 24: 7729–7745, **2005**.

Andrews, C.A., Shah, K.V., Daniel, R.W., Hirsch, M.S., and Rubin, R.H. A serological investigation of BK virus and JC virus infections in recipients of renal allografts. *J. Infect. Dis.* 158: 176–181, **1988**.

Apperley, J.F., Rice, S. J., Bishop, J.A., Chia, Y.C., Krausz, T., Gardner, S. D., and Goldman, J.M. Late-onset hemorrhagic cystitis associated with urinary excretion of polyomaviruses after bone marrow transplantation. *Transplantation* 43: 108–112, **1987**.

Arroyo, J.D. and Hahn, W.C. Involvement of PP2A in viral and cellular transformation. *Oncogene* 24: 7746–7755, **2005**.

Arthur, R.R., Shah, K.V., Baust, S. J., Santos, G.W., and Saral, R. Association of BK viruria with hemorrhagic cystitis in recipients of bone marrow transplants. *N. Engl. J. Med.* 315: 230–234, **1986**.

Arthur, R.R., Grossman, S. A., Ronnett, B.M., Bigner, S. H., Vogelstein, B., and Shah, K.V. Lack of association of human polyomaviruses with human brain tumors. *J. Neurooncol.* 20: 55–58, **1994**.

Beggs, A.H., Miner, J.H., and Scangos, G.A. Cell type-specific expression of JC virus T antigen in primary and established cell lines from transgenic mice. *J. Gen. Virol.* 71: 151–164, **1990**.

Bergsagel, D.J., Finegold, M.J., Butel, J.S., Kupsky, W.J., and Garcea, R.L. DNA sequences similar to those of simian virus 40 in ependymomas and choroid plexus tumors of childhood. *N. Engl. J. Med.* 326: 988–993, **1992**.

Boldorini, R., Caldarelli-Stefano, R., Monga, G., Zocchi, M., Mediati, M., Tosoni, A., and Ferrante, P. PCR detection of JC virus DNA in the brain tissue of a 9-year-old child with pleomorphic xanthoastrocytoma. *J. Neurovirol.* 4: 242–245, **1998**.

Boldorini, R., Pagani, E., Car, P.G., Omodeo-Zorini, E., Borghi, E., Tarantini, L., Bellotti, C., Ferrante, P., and Monga, G. Molecular characterisation of JC virus strains detected in human brain tumours. *Pathology* 35: 248–253, **2003**.

Brade, L., Müller-Lantzsch, N. and zur Hausen, H. B-lymphotropic papovavirus and possibility of infections in humans. *J. Med. Virol.* 6: 301–308, **1981**.

Bright, R.K., Kimchi, E.T., Shearer, M.H., Kennedy, R.C., and Pass, H.I. SV40 Tag-specific cytotoxic T lymphocytes generated from the peripheral blood of malignant pleural mesothelioma patients. *Cancer Immunol. Immunother.* 50: 682–690, **2002**.

Brousset, P., de Araujo, V., and Gascoyne, R.D. Immunohistochemical investigation of SV40 large T antigen in Hodgkin and non-Hodgkin's lymphoma. *Int. J. Cancer* 112: 533–535, **2004**.

Butel, J.S., Jafar, S., Stewart, A.R., and Lednicky, J.A. Detection of authentic SV40 DNA sequences in human brain and bone tumours. *Dev. Biol. Stand.* 94: 23–32, **1998**.

Carbone, M., Pass, H.I., Rizzo, P., Marinetti, M., Di Muzio, M., Mew, D.J., Levine, A.S., and Procopio, A. Simian virus 40-like DNA sequences in human pleural mesothelioma. *Oncogene* 9: 1781–1790, **1994**.

Carbone, M., Rizzo, P., Procopio, A., Giuliano, M., Pass, H.I., Gebhardt, M.C., Mangham, C., Hansen, M., Malkin, D.F., Bushart, G., Pompetti, F., Picci, P., Levine, A.S., Bergsagel, J.D., and Garcea, R.L. SV40-like sequences in human bone tumors. *Oncogene* 13: 527–535, **1996**.

Carter, J.J., Madeleine, M.M., Wipf, G.C., Garcea, R.L., Pipkin, P.A., Minor, P.D., and Galloway, D.A. Lack of serologic evidence for prevalent simian virus 40 infection in humans. *J. Natl. Cancer Inst.* 95: 1522–1530, **2003**.

Casini, B., Borgese, L., Del Nonno, F., Galati, G., Izzo, L., Caputo, M., Perrone Donnorso, R., Castelli, M., Risuleo, G., and Visca, P. Presence and incidence of DNA sequences of human polyomaviruses BKV and JCV in colorectal tumor tissues. *Anticancer Res.* 25: 1079–1085, **2005**.

Castaigne, P., Rondot, P., Escourolle, R., Ribadeau Dumas, J.L., Cathala, F., and Hauw, J.J. Leucoencephalopathie multifocale progressive et gliomes multiples. *Rev Neurol (Paris)* 130: 379–392, **1974**.

Chapman, C., Flower, A.J., and Durrant, S. T. The use of vidarabine in the treatment of human polyomavirus associated acute haemorrhagic cystitis. *Bone Marrow Transplant.* 7: 481–483, **1991**.

Coleman, D.V., Wolfendale, M.R., Daniel, R.A., Dhanjal, N.K., Gardner, S. D., Gibson, P.E., and Field, A.M. A prospective study of human polyomavirus infection in pregnancy. *J. Infect. Dis.* 142: 1–8, **1980**.

Corallini, A., Barbanti-Brodano, G., Bortoloni, W., Nenci, I., Cassai, E., Tampieri, M., Portolani, M. and Borgatti, M. High incidence of ependymomas induced by BK virus, a human papovavirus: brief communication. *J. Natl. Cancer Inst.* 59: 1561–1564, **1977**.

Corallini, A., Altavilla, G., Cecchetti, M.G., Fabris, G., Grossi, M.P., Balboni, P.G., Lanza, G., and Barbanti-Brodano, G. Ependymomas, malignant tumors of pancreatic islets, and osteosarcomas induced in hamsters by BK virus, a human papovavirus. *J. Natl. Cancer Inst.* 61: 875–883, **1978**.

Corallini, A., Altavilla, G., Carra, L., Grossi, M.P., Federspil, G., Caputo, A., Negrini, M., and Barbanti-Brodano, G. Oncogenicity of BK virus for immunosuppressed hamsters. *Arch Virol.* 73: 243–253, **1982**.

Corallini, A., Altavilla, G., Pozzi, L., Bignozzi, F., Negrini, M., Rimessi, P., Gualandi, F., and Barbanti-Brodano, G. Systemic expression of HIV-1 tat gene in transgenic mice induces endothelial proliferation and tumors of different histotypes. *Cancer Res.* 53: 5569–5575, **1993**.

Cristaudo, A., Foddis, R., Vivaldi, A., Buselli, R., Gattini, V., Guglielmi, G., Cosentino, F., Ottenga, F., Ciancia, E., Libener, R., Filiberti, R., Neri, M., Betta, P., Tognon, M., Mutti, L., and Puntoni, R. SV40 enhances the risk of malignant mesothelioma among people exposed to asbestos: a molecular epidemiologic case-control study. *Cancer Res.* 65: 3049–3052, **2005**.

Dalrymple, S. A. and Beemon, K.L. BK virus T antigens induce kidney carcinomas and thymoproliferative disorders in transgenic mice. *J. Virol.* 64: 1182–1191, **1990**.

David, H., Mendoza, S., Konishi, T., and Miller, C.W. Simian virus 40 is present in human lymphomas and normal blood. *Cancer Lett.* 162: 57–64, **2001**.

Del Valle, L., Gordon, J., Assimakopoulou, M., Enam, S., Geddes, J.F., Varakis, J.N., Katsetos, C.D., Croul, S., and Khalili, K. Detection of JC virus DNA sequences and expression of the viral regulatory protein T-antigen in tumors of the central nervous system. *Cancer Res.* 61: 4287–4293, **2001**.

Del Valle, L., Gordon, J., Enam, S., Delbue, S., Croul, S., Abraham, S., Radhakrishnan, S., Assimakopoulou, M., Katsetos, C.D., and Khalili, K. Expression of human neurotropic polyomavirus JCV late gene product agnoprotein in human medulloblastoma. *J. Natl. Cancer Inst.* 94: 267–273, **2002**.

De Rienzo, A., Tor, M., Sterman, D.H., Aksoy, F., Albelda, S. M., and Testa, J.R. Detection of SV40 DNA sequences in malignant mesothelioma specimens from the United States, but not from Turkey. *J. Cell. Biochem.* 84: 455–459, **2002** .

de Sanjose, S., Shah, K.V., Domingo-Domenech, E., Engels, E.A., Fernandez de Sevilla, A., Alvaro, T., Garcia-Villanueva, M., Romagosa, V., Gonzalez-Barca, E., and Viscidi, R.P. Lack of serological evidence for an association between simian virus 40 and lymphoma. *Int. J. Cancer* 104: 522–524, **2003**.

Eddy, B.E., Borman, G.S., Berkeley, W.H., and Young, R.D. Tumors induced in hamsters by injection of rhesus monkey kidney cell extracts. *Proc. Soc. Exp. Biol. Med.* 107: 191–197, **1961**.

Eddy, B.E., Borman, G.S., Grubbs, G.E., and Young, R.D. Identification of the oncogenic substance in rhesus monkey kidney cell cultures as Simian Virus 40. *Virology* 17: 65–75, **1962**.

Emri, S., Kocagoz, T., Olut, A., Gungen, Y., Mutti, L., and Baris, Y.I. Simian virus 40 is not a cofactor in the pathogenesis of environmentally induced malignant pleural mesothelioma in Turkey. *Anticancer Res.* 20: 891–894, **2000** .

Engels, E.A. Cancer risk associated with receipt of vaccines contaminated with simian virus 40: epidemiologic research. *Expert Rev. Vaccines* 4: 197–206, **2005**.

Engels, E.A., Sarkar, C., Daniel, R.W., Gravitt, P.E., Verma, K., Quezado, M., and Shah, K.V. Absence of simian virus 40 in human brain tumors from northern India. *Int. J. Cancer* 101: 348–352, **2002**.

Engels, E.A., Katki, H.A., Nielsen, N.M., Winther, J.F., Hjalgrim, H., Gjerris, F., Rosenberg, P.S., and Frisch, M. Cancer incidence in Denmark following exposure to poliovirus vaccine contaminated with simian virus 40. *J. Natl. Cancer Inst.* 95: 532–539, **2003**.

Engels, E.A., Viscidi, R.P., Galloway, D.A., Carter, J.J., Cerhan, J.R., Davis, S., Cozen, W., Severson, R.K., de Sanjose, S., Colt, J.S., and Hartge, P. Case-control study of simian virus 40 and non-Hodgkin lymphoma in the United States. *J. Natl. Cancer Inst.* 96: 1368–1374, **2004**.

Feigenbaum, L., Hinrichs, S. H., and Jay, G. JC virus and simian virus 40 enhancers and transforming proteins: role in determining tissue specificity and pathogenicity in transgenic mice. *J. Virol.* 66: 1176–1182, **1992**.

Flaegstad, T., Andresen, P.A., Johnsen, J.I., Asomani, S. K., Jorgensen, G.E., Vignarajan, S., Kjuul, A., Kogner, P., and Traavik, T. A possible contributory role of BK virus infection in neuroblastoma development. *Cancer Res.* 59: 1160–1163, **1999**.

Franks, R.R., Rencic, A., Gordon, J., Zoltick, P.W., Curtis, M., Knobler, R.L., and Khalili, K. Formation of undifferentiated mesenteric tumors in transgenic mice expressing human neurotropic polyomavirus early protein. *Oncogene* 12: 2573–2578, **1996**.

Frisque, R.J., Rifkin, D.B., and Walker, D.L. Transformation of primary hamster brain cells with JC virus and its DNA. *J. Virol.* 35: 265–269, **1980**.

Galateau-Salle, F., Bidet, P., Iwatsubo, Y., Gennetay, E., Renier, A., Letourneux, M., Pairon, J.C., Moritz, S., Brochard, P., Jaurand, M.C., and Freymuth F. SV40-like DNA sequences in pleural mesothelioma, bronchopulmonary carcinoma, and nonmalignant pulmonary diseases. *J. Pathol.* 184: 252–257, **1998**.

Gardner, S. D., Field, A.M., Coleman, D.V., and Hulme, B. New human papovavirus (B.K.) isolated from urine after renal transplantation. *Lancet* 1: 1253–1257, **1971**.

Gardner, S. D., MacKenzie, E.F., Smith, C., and Porter, A.A. Prospective study of the human polyomaviruses BK and JC and cytomegalovirus in renal transplant recipients. *J. Clin. Pathol.* 37: 578–586, **1984**.

Goudsmit, J., Wertheim-van Dillen, P., van Strien, A., and van der Noordaa, J. The role of BK virus in acute respiratory tract disease and the presence of BKV DNA in tonsils. *J. Med. Virol.* 10: 91–99, **1982**.

Greenlee, J.E., Narayan, O., Johnson, R.T., and Herndon, R.M. Induction of brain tumors in hamsters with BK virus, a human papovavirus. *Lab. Invest.* 36: 636–641, **1977**.

Greenlee, J.E., Becker, L.E., Narayan, O., and Johnson, R.T. Failure to demonstrate papovavirus tumor antigen in human cerebral neoplasms. *Ann. Neurol.* 3: 479–481, **1978**.

Griffiths, D.J., Nicholson, A.G., and Weiss, R.A. Detection of SV40 sequences in human mesothelioma. *Dev. Biol. Stand.* 94: 127–136, **1998**.

Grossi, M.P., Meneguzzi, G., Chenciner, N., Corallini, A., Poli, F., Altavilla, G., Alberti, S., Milanesi, G., and Barbanti-Brodano, G. Lack of association between BK virus and ependymomas, malignant tumors of pancreatic islets, osteosarcomas and other human tumors. *Intervirology* 15: 10–17, **1981**.

Gullotta, F., Masini, T., Scarlato, G., and Kuchelmeister, K. Progressive multifocal leukoencephalopathy and gliomas in a HIV-negative patient. *Pathol. Res. Pract.* 188: 964–972, **1992**.

Hayashi, H., Endo, S., Suzuki, S., Tanaka, S., Sawa, H., Ozaki, Y., Sawamura, Y., and Nagashima, K. JC virus large T protein transforms rodent cells but is not involved in human medulloblastoma. *Neuropathology* 21: 129–137, **2001**.

Heilbronn, R., Albrecht, I., Stephan, S., Bürkle, A., and zur Hausen, H. Human cytomegalovirus induces JC virus DNA replication in human fibroblasts. *Proc. Natl. Acad. Sci. USA* 90: 11 406–11 410, **1993**.

Heinsohn, S., Scholz, R.B., Weber, B., Wittenstein, B., Werner, M., Delling, G., Kempf-Bielack, B., Setlak, P., Bielack, S., and Kabisch, H. SV40 sequences in human osteosarcoma of German origin. *Anticancer Res.* 20: 4539–4545, **2000** .

Herbarth, B., Meissner, H., Westphal, M., and Wegner, M. Absence of polyomavirus JC in glial brain tumors and glioma-derived cell lines. *Glia* 22: 415–420, **1998**.

Hirvonen, A., Mattson, K., Karjalainen, A., Ollikainen, T., Tammilehto, L., Hovi, T., Vainio, H., Pass, H.I., Di Resta, I., Carbone, M., and Linnainmaa, K. Simian virus 40 (SV40)-like DNA sequences not detectable in Finnish mesothelioma patients not exposed to SV40-contaminated polio vaccines. *Mol. Carcinog.* 26: 93–99, **1999**.

Hogan, T.F., Borden, E.C., McBain, J.A., Padgett, B.L., and Walker, D.L. Human polyomavirus infections with JC virus and BK virus in renal transplant patients. *Ann. Intern. Med.* 92: 373–378, **1980**.

Huang, H., Reis, R., Yonekawa, Y., Lopes, J.M., Kleihues, P., and Ohgaki, H. Identification in human brain tumors of DNA sequences specific for SV40 large T antigen. *Brain Pathol.* 9: 33–42, **1999**.

Hubner, R. and Van Marck, E. Reappraisal of the strong association between simian virus 40 and human malignant mesothelioma of the pleura (Belgium). *Cancer Causes Control* 13: 121–129, **2002**.

Jin, M., Sawa, H., Suzuki, T., Shimizu, K., Makino, Y., Tanaka, S., Nojima, T., Fujioka, Y., Asamoto, M., Suko, N., Fujita, M., and Nagashima, K. Investigation of simian virus 40 large T antigen in 18 autopsied malignant mesothelioma patients in Japan. *J. Med. Virol.* 74: 668–676, **2004**.

Johne, R., Enderlein, D., Nieper, H., and Müller, H. Novel polyomavirus detected in the feces of a chimpanzee by nested broad-spectrum PCR. *J. Virol.* 79: 3883–3887, **2005**.

Kim, J.Y., Koralnik, I.J., LeFave, M., Segal, R.A., Pfister, L.A., and Pomeroy, S. L. Medulloblastomas and primitive neuroectodermal tumors rarely contain polyomavirus DNA sequences. *Neuro-oncology* 4: 165–170, **2002**.

Kouhata, T., Fukuyama, K., Hagihara, N., and Tabuchi, K. Detection of simian virus 40 DNA sequence in human primary glioblastomas multiforme. *J. Neurosurg.* 95: 96–101, **2001**.

Krainer, M., Schenk, T., Zielinski, C.C., and Müller, C. Failure to confirm presence of SV40 sequences in human tumours. *Eur. J. Cancer* 31 A: 1893, **1995**.

Krieg, P., Amtmann, E., Jonas, D., Fischer, H., Zang, K., and Sauer, G. Episomal simian virus 40 genomes in human brain tumors. *Proc. Natl. Acad. Sci. USA* 78: 6446–6450, **1981**.

Krynska, B., Gordon, J., Otte, J., Franks, R., Knobler, R., DeLuca, A., Giordano, A., and Khalili, K. Role of cell cycle regulators in tumor formation in transgenic mice expressing the human neurotropic virus, JCV, early protein. *J. Cell. Biochem .* 67: 223–230, **1997**.

Krynska, B., Otte, J., Franks, R., Khalili, K., and Croul, S. Human ubiquitous JCV(CY) T-antigen gene induces brain tumors in experimental animals. *Oncogene* 18: 39–46, **1999a**.

Krynska, B., Del Valle, L., Croul, S., Gordon, J., Katsetos, C.D., Carbone, M., Giordano, A., and Khalili, K. Detection of human neurotropic JC virus DNA sequence and expression of the viral oncogenic protein in pediatric medulloblastomas. *Proc. Natl. Acad. Sci. USA* 96: 11 519–11 524, **1999b**.

Laghi, L., Randolph, A.E., Chauhan, D.P., Marra, G., Major, E.O., Neel, J.V., and Boland, C.R. JC virus DNA is present in the mucosa of the human colon and in colorectal cancers. *Proc. Natl. Acad. Sci. USA* 96: 7484–7489, **1999**.

Lavia, P., Mileo, A.M., Giordano, A., and Paggi, M.G. Emerging roles of DNA tumor viruses in cell proliferation: new insights into genomic instability. *Oncogene* 22: 6508–6516, **2003**.

Lazutka, J.R., Neel, J.V., Major, E.O., Dedonyte, V., Mierauskine, J., Slapsyte, G., and Kesminiene, A. High titers of antibodies to two human polyomaviruses, JCV and

BKV, correlate with increased frequency of chromosomal damage in human lymphocytes. *Cancer Lett.* 109: 177–183, **1996**.

Lednicky, J.A., Stewart, A.R., Jenkins. J.J., III, Finegold, M.J., and Butel, J.S. SV40 DNA in human osteosarcomas shows sequence variation among T-antigen genes. *Int. J. Cancer* 72: 791–800, **1997**.

Leithner, A., Weinhaeusel, A., Windhager, R., Schlegl, R., Waldner, P., Lang, S., Dominkus, M., Zoubek, A., Popper, H.H., and Haas, O.A. Absence of SV40 in Austrian tumors correlates with low incidence of mesotheliomas. *Cancer Biol. Ther.* 1: 375–379, **2002**.

London, W.T., Houff, S. A., Madden, D.L., Fuccillo, D.A., Gravell, M., Wallen, W.C., Palmer, A.E., Sever, J.L., Padgett, B.L., Walker, D.L., ZuRhein, G.M., and Ohashi, T. Brain tumors in owl monkeys inoculated with a human polyomavirus (JC virus). *Science* 201: 1246–1249, **1978**.

Lopez-Rios, F., Illei, P.B., Rusch, V., and Ladanyi, M. Evidence against a role for SV40 infection in human mesotheliomas and high risk of false-positive PCR results owing to presence of SV40 sequences in common laboratory plasmids. *Lancet* 364: 1157–1166, **2004**.

MacKenzie, J., Wilson, K.S., Perry, J., Gallagher, A., and Jarrett, R.F. Association between simian virus 40 DNA and lymphoma in the United Kingdom. *J. Natl. Cancer Inst.* 95: 1001–1003, **2003**.

Major, E.O., Mourrain, P., and Cummins, C. JC virus-induced owl monkey glioblastoma cells in culture: biological properties associated with the viral early gene product. *Virology* 136: 359–367, **1984**.

Malkin, D., Chilton-MacNeill, S., Meister, L.A., Sexsmith, E., Diller, L., and Garcea, R.L. Tissue-specific expression of SV40 in tumors associated with the Li-Fraumeni syndrome. *Oncogene* 20: 4441–4449, **2001**.

Mandl, C., Walker, D.L., and Frisque, R.J. Derivation and characterization of POJ cells, transformed human fetal glial cells that retain their permissivity for JC virus. *J. Virol.* 61: 755–763, **1987**.

Manfredi, J.J., Dong, J., Liu, W.J., Resnick-Silverman, L., Qiao, R., Chahinian, P., Saric, M., Gibbs, A.R., Phillips, J.I., Murray, J., Axten, C.W., Nolan, R.P., and Aaronson, S. A. Evidence against a role for SV40 in human mesothelioma. *Cancer Res.* 65: 2602–2609, **2005**.

Mantyjärvi, R.A., Meurman, O.H., Vihma, L., and Berglund, B. A human papovavirus (B.K.), biological properties and seroepidemiology. *Ann. Clin. Res.* 5: 283–287, **1973**.

Martini, F., Iaccheri, L., Lazzarin, L., Carinci, P., Corallini, A., Gerosa, M., Iuzzolino, P., Barbanti-Brodano, G., and Tognon, M. SV40 early region and large T antigen in human brain tumors, peripheral blood cells, and sperm fluids from healthy individuals. *Cancer Res.* 56: 4820–4825, **1996**.

Martini, F., Dolcetti, R., Gloghini, A., Iaccheri, L., Carbone, A., Boiocchi, M., and Tognon, M. Simian-virus-40 footprints in human lymphoproliferative disorders of HIV- and HIV+ patients. *Int. J. Cancer* 78: 669–674, **1998**.

Martini, F., Lazzarin, L., Iaccheri, L., Vignocchi, B., Finocchiaro, G., Magnani, I., Serra, M., Scotlandi, K., Barbanti-Brodano, G., and Tognon, M. Different simian virus 40 genomic regions and sequences homologous with SV40 large T antigen in DNA of human brain and bone tumors and of leukocytes from blood donors. *Cancer* 94: 1037–1048, **2002**.

Mason, D.H., Jr. and Takemoto, K.K. Transformation of rabbit kidney cells by BKV(MM) human papovavirus. *Int. J. Cancer* 19: 391–395, **1977**.

Mayall, F.G., Jacobson, G., and Wilkins, R. Mutations of p53 gene and SV40 sequences in asbestos associated and non-asbestos-associated mesotheliomas. *J. Clin. Pathol.* 52: 291–293, **1999**.

McLaren, B.R., Haenel, T., Stevenson, S., Mukherjee, S., Robinson, B.W., and Lake, R.A. Simian virus (SV) 40 like sequences in cell lines and tumour biopsies from Australian malignant mesotheliomas. *Aust. N. Z. J. Med.* 30: 450–456, **2000**.

Mendoza, S. M., Konishi, T., and Miller, C.W. Integration of SV40 in human osteosarcoma DNA. *Oncogene* 17: 2457–2462, **1998**.

Montesinos-Rongen, M., Besleaga, R., Heinsohn, S., Siebert, R., Kabisch, H., Wiestler, O.D., and Deckert, M. Absence of simian virus 40 DNA sequences in primary central nervous system lymphoma in HIV-negative patients. *Virchows Arch.* 444: 436–438, **2004**.

Mulatero, C., Surentheran, T., Breuer, J., and Rudd, R.M. Simian virus 40 and human pleural mesothelioma. *Thorax* 54: 60–61, **1999**.

Nagashima, K., Yasui, K., Kimura, J., Washizu, M., Yamaguchi, K., and Mori, W. Induction of brain tumors by a newly isolated JC virus (Tokyo-1 strain). *Am. J. Pathol.* 116: 455–463, **1984**.

Nakatsuka, S., Liu, A., Dong, Z., Nomura, S., Takakuwa, T., Miyazato, H., Aozasa, K.; Osaka Lymphoma Study Group. Simian virus 40 sequences in malignant lymphomas in Japan. *Cancer Res.* 63: 7606–7608, **2003**.

Neel, J.V., Major, E.O., Awa, A.A., Glover, T., Burgess, A., Traub, R., Curfman, B., and Satoh, C. Hypothesis: "Rogue cell"-type chromosomal damage in lymphocytes is associated with infection with the JC human polyoma virus and has implications for oncogenesis. *Proc. Natl. Acad. Sci. USA* 93: 2690–2695, **1996**.

Negrini, M., Rimessi, P., Mantovani, C., Sabbioni, S., Corallini, A., Gerosa, M.A., and Barbanti-Brodano, G. Characterization of BK virus variants rescued from human tumours and tumour cell lines. *J. Gen. Virol.* 71: 2731–2736, **1990**.

Newcomb, P.A., Bush, A.C., Stoner, G.L., Lampe, J.W., Potter, J.D., and Bigler, J. No evidence of an association of JC virus and colon neoplasia. *Cancer Epidemiol. Biomarkers Prev.* 13: 662–666, **2004**.

Ohsumi, S., Motoi, M., and Ogawa, K. Induction of undifferentiated tumors by JC virus in the cerebrum of rats. *Acta Pathol. Jpn.* 36: 815–825, **1986**.

Okamoto, H., Mineta, T., Ueda, S., Nakahara, Y., Shiraishi, T., Tamiya, T., and Tabuchi, K. Detection of JC virus DNA sequences in brain tumors in pediatric patients. *J. Neurosurg.* 102 (3 Suppl): 294–298, **2005**.

Olin, P. and Giesecke, J. Potential exposure to SV40 in polio vaccines used in Sweden during 1957: no impact on cancer incidence rates 1960 to **1993**. *Dev. Biol. Stand.* 94: 227–233, **1998**.

Padgett, B.L., Walker, D.L., ZuRhein, G.M., Eckroade, R.J., and Dessel, B.H. Cultivation of papova-like virus from human brain with progressive multifocal leucoencephalopathy. *Lancet* 1: 1257–1260, **1971**.

Padgett, B.L., Walker, D.L., Desquitado, M.M., and Kim, D.U. BK virus and non-haemorrhagic cystitis in a child. *Lancet* 1: 770, **1983**.

Pepper, C., Jasani, B., Navabi, H., Wynford-Thomas, D., and Gibbs, A.R. Simian virus 40 large T antigen (SV40LTAg) primer specific DNA amplification in human pleural mesothelioma tissue. *Thorax* 51: 1074–1076, **1996**.

Pilatte, Y., Vivo, C., Renier, A., Kheuang, L., Greffard, A., and Jaurand, M.C. Absence of SV40 large T-antigen expression in human mesothelioma cell lines. *Am. J. Respir. Cell. Mol. Biol.* 23: 788–793, **2000**.

Portolani, M. and Borgatti, M. Stable transformation of mouse, rabbit and monkey cells and abortive transformation of human cells by BK virus, a human papovavirus. *J. Gen. Virol.* 38: 369–374, **1978**.

Procopio, A., Strizzi, L., Vianale, G., Betta, P., Puntoni, R., Fontana, V., Tassi, G., Gareri, F., and Mutti, L. Simian virus-40 sequences are a negative prognostic cofactor in patients with malignant pleural mesothelioma. *Genes Chromosomes Cancer* 29: 173–179, **2000**.

Purchio, A.F. and Fareed, G.C. Transformation of human embryonic kidney cells by human papovavirus BK. *J. Virol.* 29: 763–769, **1979**.

Rencic, A., Gordon, J., Otte, J., Curtis, M., Kovatich, A., Zoltick, P., Khalili, K., and Andrews, D. Detection of JC virus DNA sequence and expression of the viral oncoprotein, tumor antigen, in brain of immunocompetent patient with oligoastrocytoma. *Proc. Natl. Acad. Sci. USA* 93: 7352–7357, **1996**.

Rollison, D.E., Helzlsouer, K.J., Alberg, A.J., Hoffman, S., Hou, J., Daniel, R., Shah, K.V., and Major, E.O. Serum antibodies to JC virus, BK virus, simian virus 40, and the risk of incident adult astrocytic brain tumors. *Cancer Epidemiol. Biomarkers Prev.* 12: 460–463, **2003**.

Rollison, D.E., Page, W.F., Crawford, H., Gridley, G., Wacholder, S., Martin, J., Miller, R., and Engels, E.A. Case-control study of cancer among US Army veterans exposed to simian virus 40-contaminated adenovirus vaccine. *Am. J. Epidemiol.* 160: 317–324, **2004**.

Rollison, D.E., Utaipat, U., Ryschkewitsch, C., Hou, J., Goldthwaite, P., Daniel, R., Helzlsouer, K.J., Burger, P.C., Shah, K.V., and Major, E.O. Investigation of human brain tumors for the presence of polyomavirus genome sequences by two independent laboratories. *Int. J. Cancer* 113: 769–774, **2005 a**.

Rollison, D.E., Helzlsouer, K.J., Halsey, N.A., Shah, K.V., and Viscidi, R.P. Markers of past infection with simian virus 40 (SV40) and risk of incident non-Hodgkin lymphoma in a Maryland cohort. *Cancer Epidemiol. Biomarkers Prev.* 14: 1448–1452, **2005 b**.

Saitoh, K., Sugae, N., Koike, N., Akiyama, Y., Iwamura, Y., and Kimura, H. Diagnosis of childhood BK virus cystitis by electron microscopy and PCR. *J. Clin. Pathol.* 46: 773–775, **1993**.

Schuler, F., Dölken, S. C., Hirt, C., Dölken, M.T., Mentel, R., Gurtler, L.G., Dölken, G. No evidence for simian virus 40 DNA sequences in malignant non-Hodgkin lymphomas. *Int. J. Cancer* 118: 498–504, **2005**.

Seehafer, J., Downer, D.N., Salmi, A., and Colter, J.S. Isolation and characterization of BK virus-transformed rat and mouse cells. *J. Gen. Virol.* 42: 567–578, **1979**.

Shah, K.V. Polyomaviruses. In: Fields, B.N, Knipe, D.M., Howley, P.M. (Eds.), *Fields Virology*. Lippincott-Raven Publishers, Philadelphia, Chapter 64, pp. 2027–2043, **1996**.

Shah, K.V. and Nathanson, N. Human exposure to SV40: review and comment. *Am. J. Epidemiol.* 103: 1–12, **1976**.

Shah, K.V., Galloway, D.A., Knowles, W.A., and Viscidi, R.P. Simian virus 40 (SV40) and human cancer: a review of the serological data. *Rev. Med. Virol.* 14: 231–239, **2004**.

Shivapurkar, N., Wiethege, T., Wistuba, I.I., Salomon, E., Milchgrub, S., Muller, K.M., Churg, A., Pass, H., and Gazdar, A.F. Presence of simian virus 40 sequences in malignant mesotheliomas and mesothelial cell proliferations. *J. Cell. Biochem.* 76: 181–188, **1999**.

Shivapurkar, N., Harada, K., Reddy, J., Scheuermann, R.H., Xu, Y., McKenna, R.W., Milchgrub, S., Kroft, S. H., Feng, Z., and Gazdar, A.F. Presence of simian virus 40 DNA sequences in human lymphomas. *Lancet* 359: 851–852, **2002**.

Shivapurkar, N., Takahashi, T., Reddy, J., Zheng, Y., Stastny, V., Collins, R., Toyooka, S., Suzuki, M., Parikh, G., Asplund, S., Kroft, S. H., Timmons, C., McKenna, R.W., Feng, Z., and Gazdar, A.F. Presence of simian virus 40 DNA sequences in human lymphoid and hematopoietic malignancies and their relationship to aberrant promoter methylation of multiple genes. *Cancer Res.* 64: 3757–3760, **2004**.

Shollar, D., Del Valle, L., Khalili, K., Otte, J., and Gordon, J. JCV T-antigen interacts with the neurofibromatosis type 2 gene product in a transgenic mouse model of malignant peripheral nerve sheath tumors. *Oncogene* 23: 5459–5467, **2004**.

Sima, A.A., Finkelstein, S. D., and McLachlan, D.R. Multiple malignant astrocytomas in a patient with spontaneous progressive multifocal leukoencephalopathy. *Ann. Neurol.* 14: 183–188, **1983**.

Simsir, A., Fetsch, P., Bedrossian, C.W., Ioffe, O.B., and Abati, A. Absence of SV-40 large T antigen (Tag) in malignant mesothelioma effusions: an immunocytochemical study. *Diagn. Cytopathol.* 25: 203–207, **2001**.

Small, J.A., Khoury, G., Jay, G., Howley, P.M., and Scangos, G.A. Early regions of JC virus and BK virus induce distinct and tissue-specific tumors in transgenic mice. *Proc. Natl. Acad. Sci. USA* 83: 8288–8292, **1986 a**.

Small, J.A., Scangos, G.A., Cork, L., Jay, G., and Khoury, G. The early region of human papovavirus JC induces dysmyelination in transgenic mice. *Cell* 46: 13–18, **1986 b**.

Stewart, A.R., Lednicky, J.A., and Butel, J.S. Sequence analyses of human tumor-associated SV40 DNAs and SV40 viral isolates from monkeys and humans. *J. Neurovirol.* 4: 182–193, **1998**.

Stolt, A., Kjellin, M., Sasnauskas, K., Luostarinen, T., Koskela, P., Lehtinen, M., and Dillner, J. Maternal human polyomavirus infection and risk of neuroblastoma in the child. *Int. J. Cancer* 113: 393–396, **2005**.

Stoner, G.L., Ryschkewitsch, C.F., Walker, D.L., Soffer, D., and Webster, H.D.A monoclonal antibody to SV40 large T-antigen labels a nuclear antigen in JC virus-transformed cells and in progressive multifocal leukoencephalopathy (PML) brain infected with JC virus. *J. Neuroimmunol.* 17: 331–345, **1988**.

Strayer, D.S., Cordelier, P., Kondo, R., Liu, B., Matskevich, A.A., McKee, H.J., Nichols, C.N., Mitchell, C.B., Geverd, D.A., White, M.K., and Strayer, M.S. What they are, how they work and why they do what they do? The story of SV40-derived gene therapy vectors and what they have to offer. *Curr. Gene Ther.* 5: 151–165, **2005**.

Strickler, H.D., and the International SV40 Working Group. A multicenter evaluation of assays for detection of SV40 DNA and results in masked mesothelioma specimens. *Cancer Epidemiol. Biomarkers Prev.* 10: 523–532, **2001**.

Strickler, H.D. and Goedert, J.J. Exposure to SV40-contaminated poliovirus vaccine and the risk of cancer – a review of the epidemiological evidence. In: Brown, F. and Lewis, A.J. (Eds.), *A Possible Human Polyomavirus*. Karger-Verlag, Basel, Switzerland, pp. 235–244, **1998**.

Strickler, H.D., Goedert. J.J., Fleming, M., Travis, W.D., Williams, A.E., Rabkin, C.S., Daniel, R.W., and Shah, K.V. Simian virus 40 and pleural mesothelioma in humans. *Cancer Epidemiol. Biomarkers Prev.* 5: 473–475, **1996**.

Strickler, H.D., Rosenberg, P.S., Devesa, S. S., Hertel, J., Fraumeni, J.F., Jr., Goedert, J.J. Contamination of poliovirus vaccines with simian virus 40 (1955–1963) and subsequent cancer rates. *JAMA* 279: 292–295, **1998**.

Strickler, H.D., Goedert, J.J., Devesa, S. S., Lahey, J., Fraumeni, J.F., Jr., and Rosenberg. P.S. Trends in U.S. pleural mesothelioma incidence rates following simian virus 40 contamination of early poliovirus vaccines. *J. Natl. Cancer Inst.* 95: 38–45, **2003**.

Sui, L.F., Williamson, J., Lowenthal, R.M., and Parker, A.J. Absence of simian virus 40 (SV40) DNA in lymphoma samples from Tasmania, Australia. *Pathology* 37: 157–159, **2005**.

Suzuki, S. O., Mizoguchi, M., and Iwaki, T. Detection of SV40T antigen genome in human gliomas. *Brain Tumor Pathol.* 14: 125–129, **1997**.

Takemoto, K.K., Linke, H., Miyamura, T., and Fareed, G.C. Persistent BK papovavirus infection of transformed human fetal brain cells. I. Episomal viral DNA in cloned lines deficient in T-antigen expression. *J. Virol.* 29: 1177–1185, **1979**.

Testa, J.R., Carbone, M., Hirvonen, A., Khalili, K., Krynska, B., Linnainmaa, K., Pooley, F.D., Rizzo, P., Rusch, V., and Xiao, G.H. A multi-institutional study confirms the presence and expression of simian virus 40 in human malignant mesotheliomas. *Cancer Res.* 58: 4505–4509, **1998**.

Theodoropoulos, G., Panoussopoulos, D., Papaconstantinou, I., Gazouli, M., Perdiki, M., Bramis, J., and Lazaris, A.C. Assessment of JC polyoma virus in colon neoplasms. *Dis. Colon Rectum* 48: 86–91, **2005**.

Thu, G.O., Hem, L.Y., Hansen, S., Moller, B., Norstein, J., Nokleby, H., and Grotmol, T. Is there an association between SV40 contaminated polio vaccine and lymphoproliferative disorders? An age-period-cohort analysis on Norwegian data from 1953 to 1997. *Int. J. Cancer* 118: 2035–2039, **2006**.

Uchida, S., Watanabe, S., Aizawa, T., Kato, K., and Furuno, A. Induction of papillary ependymomas and insulinomas in the Syrian golden hamster by BK virus, a human papovavirus. *GANN* 67: 857–865, **1976**.

Vera, M. and Fortes, P. Simian virus-40 as a gene therapy vector. *DNA Cell Biol.* 23: 271–282, **2004**.

Vilchez, R.A., Lednicky, J.A., Halvorson, S. J., White, Z.S., Kozinetz, C.A., and Butel, J.S. Detection of polyomavirus simian virus 40 tumor antigen DNA in AIDS-related systemic non-Hodgkin lymphoma. *J. Acquir. Immune Defic. Syndr.* 29: 109–116, **2002a**.

Vilchez, R.A., Madden, C.R., Kozinetz, C.A., Halvorson, S. J., White, Z.S., Jorgensen, J.L., Finch, C.J., and Butel, J.S. Association between simian virus 40 and non-Hodgkin lymphoma. *Lancet* 359: 817–823, **2002b**.

Vilchez, R.A., Lopez-Terrada, D., Middleton, J.R., Finch, C.J., Killen, D.E., Zanwar, P., Jorgensen, J.L., and Butel, J.S. Simian virus 40 tumor antigen expression and immunophenotypic profile of AIDS-related non-Hodgkin's lymphoma. *Virology* 342: 38–46, **2005**.

Völter, C., zur Hausen, H., Alber, D., and de Villiers, E.M. Screening human tumor samples with a broad-spectrum polymerase chain reaction method for the detection of polyomaviruses. *Virology* 237: 389–396, **1997**.

Völter, C., zur Hausen, H., Alber, D., and de Villiers, E.M. A broad spectrum PCR method for the detection of polyomaviruses and avoidance of contamination by cloning vectors. *Dev. Biol. Stand.* 94: 137–142, **1998**.

Weggen, S., Bayer, T.A., von Deimling, A., Reifenberger, G., von Schweinitz, D., Wiestler, O.D., and Pietsch, T. Low frequency of SV40, JC and BK polyomavirus sequences in human medulloblastomas, meningiomas and ependymomas. *Brain Pathol.* 10: 85–92, **2000**.

White, M.K. and Khalili, K. Polyomaviruses and human cancer: molecular mechanisms underlying patterns of tumorigenesis. *Virology* 324: 1–16, **2004**.

Winklhofer, K.F., Albrecht, I., Wegner, M., and Heilbronn, R. Human cytomegalovirus immediate-early gene 2 expression leads to JCV replication in nonpermissive cells via transcriptional activation of JCV T antigen. *Virology* 275: 323–334, **2000**.

Woloschak, M., Yu, A., and Post, K.D. Detection of polyomaviral DNA sequences in normal and adenomatous human pituitary tissues using the polymerase chain reaction. *Cancer* 76: 490–496, **1995**.

Yamamoto, H., Nakayama, T., Murakami, H., Hosaka, T., Nakamata, T., Tsuboyama, T., Oka, M., Nakamura, T., and Toguchida, J. High incidence of SV40-like sequences detection in tumour and peripheral blood cells of Japanese osteosarcoma patients. *Br. J. Cancer* 82: 1677–1681, **2000**.

Yogo, Y., Hondo, R., Uchida, S., Watanabe, S., Furuno, A., and Yoshiike, K. Presence of viral DNA sequences in hamster tumors induced by BK virus, a human papovavirus. *Microbiol. Immunol.* 24: 861–869, **1980**.

Zhen, H.N., Zhang, X., Bu, X.Y., Zhang, Z.W., Huang, W.J., Zhang, P., Liang, J.W., and Wang, X.L. Expression of the simian virus 40 large tumor antigen (Tag) and formation of Tag-p53 and Tag-pRb complexes in human brain tumors. *Cancer* 86: 2124–2132, **1999**.

zur Hausen, H. Proliferation-inducing viruses in non-permissive systems as possible causes of human cancers. *Lancet* 357: 381–384, **2001**.

zur Hausen, H. SV40 in human cancers – an endless tale? *Int. J. Cancer* 107: 687, **2003**.

zur Hausen, H. and Gissmann, L. Lymphotropic papovaviruses isolated from African green monkey and human cells. *Med. Microbiol. Immunol. (Berl.)* 167: 137–153, **1979**.

10
Helicobacter, Chronic Inflammation, and Cancer

James G. Fox, Timothy C. Wang, and Julie Parsonnet

10.1
Discovery, Taxonomy, and Genomics

10.1.1
Discovery

10.1.1.1 Gastric Helicobacters

Despite the inevitable controversy that heralds any new discovery, *Helicobacter pylori* is firmly established as a human pathogen. The bacterium is found in the antral and fundic gastric mucosa of infected humans. The bacteria are always associated with histopathological lesions usually consisting of infiltrates of mononuclear cells and polymorphonuclear leucocytes. When the patient is treated with a regimen of antimicrobials known to eradicate *H. pylori*, the inflammation regresses over time. However, if the patient relapses and the organism is recultured, the gastritis is again observed.

Acute symptoms associated with natural infection also have been reported (Frommer et al., 1988). Initial *H. pylori* infections can cause profuse vomiting and epigastric pain associated with a marked acute inflammatory response. This inflammation changes to a more chronic type, although polymorphonuclear cells are still present. This active, chronic gastritis persists in most cases indefinitely and usually is not associated with symptoms.

It is now known that *H. pylori* is directly linked to peptic ulcer disease and, importantly, the World Health Organization (WHO) has listed *H. pylori* as a Class I carcinogen. While these diseases have been recognized for centuries, an infectious cause was not actively pursued until the latter part of the twentieth century. Prior to 1982, peptic ulcer disease was attributed to excessive acid or stress, while gastric cancer was linked to a variety of dietary factors documented by extensive epidemiological surveys. Both were known to be associated with chronic inflammation of the stomach, but this association remained unexplained. Nevertheless, the existence of gastric bacteria and a possible association with ulcer disease had been reported by investigators dating as far back as the nineteenth century.

Infections Causing Human Cancer. Harald zur Hausen
Copyright © 2006 WILEY-VCH Verlag GmbH & Co. KGaA, Weinheim
ISBN: 3-527-31056-8

Rappin in 1881 (Rappin, 1948), and Bizzozero in 1893 (Bizzozero, 1893) in more limited studies, are credited with the first observations of gastric spiral-shaped bacteria in animals (Balfour, 1906). The most extensive early investigation of bacteria in animal stomachs was that of Hugo Salomon in 1896 (Salomon, 1896) who observed spiral-shaped organisms in the stomachs of dogs, cats and the brown Norway rat, but failed to find bacteria in humans, monkeys, cattle, pigs, mice, pigeons, and crows.

Spiral-shaped bacteria were observed initially in the stomach of humans as early as 1874, and reported sporadically for the next several decades, sometimes in association with gastric carcinoma (Krienitz, 1906; Celler and Thalheimer, 1916).

In 1875, Bottcher and Letulle were able to demonstrate the presence of bacteria within the floor and margins of ulcers (Bottcher, 1874), and Jaworski in 1889 described the presence of spiral organisms in the sediment of gastric washings. In 1924, Luck detected the presence of urease activity within the gastric mucosa. These findings were confirmed by Conway and Fitzgerald, who also concluded that urease was produced endogenously by gastric epithelial cells and probably functioned as a mucosal protective agent to neutralize gastric acid (Modlin and Sachs, 1998).

In 1938, Doenges studied 242 human gastric autopsy specimens, and found "spirochaetes" in 43% of cases, but was unable to reach any conclusions because of the presence of significant autolysis (Doenges, 1939). He also concluded that the normal rhesus monkey harbored gastric bacterial after observing "spirochetes" in 100% of 43 animals (Doenges, 1939).

This observation was followed by a study in 1941 by Freedburg and Barron of 35 partial gastrectomy specimens, in which they detected "spirochaetes" in 37% of the samples analyzed (Freedburg and Barron, 1940). Even with the aid of silver-staining methodologies, these investigators found the organism extremely difficult to detect; nevertheless, they noted that the bacteria were more often associated with ulcers, both benign and malignant. Finally, during the early 1950s, Palmer conducted an extensive survey of 1140 gastric biopsy specimens which were examined histologically, but without the use of silver stains. Nonetheless, Palmer reported the finding that "…no structure which could reasonably be considered to be of a spirochaetal nature" (Palmer, 1954). Consequently, the previous reports of spiral bacteria were interpreted as oral contaminants which multiplied in postmortem gastric tissue. During the 1950s, the principle was established that because of the stomach's low pH, bacteria could not survive there, and the organ was, for the most part, considered to be sterile.

During the 1970s, upper endoscopy became established at many medical centers, leading to more frequent mucosal sampling of the gastric epithelium through endoscopic biopsy (Steer, 1975; Steer and Colin-Jones, 1975). In 1975, Steer and Colin-Jones reported the finding of bacterial closely related to the gastric mucosa in association with biopsy specimens showing gastritis, but not in biopsies from normal stomachs (Steer, 1975; Steer and Colin-Jones, 1975). The bacteria in their samples appeared to locate under the mucus layer and in close contact with surface mucous cells. They observed the presence of flagellae – "…at least one filum projecting from one end of the bacterium…" – and their ultrastructural studies actually revealed that the bacteria were spiral, although this was not highlighted in their reports. They hypothesized that the polymorphonuclear leukocytes present in the mucosa may have migrated in response to the presence of these bacteria, and believed that they were not contaminants.

In 1984, Steer published scanning electron micrographs depicting curved and spiral bacteria in large numbers on the surface of the gastric epithelium and antrum, and in areas of gastric metaplasia in the duodenal bulb. The organisms were observed in 73% of patients with duodenal ulceration (Steer, 1984). Unfortunately, cultures only yielded *Pseudomonas aeruginosa*, a non-spiral bacterium, which was most likely a contaminant.

The observation that there were spiral bacteria present in the gastric mucosa was concurrently pursued in Western Australia by a pathologist, Dr. J. Robin Warren, at the Royal Perth Hospital. Warren had also observed for many years the presence of bacteria in the stomachs of gastritis patients, and in 1980 began compiling a series of cases in which he performed both hematoxylin and eosin (H&E) and silver stains. In 1982, he was joined in his studies by a gastroenterology fellow, Barry Marshall. In 1983, Warren reported his pathological studies, and his finding that "unidentified curved bacilli" were present in about half of all routine gastric biopsies, and were strongly associated with the presence of "active, chronic gastritis" (Marshall and Warren, 1984). He stated his belief that, "...these organisms should be recognized and their significance investigated". In an accompanying letter in the same issue of the *Lancet*, Marshall reported that he was able (after 34 previous failures) to culture the organisms (that bore some resemblance to campylobacters) on chocolate agar using *Campylobacter* isolation techniques, and that he identified as spiral bacteria. They were about 2.5 mμ in length but, unlike campylobacters, the gastric bacteria had up to five sheathed flagellae (Marshall and Warren, 1983). Although these initial studies did not address the possible pathogenic role of these bacteria, the authors concluded that "...they may have a part to play in other poorly understood, gastritis associated diseases (i.e., peptic ulcer and gastric cancer)".

Over the next few years the bacteria were isolated and cultured in several countries (United Kingdom, Holland, Germany, USA, Canada, Japan, and Peru), and characterized in much greater detail.

To demonstrate more convincingly that *H. pylori* could directly produce gastritis and/or symptoms (and thus fulfill Koch's postulates), Marshall ingested an isolate obtained from a 66-year-old man with nonulcer dyspepsia (Marshall et al ., 1985). Prior to self-inoculation, he underwent upper endoscopy. A biopsy taken from his gastric mucosa revealed no ulceration, gastritis, or evidence of infection. After premedication with cimetidine, Marshall dosed himself orally with ~10^9 colony-forming units (cfu) of *H. pylori*. Over the next few days, he had symptoms of indigestion, bloating, nausea, vomiting, headache, and irritability, and described his breath as "putrid". At 10 days post-inoculation, gastroscopy revealed active gastritis; however, at 14 days post-inoculation the symptoms resolved and gastroscopy indicated resolution of gastritis. Shortly thereafter, Arthur Morris, a young New Zealand gastroenterologist ingested 3×10^5 cfu of a different *H. pylori* strain, originally isolated from a 69-year-old woman with dyspepsia and chronic gastritis. Morris developed moderate to severe attacks of epigastric pain, acute achlorhydria, and had evidence of histological gastritis (Morris and Nicholson, 1987). His symptoms evolved into a chronic dyspepsia that persisted despite three varied courses of antibiotics. Three years later, after a course of triple therapy consisting of bismuth/metronidazole/tetracycline (Morris et al. , 1991), *H. pylori* was eradicated and his symptoms and gastritis resolved.

10.1.1.2 Enterohepatic Helicobacters

Helicobacter cinaedi, previously classified as *C. cinaedi* (CLO-1 A), was first isolated from the lower bowel of homosexuals with proctitis and colitis (Totten et al., 1985; Vaira et al., 1990). Similar to *H. cinaedi* , *H. fennelliae* previously known as *C. fennelliae* (CLO-2), was first isolated from HIV-infected homosexuals with colitis and proctitis (Fennell et al., 1984; Totten et al., 1985).

   Since then, an increasing number of *Helicobacter* spp. have been isolated from the intestinal tracts of rodents, birds, cats, dogs, primates, and humans (Lee et al., 1992; Stanley et al., 1993, 1994; Fox et al., 1994, 1995, 1996 a; Seymour et al., 1994; Ward et al., 1994 b; Franklin et al., 1996; Mendes et al., 1996; Shen et al., 1997). Several of these intestinal *Helicobacter* spp. appear to be part of the autochthonous microbiota of animal hosts (Gebhart et al., 1989; Mendes et al., 1996; Shen et al., 1997), while others have been implicated as etiological agents in diseases involving the gastrointestinal and reproductive tracts of infected hosts (Table 10.1). Indeed, intestinal *Helicobacter* spp. have been isolated from inflammatory lesions in the lower bowel of immunocompromised humans (Fennell et al., 1984) and mice (Cahill et al., 1997; Foltz et al., 1998; Fox et al., 1999 b; Franklin et al., 1999) and with chronic hepatitis (Ward et al., 1994 a,b; Fox et al., 1996 b; Franklin et al., 1998; Whary et al., 1998; Ihrig et al., 1999), hepatocellular carcinoma (Ward et al., 1994 b; Ihrig et al., 1999), biliary cancer (Matsukura et al., 2002), colon adenocarcinoma (Erdman et al., 2003 a,b), and cholecystitis (Franklin et al., 1996; Fox et al., 1998; Maurer et al., 2005).

Table 10.1 Non-*H. pylori* helicobacters isolated or identified by DNA analysis from humans (as of 2005).

Species	Other hosts	Primary site	Other sites	Reference(s)
"*H. rappini*"[a]	Sheep, dog, mice	Intestine	Blood (humans) Liver (sheep, humans[b]), stomach (dogs)	Archer et al., 1988; Kirkbride et al., 1985; Lockard and Boler, 1970; Sorlin et al., 1999; Weir et al., 1999
H. bilis	Mice, dog, gerbils	Intestine	Liver (mice, humans[b])	Fox et al., 1998; Matsukura et al., 2002

Table 10.1 (Continued)

Species	Other hosts	Primary site	Other sites	Reference(s)
H. canis[a]	Dog, cat	Intestine	Blood (humans) Liver (dog)	Foley et al., 1999; Fox et al., 1996a; Shen et al., 2001; Stanley et al., 1993
H. cinaedi[a]	Hamster, rhesus monkey, dog	Intestine	Blood, soft tissue, joints (humans) Liver (monkey)	Flores et al., 1990; Fox et al., 2001; Gebhart et al., 1989; Orlicek et al., 1993; Tee et al., 1987; Vandamme et al., 1990
H. fennelliae	Dog, macaque	Intestine	Blood	Fennell et al., 1984; Kiehlbauch et al., 1994; Totten et al., 1985
H. ganmani	Mice	Intestine	Liver[b]	Tolia et al., 2004
H. pullorum[a]	Chicken	Intestine	Liver (chicken), humans[b]	Burnens et al., 1994; Stanley et al., 1994
H. canadensis	Geese	Intestine	NR	Fox et al., 2000b
H. westmeadii	NR	NR	Blood	Trivett-Moore et al., 1997
H. winghamensis	NR	Intestine	NR	Melito et al., 2001
H. heilmannii[a]	Dogs, cats, monkeys, cheetahs, wild rats, swine	Stomach	NR	Heilmann and Borchard, 1991; Lockard and Boler, 1970; Otto et al., 1994; Sato and Takeuchi, 1982
H. felis[a]	Dogs, cats, cheetahs	Stomach	NR	Lavelle et al., 1994; Lee et al., 1988

[a] Some data suggest zoonotic potential.
[b] Organism identified by DNA analysis.
** NR, not reported.

10.1.2
Taxonomy

10.1.2.1 Gastric Helicobacters

The bacteria identified by Marshall and Warren were initially named *Campylobacter pyloridis*, because of their similarities to other *Campylobacter* species. The gastric organisms were observed to be microaerobic, Gram-negative, spiral-shaped bacteria that morphologically resembled bacteria of the *Campylobacter* genus. Given this similarity, these "campylobacter-like organisms" achieved official recognition in 1985 as *Campylobacter pyloridis* (Anonymous, 1985) and in 1987, the name was changed to *Campylobacter pylori*. A second small, rod-shaped bacterium that colonized primarily the inflamed antrum of ferrets was first cultured in 1985 by Fox et al. and named *C. pylori* ss. *mustelae*, later amended to *C. mustelae* (Fox et al., 1986, 1988 b, 1989). However, both the human and ferret gastric bacteria had a flagellar morphology that were distinct from bacteria in the *Campylobacter* genus (Marshall and Warren, 1984). The campylobacters had a single unsheathed flagellum, whereas the gastric bacteria were characterized by four sheathed flagella at one end, and the ferret organism had multiple bipolar sheathed flagella. In addition, the DNA:DNA homology, the 16 S RNA analysis and the cell wall components of the gastric bacteria differed substantially from those of *Campylobacter* spp. Finally, antibodies to the gastric bacteria showed little cross-reactivity with *C. jejuni* and other pathogenic *Campylobacter* species, indicating significant antigenic diversity. Marshall's and Warren's bacteria, and the bacteria isolated from ferrets by Fox, were therefore recognized in 1989 as belonging to a separate genus, and the organisms were renamed *Helicobacter pylori* and *H. mustelae*, respectively (Goodwin et al., 1989).

In terms of gastric helicobacters, *H. mustelae* was the second gastric organism to be isolated, characterized, and named (Fox et al., 1986, 1988 b, 1989). This organism is now linked to peptic ulcer disease and gastric adenocarcinoma, and to MALT lymphoma in ferrets (Fox et al., 1993 b, 1997; Erdman et al., 2003 a). *Helicobacter felis*, the third named gastric helicobacter was isolated from the gastric mucosa of both cats and dogs (Lee et al., 1988). "*Gastrospirillum hominis*", which has been renamed "*Helicobacter heilmannii*", has been observed to have a wide distribution and can be found in a large number of different hosts, including cats, dogs, pigs, cheetahs, nonhuman primates, and humans. In humans, "*H. heilmannii*" has been observed in association with chronic gastric inflammation, MALT lymphoma and rarely gastric adenocarcinoma, and thus is the only other gastric helicobacter (except for isolated case reports of *H. felis*) which has been associated with stomach diseases in human patients (Lee et al., 1993; Lee and O'Rourke, 1993; Fox, 1997). *H. acinonychis*, isolated from the stomachs of cheetahs, appears to be the most similar phylogenetically to *H. pylori* (Eaton et al., 1993). Another closely related organism, *H. cetorum*, has been isolated from the inflamed stomachs of dolphins and whales (Harper et al., 2002, 2003).

10.1.2.2 Enterohepatic *Helicobacter* spp.

In 1984, a group of microaerobic *Campylobacter*-like organisms (CLOs) were isolated from rectal swabs of male homosexuals suffering from protocolitis and enteritis (Fennell et al., 1984; Totten et al., 1985). These bacteria could be broadly classified into three major DNA homology groups. One of these was *H. cinaedi*, previously classified as *C. cinaedi* (CLO-1 A) (Table 10.1). The second CLO2 was named

C. fennelliae, and the third (still unnamed) organism was classified as CLO3 (On and Holmes, 1995). These organisms were later classified as Helicobacter spp., in part because they had sheathed flagella, but primarily because of DNA/DNA hybridization data and 16 S ribosomal RNA (rRNA) analysis.

Over the past two decades, many additional members of the Helicobacter genus have been identified, which have included both gastric Helicobacter spp. and enterohepatic Helicobacter spp. Several of these enterohepatic helicobacters are linked with chronic inflammatory diseases of the bowel and liver, and in some cases are directly associated with gastrointestinal cancers. All together, over 26 novel species have been identified and assigned to the Helicobacter genus, mainly on the basis of 16 S rRNA sequencing data (Fox, 2002). Ribosomal RNA codes for proteins which facilitate protein synthesis, and these sequences have been highly conserved over the course of bacterial evolution. The degree of 16 S rRNA sequence similarity is thought to correlate closely with the ancestry of bacterial species, and bacteria with sequences that are more than 90% homologous to H. pylori have been assigned to the genus Helicobacter.

10.1.3
Genomic Analysis

10.1.3.1 *H. pylori*

The two H. pylori strains that have been sequenced H. pylori 26695 and H. pylori J99 were isolated from a United Kingdom patient with gastritis in the early 1980s, and from a patient with duodenal ulcer living in the United States in 1994, respectively (Tomb et al., 1997; Alm and Noonan, 2001). Although the genome of 26695 is 24 kb larger than that of J99 (1667 versus 1643), both possess a total (G+C) % of 39%. Both strains have similar average lengths of coding sequences coding density and contain two copies of the 16 S and 23 S-5 S rRNA loci in the same relative positions (Alm and Noonan, 2001).

Table 10.2 Prevalence of *H. pylori* infection in large ($>$ 500 individual) population-based surveys (adapted from de Martel and Parsonnet, 2006).

Continent	Country	Year	Age group	No. of subjects	HP prevalence [%]	Reference
Studies in adults						
Europe	Helsinki, Finland	1990	>70	618	65	Strandberg et al., 1997
	Germany	1987	18–89	1785	39	Brenner et al., 1999
	Leicestershire, UK	1997	21–55	1431	15	Stone et al., 1998

Table 10.2 (Continued)

Continent	Country	Year	Age group	No. of subjects	HP prevalence [%]	Reference
Studies in adults						
	East Anglia, UK	1992	20–44	841	22	Jarvis et al., 2004
	Bristol, UK	1996	20–59	10 535	16	Lane et al., 2002
	North England, UK	1998	40–49	7452	27	Moayyedi et al., 2002
	Glasgow, UK	1995	25–64	5749	68	Woodward et al., 2000
	Bruneck, Italy	1990	40–79	826	86	Mayr et al., 2000
	Italy	1996	35–74	930	45	Palli et al., 1993
	Northern Ireland	1986	26–64	3511	58	Murray et al., 1997
	Ankara, Turkey	1998	25–64	1089	77	Akin et al., 2004
Asia	Shandong, China	1997	35–69	3013	66	Brown et al., 2002
	Japan	1990	45–65	1322	81	Montani et al., 2003
	Kuala Lumpur, Malaysia	NA	19–54	548	26	Goh and Parasakthi, 2001
Oceania	Christchurch, New Zealand	1997	18–91	1045	21	Collett et al., 1999
Americas	Mexico	1987	20–90	5996	81	Torres et al., 1998
	United States	1991	≥ 20	7465	33	Everhart et al., 2000
Studies in children						
Europe	Leipzig, Germany	1997	6–7	2487	6	(Herbarth et al., 2001)
	Ulm, Germany	1996	5–8	945	13	(Rothenbacher et al., 1998)
	Pavia, Italy	NA	6–19	807	12	(De Giacomo et al., 2002)
	Sardinia, Italy	1997	5–16	2810	22	(Dore et al., 2002 a)
	Northern Ireland	1986	12–24	1231	29	(Murray et al., 1997)
Asia	Seoul, South Korea	NA	6–12	753	5	(Seo et al., 2002)

Table 10.2 (Continued)

Continent	Country	Year	Age group	No. of subjects	HP prevalence [%]	Reference
Studies in children						
Americas	Southern Andes, Colombia	1992	2–9	2801	69	(Goodman et al., 1996)
	San Juan Sacatepeques, Guatemala	1999	0–3	522	22	(Steinberg et al., 2004)
	Mexico	1987	1–19	5606	51	(Torres et al., 1998)
	United States	1991	6–19	2581	33	(Everhart et al., 2000)

In addition to allelic diversity, *H. pylori* strains also differ in their gene content. The two completely sequenced genomes of *H. pylori* strains 26 695 and J99 share only 94% of their genes (Alm et al., 1999), and 6–7% of the genes are unique for each strain (Tomb et al., 1997). A comparison of 15 strains with DNA microarrays showed that in this set of strains, 1281 of 1643 genes present on the array (combined from 26 695 and J99 genomes) were shared by all strains; however, only 22% of genes were present in some of the strains (Salama et al., 2000).

Indeed, it is increasingly evident that *H. pylori* has remarkable genetic variability and intraspecies diversity. Allelic diversity is so marked that nearly all unrelated isolates of *H. pylori* have a unique sequence when a fragment of several hundred base pairs fragments are sequenced from housekeeping or virulence genes (Kansau et al., 1996; Falush et al., 2003). This allelic diversity is the result of the combination of a high (mutator-type) mutation rate (Bjorkholm et al., 2001), a high frequency of recombination between strains during mixed colonization (Go et al., 1996; Suerbaum et al., 1998; Kersulyte et al., 1999), and the ability of *H. pylori* to integrate small fragments of exogenous DNA into its chromosome (Suerbaum et al., 1998; Falush et al., 2003).

To investigate how this variability arises, investigators recently compared the genome content of 21 closely related pairs of isolates taken from the same patient at different time points (Kraft et al., 2006). The comparisons were performed by hybridization with whole-genome DNA microarrays. Their analysis indicated that the great majority of genetic changes were due to homologous recombination, suggesting that adaptation of *H. pylori* to the host individual occurs principally through sequence changes rather than loss or gain of genes (Kraft et al., 2006).

10.1.3.2   *H. hepaticus*

H. hepaticus is currently the best studied of the enterohepatic *Helicobacter* species, a diverse group that comprises bacteria that colonize the intestinal tracts and/or livers of susceptible hosts and that includes several human diarrheal pathogens including *Helicobacter fennelliae* and *Helicobacter cinaedi* (Solnick and Schauer, 2001) (Table 10.2). DNA from enterohepatic *Helicobacter* species has been found in patients with hepatobiliary diseases including hepatocellular carcinoma and biliary tract cancer, but a causal role of these bacteria in human liver disease has not been firmly established (Fox et al., 1998; Solnick and Schauer, 2001).

   H. hepaticus has many features in common with *H. pylori*: both persistently infect their hosts, leading to chronic inflammation, and in both cases this inflammation can progress to carcinoma (Suerbaum and Michetti, 2002). However, *H. hepaticus* does not colonize the stomach, but instead shares the same lower bowel habitat with *C. jejuni*, the most frequent bacterial cause of diarrhea in humans.

   The complete genome sequence of *H. hepaticus* ATCC51449 was recently sequenced (Suerbaum et al., 2003). *H. hepaticus* has a circular chromosome of 1 799 146 bp, predicted to encode 1875 proteins. A total of 938, 953, and 821 proteins have orthologues in *H. pylori*, *C. jejuni*, and both pathogens, respectively. *H. hepaticus* lacks orthologues of most known *H. pylori* virulence factors, including adhesins, the VacA cytotoxin, and almost all *cag* pathogenicity island proteins, but has orthologues of the *C. jejuni* adhesin PEB1 and the cytolethal distending toxin (CDT). The genome contains a 71-kb genomic island (HHGI1) and several genomic islets, the G+C contents of which differ from the remainder of the genome. HHGI1 encodes three basic components of a type IV secretion system and other virulence protein homologues, suggesting a role of HHGI1 in pathogenicity. *H. hepaticus*, as well as other enterohepatic *Helicobacter* spp., also encodes for a CDT which plays an important role in cell cycle arrest (Chien et al., 2000; Young et al., 2000b; Taylor et al., 2003).

   The flagellar biosynthesis system of *H. hepaticus* is similar to that of *H. pylori*, with genes encoding two flagellin types FlaA and FlaB under control of respective σ^{28} and σ^{54} promoters. Remarkably, there are two identical copies of *flaA*, including the promoter (HH1364 and HH1653), indicating a relatively recent duplication.

   In contrast to *H. pylori*, with its very large number of restriction – modification systems, *H. hepaticus* has only two complete restriction – modification systems (HH238/239 and HH1050/1051). Like *H. pylori*, *H. hepaticus* is naturally transformable (Suerbaum et al., 2003).

10.2
Life Cycle, Specificity, and Virulence Determinants in Cancer Development

10.2.1
Epidemiology of *H. pylori*

Soon after the discovery of *H. pylori* by Marshall and Warren, serological tests for the bacterium were developed by a number of investigators, and proved useful for studies of its epidemiology. Studies worldwide verified the association of *H. pylori* infection with peptic ulcer disease, and follow-up studies showed unequivocally that triple antibiotic treatment of *H. pylori* resulted in decreased recurrences of peptic ulcer disease, and cure of ulcer disease in patients in whom *H. pylori* was eradicated (Graham et al., 1992; Hentschel et al., 1993; Sung et al., 1995; Van der Hulst et al., 1997). Moreover, while epidemiological investigations confirmed that *H. pylori* infection was more common in ulcer disease, these studies also revealed that infection was extremely common even in asymptomatic individuals, and that infection rates were significantly higher in underdeveloped countries. While *H. pylori* infection was found to be present by serological testing in 30–40% of asymptomatic individuals in the U.S., it was present in 70% or more of asymptomatic individuals in underdeveloped countries.

The association of *H. pylori* with chronic superficial gastritis was followed later by studies indicating that *H. pylori* gastritis may progress over several decades to chronic atrophic gastritis. This histopathological condition is a precursor of gastric carcinoma, and is characterized by a loss of specialized glandular tissue, including both parietal and chief cells (Kuipers et al., 1995) (Fig. 10.1). The association with this preneoplastic lesion, and the epidemiological parallel between *H. pylori* infection rates and gastric cancer prevalence, suggested a possible role for *H. pylori* in the pathogenesis of gastric cancer. Gastric cancer was known to be extremely prevalent in regions of the world (Peru, Mexico, Columbia, and parts of Asia) where virtually all adults were infected with *H. pylori*, and infection was commonly present early in childhood. Three prospective, case-controlled studies by three groups based on stored sera obtained between six and years prior to cancer diagnosis, showed clearly that *H. pylori* infection was significantly more common in gastric cancer patients compared to controls, with an odds ratio (OR) of approximately 4.0 (Forman et al., 1991; Nomura et al., 1991; Parsonnet et al., 1991). The studies by Forman et al. showed that the OR increased to approximately 9.0 when cancer cases were limited to those diagnosed more than 15 years after testing positive for *H. pylori* (Forman, 1996). Based on this epidemiological evidence, a Working Group of the International Agency for Research on Cancer (IARC) concluded that infection increased the risk of cancer, and classified *H. pylori* infection as representing a group I carcinogenic exposure (IARC working group on the evaluation of carcinogenic risks to humans, 1994).

In addition, *H. pylori* was strongly linked to other stomach diseases, including gastric MALT lymphoma, a rare disorder in which there is transformation of a clonal B-cell population within the gastric mucosa (Parsonnet et al., 1994). Finally, *H. pylori*

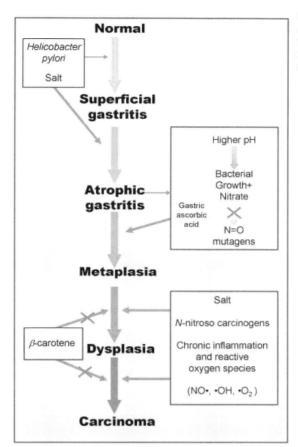

Fig. 10.1 Proposed Correa's cascade of pathologic events in gastric adenocarcinoma. An X through an arrow indicates inhibition of the process.

from Fox and Wang, NEJM, 2001

was also associated strongly with Menetrier's hypertrophic gastropathy (Bayerdorffer et al., 1994) and hyperplastic gastric polyps (Ohkusa et al., 1998).

Thus, *H. pylori* infection is extremely common, affecting approximately 50% of the world's population (Table 10.2) (Hunt, 1996). As with other enteric pathogens, however, the distribution of infection falls most heavily in the developing world. In poorer countries, *H. pylori* may be found in almost all adults and the majority of children by the age of 10 years. In contrast, *H. pylori* is now increasingly less common in the industrialized world, with studies from Europe, the U.S. and Australia indicating a decline in infection incidence of 25% per decade (Parsonnet et al., 1991; Roosendaal et al., 1997). Infection in children in these countries is now rare, except in immigrants from poorer regions of the world.

"*H. heilmannii*" ("*H. bizzozeronii*"), and to a lesser extent *H. felis,* colonize a small percentage of humans with gastritis, and peptic ulcer disease. Given that no environmental source for these bacteria have been recognized, pets have been implicated in zoonotic transmission of the organisms. The eradication of "*H. heilmannii*" by antimicrobial therapy has also resulted in the resolution of gastritis and peptic ulcer disease (Heilmann and Borchard, 1991; Hilzenrat et al., 1995; Goddard et al., 1997). In addition, the recent observation that *H. felis* infection in INS/GAS transgenic and C57/BL mice induces gastric cancer adds credence to isolated case reports of "*H. heilmannii*"-associated gastric carcinoma (Morgner et al., 1995; Yang et al., 1995; Wang et al., 2000).

10.2.1.1 Transmission of *H. pylori*

H. pylori is most likely spread via human-to-human transmission. Humans appear to be the only natural host for the organism, and no significant animal reservoir of infection has been identified. Early reports suggested that gastric *Helicobacter*-like organisms (GHLO) colonized the gastric mucosa of pigs (Ho et al., 1991). However, others have failed to identify or isolate *H. pylori* in abattoir pigs from Brazil and Germany using serology and culture techniques (Rocha et al., 1992; Korber-Golze and Scupin, 1993). Studies to identify the pig as a natural reservoir for *H. pylori* have been complicated by the florid gastric microbiota because of the pig's copraphagic habits, making GHLO isolation attempts difficult. "*H. suis*", which is closely related to "*H. heilmannii*" type 1, has been identified in the stomach of pigs (Queiroz et al., 1990; Solnick et al., 1993; Mendes et al., 1994). Thus, detailed molecular analysis of *Helicobacter*-like organisms isolated from pigs continues to be required for identity, although at present there is no convincing evidence that pigs are a reservoir for *H. pylori*. Similarly, sheep have been incriminated as a source of *H. pylori*, but these data require further confirmation (Dore et al., 2001). Data have shown that cats from one commercial source were infected with *H. pylori* (Handt et al., 1994); however, most domestic cats do not appear to represent a significant vector for transmission of the infection. *Helicobacter pylori* and "*H. heilmannii*" are the most common species reported in monkeys. *H. pylori* has been recovered from two species of Old World macaques: rhesus (*Macaca mulatta*) and cynomolgus macaques (*Macaca fascicularis*) (Baskerville and Newell, 1988; Bronsdon and Schoenknecht, 1988; Dubois et al., 1994; Reindel et al., 1999). Rhesus macaques and Japanese macaques (*M. fuscata*) have been experimentally infected with human strains of *H. pylori* (Fukuda et al., 1992; Fujioka et al., 1993; Shuto et al., 1993). Based on biochemical, phenotypic and molecular analysis (and in limited studies using molecular techniques), it is believed that *H. pylori* isolated from macaques is highly related or identical to isolates from humans. However, their limited numbers and minimal direct contact with humans renders them an unlikely source for human infection.

It has been difficult to demonstrate the presence of *H. pylori* in the environment, in contrast to most other enteric bacteria. Although water has also been implicated as a source of *H. pylori* infection (Klein et al. , 1991; Goodman et al., 1996; Brown, 2000) and the organism has been amplified (and very rarely cultured) from water (Hulten et al., 1996; Lu et al., 2002), the epidemiology of infection is not consistent with water being a prominent mode of transmission in most parts of the world. The possibility has been raised that a contaminated water supply could serve as a source of *H. pylori* infection, and *H. pylori* DNA has been detected in water samples from Lima, Peru using PCR techniques (Hulten et al., 1996). The municipal water supply (versus well water) was incriminated as an important source of *H. pylori* infection, irrespective of whether the families were of high or low socioeconomic status (Hulten et al., 1996). However water sources were linked within the neighborhood of residence and variables including population density, family age distribution, household density, and frequency of drinking untreated water were not considered (Hulten et al., 1996). Interestingly, epidemiological data collected concerning 684 children residing in the southern Colombian Andes indicated that there was a strong association of infection with swimming in rivers or streams a few times a year (Goodman et al., 1996). In another cross-sectional study, *H. pylori* infection was best predicted by childhood living conditions such as lack of fixed hot water supply (Mendall et al., 1992). Studies in southern China showed no correlation to exist between fecal contamination (using fecal coliform counts) of the water supply and the prevalence of *H. pylori* infection. However, it was determined that most subjects boiled their drinking water, irrespective of origin, and stored the water in vacuum flasks, prior to ingestion. Based on these results, the authors concluded that water was not an important source of transmission of *H. pylori* in this region of China (Mitchell et al., 1992 a).

A large epidemiological study in 1815 young adult Chileans aged under 35 years showed an association of ingestion of uncooked vegetables to increased *H. pylori* infection (Hopkins et al., 1993). These authors speculated that contamination of vegetables by raw sewage could have played a role in *H. pylori* transmission. Confounding factors such as measuring socioeconomic status on a dichotomized scale without taking into consideration that three of the 14 items – water supply, sewage disposal and indicators of residential crowding – are directly related to disease transmission (Hopkins et al., 1993). In the Colombian study, children who frequently consumed raw vegetables in general – and lettuce in particular – were more likely to be infected with *H. pylori* (Goodman et al., 1996). Children eating lettuce several times a week had a higher risk of infection (Goodman et al., 1996).

There has been a great deal of speculation regarding whether the coccoid form of *H. pylori* might play a role in the organism's survival outside its host (Jones and Curry, 1990; Mai et al., 1991; Bode et al., 1993 a,b). Experimental data indicate that *H. pylori* coccoid forms can survive for more than one year in river water, and that *H. pylori* could be cultured at 10 days from river water at 40 °C (Karim and Maxwell, 1989; West et al., 1990). *H. pylori* can also survive in milk for several days (Karim and Maxwell, 1989), implying that milk contaminated with feces containing *H. pylori* could potentially be infectious to humans. In order to test definitively the relevance of the coccoid forms, *in-vivo* experiments must be performed – that is, coccoid (unculturable) forms should be inoculated into a suitable animal model to ascertain whether indeed they are infectious. Until this is accomplished the importance of coccoidal forms in transmission of the organism from host to host will be unknown.

Declines in *H. pylori* prevalence over time are presumed to be due to corresponding improvements in sanitation and hygiene. *H. pylori* is most readily transmitted in environments where many people share living space (Teh et al ., 1994; Goodman et al., 1996). Because household crowding has been so consistently linked with infection, it has been presumed that *H. pylori* is transmitted from person to person. In support of this hypothesis, *H. pylori* has been cultured from saliva, diarrheal stools and, most consistently, from vomitus, of infected hosts (Leung et al., 1999; Parsonnet et al., 1999). Moreover, several studies have indicated that the organism is transmitted to close contacts when an infected host develops gastroenteritis (Mitchell et al., 1992 b). Thus, poorer countries, which have crowded households and higher incidence of gastroenteritis, would also be more likely to sustain transmission.

Although *H. pylori* DNA has been detected by RT-PCR in dental plaque, there are few earlier reports of viable organisms within the oral cavity, and thus an oral source of transmission is still debated (Shames et al., 1989). Recent data however, indicate an increasing number of publications where *H. pylori* has been identified by culture or PCR from dental samples (Dowsett and Kowolik, 2003; Umeda et al., 2003; Matsuda and Morizane, 2005). Also, cats colonized with *H. pylori* had the organism cultured from their saliva (Fox et al., 1996 c).

H. pylori has been detected within the feces in both children (Thomas et al., 1992) and dyspeptic adults (Kelly et al., 1994), and ability to culture *H. mustelae* in ferrets colonized with *H. mustelae* have supported the notion that fecal-oral transmission, particular during the acute achlorhydric stage (Fox et al., 1992, 1993 a). Since early childhood (age < 3 years) appears to be the most frequent age of acquisition of infection, and diarrhea is particularly frequent in this age group, a fecal-oral route seems plausible. For example, *H. pylori* was cultured from the feces of humans administered a cathartic (Parsonnet et al., 1999). Nevertheless, definitive evidence that fecal-oral transmission occurs routinely is still lacking, and many questions remain regarding the mechanisms involved in acquisition of *H. pylori* infection (Cave, 1997).

10.2.1.2 Age of Acquisition

In populations of lower socioeconomic status, infection with *H. pylori* most frequently occurs in childhood. Cohort studies of young children in the U.S. border region with Mexico, immigrants from Latin America in California, Alaskan native Americans and in Peru indicate that children have infection rates that are threefold those of adults in the same communities (Parsonnet, 1995). Several investigators report that young children are infected recurrently, losing infection and then acquiring it again until it eventually becomes a persistent infection. These conclusions, however, are confounded by imperfect sensitivity and specificity of diagnostic tests. For example, a breath test which has 95 % specificity would, by chance alone, yield a false new infection rate of 5 % with serial testing. In one study that required PCR confirmation of positive stool antigen testing, 46 % of transiently positive stools were positive for *H. pylori*, indicating that some true transient infections do occur (Haggerty et al., 2005). Regardless of the frequency of transient infection, however, in high-risk regions of the world, sustained infection typically begins before age 10 years, and often before age 5 years. In industrialized regions of the world, infection is acquired more evenly among age groups. In that respect, *H. pylori*'s epidemiology parallels that of other enteric infections – that is, *Shigella* and hepatitis A – which cause childhood infections in the developing world, but in areas of low incidence, are less age-discriminatory. Regardless of age at onset, because *H. pylori* infection persists throughout life, its prevalence universally increases with age. For unknown reasons, men also have somewhat higher prevalence of *H. pylori* than women (de Martel et al., 2005).

The duration of *H. pylori* infection and age of acquisition have also been linked to variability in *H. pylori* disease outcome. Unfortunately, these risk factors have been difficult to prove observationally because the time of *H. pylori* acquisition is rarely known. Through analogy to other tumors, however, this idea gains credence. Studies of experimentally induced cancers indicate that chronic inflammation results in random CpG mutations that accumulate over time, increasing risk for cancer with duration of inflammation. Such CpG mutations have been observed in gastric tissue of individuals with *H. pylori* infection, suggesting that the longer infection persists, the greater the probability of accumulating the deleterious mutations that lead to cancer (Shibata et al., 2002). In humans, however, only indirect evidence supports the duration/age hypothesis (Blaser et al., 1995).

As described above, *H. pylori* is genetically diverse. This diversity is so informative to have been used to geographically map human migrations (Falush et al., 2003). Because *H. pylori*'s genetic variability also influences disease pathogenesis (see below), the geography of strain type informs disease epidemiology (Covacci et al., 1999). In broad epidemiological strokes, virtually all strains of *H. pylori* in Korea and Japan contain the pathogenicity island (PAI), whereas in Europe and the U.S., the proportion is closer to 60%. In northern Europe, most strains of *H. pylori* have a *vacA* signal peptide sequence of the s1a genotype, whereas in Iberia (and Latin America), s1b predominates; in both regions the m2 genotype of the *vacA* middle sequence exceeds m1. In contrast, in Asia, *vacA* typically is of s1c type with m2 exceeding m1. In Egypt, the less virulent s2 genotype predominates (Van Doorn et al., 1999). Within countries, there are also population differences in infecting strains. For example, in California, strains with the PAI are more common in blacks and in immigrants than in other populations (Parsonnet et al., 1997b). It is not clear how much these regional differences in bacterial genotype prevalence influence disease incidence.

Once *H. pylori* infection occurs, it persists in the stomach for the host's life, or until advanced preneoplasia in the stomach makes the gastric environment inhospitable to further colonization. Typically, the host will die never knowing the infection was present. In a considerable number of individuals, however, one of four adverse outcomes might occur: gastric ulcer, duodenal ulcer, gastric adenocarcinoma, or gastric MALT lymphoma. As would be expected for a major risk factor for disease, the epidemiology of these diseases parallels *H. pylori*'s epidemiology (although MALT lymphoma is too rare and too poorly reported to monitor trends over time).

10.2.1.2.1 Epidemiology of Gastric Cancer and *H. pylori*

Gastric cancer was the leading cause of cancer death in the U.S. and Western Europe through the mid-twentieth century, with incidence rates in men in 1930 exceeding 45/100 000 per year. Over the century, the incidence of gastric cancer has plummeted, however. In the U.S., the age-adjusted incidence rates between 1998 and 2002 was 8.8/100 000 per year (Ries et al., 2005). Despite the aging of the U.S. population (the majority of gastric cancers occur in the elderly), the National Cancer Institute estimates that less than 1% of U.S. residents born now would be expected to develop stomach cancer in their lifetime. This mortality rate of 4.5/100 000 per year represents a tenfold drop since 1930; mortality rates have continued to decline 25% during the past decade. Unfortunately, due to the late stage at which most tumors are discovered, however, the case-fatality rate remains high, with a five-year survival of only 23% and 11 500 people in the U.S. dying of stomach cancer in 2005.

Worldwide, there is great variability in gastric cancer rates (Ferlay et al., 2004) (Fig. 10.2). In 2002, the age-adjusted incidences of gastric cancer in European men ranged from 7.9/100 000 in Denmark to 41.9/100 000 in Belarus. In Latin America

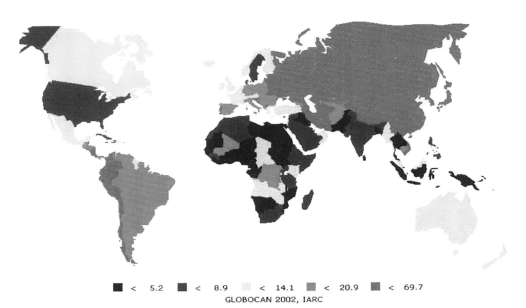

Stomach, Males
Age-Standardized incidence rate per 100,000

■ < 5.2   ■ < 8.9   ▨ < 14.1   ▨ < 20.9   ▥ < 69.7
GLOBOCAN 2002, IARC

Fig. 10.2 Age-standardized incidence of stomach cancer worldwide demonstrates variability within regions (from Ferlay et al., 2004). Although low reported low rates of cancer in Africa have led some to pursue physiological mechanisms for the "African enigma", incomplete cancer registries and limited cancer diagnostics in some countries may make comparisons misleading.

and East Asia, rates of stomach cancer remain consistently high, with peak rates in men in Chile (46.1/100 000) and Korea (69.7/100 000), respectively, and lowest rates in Mexico (13.1/100 000) and Mongolia (39.2/100 000), respectively. Other regions of the world have considerable variability in cancer rates, although registries are of inconsistent coverage and quality to make broad conclusions (Parkin et al., 1999). These geographical patterns are similar for men and women, although in any given location men consistently have twice the rates of cancer as women.

Overall, IARC data indicate a decline in gastric cancer incidence and mortality in virtually every country in which cancer registries monitor trends. In, Japan, where gastric cancer is infamous for its high incidence, rates are also declining dramatically – in some areas by almost 50% between 1966 and 2001 (Fig. 10.3) (Osaka Cancer Registry, 2004). Despite this unplanned, international "triumph" (Howson et al., 1986), gastric cancer remains a blight in much of the world. In the year 2001, 522 000 men and 328 000 women died from stomach cancer, making it the second leading cause of cancer death worldwide (Table 10.3). Even within low-risk countries, certain racial/ethnic groups retain higher rates of disease than others. In the U.S., cancer statistics indicate that gastric cancer remains the sixth leading cause of cancer death among Asians, the eighth among Native Americans, and the tenth among Blacks and Hispanics (U.S. Cancer Statistics Working Group, 2005). In Malayasia, gastric cancer is more common among Chinese and Indians, and less common in Malays (Kandasami et al., 2003). Furthermore, although worldwide gastric cancer mortality rates declined 5% between 1985 and 1990, due to aging of the world's population the number of cases actually increased 6% (Parkin et al., 1999).

Table 10.3 Estimated cancer deaths globally (2000), at the most common organ/tissue sites (from Parkin et al., 2001).

Cancer	Male	Female	Both sexes	%
Lung	810 000	293 000	1 103 000	17.8
Stomach	405 000	241 000	647 000	10.4
Liver	384 000	165 000	549 000	8.8
Colon/rectum	255 000	238 000	492 000	7.9
Breast	0	373 000	373 000	6.0
Esophagus	227 000	111 000	338 000	5.4
Cervix uteri	0	233 000	233 000	3.8
Pancreas	112 000	101 000	213 000	3.4
Prostate	204 000	0	204 000	3.3
Leukemia	109 000	86 000	195 000	3.1

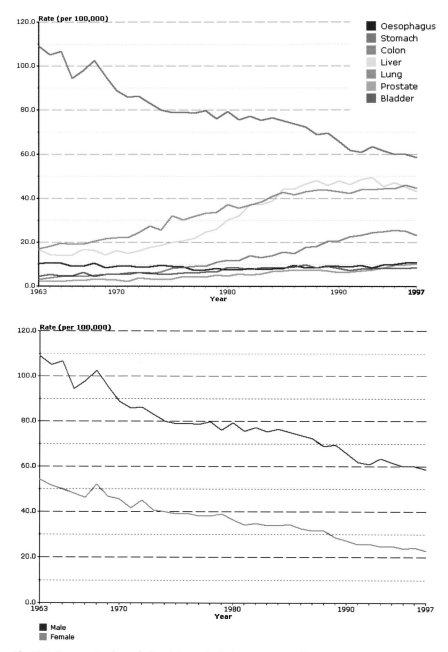

Fig. 10.3 Cancer rates have declined dramatically in many parts of the world, including Japan. Graphs representing cancer incidence rates in Japan adjusted to the world population (Osaka Cancer Registry, 2004).

It is well established that gastric cancer is preceded by chronic and acute gastric inflammation or gastritis (see Section 10.2.6). During the early 1980s, Marshall and Warren, as well as many other investigators, established that *H. pylori* was the preeminent cause of this gastritis, making it a leading suspect in gastric carcinogenesis. Subsequently, hundreds of epidemiological studies have been conducted to investigate this possible link. The strongest among these studies were those with prospective types of designs. These include nested case-control studies with greater than 10 years of follow-up (summary OR for gastric cancer = 5.9) and a prospective study in Japan which, after eight years of follow-up found cancer only in *H. pylori* -infected subjects (infinite OR) (Helicobacter and Cancer Collaborative, 2001; Uemura et al., 2001). The strong associations observed led the International Agency for Cancer Research to categorize *H. pylori* as a definite cause of cancer in humans, its strongest risk factor category (International Agency for Research on Cancer, 1994). In fact, *H. pylori* must be considered among the strongest risk factors identified for any cancer. Based on the OR above, and the high prevalence of infection, it can be crudely estimated that in high-risk areas, the proportion of gastric cancers attributable to *H. pylori* exceeds 80%.

Given the continued high rates of gastric cancer worldwide and the high attributable proportion, understanding and modulating *H. pylori*'s role in carcinogenesis remains imperative. As studies of cancer prevention continue, another critical issue being addressed is why a small minority of infected hosts (estimated at <5%) develop gastric cancer, while the great majority do not. Among theories being actively pursued are variability in bacterial genetics, variability in host genetics, age at acquisition of infection, diet, co-infection with other pathogens, and noninfectious environment exposures (Menaker et al., 2004). Of these, the strongest support for a role in outcome exist for bacterial and host genetics (Blaser, 2002; Basso and Plebani, 2004).

Several bacterial genes impart higher risk of cancer than others. A number of investigators have observed that *H. pylori* which contain the PAI of genes confer a higher risk for gastric cancer than those that do not (Parsonnet et al., 1997 a; Enroth et al., 2000). Accumulating data suggest that monitoring for *H. pylori* by a single method such as a serological test markedly underestimates the prevalence of *H. pylori* infection. A Swedish study used not only a conventional ELISA but also used Western blot analysis for antibodies against the CagA protein of *H. pylori,* the presence of which signifies prior or active infection. A high prevalence of infection in patients with gastric cancer was found, and a much higher OR was associated with *H. pylori* infection (Ekstrom et al., 2001). Also, in a recent study conducted in Germany (Brenner et al., 2004), the investigators applied three exclusion criteria to minimize bias against possible clearance of *H. pylori* during progression of the disease, and documented that this increased the OR of noncardia gastric cancer from 3.7 [95% confidence interval (CI) 1.7–7.9] to 18.3 (95% CI 2.4–136.7) for any *H. pylori* infection, and from 5.7 (95% CI 2.6–12.8) to 28.4 (95% CI 3.7–217.1) for *H. pylori* CagA$^+$ strains-infected patients (Brenner et al., 2004).

A meta-analysis that included 16 studies with 2284 cases and 2770 controls has recently confirmed the increased risk of gastric cancer in patients infected with cagA$^+$

H. pylori. Infection with the latter strains increased the risk for gastric cancer over the risk associated with *H. pylori* infection alone (2.87- and 2.28-fold, respectively (Huang et al., 2003).

Nevertheless, the almost universal prevalence of PAI-positive strains in some parts of the world can obscure this finding. The association between the PAI and cancer is particularly manifest for the "intestinal type" of gastric cancer that retains morphological similarity to intestinal tissue. PAI-positive strains have also been closely linked to p53 mutations found in intestinal cancers (Shibata et al., 2002) (Table 10.4). The diffuse type of gastric cancer, though still strongly associated with *H. pylori,* has equal association with PAI-positive and -negative strains (Parsonnet et al., 1997 a). Additionally, polymorphisms in the vaculolating cytotoxin (*vacA*) gene of infecting *H. pylori* strains may impart a higher risk for malignancy. Among the polymorphisms studied, the s1 and m1 *vacA* alleles (these alleles are associated with augmented inflammation) have been most consistently linked to a higher cancer risk (Bravo et al., 2002; Figueiredo et al., 2002; Garza-Gonzalez et al., 2004; Perez-Perez et al., 2005). Host genetics also play a role in disease outcome. Numerous studies have now confirmed El-Omar's landmark report which indicated that the host's interleukin (IL) 1β genotype and the genotype of the IL-1β endogenous receptor antagonist (IL-1 RN) influenced disease outcome (El-Omar et al., 2000). In case-control studies of *H. pylori*- infected subjects with and without cancer, biallelic C/C

Table 10.4 Genetic changes in gastric adenocarcinoma.[a]

Changes	Gene	Frequency [%]
Suppression/Loss	P53	60–70
	FHIT	60
	APC	50
	DCC	50
	E-cadherin	<5
Amplification/Up-regulation	COX-2	70
	HGF/SF	60
	VEGF	50
	c-Met	45
	AIB-1	40
	β-catenin	25
	K-sam	20
	Ras	10–15
	c-erb B2	5–7
Microsatellite instability (MSI)		25–40
DNA aneuploidy		60–75

[a] Data from Kounouras et al. (2005).

at either base 31 or 511 increases the risk of cancer 2.5-fold compared to the T/T alleles. Similarly, the presence of an allele of IL-1 RN with only two tandem repeats increases the cancer risk. These findings have been reproduced in other, but not all, countries (Perez-Perez et al., 2005). Combinations of these detrimental alleles increases the risk of cancer further (Figueiredo et al., 2002). Host tumor necrosis factor (TNF)-α and IL-10 allelic variation has also been linked to disease, though with somewhat smaller and more variable effect sizes (Perez-Perez et al., 2005); in conjunction with a PAI+ *H. pylori* infection, this effect is even more marked (El-Omar et al., 2003). In addition, several reports have implicated HLA genotypes as either detrimental or beneficial in protecting against cancer, though no consistent pattern has emerged.

Prior to the discovery of *H. pylori*, diet had been studied extensively as a cause of gastric cancer. In 1997, a panel of experts met to review the entirety of dietary data and to weigh the risk of cancer associated with foods. Foods were categorized as convincing, probable, possible, and insufficient risk factors for malignancy. For stomach cancer, only a few items were considered convincing or probable in their association with disease: these included salt (convincingly deleterious) and fruits, vegetables, and vitamin C (probably protective) (World Cancer Research Fund, 1997). A number of other factors were deemed to have no probable relationship with stomach cancer, including alcohol, black tea, coffee, and nitrates from vegetables. The panel did not consider dietary factors in conjunction with *H. pylori* infection however, and data in this area are slim. Data on salt are particularly unconvincing. Although salt has been identified as a risk factor for gastric cancer in a population with relatively high *H. pylori* prevalence (Tsugane et al., 2004), no study has compared the effects of salt in *H. pylori*-infected and uninfected humans. In animal models, salt has variable effects on carcinogenesis with *H. pylori*, accelerating progression of preneoplasia in infected C57/BL6 mice but not B6129 or hypergastrinemic INS-GAS mice (Fox et al., 1999 a, 2003 a; Rogers et al., 2005)

Some of the most intriguing cofactors of gastric cancer that are being actively pursued are other infectious agents. With advanced gastric atrophy consequent to *H. pylori* infection, gastric acid secretion diminishes. This loss of acid permits colonization of the gastric mucosa by nitrosating bacteria that can convert nitrates to mutagenic *N*-nitrosamines. In contrast, another co-infection – intestinal helminth infection – may diminish cancer risk by limiting host inflammatory responses. This is accomplished by shifting the normal proinflammatory Th1 response induced by *H. pylori* to a noninflammatory Th2 response promoted by the helminth infection. In children, in Colombia and South Africa, investigators have observed higher levels of Th2-dependent IgG1 to *H. pylori* than in children without helminths (Mitchell et al., 2002; Whary et al., 2005). Physiologically, persons with *H. pylori* in conjunction with *Schistosoma mansoni* infection, have been found to have reduced apoptosis and cell proliferation than persons with *H. pylori* alone (Elshal et al., 2004). It has been postulated that these effects explain the paradoxically low rates of gastric cancer in impoverished areas with high prevalence of *H. pylori*. Alternative explanations, however, such as low overall life expectancy and limited cancer registries and diagnostics, have not been excluded as reasons for the "African enigma". Epstein–Barr virus (EBV), which is a known risk factor for a rare form of gastric cancer – lymphoepithelioma-like carcinoma – has not been shown to interact with *H. pylori* to increase cancer risk.

10.2.1.2.2 Gastric Non-Hodgkin's Lymphoma

Primary gastric non-Hodgkin's lymphoma (NHL) is a rare disease. In studies from Europe, North America and the Middle East, this tumor affected a mere 0.2 to 0.9 per 100 000 population per year (Ullrich et al., 2002; Bani-Hani et al ., 2005). Incidence rates increase with age, with gastric lymphomas being vanishingly rare before the age of 30 years (Claviez et al., 2005). They are also somewhat more common in men than in women. Although rates of gastric lymphoma are quite low, the stomach is the most common extranodal site for NHL.

Gastric lymphomas may be of several histological types, the most common of which are marginal-zone B-cell lymphomas arising from lymphoid follicles known as mucosal-associated lymphoid tissue (MALT) and diffuse large B-cell lymphomas. The proportions in each category vary from study to study, probably due both to aggressiveness in diagnosis and the skill of the pathologist. Because MALT is a known consequence of *H. pylori* infection (30% of infected persons have MALT; Marshall and Windsor, 2005), interest in infection as a cause of MALT lymphoma naturally followed its discovery. The first case-series revealed well over 92% prevalence of *H. pylori* in 110 patients with gastric lymphoma (Wotherspoon et al., 1991), while one early study reported the regression of lymphoma with *H. pylori* eradication (Wotherspoon et al., 1993). In an epidemiological survey of 33 American and Swedish gastric lymphoma cases and matched controls, antecedent *H. pylori* was associated with a 6.3-fold increased risk of gastric lymphoma; the great majority of these lymphomas were diffuse large-cell lymphomas (Parsonnet et al., 1994). The most compelling data linking *H. pylori* and cancer, however, are derived from treatment trials. In these studies, early-stage gastric MALT lymphomas show remarkable response to *H. pylori* eradication, with 80% of patients going into complete remission (Stolte et al., 2002). Unfortunately, approximately 5% will relapse annually after achieving remission. Those who do relapse or have recurring *H. pylori* infection are more likely to have t(11:18) rearrangements of the immunoglobulin heavy chain than those not relapsing (Liu et al., 2002; Wundisch et al., 2005). Moreover, among those patients who remain in remission for an extended period, approximately 30% will have evidence of gastric lymphocyte monoclonality on molecular analysis. Thus, although there is clinical evidence that *H. pylori* provides a proliferative drive to lymphocytes, longer-term follow-up is necessary to assess the true "cure".

Why gastric lymphoma occurs in a vanishingly small proportion of *H. pylori*-infected hosts remains a mystery. As with gastric cancer, host polymorphisms in genes related to inflammation – specifically IL-1 L receptor antagonist and glutathione S-transferase genes –may play a role in outcome (Rollinson et al., 2003). Unlike gastric cancer, however, microbial polymorphisms have only been weakly linked to lymphomagenesis (Witherell et al., 1997; Delchier et al ., 2001).

"*H. heilmannii*" has also been associated with primary gastric low-grade lymphoma in humans (Regimbeau et al., 1998; Morgner et al., 2000). Similar to *H. pylori*-associated lymphoma, clinical remission of the lymphoma was noted in five patients after antibiotic eradication of the gastric *Helicobacter* (Roggero et al., 1995; Hussell et al., 1996; Morgner et al., 2000).

10.2.2
Bacterial Factors Responsible for Cell Specificity and Virulence

Helicobacter pylori is highly adapted to survive in the highly acidic environment of the stomach. In addition, the organism has specific tropism for gastric epithelial cells. Thus, in addition to colonizing the stomach, the organism can be found in areas of gastric metaplasia that occur in the duodenum, in Barrett's esophagus (Borhan-Manesh and Farnum, 1993), and even in the jejunum (within Meckel's diverticulum) and in isolated gastric metaplasia of the rectum, though in the latter two cases this appears to be a rare event (Hunt, 1996; Hill and Rode, 1998). Within the environment of the stomach, the organism is actively motile and free-living, existing just beneath the mucus layer of the stomach overlaying the gastric epithelial cells. Motility is clearly important for colonization of the stomach; this ability to colonize the gastric milieu is achieved through the organism's spiral shape and the unipolar flagella which allow movement through and below the mucus layer of the stomach. A recent elegant study performed in gerbils, indicates that *H. pylori* utilizes the gastric mucus pH gradient for precise spatial orientation in the mucus layer of the stomach (Schreiber et al., 2004).

For the most part, *H. pylori* are not invasive organisms, and the vast majority of the bacteria exist in an nonadherent, extracellular, mucous environment, which may account for many of the difficulties in immune clearance by the host, or antibiotic eradication. A small number of organisms have been shown to adhere to gastric epithelial cells (perhaps ~10%), and rare organisms may be found intracellularly, suggesting actual invasion (Wilkinson et al., 1998; Semino-Mora et al., 2003; Oh et al., 2005). Adherence of *H. pylori* to the gastric epithelium is a complicated process which most likely involves a number of surface receptors including Lewis B-binding adhesin, BabA (Ilver et al. , 1998) (which binds to surface mucus cell receptor Lewis B histoblood group antigen, and Lewis X, a glycosphingolipid which recognizes and binds to Sab A (sialic acid binding adhesin) of *H. pylori* (Mahdavi et al., 2002). The distribution mirrors the expression of trefoil factor 1, which also serves as binding factor for *H. pylori*, as does Muc5 AC (Linden et al., 2002; Clyne et al., 2004). In addition, *H. pylori* has been found to adhere preferentially, within the gastric units, to the surface mucous cells of the gastric pits, and generally not to adhere to the mucous neck, parietal or chief cells (Falk et al., 1993). However, the organism is able to invade deeply within the gastric glands, particularly within the non-acid-secreting mucosa of the gastric antrum (Thomsen et al., 1990).

The bacterial factors which allow for persistence of *H. pylori* within the gastric lumen are still being investigated, but several critical factors have been determined. Some of this information derives from animal models and the creation of *H. pylori* isogenic mutants. The most critical factor which allows *H. pylori* survival is the abundant production of urease, enabling hydrolysis of urea to ammonia and carbon dioxide. *H. pylori* synthesizes extremely high quantities of urease, which in total contribute to over 5% of the bacterial protein (Mobley, 1997). The generation of urease, among other effects, assists in neutralizing gastric acidity and allows the organism to withstand the low pH of the stomach. *H. pylori* is an acid-tolerant neutrophile (Rektorschek et al., 1998), and isogenic mutants of *H. pylori* which are deficient in urease are unable to colonize the gastric mucosa of the gnotobiotic piglet (Eaton et al., 1991). Motility by *H. pylori* is also critical to the organism's survival, and isogenic mutants of *H. pylori* lacking flagella have also been unable to colonize the gnotobiotic piglet (Eaton et al., 1992, 1996). *H. pylori* also produces a number of enzymes (e.g., phopholipase A2) which are involved in the breakdown of the surfactant layer overlying the gastric epithelium. Isogenic mutants of the gene *pldA*, which encodes for an outer member phospholipase, are also unable to colonize mouse models of *Helicobacter* infection.

The two genetic loci linked with virulence that have received the greatest amount of study are the *cag* locus and the *vacA* gene which encode for the vacuolating cytotoxin. The vacuolating cytotoxin first described by Leunk et al. (1988) induces a vacuolating effect in several cell lines, including gastric cell lines. The vacuolating toxin of *H. pylori* has been identified and characterized as a secreted protein; isogenic mutants lacking the toxin do not induce a vacuolating effect on cell lines (Harris et al., 1996; Smoot et al., 1996).

It has been established that there is considerable genetic diversity in *Vac* alleles, the most extensively studied having been the s1/m1 *vacA* allele. This typically encodes vacA protein which has a high level of vacuolating cytotoxin activity *in vitro* (Atherton et al., 1995). Other forms of vacA are associated with either a lower cytotoxin activity or no activity at all (Atherton, 2002). In one study, Tox⁻ *H. pylori* strains did not induce gastric cell damage *in vivo*, whereas Tox⁺ *H. pylori* strains caused gastric damage in a mouse model (Marchetti et al., 1995). Oral dosing of vacA also caused damage to gastroduodenal epithelia, including superficial erosions (Telford et al., 1994; Ghiara et al., 1995). Results in gerbils and gnotobiotic piglets dosed experimentally with wild-type toxigenic strains of *H. pylori* or their null mutants, showed no differences between gastric lesions produced by both strains, however (Eaton et al., 1997; Wirth et al., 1998). Nevertheless, it is important to remember that although ca. 50% of *H. pylori* strains are Tox⁻, they are still capable of inducing gastritis in humans (Cover, 1996; Gebert et al., 2003).

Recent data with direct relevance to the role of vacA in pathogenesis and the persistence of *H. pylori* infection indicate that VacA efficiently blocks the proliferation of T cells by inducing a G_1/S cell cycle arrest (Gebert et al., 2003). These authors concluded that VacA interfered with the T-cell receptor/IL-2 signaling pathway at the level of the Ca^{2+}-calmodulin-dependent phosphatase, calcineurin. Nuclear translocation of the nuclear factor of activated T cells (NFAT), a transcription factor which acts as a global regulator of immune response genes, was abrogated. This manifested in down-regulation of IL-2 transcription. The immunosuppressive drug FK506 partially mimicked vacA activities; thus, they likely shared a mechanism which could account for a local host immune suppression. These data could in part explain the often life-long chronicity of *H. pylori* infections (Gebert et al ., 2003). It is interesting to note that *C. jejuni*, as well as several enterohepatic helicobacters, produces a CDT which also inhibits cell cycle progression in epithelial cells, including T cells (Whitehouse et al. , 1998; Chien et al., 2000; Young et al., 2000b).

The cytotoxin-associated (*cagA*) gene was initially considered a prerequisite for vacuolating toxin activity due to the high degree of correlation between the presence of cagA and the ability of *H. pylori* to express the toxin (Tummuru et al., 1993). However, subsequent data showed that isogenic mutants of cagA still were still able to produce the toxin (Tummuru et al., 1994; Crabtree et al., 1995; Xiang et al., 1995).

The *cagA* is now known to be part of the cag locus, considered an important virulence determinant. This 40-kb DNA fragment is considered to be a PAI, and consists of a cluster of genes (more than 25). This PAI is more commonly found in *H. pylori* strains isolated from peptic ulcer and gastric cancer patients (Censini et al., 1996).

A functional *cag* PAI is required for the internalization of CagA within gastric epithelial cells. Once internalized, CagA becomes phosphorylated by members of the Src family of kinases, implicated in other malignancies. The phosphorylated CagA then activates SHP2 (a eucaryotic phosphatase), as well as ERK (a member of the MAPK family). This process results in morphological derangement of epithelial cells (Higashi et al., 2002b; Tsutsumi et al., 2003). More recently, investigators have studied the possible biological activities of CagA proteins in relation to tyrosine phosphorylation motifs (TPMs). Interestingly, the number of TPMs in *H. pylori* strains in patients from Western countries varies, as does the number of motifs resulting in variability in SHP2 binding affinity. This contrasts with the TPMs of *H. pylori* strains isolated from patients living in eastern Asian countries, wherein the TPMs match the consensus SHP2 binding site, resulting in increased SHP2 binding and cell derangements similar to that noted when cells are stimulated by growth factors (Higashi et al., 2002a). These differences in TPMs between Western and Eastern strains may in part explain the marked differences in gastric cancer noted in these different geographic regions.

It is proposed that the cag PAI is involved in the delivery of effector molecules into host cells (Odenbreit et al., 2000; Stein et al., 2000). Other cag PAI-related proteins are also required for the activation in gastric epithelial cells of NF-κB, which plays a key role in host immune responses and inflammation (Keates et al., 1997; Sharma et al., 1998).

Strains of *H. pylori* with the cag PAI (Covacci et al., 1993), the so-called *H. pylori* type I, versus *H. pylori* type II strains which lack the cag island (Xiang et al., 1995), are capable of inducing IL-8 expression and tyrosine phosphorylation of a 145-kDa protein from gastric epithelial cells (Crabtree et al., 1994; Segal et al., 1997). Furthermore, isogenic mutants lacking numerous genes of the *cag* PAI abolish these *in-vitro* effects (Tummuru et al., 1995; Censini et al., 1996; Segal et al., 1997). Importantly however, *H. pylori* isogenic mutants lacking either cagA, cagF or cagN failed to abolish IL-8 production.

Recently, investigators have shown that *H. pylori* was recognized by epithelial cells via Nod1, an intracellular pathogen-recognition molecule with specificity for peptidoglycan of Gram-negative bacteria (Viala et al., 2004). These authors demonstrated that Nod1 detection of *H. pylori* depended on the delivery of peptidoglycan to host cells by the *H. pylori* type IV secretion system, encoded by *cag* PAI. Consistent with the involvement of Nod1 in host defense, Nod1-deficient mice were more susceptible to infection by *cag* PAI-positive *H. pylori* than were wild-type mice (Viala et al., 2004). Thus, it appears that Nod1 may represent a key molecule in the innate immune sensing of *cag* PAI-positive *H. pylori* by epithelial cells. Nevertheless, it remains unclear how such cells might sense and respond to *H. pylori* that do not possess a *cag* PAI, or in which the *cag* PAI is non-functional (Philpott et al., 2002).

The recent sequencing of the entire genome of two strains of *H. pylori* will allow investigators to explore more fully the virulence factors already described, as well as to determine the presence of others (Tomb et al., 1997; Alm et al., 1999).

10.2.3
Host Factors Playing a Role in Gastric Diseases

Although worldwide, half of the population is infected with *H. pylori*, only a small percentage of individuals (e.g., 1–3%) progress to gastric cancer. There has been extensive debate as to whether bacterial or host factors can account for the diverse outcomes (asymptomatic, duodenal ulcer or gastric cancer) of *H. pylori* infection. While bacterial factors likely play an important role in disease pathogenesis, a true "carcinogenic strain" has not been identified, and the bulk of evidence suggests that host factors are paramount in determining progression to gastric cancer. As detailed below, murine models of *Helicobacter* infection indicate that certain inbred murine strains (e.g., C57 BL/6) are highly susceptible to cancer progression, while other inbred strains (e.g., BALB/c) are very resistant to gastric adenocarcinoma and its precursor lesions. In addition, *Cag*-negative strains such as *H. felis* appear to be as carcinogenic (if not more so) in mice as *Cag*-positive strains. In every model system studied, the progression to gastric cancer correlates strongly with the intensity and type of immune response, which is strongly governed by host genetic factors.

During the past few decades, a number of studies have indicated a strong role for genetic factors in gastric cancer. Gastric cancer risk is increased up to threefold in individuals with a first-degree relative with gastric cancer, and 10% of cases appear to exhibit familial clustering. While *H. pylori* infection also runs in families, family history remains a risk factor even after control for *H. pylori* infection. Nevertheless, only a small part of the familial clustering of gastric cancer could be attributable to known family cancer syndromes.

The search for other genetic factors began with the observation that relatives of patients with gastric cancer had a higher prevalence of atrophy and hypochlorhydria (see Table 10.3). This increased prevalence of atrophy was limited only to those patients who were also infected with *H. pylori*, suggesting (hypothetically) that genetic factors led to more intense immunity to *H. pylori*. In addition, the search for genetic factors also built upon the observation that patients who progressed to atrophy and cancer appeared to secrete lower levels of acid compared to patients with duodenal ulcer disease. Thus, the initial genetic study of families with an increased incidence of precancerous changes focused on IL-1β, a well-known proinflammatory cytokine that is also a powerful inhibitor of acid secretion. The IL-1β gene cluster includes both IL-1β and IL-1RN, its naturally occurring receptor antagonist. The study conducted by El-Omar et al. of a Caucasian population from Poland and Scotland showed that individuals with the IL-1β-31*C or -511*T and IL-1RN*2/*2 genotypes had a two- to threefold increased risk of developing atrophy and gastric cancer in the setting of *H. pylori* infection (El-Omar et al., 2000). This was quickly confirmed by Portuguese and Japanese groups, who also showed a strong association between IL-1 gene cluster (IL-1β and IL-1RN) proinflammatory polymorphisms and an increased risk of gastric cancer (Machado et al., 2001; Furuta et al., 2004). The basic finding that an increased risk for gastric cancer is associated with proinflammatory IL-1β polymorphisms has been confirmed in many populations, including those in China, Taiwan, Mexico, Korea, Germany, and Brazil, as recently reviewed (Furuta et al., 2004; Palli et al., 2005; Perez-Perez et al., 2005), although a smaller number of studies have not found any such association. Later studies by El-Omar combined genetic polymorphisms in TNF-α and IL-10, resulting in a high-risk genotype with a 27-fold or greater risk of gastric cancer (El-Omar et al., 2003). A study by Machado and colleagues also noted the importance of the TNF-α-308 polymorphism, and found that a combination of IL-1 and TNF-α gene polymorphisms markedly increased the risk for atrophy and gastric cancer (Machado et al., 2001). More recent studies have identified the -251 T allele in the IL-8 promoter as being significantly associated with an increased risk of gastric cancer (Lee et al., 2005; Taguchi et al., 2005). These observations provide strong evidence for host genetics in determining the progression to gastric cancer, and have strengthened the connection the inflammatory response and gastric carcinogenesis.

10.2.4
Environmental Factors

While almost all patients infected with *H. pylori* develop some degree of chronic active gastritis, most will remain free of symptoms or adverse consequences to their health and well-being. Prior to the recent focus on host genetic polymorphisms, a number of studies investigated the role of diet and other environmental cofactors in contributing to the development of gastric cancer. Migration studies in particular point to the importance of the local environment in dictating gastric cancer risk, and while much of this environmental risk was likely due to *H. pylori* infection, the infection rates alone do not account for the vast geographical differences in gastric cancer rates in Japan compared to Africa and other countries. Thus, a recent assessment regarding the role of diet, parasite co-infection and bacterial overgrowth will be discussed in the following sections.

10.2.4.1 **Diet**

Several decades ago, there was a tremendous interest in the relationship between dietary composition and the overall risk of gastric cancer. Epidemiological studies had pointed to a possible risk associated with diets high in salt and nitrates, and low in fresh fruits and vegetables. The greatest attention was given to the effect of high nitrate intake, under the notion that nitrates can be reduced to nitrite and then react with other nitrogenated substances to produce *N*-nitroso compounds which are known carcinogens. However, large prospective cohort studies failed to confirm an increased risk (van Loon et al., 1998). A high salt intake has been even more strongly linked epidemiologically to gastric cancer risk, and has been shown in some animal studies to induce more severe gastric lesions. However, long-term murine studies have not demonstrated any acceleration of gastric cancer in *Helicobacter*-infected mice (Rogers et al., 2005). The protective effect of a high consumption of fresh fruits and vegetables led to a number of chemoprevention studies involving treatment with antioxidants such as selenium, beta-carotene, alpha-tocopherol, and ascorbic acid. However, these studies have also been largely inconclusive. A recent meta-analysis confirmed this general lack of efficacy, with the possible exception of selenium (Bjelakovic et al., 2004). In long-term interventional studies, such as that conducted by Correa and colleagues, the beneficial effects of antioxidants, while present at six years of follow-up, were not evident at 12 years of follow up, in contrast to the effects of antibiotic eradication which were long-lasting (Mera et al., 2005).

10.2.4.2 **Co-Infection**

While most of the focus has been on diet as a cofactor for gastric cancer, a number of recent studies have pointed to parasitic co-infection as possibly important in modulating cancer risk. Gastric atrophy and cancer have been clearly linked to a vigorous Th1 immune response to *H. pylori*. In contrast, many parasitic infections, particularly infections with intestinal helminths, lead to a strong Th2 immune response. The "hygiene hypothesis" has suggested that improvements in sanitation leading to decreased parasitic infections has led to an increase in Th1 immune-mediated diseases. In addition, it was postulated by Fox et al. that the African enigma could be due in part to a higher level of parasitic infections in some areas of the world (Fox et al ., 2000 a). Childhood infection with Th2-polarizing helminthic infection, in areas of the world where climate and poor sanitation favor the life cycle and transmission of parasites, could in theory promote a Th2 response to *H. pylori* . In order to test this as a possible mechanism, Fox's group carried out a co-infection study in mice, which demonstrated amelioration of gastric atrophy co-infected with *H. felis* and *Heligmosomoides polygyrus*, a murine intestinal nematode (Fox et al., 2000 a). The decrease in risk for gastric atrophy in mice dually infected with *H. felis* and the nematode was supported by a shift in the Th1-biased response to *H. felis* toward a Th2-like phenotype of gastritis. Co-infection with *H. polygyrus* also led to a marked increase in anti-inflammatory cytokines IL-4, IL-10 and TGF-β, and lower levels of proinflammatory interferon (IFN)-γ, TNF-α and IL-1β. More direct experimental evidence that T-cell immune responses lead directly to preneoplastic changes in the gastric mucosa have come from the *H. felis* model of adoptive transfer gastritis, whereby adoptive transfer of C57 BL/6 splenocytes or CD4+ lymphocytes or Th1 cells to immunodeficient recipients results in enhanced gastritis and decreased bacterial colonization after *H. felis* infection (Mohammadi et al., 1997; McCracken et al., 2005). In addition, studies by Yamori et al. have employed a noninfectious gastritis model employing mice transgenic for T-cell receptors specific to ovalbumin, and using the adoptive transfer of T cells, with or without deficiency of IL-4, IFN-γ or IL-12, and injections of oval-bumin into the gastric mucosa (Yamori et al., 2004). These studies demonstrate clearly that antigenic activation of Th1-type T cells infiltrating into the gastric mucosa enhance dysregulated apoptosis and epithelial cell turnover.

Support for this Th1/Th2 paradigm as the best explanation for geographic variations in gastric cancer rates has come from measurement of IgG subclass responses as a surrogate marker for polarization of T-helper cell function (Mitchell et al., 2002). These studies suggested that adults in undeveloped areas of the world tend to show predominantly Th2-associated IgG2 response to *H. pylori*, rather than the Th1-associated IgG2 responses observed in developed countries. Thus, the host immune response to *H. pylori* infection in an African population differs from that observed in subjects from developed countries (such as Germany) (Mitchell et al., 2002). More recently, the Th2 responses to *H. pylori* have been linked more directly to intestinal helminth infections. In a study of children living in two different regions of Columbia, Whary et al. showed that there was a higher rate of intestinal helminthiasis and higher Th2-associated IgG1 responses to *H. pylori* in children from the region (Tumaco) showing lower gastric cancer rates (Whary et al., 2005). Overall, parasitic co-infection is likely to be strongly protective against gastric cancer development, recognizing that other factors are also important.

10.2.4.3 Bacterial Overgrowth

While *H. pylori* is clearly the major trigger leading to chronic gastritis and the development of gastric atrophy, *H. pylori* colonization actually declines in patients with severe hypochlorhydria. At the time of diagnosis of gastric cancer, *H. pylori* infection is often difficult to appreciate or detect, even with multiple methodologies. Thus, questions have been raised as to whether *H. pylori* is important in the advanced stages of preneoplasia, or simply a trigger for the development of gastric atrophy. Indeed, reports from several groups have shown that in mice, bacteria other than *H. pylori*, such as *Acinetobacter iwoffii*, can induce atrophic gastritis (Rathinavelu et al ., 2003). Furthermore, there is evidence from a number of model systems that, in general, gastric cancer is preceded by a long period of achlorhydria, and reduced gastric acid consistently predisposes the stomach to colonization by bacteria and inflammation. The number and diversity of bacterial organisms in the stomach rises as the intragastric pH rises, and bacterial overgrowth in theory leads to increased formation of *N*-nitroso compounds. Thus, gastrin-deficient mice housed in a conventional (non-SPF) facility develop bacterial overgrowth, chronic gastritis, and progress to gastric cancer (Zavros et al., 2002, 2005). Similar antral tumors develop in *H. felis*-infected wild-type mice, again after longstanding achlorhydria and after *Helicobacter* organisms are nearly undetectable (Cai et al., 2005). Consequently, one can hypothesize that the primary role of *H. pylori* in gastric cancer is in the induction of atrophic gastritis and hypochlorhydria, leading to bacterial overgrowth. While acid-suppressing drugs can result in bacterial overgrowth and possibly increased formation of *N*-nitroso compounds, there is currently no supportive evidence for an increased risk of gastric cancer in patients receiving these medications, particularly in the absence of *H. pylori* infection. Recent studies have shown beneficial effects of antibiotic eradication regimens on gastric cancer progression in *H. pylori*-infected patients (Wong et al. , 2004); however, the possibility must be considered that the beneficial effect of antibiotics might be as much from the eradication of non-*H. pylori* organisms as it is from *H. pylori* eradication.

10.2.5
Natural History and Stages of Infection

Helicobacter pylori, as the second most common chronic bacterial infection in humans, infects almost half of the world's population. However, the natural history of this infection is extremely variable and the vast majority of infected individuals – perhaps 75 % or more – will remain asymptomatic and experience no adverse consequences from the infection. Thus, with respect to gastric cancer, it is clear that *H. pylori* infection on its own is not sufficient, and that other factors – bacterial, host or unknown cofactors – are required. Infection is typically acquired early in life, either through a fecal-oral or oral-oral route of transmission, followed by a long quiescent phase where there is a chronic gastritis of variable intensity and minimal symptoms. Peptic ulcer disease tends to develop when patients are in their twenties and thirties, whereas gastric cancer arises several decades or more later. Perhaps only 10–15 % of infected patients will develop peptic ulcer disease, while the risk of gastric cancer is estimated at approximately 1 % (though it may be 3 % or more in Japan and other high-risk countries). Interestingly, patients who develop duodenal ulcer (DU) disease appear to be somewhat protected from gastric cancer, with a lower overall risk of developing malignancy of the stomach (Hansson et al., 1996). This is thought to be due to a higher basal level of acid secretion, which in some instances could be related to a low-expressing IL-1β genotype. The notion that patients with DU are protected has been supported by endoscopic studies, where such patients had a low risk of cancer progression, while those with non-ulcer dyspepsia had a relatively high risk (e.g., 5 %) of progression (Uemura et al., 2001). Based on the results of this and other studies, it has been suggested that the location and severity of gastritis could be predictive of the risk of progression to gastric cancer, with antral gastritis alone representing a lower risk while "corpus gastritis" (gastritis involving the body and proximal portions of the stomach) represented a greater risk. In any case, it appears that progression to atrophy/cancer, duodenal ulcer, or asymptomatic status represent relatively distinct pathways for long-term infected patients.

H. pylori has been associated with an increased risk of both "intestinal-type" and "diffuse-type" gastric cancer – two histological types of gastric cancer according to the Lauren classification. While little is known regarding the histological progression leading to diffuse gastric cancer, that leading to intestinal-type gastric cancer has been studied for several decades and has been organized into a series of discrete steps known as the Correa pathway (Correa, 1995) (see Fig. 10.1). According to this model, intestinal-type gastric cancer arises from chronic *Helicobacter* infection, through a multistep pathway involving stages of superficial gastritis, atrophic gastritis, metaplasia, dysplasia and finally carcinoma (Fox and Wang, 2001). While the terms "atrophy" and "intestinal metaplasia" have been confusing and at times used synonymously, accumulating evidence suggests that intestinal metaplasia (IM) is less consistently associated with gastric cancer than gastric atrophy. Gastric atrophy – defined in the corpus as loss of specialized cell types such as parietal and chief cells – has also been recognized as being associated with replacement of the stomach by pseudopyloric metaplasia (El-Zimaity et al., 2002), also known as mucous metaplasia or spasmolytic polypeptide-expressing metaplasia or SPEM (Schmidt et al., 1999). Accumulating data suggest that SPEM is more strongly associated than IM with gastric cancer, and is more likely to be the precursor lesion (Halldorsdottir et al., 2003). At the present time, it is difficult to determine precisely what histological stage constitutes the "point of no return" for gastric cancer progression. While human studies suggest that, at the stage of atrophy/metaplasia, the lesion is only partially reversible and cancer not preventable with antibiotic eradication (Wong et al., 2004), studies in mice (see below) have suggested that atrophy/SPEM can regress significantly with antibiotic eradication (Cai et al., 2005).

10.2.6
Chronic Inflammation and Cancer

While a number of factors are likely involved in the predisposition and progression to gastric cancer, it is clear that chronic inflammation is a paramount feature that links gastric cancer to many other types of cancer. The link between inflammation and cancer dates back several millennia, but is commonly attributed to Virchow who in 1863 first demonstrated the abundant presence of leukocytes in neoplastic tissues. Epidemiological studies show a clear association between chronic inflammatory conditions and subsequent malignant transformation of the tissues, and the gastrointestinal tract is commonly affected with inflammation associated neoplasia (Philip et al., 2004). *Helicobacter pylori*-associated gastritis is perhaps the best example of a more widespread association, but one that has generated remarkable new insights into the mechanisms of carcinogenesis. Chronic inflammation is typically derived from acute inflammation, but in fact is qualitatively different from the more acute process. Indeed, several studies have suggested that while chronic inflammation predisposes to cancer, acute inflammation may actually protect the host from cancer (Philip et al., 2004). Some of the factors that distinguish chronic inflammation, particularly in the setting of *Helicobacter*-associated gastritis, are highlighted in the following sections.

10.2.6.1 Reactive Oxygen/Nitrogen Species

One of the hallmarks of chronic inflammation, such as *H. pylori*-associated gastritis, is an increase in oxidative stress induced by reactive oxygen species (ROS) such as superoxide anion O_2^-, hydroxyl radical OH•, and H_2O_2, are generated in cells as physiological byproducts of electron transfer reactions and arachidonic acid metabolism (Hocker et al., 1998). The inflamed stomach is also characterized by increased production of nitric oxide (NO) through up-regulation of the inducible nitric oxide synthase (iNOS); NO subsequently reacts with superoxide to form a variety of nitrosated species that can exert oncogenic effects. Indeed, it has been recognized that *H. pylori* arginase, encoded by rocF, competitively inhibits NO production in macrophages by consuming l-arginine (Viala et al., 2004). In the case of gastritis, the majority of ROS and NOS is likely generated by infiltrating inflammatory cells such as neutrophils and macrophages, but ROS and NOS can also be produced by epithelial cells and *H. pylori* itself. For example, spermine oxidase is induced in gastric epithelia by *H. pylori* which, via generation of H_2O_2 by oxidation of polyamines, can cause apoptosis and DNA damage (Xu et al., 2004).

While ROS and NOS can be elevated in acute pathological states, greater damage is associated with long-term increases in ROS and NOS associated with chronic inflammation. While the host does have a complex antioxidant system (catalase, superoxide dismutase, glutathione peroxidase, and thioredoxin) with which to battle the oxidative stress, over time this protective system can be overcome or depleted, leading to disorders such as peptic ulcer disease and gastric cancer.

Although oxidative stress can have cytotoxic effects, and function as a trigger for programmed cell death (apoptosis), it can also modulate the expression of a variety of genes involved in immune and inflammatory responses (such as NF-κB), as well as the expression of growth factor-regulated genes (Hocker et al., 1998). Oxidative stress can result in up-regulation of a variety of cytokines, adhesion molecules, cyclooxygenase (COX)-2 and angiogenic factors (such as VEGF).While there are likely many downstream targets, the most important target of ROS and NOS is DNA (Toyokuni et al., 1995). ROS and nitrosating species such as NO can induce several kinds of DNA damage, including strand breakage, base modification and DNA–protein crosslinking; however, the end result is the likelihood of mutation of DNA. In the classical model linking inflammation and cancer, the combination of increased cell damage and turnover, increased cell proliferation, and increased mutagenesis are sufficient to lead to initiate and promote cancer formation (Parsonnet, 1993). Indeed, many chemoprevention trials employing antioxidants have attempted to lever this model to inhibit or prevent gastric cancer development by reducing ROS and NOS. While antioxidant supplementation has had mixed results, studies in mouse models involving overexpression of thioredoxin-1 (TRX-1), as a redox-active protein involved in scavenging ROS, has been successful. Transgenic mice overexpressing TRX-1 showed decreased oxidative stress and decreased atrophic gastritis compared to wild-type mice, thereby validating to a large extent the importance of ROS in gastric preneoplasia (Kawasaki et al., 2005). Similarly, iNOs$^{-/-}$ knockout mice on a C57 BL background infected with *H. felis* have a predominant Th2 immune response with only a modest inflammatory response (Ihrig et al., 2005).

10.2.6.2   **Epithelial Cell Proliferation and Apoptosis**

While chronic inflammation clearly has many procarcinogenic effects, a critical factor in the cascade leading to gastric cancer is likely the induction of cellular apoptosis in the gastric mucosa. An altered rate of apoptosis and proliferation has for many years been considered an important biomarker for increased risk of neoplasia. The observation that *H. pylori* infection is associated with increased apoptosis was first reported in human patients by Moss et al. (1996), and this has since been confirmed by many groups. Increased apoptosis secondary to gastric *Helicobacter* infection was shown for the first time by Wang et al. in the *H. felis*-infected C57BL/6 mouse (Wang et al., 1998). These findings were confirmed by others in both the mouse model and in a Mongolian gerbil model (Peek et al., 2000). Importantly, in the *Helicobacter* mouse model, mucosal apoptosis occurs over a narrow time window and is associated closely with a marked decline in parietal and chief cells in the fundic mucosa. In addition, this apoptotic phase is followed by rebound hyperproliferation and the appearance of metaplasia.

While *H. pylori* may induce apoptosis in part through direct interactions with epithelial cells, the organism is largely confined to the gastric pits, while the apoptotic zone clearly extends deeper into the neck region and beyond the gastric glands. In addition, a number of studies have pointed to the effects of inflammatory cytokines such as TNF-α, IFN-γ, and IL-1β that can all have proapoptotic effects. However, studies by Houghton et al. have pointed to the Fas/FasL system as being primarily responsible for the induction of gastric epithelial apoptosis. *H. pylori* infection is associated with increased expression of Fas receptors – due in part to upregulation by IL-1β and TNF-α – and an influx of T lymphocytes that express FasL (Houghton et al., 2000a). *Helicobacter* infection of Fas-deficient mice did not result in any significant increases in apoptosis, proliferation or atrophy, underscoring again the link between the induction of apoptosis and the proliferative response (Houghton et al., 2000b).

Mucosal apoptosis may be very important in extending or amplifying the inflammatory response, and likely plays a role in the recruitment of cells from the circulation. In addition, many – if not most – carcinogens appear to induce apoptosis early on in the tissues most susceptible to the development of cancer. In the case of *H. felis*-infected C57 BL/6 mice, this field of increased apoptosis extends through the isthmus/progenitor cell zone of the fundic mucosa (Wang et al., 1998). The implications of apoptosis in the stem cell zone of the stomach, which would lead to stem cell deficiency or failure, have not previously been considered.

10.2.6.3   **Role of Specific Cytokines**

Another important feature of chronic inflammation – which may distinguish it from acute inflammation – is the sustained elevation of specific proinflammatory cytokines. In patients with chronic *H. pylori* infection, the increase in local levels of chemokines and cytokines may be quite marked, and may on their own result in specific effects as well as contributing to the recruitment and activation of immune cells. Much remains to be discovered regarding the pathways leading to initial immune recognition and antigen presentation by *H. pylori*, but it seems clear that the initial interaction involves the innate immune system. Macrophages and monocytes respond to *H. pylori* and other gastric helicobacters through the Toll-like receptor-2 (TLR2) (Mandell et al., 2004). A role for other Toll-like receptors, such as TLR4, 5, and 9, has been suggested but remain less well established. Signaling through TLR2 leads to NF-κB activation and release of early proinflammatory cytokines, such as IL-1β, followed later by activation of an adaptive immune response, which in the case of *H. pylori* is typically of a Th1-polarized cytokine pattern. The importance of a Th1 immune response in the induction of gastric cancer is discussed above. In any case, it is clear that the development of gastric atrophy, metaplasia, dysplasia and cancer is largely the result of the immune response to gastric *Helicobacter* infection, rather than representing direct effects of the bacteria. Immunodeficient mice, including both RAG-deficient mice and T-cell-deficient mice, are protected from *Helicobacter*-dependent atrophy and dysplasia, despite high levels of colonization (Roth et al., 1999; Houghton et al., 2002). Mice that are susceptible to gastric cancer, such as C57 BL/6 mice, have very strong Th1 immune responses, characterized by high levels of cytokines such as IFN-γ, TNF-α, IL-1β and IL-6 (Fox et al., 2000a). This has led to the hypothesis that much of the preneoplastic epithelial changes that arise in the gastric mucosa are due to increases in these proinflammatory cytokines. This hypothesis has been supported by the findings of several recent studies which have involved the infusion of proinflammatory cytokines. First, Cui et al. presented a study in which they examined the effect of short-term infusions of cytokines on the gastric mucosa of two strains of mice (C57 BL/6 and BALB/c). The cytokines – which were given using Alzet osmotic pumps at equimolar doses of 5 mg kg^{-1} per day (IL-1β), 10 mg kg^{-1} per day (TNF-α), and 20 mg kg^{-1} per day (IFN-γ) for two weeks along with bovine serum albumin (BSA) controls – reproduced many of the epithelial changes observed with chronic *Helicobacter* infection. The infusion of cytokines, including IL-1β, resulted in a reproduction of the atrophy model and in measurable increases in apoptosis as measured by caspase-3 staining, decreased parietal cell number and induction of mucous metaplasia (Cui et al., 2003). Interestingly, the infusion of cytokines had no significant effect in BALB/c mice, which were previously shown to be resistant to *H. felis*-dependent gastric atrophy (Wang et al., 1998). In more recent studies, Kang et al. have also reported that infusion into mice of IFN-γ recapitulated the mucous metaplasia observed in *H. felis*-infected mice (Kang et al., 2005). More recent preliminary studies suggest that transgenic overexpression of IL-1β can induce gastric atrophy and neoplasia in the absence of *Helicobacter* infection (Tu et al., 2005). Taken together, these results strongly support a model in which progression to gastric cancer is primarily a cytokine-driven and immune-mediated disease.

Recent studies by Mueller et al. using laser capture microdissection and transcriptome analysis of chief, parietal, and mucus epithelial cells in *H. pylori*-infected mice indicated that the mucous cell of the infected stomach orchestrated a complex interaction (Mueller et al., 2004, 2005a). Interestingly, neither chief nor parietal cell genes were deregulated at either two time points of the experiment – that is, at 2 and 28 wks post *H. pylori* infection. The mucous cell plays a role in sampling and sensing the gastric environment as well as initiation of host defense responses. Cytokines, chemokines and genes involved in antigen processing were up-regulated in the mucous cell in *H. pylori* -infected mice (Mueller et al., 2005 a). In the mucus-producing cell, the authors found strong evidence for a proinflammatory response: the cytokines IL-1β, TNF-α, and IFN-γ or their downstream target genes, as well as the two chemokines, granulocyte macrophage colony-stimulating factor and RANTES, were up-regulated (Mueller et al., 2005 a). The mucous cell transcriptome was also highly enriched for cytoskeletal and cell-junctional proteins – factors that probably play an important role in maintaining cell polarity and forming a tight barrier that protects against the host gastric contents. Most genes in the tumor suppressor category were repressed, compared with uninfected mice, suggesting that tumor suppression was dampened. These data support the proposal that, at least in the timeframe of the experiment, *H. pylori* affects growth control and apoptosis as early as the first week of infection (Mueller et al., 2004, 2005 a).

10.2.6.4 Link to T Cells and Macrophages

The link between gastric cancer and specific types of cytokines again points to the importance of specific immune cell subsets in the pathogenesis and progression of cancer. In the case of gastric cancer, as well as many other types of solid cancer, the key culprits appear to be macrophages and T cells. The data regarding T cells has been discussed above, and relates to the critical role played by IFN-γ-producing CD4+ T cells in *Helicobacter*-dependent atrophic gastritis. The predominant immune cell present in *H. pylori*-gastritis is the Th1-polarized CD4+ T cell, and in murine models, transfer of this cell enhances gastritis while deletion of IFN-γ inhibits progression to preneoplasia (Mohammadi et al., 1997; Itoh et al., 1999; Sawai et al., 1999). CD4+ T cells have also been shown to play a key role in immune enhancement of skin carcinogenesis (Daniel et al., 2003). However, while these studies demonstrate that CD4+ T lymphocytes are essential, they do not provide that they are the only cell type involved in the initiation and progression of gastric cancer. Indeed, growing evidence supports a key role for other immune cell populations, particularly macrophages.

As suggested above, macrophages are the main source of growth factors and cytokines as the site of inflammation, and macrophages have a central role in not only the initiation of inflammation but also in the resolution of inflammation. Recent studies indicate that the primary cells expressing IL-8 and IL-1β – macrophages and related myeloid lineages such as tumor-associated macrophages (TAM) – play a critical pathogenic role in many tumors. These inflammatory cells of the innate immune system are recruited to the tumor microenvironment, where they contribute to the regenerative "niche" (Pull et al., 2005) and exert protumorigenic effects (Balkwill and Mantovani, 2001; Coussens and Werb, 2002). Accordingly, in many human tumors the infiltration of macrophages is associated with a poor prognosis.

Evidence from Pollard's group indicates that infiltration with macrophages promotes both the development of breast cancers and their eventual spread to other sites in the body (Lin et al., 2001). The elimination of macrophages using CSF-1 null mice showed that macrophage recruitment is important for progression of mammary gland tumors, since invasive growth and metastasis were significantly attenuated (Lin et al., 2001; Wyckoff et al., 2004). A number of studies now suggest that macrophages promote the growth and invasiveness of cancer cells via NF-κB (Hagemann et al., 2005). In addition to enhancing vascularity and growth, these macrophages may suppress local T-cell responses (Kusmartsev and Gabrilovich, 2005). Another downstream target of IL-1β, the cytokine IL-6, is mainly produced by myeloid cells during the promotion stage of colon cancer (Greten et al., 2004). Macrophages appear to be particularly important in cancer progression, because of their production, in addition to IL-1β and IL-8, of many factors that can promote cancer, including reactive oxygen intermediates, growth factors, and metalloproteinases. Numerous studies have shown a correlation between macrophage infiltration and tumor vascularity and progression, including studies in gastric cancer (Ohno et al., 2003). In a transgenic model of preneoplasia involving overexpression of both COX-2 and mPGES-1 in the gastric mucosa, Oshima et al. showed that prostaglandin E_2 enhanced the recruitment of tissue macrophages and demonstrated more directly a link between macrophage activation and preneoplasia of the stomach (Oshima et al., 2004, 2005).

10.2.6.5 Bone Marrow Stem Cell Recruitment

While chronic inflammation leads to up-regulation of many chemokines and cytokines, and recruitment to the stomach of a number of immune cell populations, only recently has attention focused on the recruitment of progenitor cell populations. Studies conducted by Wang and colleagues led to observations that gastric cancer in the *H. felis*-infected C57 BL/6 mouse is preceded by the development of mucous metaplasia and expansion of an aberrant cellular lineage that expressed TFF2 (Wang et al., 1998). This lineage, termed SPEM for spasmolytic polypeptide-expressing metaplasia, is distinct from the normal mucous neck cells of the stomach, but clearly gives rise to the dysplasia and cancer that later develops in the stomach (Schmidt et al., 1999; Lee et al., 2003). Transcriptional profiling of this SPEM population, obtained using laser capture microdissection of C57 BL *H. felis*-infected mice, indicated the presence of transcripts such as Xist that were not normally expressed in adult epithelial tissues, but were normally expressed early in embryonic development and in stem cells (Nomura et al., 2004).

Classically, epithelial cancers such as gastric carcinoma are believed to originate from the transformation of tissue stem cells. However, based on the unusual nature of this metaplasia, our laboratory set out to test the hypothesis that gastric cancer might originate from a circulating bone marrow-derived stem cell (BMDC) population (Houghton et al., 2004). The model used was a lethally irradiated wild-type C57 BL/6 mouse transplanted with tagged bone marrow from donor mice. These included transplantation with gender-matched or gender-mismatched bone marrow from C57 BL/6 JGtrosa26 (ROSA 26) mice that express a non-mammalian beta-galactosidase enzyme, C57 BL/6 J-*beta-actin-EGFP* (GFP) mice, or C57 BL/6 J controls.

In the initial studies, transplantation was carried out with ROSA26 donors, and BMDCs were tracked with X-gal staining. Under the usual experimental conditions used of lethal irradiation and rescue with bone marrow transplantation, long-term BMDC engraftment in the stomach was observed to be an extremely unusual event. In addition, acute injury or selective gastric cell loss was not sufficient for engraftment of the stomach. ROSA26-transplanted C57 BL/6 mice with ulcers generated by cryoinjury or submucosal acetic acid injections showed no evidence of mucosal engraftment by BMDCs (Houghton et al., 2004). Similarly, complete parietal cell loss induced by the chemical compound DMP777 (a protonophore with specificity for acid secretory membranes) led to proliferation and regeneration but not to BMDC engraftment in the stomach. Acute short-term (3 weeks) *H. felis* infection, which is associated with a severe, acute inflammatory response, was also insufficient. However, chronic (20–52 weeks) *H. felis* infection led to substantial BMDC engraftment which was revealed by X-gal staining of epithelial cells in the body and corpus of the stomach, and also by immunocytochemistry for *E. coli*-specific beta-galactosidase. The vast majority – if not all – of the metaplasia, dysplasia and cancer was shown to be derived from BMDCs. Double-label immunofluorescence studies showed that the metaplastic and dysplastic BMDCs were clearly epithelial in origin, as indicated by the expression of cytokeratins (CK19) and the absence of CD45 expression. The donor origin of the cancers in these mice was thus demonstrated using a variety of methodologies, including: (i) X-gal staining; (ii) immunocytochemistry for *E. coli* beta-galactosidase; (iii) immunofluorescence of GFP; (d) immunostaining for GFP; (iv) laser capture microdissection and PCR for the Rosa26 transgene; and (v) Y-FISH for the donor-specific Y chromosome in gender-mismatched transplants. Finally, this process did not seem to involve fusion, as evidenced by the presence of a 2 N DNA content and a single X and single Y chromosome (Houghton et al., 2004).

Overall, these data have suggested a new paradigm for the development of adenocarcinoma of the stomach, and a new explanation for the link between chronic inflammation and cancer (Houghton and Wang, 2005). In this model, the carcinogenic stimulus –in this case a combination of *H. pylori* infection and the associated inflammatory response – results in recruitment and engraftment of BDMCs to the gastric mucosa, where they give rise over time to metaplasia, dysplasia, and cancer. The model encompasses a number of discrete steps that include: (i) inflammation-mediated alterations in the gastric stem cell niche; (ii) damage or failure of endogenous tissue stem cells; (iii) mobilization into the circulation of progenitor cells; (iv) recruitment and engraftment of BMDCs into the gastric stem cell niche; and (v) continued proliferation and aberrant differentiation of BMDCs in the altered niche.

10.3
Prevention of *H. pylori*-Induced Cancer

10.3.1
Interrupting Transmission in Children

Clearly, epidemiological data strongly support the key role that socioeconomic conditions play in determining the prevalence of *H. pylori* infections in various countries. Thus, personal hygiene, sanitary standards and reduction of high-density living conditions combine to reduce transmission of *H. pylori* in children.

Prophylactic vaccine strategies have been proposed as an ideal method to interrupt *H. pylori* transmission in children. The feasibility of this approach has been proven in mouse models, but successful vaccine candidates have not been forthcoming despite considerable effort.

10.3.2
Treatment Strategies of *H. pylori* in Populations at Risk

With respect to dietary antioxidants, some observational data in humans suggest that ascorbic acid and beta-carotene can protect against cancer in *H. pylori*-infected hosts (Ekstrom et al., 2000). Intervention studies, however, have been less promising. In one study, the six-year administration of supplemental ascorbic acid and beta-carotene prevented progression of preneoplasia in less than 20% of infected subjects immediately after supplementation was completed; however, these benefits were not maintained six years later (Correa et al., 2000; Mera et al., 2005).

The recognition that *H. pylori* represented a significant risk factor for gastric cancer raised the possibility that antibiotic treatment might reduce the overall risk of the condition. Decision analysis studies indicated that, if *H. pylori* eradication could reduce gastric cancer risk by 30% or more, a strategy of screening and treating patients for *H. pylori* infection could in theory be cost-effective (Parsonnet et al., 1996). However, the critical question continues to be whether *H. pylori* eradication can reduce gastric cancer risk, and at what stage the histopathological progression is reversible. Initial studies from Japan involving *H. pylori* eradication in patients who had undergone partial gastrectomy for early gastric cancer suggest a reduction in risk of recurrent gastric cancer (Uemura et al., 1997). The study by Uemura et al. (2001) was one of the first long-term, prospective studies of infected and uninfected patients with dyspepsia who underwent endoscopy and in whom the development of gastric cancer was the end point. It is important to note that *H. pylori* infection was assessed by three different methods. In this study of 1526 Japanese patients, gastric cancer developed in approximately 3% of the infected patients but in none of the uninfected patients. The risk was increased in all subgroups of patients (those with gastric ulcers, hyperplastic polyps, and nonulcer dyspepsia) except for patients with duodenal ulcers. Although the study was limited by histological analysis of only two gastric-biopsy specimens at each time point, the risk of gastric cancer was also clearly related to specific histological features found on the initial endoscopy, which included severe gastric atrophy, corpus-predominant gastritis, and intestinal meta-plasia (Uemura et al., 2001).

One of the most tantalizing and provocative findings in the study by Uemura and colleagues is that eradication of *H. pylori* prevented or delayed the development of gastric cancer. However, the question of who should undergo *H. pylori* eradication remains unresolved. The ideal treatment for nonulcer dyspepsia has been hotly de-bated, with the focus largely on the efficacy of anti-*H. pylori* therapy for the relief of upper abdominal symptoms (McColl et al., 1998; Talley et al., 1999). Uemura et al. suggest that patients with nonulcer dyspepsia have the highest risk of cancer (4.7%), and it can now be argued that these patients should have anti-*H. pylori* therapy on the basis of the risk of cancer alone. However, most patients with chronic *H. pylori* infection have no symptoms, which raises questions about the need for population-based screening for infection or predictive gastric pathological features. Complete resolution of this question will require large randomized controlled trials with long-term follow-up, most likely carried out in countries where gastric cancer rates are high. One such randomized clinical trial of *H. pylori* eradication as cancer preven-tion has been completed to date. Conducted in China, the results were inconclusive. Over 7.5 years (an interval that may have been too short), *H. pylori* eradication did not prevent cancer, although the trend was towards some diminution in cancer risk (Wong et al., 2004). In a subset of those without preneoplastic lesions, *H. pylori* erad-ication appeared to provide a significant reduction in cancer. Unfortunately, since the group without preneoplasia is at relatively low risk of cancer, this finding pro-vides little insight into cancer prevention. Studies of *H. pylori* 's effects on preneo-plastic conditions themselves are conflicting (Hojo et al., 2002). Acute inflammation has typically been deemed reversible, whereas intestinal metaplasia has not. Moreover, atrophic gastritis variably regressed. The most promising study evaluated the effects of *H. pylori* eradication 12 years after randomized treatment or placebo (Mera et al., 2005). In that study, the benefits of *H. pylori* eradication on preneoplasia score accrued over time, suggesting that shorter-term studies were inadequate to discern potential benefits.

The approach of widespread eradication of *H. pylori* for the purpose of reducing gastric cancer risk has been complicated by recent speculation that *H. pylori* may ac-tually be protective against gastroesophageal (GE) junction tumors (Blaser, 1999 a,b). The prevalence of *H. pylori* has clearly been declining in most developed countries such as the U.S., in concert with declining rates of well-differentiated, in-testinal adenocarcinomas. However, the rates of cancers involving the esophagus or gastric cardia, the so-called GE junction cancers, have been rapidly increasing over the past decade. Eradication of *H. pylori* was shown in some studies to result in in-crease rates of GE reflux, a known factor in the pathogenesis of Barrett's esophagus and esophageal cancer (Labenz et al., 1997; Vicari et al., 1998). In addition, reports from one group have indicated that infection with *H. pylori*, particularly cagA[+] strains, was inversely associated with GE junction cancers, suggesting that it may be protective (Chow et al., 1998). Thus, many questions remain with respect to the role of *H. pylori* in specific gastric diseases and the precise recommendations regarding diagnosis and treatment of *H. pylori* in asymptomatic patients.

10.4
Animal Models

10.4.1
Animal Models for *Helicobacter*-Induced Gastric Cancer

10.4.1.1 Gerbil

The gerbil has been shown to have particular relevant features which can be used to address the question of the potential of *H. pylori* to induce gastric cancer. Gerbils were first reported as a model for experimental *H. pylori* infection in 1991 (Yokota et al., 1991). Subsequently, Japanese investigators noted intestinal metaplasia, atrophy, and gastric ulcer in gerbils after experimental infection with *H. pylori* (Hirayama et al., 1996; Honda et al., 1998a). In one study, acute gastritis with erosions of the gastric mucosa occurred shortly after infection, whereas gastric ulcers, cystica profunda, and atrophy with intestinal metaplasia were observed at 3–6 months after *H. pylori* infection (Honda et al., 1998a). Following these findings, two separate research groups have noted that gerbils infected with *H. pylori* from periods ranging from 15 to 18 months develop gastric adenocarcinoma (Honda et al., 1998b; Watanabe et al., 1998) (Table 10.5).

In one study, gerbils were observed for up to 62 weeks, and 37% were found to develop adenocarcinoma in the pyloric region (Watanabe et al., 1998). The gastric cancers were clearly documented histologically. Vascular invasion and metastases were not observed; it is possible, however, that they may develop with longer periods of observation. In another report, *H. pylori* induced adenocarcinoma at 15 months post inoculation, but the authors did not record metastases or vascular invasion (Honda et al., 1998b). Interestingly, the development of cancer is preceded by a cystica profunda; this is an invagination of atypical glands into the submucosa and is considered by some to be a premalignant lesion. The histological progression in the gerbil closely resembled that observed in humans, in terms of the early appearance of intestinal metaplasia, well-differentiated histological patterns of the gastric malignancy, and antral location of the gastric cancers. As for the association with gastric ulcers and gastric cancer in humans, the gerbils also had gastric ulcer disease in conjunction with gastric cancer (Hansson et al., 1996). The development of metaplasia with production of predominantly acid sialomucins was associated with tumor development. Whether the cancers arose directly form these metaplastic cells is unknown, but the tumors clearly originated deep in the gastric glands, in close proximity to these metaplastic cells (Watanabe et al., 1998).

Although most of the tumors in this *H. pylori* gerbil model originated in the pyloric region of the stomach, significant changes in the oxyntic mucosa consistent with chronic atrophic gastritis were seen (Watanabe et al., 1998). Glandular tissue in the gastric body and fundus were atrophied and replaced by hyperplastic epithelium of the pseudopyloric type. The differences between this lesion and gastric atrophy in human patients is that the gerbil corpus is not "thinner" consequent to the pseudopyloric hyperplasia (Wang et al., 1998; Watanabe et al., 1998). Thus, the diagnosis of

Table 10.5 Summary of key rodent models of infectious gastrointestinal and liver cancer.[a]

Rodent	Infectious agent/ transgene	Tumor	Comment
C57 BL mice	*H. felis*	Gastric adenocarcinoma	Natural gastric pathogen, but lacks *cag* and *vacA*
INS-GAS FVB mice[b]	*H. felis* and *H. pylori*	Gastric adenocarcinoma	Constitutive hypergastrinemia promotes tumorigenesis
Mongolian gerbil	*H. pylori*	Gastric adenocarcinoma	Closely mimics human disease, but few reagents
BALB/c mice	Several *Helicobacter* spp.	Gastric MALT lymphoma	Usually requires 18–24 months
Genetically engineered mice: IL-10-, IL-2-, Gα$_{i2}$-, Muc2-, Smad3$^{-/-}$, etc. -deficient; especially on 129 Sv background	„Endogenous microbiota" or *H. hepaticus, H. bilis*	Lower bowel carcinoma	Bacteria in endogenous microbiota models not well defined; *H. hepaticus* or *H. bilis* reliably induces disease
Lymphocyte-deficient mice: SCID or Rag$^{-/-}$; especially on 129 Sv background	„Endogenous microbiota" or *H. hepaticus*	Lower bowel carcinoma	Often used for adoptive transfer studies; *H. hepaticus* induces tumors in untreated Rag2$^{-/-}$ mice
Transgenic mice[b]	HBV or HCV transgene(s)	HCC	Prove tumorigenic potential of viral gene products; adoptive transfer or inducible gene strategies required for hepatitis
A/JCr and other mice[b]	*H. hepaticus*	HCC	Natural murine pathogen induces chronic active hepatitis and HCC

[a] Data modified from Rogers and Fox (2004).
[b] Male predominant. HBV, hepatitis B virus; HCC, hepatocellular carcinoma; HCV, hepatitis C virus; MALT, mucosal-associated lymphoid tissue; PAI, pathogenicity-associated islands.

atrophy is not involved with the thickness of the mucosa but rather with the loss of oxyntic (parietal and chief) cell populations within the gastric glands. Growing evidence suggests that the parietal cell may regulate key differentiation decisions within the gastric glands, and ablation of parietal cells using transgenic technology (Li et al., 1996) or their loss to infection with *H. felis* and *H. pylori* infection leads to altered glandular differentiation and neck cell proliferation as well as to changes in gastric acid and gastrin physiology.

The expansion of an aberrant neck cell ("regenerative hyperplasia" or "pseudopyloric hyperplasia") in the gerbils is similar to that observed in the *H. felis* mouse model. This lineage has been shown to be spasmolytic polypeptide (SP) -positive (Wang et al., 1998), and this SP-positive lineage also develops in *H. pylori*-associated gastric cancers in humans (Schmidt et al., 1998). The loss of oxyntic glandular tissue in response to *H. pylori* infection suggests that the gerbil becomes achlorhydric before the development of gastric cancer. Although the precise effects of chronic *H. pylori* infection on gastric acid secretion are not known, serum gastrin levels in the *H. pylori* infected gerbil are increased.

The unusual susceptibility of this animal species to gastric cancer using a fairly standard *H. pylori* strain underscores once again the overriding importance of host factors in determining the outcome from *Helicobacter* infection (Wang and Fox, 1998). It is important to note that many laboratories – particularly those outside of Japan – have been unable to document the carcinogenic potential of *H. pylori* in the gerbil model. Recently, however, investigators in the U.S. using *H. pylori* strain B128 serially passaged in gerbils documented rapid onset gastric adenocarcinoma in gerbils. This study serves to highlight the importance of bacterial factors as well as host susceptibility in cancer induction (Franco et al., 2005).

10.4.1.2 Mouse

As detailed above, most of the major advances in our understanding of gastric cancer pathogenesis have been derived from studies with mice. In particular, much insight has been derived from the *Helicobacter*-infected mouse, first described by James Fox and Adrian Lee (Lee et al., 1990). While a number of other animal models have been developed for both gastric cancer (e.g., MNNG-induced cancer in rats) and for *Helicobacter*-mediated infection (ferret, gerbil, gnotobiotic pig, primate, etc.), the mouse model has clear advantages with respect to their small size, cost, ease of infection, reproducibility, and especially the power of genetic manipulation. The *Helicobacter*-infection model has been combined now with a variety of inbred strains, transgenic and knockout mice to assess the relative contribution of host versus non-host factors in the preneoplastic process. Indeed, the combination of genetic manipulation in the setting of initiation and promotion by the authentic carcinogen (gastric *Helicobacter*) makes this model, in many respects, the best cancer model for study.

In the early investigations by a number of groups, it became clear from studies with inbred mice that progression to preneoplasia was largely determined by the host response. For example, the C57BL/6 inbred mouse strain responded to *H. felis* infection with a robust Th1 immune response, in contrast to the BALB/c inbred strain which showed a predominant Th2 response (Mohammadi et al., 1996; Sakagami et al., 1996; Wang et al., 1998). Consequently, C57BL/6 mice showed rapid progression to atrophy and metaplasia with declining colonization levels, while BALB/c mice maintained high numbers of organisms with minimal epithelial injury or atrophy. Additional studies employing RAG and SCID mice and T-cell-deficient mice pointed to the importance of T-cell responses (Roth et al., 1999), while the use of cytokine knockout mice showed *H. pylori*-induced mucosal inflammation to be Th1-mediated and exacerbated in IL-4 but not IFN-γ gene-deficient mice (Smythies et al., 2000).

However, while genetic manipulation of the various cytokine genes clarified many aspects of the immunopathogenesis of the disease, the unmanipulated C57BL/6 mouse has proved surprisingly robust as a model for cancer development. Interestingly, many of the early *H. felis* infection studies included observations periods that extended up to one year but not beyond, and described changes of atrophy and metaplasia, but not more advanced pathology. The presence of dysplasia and invasive carcinoma in the *H. felis*-infected C57BL/6 mouse was first described by Fox and Wang (Fox et al., 2002 b), when the observation period was extended out to 14 months. More recently, progression to antral carcinomas has been reported in mice in which the model has been extended out to 22 months (Cai et al., 2005). Indeed, in many of the models of gastric cancer, a long period of achlorhydria, associated with presumed bacterial overgrowth, appears to be the common denominator in mouse models of antral carcinoma (Zavros et al., 2005).

As described above, the C57BL/6 mouse model of *Helicobacter* infection has been very useful for the study of dietary cofactors (such as salt) and for manipulation of the Th1-Th2 immune response. However, another factor is likely to be the particular *H. pylori* strain, and this question has been more difficult to address using the wild-type C57BL/6 mouse. The wild-type mouse can be infected with a few "mousefied" *H. pylori* strains. The mouse commonly used strain has been the *H. pylori* Sydney strain, first described by Lee in 1997 (Lee et al., 1997). However, most *H. pylori* strains – including the Sydney strain – have shown less consistent patterns of colonization, and for the most part have proven less carcinogenic in the C57BL/6 mouse (Thompson et al., 2004), although a recent study has for the first time demonstrated high-grade dysplasia in C57BL/6 × 129 S6/SvEv (B6129) mice infected for 15 months with *H. pylori* SS1 (Rogers et al., 2005). Nevertheless, the *H. felis*-infected C57BL/6 mouse has proven for the most part to be the superior model.

A role for bacterial factors also has been demonstrated using *Helicobacter*-infected transgenic mice. The first *Helicobacter*-dependent mouse model of gastric cancer was reported by Wang et al., who showed that *H. felis* infection of insulin-gastrin (INS-GAS) transgenic mice led to the rapid appearance of atrophy, metaplasia, dysplasia and gastric cancer (Wang et al., 2000). The model has proved ideal as an accelerated model of carcinogenesis. The model leads to accelerated gastric cancer in part due to the effect of elevated circulating levels of amidated gastrin which bind to CCK-B receptors to activate a histamine pathway, leading to altered growth and immune responses (Takaishi et al., 2005), and to relatively low levels of glycine-extended gastrin which may inhibit progression to preneoplasia (Cui et al., 2004). This INS-GAS mouse model has been used to demonstrate that cagE is likely an important virulence factor, since deletion of this gene (in the B128 *H. pylori* strain) delayed the progression to carcinoma (Fox et al., 2003 b). Previous studies have also demonstrated the requirement for cagE in inducing gastric injury during the early states of *H. pylori* infection in gerbils (Israel et al., 2001).

These results are also consistent with a report demonstrating that *H. pylori* isogenic *cagE* mutant strains retain the ability to induce expression of host genes that may function in cellular recognition events (Guillemin et al., 2002). The authors co-cultured either a wild-type *H. pylori* strain or an isogenic *cagE⁻* mutant with gastric epithelial cells. Both strains induced expression of several mediators of injury, including IFN-γ, plasminogen, endothelin-1, and trefoil factor 1, as well as a number of signal transduction genes (Guillemin et al., 2002). However, these genes were not induced by an *H. pylori* mutant strain that lacked the *cag* island (Guillemin et al., 2002), indicating that host cells respond differently to strains lacking the entire *cag* island and those with a defective secretory system (e.g., *cagE⁻*). These data raise the hypothesis that the *H. pylori* B128 *cagE⁻* mutant strain still harbors portions of the *cag* secretion apparatus that allow it to engage in intimate contact with host cells and to elicit a proinflammatory response (Fox et al., 2003b).

While a number of other very useful murine model of gastric cancer have been developed (Judd et al., 2004; Rogers and Fox, 2004; Zavros et al., 2005), it is likely that the role of *Helicobacter* infection – and the associated immune response – will be critical in mimicking precisely the cancer pathways most relevant to human disease.

10.4.1.3 Ferret

H. mustelae persistently infects the inflamed mucosa of ferrets, and colonization of *H. mustelae* in ferret stomachs occurs shortly after weaning (Fox et al., 1988a). In addition, Koch's postulates have been fulfilled; that is, oral inoculation of *H. mustelae* into naive ferrets not infected with *H. mustelae* induces a chronic, persistent gastritis analogous to the gastritis associated with *H. mustelae* in naturally infected ferrets. Ferrets have also been used successfully as a suitable model to study the pathogenesis and epidemiology of *Helicobacter*-associated chronic gastritis and gastric cancer (Fox et al., 1990). The histopathological changes observed closely coincide in topography with the presence of *H. mustelae*. In the oxyntic mucosa, inflammation and *H. mustelae* are limited to the superficial portion, and as such is classified as a superficial gastritis. In the distal antrum the inflammation involves the full thickening of the mucosa, and is given the term "diffuse antral gastritis", as described in humans. *H. mustelae* are noted in the distal antrum at the surface, the superficial portion of the glands, and within the gastric pits. In the proximal antrum and the transitional mucosa, the element of focal glandular atrophy and regeneration is observed in addition to those lesions described in the distal antrum. There is also deep focal *H. mustelae* colonization of multiple antral glands. *Helicobacter*-associated gastritis in the ferret model has many similarities with the human disease, and contributes considerably to the interpretation of chronic gastritis in humans. The lesions observed in the distal antrum and the oxyntic mucosa closely resemble the diffuse antral gastritis observed in humans which, like the ferret model, is usually accompanied by superficial gastritis of the corpus. This clinicopathological entity underlies the duodenal ulcer syndrome (Fox et al., 1990; Correa, 1992), whereas histologically the proximal antrum and the transitional zone of *H. mustelae*-infected ferrets represent early stages of the multifocal atrophic gastritis of humans; this histological presentation is often linked to gastric ulcer and gastric carcinoma (Fox et al., 1990; Correa,

1992). The importance of these premalignant lesions associated with *H. mustelae* infection is highlighted by the report that naturally occurring pyloric adenocarcinoma has also been linked to *H. mustelae* in ferrets (Fox et al., 1997).

Chronic *H. pylori* infection can cause an increase in cell proliferation (Brenes et al., 1993), and many studies have indicated that abnormal cell proliferation and maturation are related to both the development and progression of neoplasia (Lipkin and Higgins, 1988). The effect of *H. mustelae* infection on gastric epithelial proliferation was studied in ferrets colonized with *H. mustelae* and specific pathogen-free (SPF) ferrets not infected with *H. mustelae* (Yu et al., 1995). PCNA-expressing gastric epithelia in the antrum and the body regions were significantly increased in the *H. mustelae*-infected ferrets versus the SPF ferrets ($P < 0.001$) (Yu et al., 1995). Comparison of the histopathology of infected ferrets indicated that PCNA positivity correlated with the histological severity of gastritis. *H. mustelae*-infected ferrets had significantly higher grades of inflammation than SPF ferrets, which had normal gastric mucosa.

In a study to define the *H. mustelae*-infected ferrets as an animal model of *H. pylori*-associated gastric cancer using MNNG (Fox et al., 1993 b), young female ferrets were given a single oral dose of MNNG (50–100 mg kg^{-1}) to ascertain whether they would develop adenocarcinoma of the stomach. Age-matched unmanipulated *H. mustelae*-infected control animals were included for comparative purposes. Nine of 10 ferrets dosed with MNNG had invasive gastric adenocarcinoma of the antrum diagnosed at necropsy (29–55 months after dosing), whereas none of the control ferrets had developed gastric cancer, when examined at an average of 63 months after the initiation of the study. The large number of gastric adenocarcinomas in the ferrets in this study may be partially due to *H. mustelae*-associated gastritis present in 100% of the MNNG-treated animals. These results indirectly implicate *H. mustelae* in MNNG-induced gastric cancer in the ferret. This hypothesis is supported by a study in our laboratory where a group of *H. mustelae*-free SPF ferrets dosed with a single dose of 100 mg kg^{-1} MNNG did not develop gastric cancer by 3.5 years post dosing (J.G. Fox, unpublished results).

The ferret stomach closely resembles that of the human stomach in its anatomy, histology, and physiology (Fox, 1988). The structure of the ferret gastric mucosa at the cellular level is remarkably similar to that of humans. Ferrets secrete gastric acid and proteolytic enzymes under basal conditions and, like humans infected with *H. pylori*, *H. mustelae*-infected ferrets have hypergastrinemia (Perkins et al., 1996). The ferret also is similar to humans in its biochemical processing of beta-carotene, making it an important model for studying the anticancer properties of this compound (Wang et al., 1992). Most recently, the *H. mustelae*-infected ferret has been used to demonstrate the protective effects of lycopene supplementation in smoke-induced changes in cell proliferation, p53, and apoptosis in the gastric mucosa (Liu et al., 2006).

10.4.2
Animal Models of MALT Lymphoma

10.4.2.1 *H. felis*-Induced MALT Lymphoma

Mucosal-associated lymphoid tissue (MALT) low-grade lymphoma (MALToma) in *H. felis*-infected BALB/c mice has been reported. These mice did not develop lymphoma until more than 20 months after infection, almost the entire life span of a mouse (Enno et al., 1995). This has particular relevance with the association of *H. pylori* and MALToma in humans (Wotherspoon et al., 1993). A genetic event has been postulated to initiate the transition from gastritis to low-grade MALToma (Calvert et al., 1995). Humans have an approximately balanced κ:λ ratio which facilitates the distinction of lymphoma from gastritis. In humans, MALToma has been distinguished from severe gastritis by evaluating clonality using κ and λ antigen markers or immunoglobulin gene probes (Wotherspoon et al., 1993; Savio et al., 1996). One disadvantage of studying the mouse gastric MALToma is the disparate 20:1 κ:λ ratio in mice, which has made comparisons to the human situation difficult. Monoclonal lesions confirmed by phenotype and genotype have regressed after antibiotic therapy for *H. pylori,* suggesting that some of these lesions may actually represent a transition to neoplasia (Savio et al., 1996). The *H. felis*-infected mouse model has helped to answer these fundamentally important questions.

These authors have used the BALB/c model to further dissect the role of *Helicobacter* spp. (*H. pylori, H. felis,* and *H. heilmannii*) in gastric lymphomagenesis (Mueller et al., 2003). They showed that the initial step in lymphoma development is marked by infiltration of reactive lymphocytes into the stomach and the initiation of a mucosal immune response. Using the microarray analysis of both the mucosa and lymphoma element of gastric tissue (employing laser capture microdissection), they reported on the molecular markers of both of these processes, including genes coding for the immunoglobulins and the small proline-rich protein Sprr 2A. In their model, a progression of the disease is characterized histologically by the antigen-driven proliferation and aggregation of B cells and the gradual appearance of lymphoepithelial lesions with increased expression of genes previously associated with malignancy, including the laminin receptor-1 and the multidrug-resistance channel MDR-1 (Mueller et al., 2003). The transition to destructive lymphoepithelial lesions and malignant lymphoma was identified by an increase in transcription of a single gene encoding calgranulin A/Mrp-8. The transcript was expressed in both the mucosal and the lymphocytic fraction, being more abundant in the mucosal tissue. Because calgranulin mainly functions extracellularly (Donato, 2001), the authors suggest that investigating the localization of the corresponding protein will be useful in shedding light on its function in MALT lymphoma development (Mueller et al., 2003).

In a more recent report using the same model, the authors have provided insight into why some *Helicobacter*-induced MALTomas relapse after apparent remission following antibiotic treatment (Mueller et al., 2005 b). They addressed the role of antigenic stimulation in the pathogenesis of the lymphoma by experimental infection with *H. felis* in BALB/C mice, followed by antibiotic eradication therapy and sub-sequent reinfection. Antimicrobial therapy was successful in 75% of mice, and led to complete histological but not "molecular" tumor remission. Although the lymphoepithelial lesions disappeared and most gastric lymphoid aggregates resolved, transcriptional profiling revealed the long-term mucosal persistence of residual B cells. After experimental reinfection with *Helicobacter*, there was a rapid recurrence of the lymphomas. These tumors were more aggressive than the original lymphomas, having higher proliferation and a more aggressive phenotype of the tumor (Mueller et al., 2005 b). Immunophenotyping of tumor cells revealed massive infiltration of lesions by CD4+ T cells, which express CD28, CD69, and IL-4 but not IFN-γ. These data suggested that tumor B-cell proliferation was driven by Th 2-polarized, immunocompetent, and activated T cells. The number of dendritic cells in the follicles also predicted the success of antibiotic therapy in the regression of the tumor (Mueller et al., 2005 b).

10.4.3
Animal Models for Enterohepatic *Helicobacter*-Induced Cancer

10.4.3.1 *Helicobacter hepaticus*-Induced Liver Cancer

A bacterium was identified in the livers of A/JCr mice with hepatitis, hepatic adenomas, and hepatocellular carcinoma (HCC) during a long-term carcinogenesis study conducted at the National Cancer Institute in 1992 (Ward et al., 1994 a). A Gram-negative bacterium isolated from these mice with diseased livers was characterized and named *H. hepaticus* (Fox et al., 1994). This organism causes a persistent infection and is prevalent in mouse colonies, both commercial and academic, throughout the world (Weghorst et al., 1989; Foltz et al., 1995; Shames et al., 1995). In addition to A/JCr mice, *H. hepaticus* also causes hepatitis in BALB/cCr, SJL/NCr, SCID/NCr, C_3 H/HeNCr, $B_6C_3F_1$ mice and AXB recombinant strains. Like AJ/Cr mice, *H. hepaticus* infection in B6C3F1, AXB and AB6F1 mice also causes liver cancer. The ecological niche of *H. hepaticus* is the lower bowel, and fecal-oral transmission is the suspected natural route (Fox et al., 1996 b). The liver lesion of mice with natural *H. hepaticus* infection progressively increases in severity.

Similar to the lesions found in acute viral hepatitis of humans, the early inflammation in livers of mice infected with *H. hepaticus* consisted of lobular infiltrates comprised predominantly of macrophages variably accompanied by fewer neutrophils and/or lymphocytes. Lobular inflammation was accompanied by spotty or confluent coagulative necrosis of hepatocytes. Portal/periportal infiltrates were comprised chiefly of mixed T and B lymphocytes as well as unlabeled lymphocytoid, presumably natural killer (NK), cells. Up-regulated expression of iNOS and COX-2 within inflammatory foci was demonstrated in both leukocytes and hepatocytes by immunohistochemistry. Immunohistochemical analysis reinforced the striking similarities in inflammatory patterns and progression between susceptible mice infected with *H. hepaticus* and human patients suffering from acute viral hepatitis (Ferrell et al., 2002).

Random and perivenular lobular necroinflammatory lesions, with spotty or confluent hepatocellular coagulative necrosis, precede lymphocyte accumulations in the portal triads in infected A/JCr mice (Ward et al., 1994 a,b; Fox et al ., 1996 b; Rogers et al., 2004). Random scattered acidophil bodies, representing apoptosis of individual hepatocytes, may be seen without overt inflammation. Kupffer and hepatic stellate (Ito) cell hyperplasia accompany lobular lesions, and oval cell proliferation with neocholangiole formation is a common sequel to portal inflammation, especially in cases of interface hepatitis (Ward et al., 1994 a; Ihrig et al., 1999; Rogers et al., 2004). It is not known whether hepatic lesions are solely attributable to bacterial invasion or whether soluble antigens or toxins gaining access from the lower bowel via the portal circulation might also contribute (Fox et al., 1996 b). Using BrdU, increased liver cell proliferation associated with *H. hepaticus* was detected (Fox et al., 1996 b). There was an age-associated increase in cell proliferation in infected animals that was not seen in uninfected control mice and was more pronounced in infected male than female mice (Fox et al., 1996 b). Increased hepatocyte proliferation indices in *H. hepaticus*-infected male mice is consistent with the observation of increased hepatomas and hepatocellular carcinomas observed in *H. hepaticus*-infected aged A/JCr male mice (Ward et al., 1994 a,b; Franklin et al., 2001). Importantly, we have induced liver lesions experimentally by intraperitoneal or oral inoculation of *H. hepaticus* into A/JCr but not C57BL mice (Ward et al., 1994 a; Ihrig et al., 1999). Persistent infection of germ-free female outbred mice with *H. hepaticus* also induced chronic hepatitis, albeit of milder severity than that seen in males and in one mouse, HCC (Fox et al., 1996 d).

Using Affymetrix gene chip microarray we recently compared uninfected versus *H. hepaticus*-infected A/JCr male mice at 3, 6, and 12 months, and also compared infected males with and without severe liver lesions (Boutin et al. , 2004). As expected, a large number of transcriptionally up-regulated genes in the livers of mice with moderate-severe hepatitis were related to inflammation. In agreement with immunohistological demonstration of histiocytic lobular hepatitis, many up-regulated genes were attributable to Kupffer cells and recruited monocyte/macrophages including MARCO, MHCII, lysozyme, LY-6, LY-117, CCR5, macrophage-expressed gene 1, and LAPTM5. Innate immunity and acute-phase responses were represented by numerous genes including serum amyloid A, and very prominently by lipocalin 2 (NGAL/24p3), and other lipocalins including orosomucoid and retinol-binding protein (Boutin et al., 2004). Lipocalins bind lipophilic molecules including lipopolysaccharide (LPS) and other bacterial cell wall products, and also are involved in mucosal immunity, chaperoning, lymphocyte apoptosis, and male scent expression (Cavaggioni and Mucignat-Caretta, 2000; Devireddy et al., 2001; Xu and Venge, 2000). Evidence of active antigen processing was documented by increases in proteasome, Ia invariant chain, cathepsin S, and MHC II transcripts. The type 1 immune response demonstrated by serum antibody subtype analysis, and documented previously (Whary et al., 1998), was corroborated by microarray analysis including increases of numerous IFN-γ-inducible GTPases, proteins, and transcripts, as well as STAT1, leukocyte-specific protein, and others. Many endogenous hepatic enzymes were significantly down-regulated in mice with lesions, suggesting decreased hepatocellular functionality in the diseased liver. Interestingly, male mice with severe disease versus both uninfected controls and infected males without disease, had significantly decreased levels of hydroxysteroid dehydrogenase-5, $\delta<5>$-3-β, the hepatic enzyme responsible for inactivating the potent androgen dihydrotestosterone. This could explain in part the gender effect. Other enzymes specifically associated with steroid metabolism were also up-or down-regulated in males with disease versus those without (Boutin et al., 2004). There is significant overlap of function in enzymes involved in sex-steroid modification and bile acid synthesis, raising two potential pathogenetic mechanisms for disease outcomes in the livers of male mice (Pirog and Collins, 1999; Schwarz et al., 2000).

10.4.3.2 *Helicobacter bilis*-Associated Hepatitis

Helicobacter bilis has been isolated from the intestines and livers of inbred mice aged 18 months or more. This organism, like *H. hepaticus*, is strongly urease-positive (Fox et al., 1995), but morphologically it is more fusiform than spiral in shape. It measures 0.4×4–5 μm in size, but has overlapping periplasmic fibers similar to those of "*H. rappini*". The livers of *H. bilis*-infected inbred mice had multifocal hepatitis. The severity of the liver lesions was strain-dependent, with CBA/CA having the most severe hepatitis, followed by DBA/2 mice, and the least severe being C57BL/6 mice. The BALB/c mice had no inflammatory lesions in the liver. *H. bilis*-associated hepatitis is also observed in outbred CD mice (Fox et al., 2004). A bacterium with this morphology has also been observed in the livers of rats experimentally infected with *Fasciola hepatica* (Foster, 1984). Unlike *H. hepaticus*, *H. bilis* has an extended host range, having been isolated from the feces of dogs, cats, and gerbils, as well as being incriminated in cholecystitis and liver cancer in humans (Fox et al., 1998; Fox, 2002; Matsukura et al., 2002). Immunogenic proteins present in *H. bilis* have also been identified in *H. hepaticus* and *H. pullorum* (Ge et al., 2001; Kornilovs'ka et al., 2002). These immunodominant proteins may be useful for the development of the serodiagnosis of these helicobacters in both humans and animals.

10.4.3.3 *Helicobacter hepaticus* and Lower Bowel Cancer

While an extensive review of animal models of inflammatory bowel disease (IBD) is beyond the scope of this chapter, it is increasingly apparent that enterohepatic *Helicobacter* spp. – particularly *H. hepaticus* and *H. bilis* – play a key role as inflammatory mediators in the onset and progression of colitis in a number of mouse models. *H. hepaticus* and *H. bilis* persistently colonize the lower bowel of mice (Fox et al., 1995, 1996 d; Maggio-Price et al., 2005) and presumably reach the liver via the portal circulation, although direct retrograde migration via the common bile duct has not been disproven. The immune response to *H. hepaticus* infection appears to be Th1-mediated, since splenocytes produced large amounts of IFN-γ when stimulated with *H.*

hepaticus antigens (Whary et al., 2000). Normally, humans and other animals remain hyporesponsive or tolerant to their own enteric flora. In patients with IBD, tolerance is disrupted as individuals become "hyper-responsive" to endogenous enteric antigens (Duchmann et al., 1995). IL-10 is a Th2 cytokine with anti-inflammatory and Th1-suppressive effects, and the lack of IL-10 manifests predictably as an unopposed Th1 immune response (Berg et al., 1996; Kullberg et al., 1998). The IL-10$^{-/-}$ mice reared conventionally (it is highly probable that these mice were infected with *Helicobacter* spp.) present with enterocolitis (Kuhn et al., 1993) and lower bowel cancer (Berg et al., 1996). Rearing IL10$^{-/-}$ mice in SPF facilities restricted the inflammation to the colon (Berg et al., 1996; Kullberg et al ., 1998), whereas in germ-free IL-10$^{-/-}$ mice there is no lower bowel inflammation. Thus, enteric bacterial antigens including *H. hepaticus* or *H. bilis* contribute to the induction of colitis (Kullberg et al ., 2002; Maggio-Price et al., 2005) and, more recently, the induction of colon cancer in RAG mice, TGFB$_1$ and Smad3$^{-/-}$ deficient mice (Engle et al., 2002; Erdman et al., 2003 a; Maggio-Price et al., 2006).

The CD4$^+$CD45$^+$Rb^{hi} model of *H. hepaticus*-induced colitis in SCID or RAG mice is well established, and has been duplicated in a number of laboratories (Cahill et al., 1997; Powrie et al ., 1997). Monoinfection of germ-free SCID mice or outbred mice with either *H. hepaticus* or *H. muridarum* and their ability to induce enterocolitis also illustrates the proinflammatory capabilities of these helicobacters (Fox et al., 1996 d; Jiang et al., 2002).

This model has been further defined in the *H. hepaticus*-infected 129 Rag mouse model which documents the progression of colitis to lower bowel adenocarcinoma (Erdman et al., 2003 a,b). Importantly, this model of lower bowel cancer fulfills all of the histological criteria for a diagnosis of colonic adenocarcinoma outbred by a panel of experts (Boivin et al., 2003). The progression of *H. hepaticus*-induced lower bowel cancer can be modulated by subsets of T cells; T-regulatory cells abrogate inflammation and cancer, while T-effector cells CD4$^+$CD45$^+$ Rb^{hi} accelerate the process (Erdman et al., 2003 a,b).

Observations that colorectal cancer can be reduced in patients receiving oral aspirin therapy or various other anti-inflammatory medications indicate the apparent role of inflammation in the pathogenesis of these tumors. Using the Apc$^{min/+}$ mouse model of colon polyps, we have demonstrated that T-regulatory cells (CD4$^+$CD45$^+$Rb^{low}) can actually induce the regression of intestine polyps in this model (Erdman et al., 2005). Surprisingly, when the Apc$^{min/+}$ Rag$^{-/-}$ mouse C57BL/6 model infected with *H. hepaticus* or administered proinflammatory lymphocytes (CD4$^+$CD45$^+$Rb^{hi}), both intestinal and mammary tumors are statistically increased in number (Roa et al. in press).

10.5
Virulence Determinants of Enterohepatic *Helicobacter* spp.

10.5.1
H. hepaticus is a Tumor Promoter in the Liver

A/JCr has a low incidence and multiplicity of liver tumors, and their susceptibility to *H. hepaticus*-induced hepatitis and development of HCC has provided a unique opportunity to dissect *Helicobacter*-associated tumorigenesis. Hepatocyte proliferation is strongly linked to tumor promotion, and presumably is the result of *H. hepaticus*-induced chronic inflammation; it is in part responsible for the increased rates of hepatocellular tumors in male A/JCr mice (Fox et al., 1996 b; Nyska et al., 1997; Ihrig et al., 1999). There is also evidence for the presence of elevated levels of oxidative stress in *H. hepaticus*-associated hepatitis, there being a time-dependent increase in 8-oxo-2'-deoxyguanosine in the liver of *H. hepaticus*-infected A/JCr mice compared to uninfected, age-matched controls (Sipowicz et al., 1997 a). The source of the ROS was determined to be the hepatocytes. Immunohistochemistry revealed an increased number of cells expressing cytochrome P450 (CYP), and co-localization of formazan and the 2A5 isoform of the enzyme (CYP2A5) suggested a possible mechanism for the production of ROS. In addition, immunohistochemistry for glutathione S-transferase indicated that the hepatocytes were attempting to produce increased amounts of reduced glutathione (GSH). GSH is involved in protecting cells from killing by NO and by ROS, and both *de-novo* synthesis of GSH and reduction of oxidized glutathione (GSSG) are important responses to increased oxidative stress (Luperchio et al., 1996). The oxidative stress associated with *H. hepaticus* infection may result in an induction of lipid peroxidation and the generation of malondialdehyde. The latter reacts with deoxyguanosine in DNA and results in the formation of the cyclic pyrimidopurinone *N*-1, *N*2 malondialdehyde – deoxyguanosine (M_1dG) adduct. This adduct can cause mutations that may ultimately lead to liver carcinogenesis. Higher levels of M_1dG were detected in the liver DNA of *H. hepaticus*-infected A/JCr mice compared to controls, with levels increasing from 3 to 12 months post infection. There was a significant age-dependent increase in the level of M_1dG in the caudate and median lobes of the A/JCr mice relative to control mice (Singh et al., 2001).

A central problem with these two studies is that a single biomarker may not be representative of the chemistry occurring at sites of *H. hepaticus*-induced inflammation. Future studies should include utilization of a series of DNA damage products as biomarkers of inflammation, including nitrosative deamination products of DNA bases (2'-deoxy-xanthosine, -oxanosine, -uridine, - and inosine), the etheno adduct of dA (believed to arise from lipid peroxidation products), and M_1G as well as sensitive methods to quantify abasic sites and strand breaks in cells.

Strain differences in *H. hepaticus* susceptibility also suggest a mechanism such as tumor promotion, because it is known that tumor promotion in the mouse liver is influenced strongly by genetics of the host (Diwan et al., 1986; Watanapa and Watanapa, 2002). A tumor promotion mechanism is also supported by a lack of mutagenic response in the Ames' assay, as well as a lack of demonstrated mutations in H-, K-, and N-ras and p53 tumor suppresser genes in liver tumors of A/JCr mice infected with *H. hepaticus* (Canella et al., 1996; Diwan et al., 1997; Sipowicz et al., 1997 b). When male A/JCr infant mice infected with *H. hepaticus* were given a single intraperitonal dose of NDMA they developed a statistically higher incidence of hepatocellular adenomas at 31–36 weeks and 51–64 weeks post infection when compared to uninfected A/JCr mice similarly treated with the carcinogen (Diwan et al., 1997). There was also a fourfold increase in multiplicity of adenomas at 31–36 weeks post infection, and a fivefold increase in both incidence and multiplicity of carcinomas after 50 weeks. These data indicate that *H. hepaticus* not only stimulates growth of tumors from initiated cells, but also enhances progression to malignancy (Diwan et al., 1997). All of these factors in combination suggest that *H. hepaticus* exerts a tumor promotion effect in the liver of A/JCr mice.

10.5.2
H. hepaticus Increases ROS and Intestinal Tumors

Gpx double knockout mice lack the two isoforms of Gpx expressed in the intestinal tract, and therefore are deficient in their ability to scavenge ROS (Chu et al., 2004). When these knockout mice are infected with *H. hepaticus* they develop a significantly higher incidence of intestinal tumors when compared to their uninfected counterpart (Chu et al., 2004).

10.5.3
H. hepaticus Pathogenicity Island

Genome sequence analysis of *H. hepaticus* revealed the presence of a genomic island with low G+C content that comprises 70 kb of sequence and 71 predicted genes. The island, in part, comprises elements that suggest a role for it in virulence. This island, termed *H. hepaticus* genomic island 1 (HHGI1), comprises three genes that encode homologues of components (VirB10, VirB4, and VirD4) of a type IV secretion system (T4SS). HHGI1 also contains a gene with homology to *Vibrio cholerae hcp*, which encodes a secreted protein co-regulated with the *V. cholerae* hemolysin, a gene cluster (HH244 to HH251) with significant homology to clusters of genes of unknown function on the small chromosome of *V. cholerae* (VCA0107 to VCA0115) and the *Yersinia pestis* genome. Unlike many pathogenicity islands, HHGI1 is not associated with a tRNA gene and not flanked by direct repeats. However, it contains a prophage P4-like integrase gene (HH0269), a feature that has been found in several pathogenicity islands. In the same study, we established by genome comparisons with a whole-genome DNA microarray that while all strains that had been associated with liver disease, including the sequenced strain 3B1 (ATCC 51449), contained the complete island, many *H. hepaticus* isolates lack parts of the island or even all HHGI1 genes. Significantly, none of these HHGI1-defective strains had caused liver disease in the mice from which they had been isolated. Taken together, these data suggested that HHGI1 might be involved in virulence of *H. hepaticus*. We therefore selected two *H. hepaticus* isolates, HhNET and HhG, with partial or complete deletions of the island and compared their virulence with that of the sequenced strain that harbors the complete island (Suerbaum et al., 2003).

We have shown that A/JCr mice infected with strains of *H. hepaticus* (HhG and HhNET) lacking all or part of a 70-kb genomic putative PAI have less-severe *Helicobacter*-associated liver disease than mice infected with the strain Hh3B1, which contains a complete HHGI1 island. While the study clearly demonstrates that isolates of *H. hepaticus* with different genomic contents differ significantly in their potential to cause liver disease in A/JCr mice, further experiments with isogenic mutants lacking the island will be required to firmly prove the role of the HHGI1 island in these differences, and attempts to construct series of such mutants are under way in our laboratories (Boutin et al., 2005).

10.5.4
Cytolethal Distending Toxin (CDT)

Candidate virulence determinants in enterohepatic *Helicobacter* species (EHS) have begun to be identified. *H. hepaticus* and a subset of the other EHS (*H. cinaedi*, *H. pullorum*, *H. bilis* and *H. marmotae*) each produce CDT (Chien et al., 2000; Young et al., 2000 a,b), a potential virulence factor elaborated by a heterogeneous group of pathogenic bacteria including *C. jejuni* and other *Campylobacter* species, certain *E. coli* strains, *Shigella dysenteriae*, *Haemophilus ducreyi*, and *Actinobacillus actinomycetemcomitans*. CDT induces progressive cell enlargement and eventual death in cultured mammalian cells. Cytotoxicity is accompanied by G_2/M cell cycle arrest. In all bacterial species (including *Helicobacter* spp.) in which CDT activity has been demonstrated, three linked genes (*cdtA*, *cdtB*, and *cdtC*) encode cytotoxic activities. CdtB has position-specific homology to type I mammalian DNases and exhibits nuclease activity *in vitro* (Lara-Tejero and Galan, 2000; Elwell et al., 2001). Mammalian cells treated with CDT have evidence of the activation of DNA repair mechanisms (Li et al., 2002; Hassane et al., 2003). There is evidence that CdtA, CdtB, and CdtC form a tripartite AB_2 toxin, with CdtB as the active A subunit and CdtA and CdtC forming a heterodimeric B subunit (Lara-Tejero and Galan, 2001).

To investigate the role of CDT in the pathogenesis of *H. hepaticus*, transposon mutagenesis was used to generate a series of isogenic mutants in and around the *cdtABC* gene cluster. An *H. hepaticus* transposon mutant with a disrupted *cdtABC* coding region no longer produced CDT activity. Conversely, a transposon insertion outside of the cluster did not affect the CDT activity. An examination of these mutants showed that CDT represents the previously described granulating cytotoxin in *H. hepaticus*. Challenge of C57BL/6 IL-10$^{-/-}$ mice with isogenic *H. hepaticus* mutants revealed that CDT expression is not required for colonization of the murine gut at 6 weeks post infection. However, a CDT-negative *H. hepaticus* mutant had a significantly diminished capacity to induce lesions in this murine model of inflammatory bowel disease (Young et al., 2004).

A cdtB-deficient *H. hepaticus* isogenic mutant (HhcdtBm7) was recently generated in our laboratory and characterized for colonization parameters in four intestinal regions (jejunum, ileum, cecum, and colon) of outbred Swiss Webster (SW) mice. Inactivation of the *cdtB* gene abolished the ability of HhcdtBm7 to colonize female mice at both 8 and 16 weeks post infection (wpi), whereas HhcdtBm7 colonized all four intestinal regions of three of five males at 8 wpi and then was eliminated by 16 wpi. Wild-type *H. hepaticus* was detected in the corresponding intestinal regions of both male and female mice at 8 and 16 wpi (Ge et al., 2005).

Infection with wild-type *H. hepaticus* at 8 wpi was associated with significantly increased mRNA levels of ileal and cecal IFN-γ in females between wild-type *H. hepaticus*-infected and sham-dosed females. This was not noted in female mice infected with the mutant Hhcdt Bm7. In contrast, the mRNA levels of IFN-γ were significantly higher in the colon and trended to be higher in the cecum in HhcdtBm7-colonized male mice versus the sham-dosed controls at 8 wpi. In addition, mRNA levels of ileal IFN-γ were significantly higher in control females than males at 8 wpi. There were significantly higher Th1-associated immunoglobulin G 2 a (IgG 2 a), Th2-associated IgG1 and mucosal IgA responses in mice infected with wild type *H. hepaticus* when compared to HhcdtBm7 at 16 wpi. Colonic IL-10 expressions at 16 wpi were significantly lower in both female and male mice colonized by wild-type *H. hepaticus*, or in males transiently colonized through 8 wpi by HhcdtBm7 versus control mice. These lines of evidence indicate that: (i) *H. hepaticus* CDT plays a crucial role in the persistent colonization of *H. hepaticus* in SW mice; (ii) SW female mice are more resistant to *H. hepaticus* colonization than SW male mice; (iii) there was persistent colonization of wild-type *H. hepaticus* in the cecum, colon, and jejunum, but only transient colonization in the ileum of female mice; and (iv) *H. hepaticus* colonization was associated with down-regulation of colonic IL-10 production (Ge et al., 2005).

10.6
Enterohepatic Helicobacter spp.: Are they Co-Carcinogens?

Almost 10% of people worldwide are infected with either hepatitis B virus (HBV) or hepatitis C virus (HCV). The estimated prevalence of HCV infection is 170 million individuals, or 3% of the global population (Kane, 1995), while the number of carriers of HBV exceeds 350 million or 6% of all people. More than one million people die from HBV-associated liver failure and cancer every year (Mast et al., 1999). About 70% of individuals exposed to HCV become chronically infected, and of those 5–10% will develop fatal cirrhosis or cancer (Mast et al., 1999). Because most HCV carriers are unaware of their infection status, the true prevalence of HCV-associated disease may exceed current estimates (Poovorawan et al ., 2002). Chronic viral hepatitis of either type B or C greatly increases the risk of HCC in humans. Indeed, the vast majority of HCC diagnoses worldwide are made in people who are seropositive for HBV, HCV, or both (Ferrell et al., 2002). Although studies using HBV- and HCV-transgenic mice clearly demonstrate that viral gene products can induce tumors *a priori* (Koike et al., 2002), most humans infected with HBV or HCV are exposed to additional agents known independently to increase the risk of HCC. Known toxins which initiate or promote HCC include the fungal-derived food contaminant aflatoxin B, alcohol abuse, and a large array of environmental and industrial chemicals (Ferrell et al., 2002). Animal models of human viral hepatitis also demonstrate additive risk for tumor development when exposed to toxins (Slagle et al., 1996; Madden et al., 2001). However, it is crucial to note that most studies involving animal models of viral hepatitis have not accounted for the possibility of confounding due to co-infection with hepatobiliary helicobacters. In recent years, enterohepatic *Helicobacter* spp. have been identified in most animal species used to model viral hepatitis, including woodchucks, mice, and nonhuman primates (Fox, 1997; Fox et al., 2001, 2002 a). To date, the only proven nonviral infectious causes of human liver tumors are biliary trematodes including *Opisthorchis viverrini* and *Clonorchis sinensis*, which increase the risk of cholangiocarcinoma (Watanapa and Watanapa, 2002).

Until recently, the potential role of bacterial infection in hepatobiliary carcinogenesis went largely unexplored. In the hepatobiliary system, an intriguing association between gall bladder cancer in Chilean women and *Helicobacter* spp. was uncovered by our group (Fox et al., 1998). This association has been reinforced by studies in our laboratory which demonstrate the pivotal role that certain enterohepatic helicobacters play in the development of cholesterol gallstones (a precursor to gall bladder cancer and noted in all patients in our Chilean study) in C57L mice fed a lithogenic diet (Maurer et al., 2005). Observational and case-control studies performed by numerous others worldwide have documented significant associations between hepatobiliary disease, including cancer, and the presence of *Helicobacter* spp. (Nilsson et al., 2000; Fan et al., 2002; Fukuda et al., 2002; Leong and Sung, 2002; Matsukura et al., 2002). Of importance, recent evidence implicates hepatobiliary *Helicobacter* spp. in severe HCV infection outcomes, including HCC (Ponzetto et al., 2000; Dore et al., 2002 b). A review of the recent literature concluded that there is strong evidence pointing to a role for human helicobacters in hepatobiliary neoplasms, but that clinical studies have been hampered by a shortage of appropriate control specimens as well as reliable biomarkers of enterohepatic *Helicobacter* infections (Leong and Sung, 2002). Intriguingly, very high rates of human HCC are reported in south-east Asia, where hepatobiliary helicobacters have also been identified (Kullavanijaya et al., 1999; Fukuda et al., 2002; Leong and Sung, 2002).

Because human studies are necessarily limited in scope, animal models can provide valuable tools for establishing etiological relationships and mechanistic pathways in the complicated step-wise progression of infection, inflammation, tissue damage, and neoplasia. There is therefore a need to characterize murine models of human co-infection with HBV, HCV or liver parasitic infections and hepatobiliary *Helicobacter* spp. Although *Helicobacter* spp. and human hepatitis viruses represent broadly divergent classes of pathogens, there are striking similarities in serum biochemical abnormalities and liver lesions between humans with viral hepatitis and mice with *H. hepaticus*, which suggests that there are similarities in the types of immune responses generated by both infections (Rogers Fox 2004). Serum transaminase activities are increased in both, though not necessarily correlated with individual disease severity. Initial random and perivenular lobular necrogranulomatous histological activity precedes portal lymphocyte aggregations and interface hepatitis (Rogers et al., 2004). Hepatocellular degeneration can be manifested by hydropic and steatotic vacuolar degeneration, apoptosis, and coagulative necrosis in both diseases. Because the disease patterns are similar, it is hypothesized that HBV or HCV and hepatic *Helicobacter* infections in humans could result in an additive or synergistic fashion resulting in more severe and rapid hepatitis and tumor induction than would be induced by either agent alone (Rogers A., Fox J.G. unpublished observations).

Results from these studies may reveal heretofore unrecognized synergism between virus, bacterium, and host immunity, and suggest new therapeutic targets for the prevention and intervention of chronic hepatitis and cancer.

References

Akin, L., Tezcan, S., Hascelik, G., and Cakir, B. (**2004**). Seroprevalence and some correlates of *Helicobacter pylori* at adult ages in Gulveren Health District, Ankara, Turkey. *Epidemiol. Infect.* 132: 847–856.

Alm, R.A. and Noonan, B. (**2001**). The genome in *Helicobacter pylori*. In: H.L.T. Mobley, G.L. Mendz, and S. L. Hazell (Eds.), *Physiology and Genetics.* ASM, Washington, pp. 295–311.

Alm, R.A., Ling, L.S., Moir, D.T., King, B.L., Brown, E.D., Doig, P.C., Smith, D.R., Noonan, B., Guild, B.C., deJonge, B.L., Carmel, G., Tummino, P.J., Caruso, A., Uria-Nickelsen, M., Mills, D.M., Ives, C., Gibson, R., Merberg, D., Mills, S. D., Jiang, Q., Taylor, D.E., Vovis, G.F., and Trust, T.J. (**1999**). Genomic-sequence comparison of two unrelated isolates of the human gastric pathogen *Helicobacter pylori*. *Nature* 397: 176–180.

Anonymous. (**1985**). Validation of publication of new names and new combinations previously published outside the IJSB. *Int. J. Syst. Bacteriol.* 85: 223–225.

Archer, J.R., Romero, S., Ritchie, A.E., Hamacher, M.E., Steiner, B.M., Bryner, J.H., and Schell, R.F. (**1988**). Characterization of an unclassified microaerophilic bacterium associated with gastroenteritis. *J. Clin. Microbiol.* 26: 101–105.

Atherton, J.C. (**2002**). Vacuolating cytotoxin. In: H.L. Mobley, G.L. Mendz, and S. Hazell (Eds.), Helicobacter pylori *Physiology and Genetics.* ASM Press, Washington, pp. 97–110.

Atherton, J.C., Cao, P., Peek, R.M., Jr., Tummuru, M.K., Blaser, M.J., and Cover, T.L. (**1995**). Mosaicism in vacuolating cytotoxin alleles of *Helicobacter pylori*. Association of specific vacA types with cytotoxin production and peptic ulceration. *J. Biol. Chem.* 270: 17 771–17 777.

Balfour, A. (**1906**). A hemogregarine of mammals and some notes on trypanosomiasis in the Anglo-Egyptian Sudan. *J. Trop. Med.* 9: 81–92.

Balkwill, F. and Mantovani, A. (**2001**). Inflammation and cancer: back to Virchow? *Lancet* 357: 539–545.

Bani-Hani, K.E., Yaghan, R.J., and Matalka, II. (**2005**). Primary gastric lymphoma in Jordan with special emphasis on descriptive epidemiology. *Leuk. Lymphoma* 46: 1337–1343.

Baskerville, A., and Newell, D.G. (**1988**). Naturally occurring chronic gastritis and *C. pylori* infection in the rhesus monkey: a potential model for gastritis in man. *Gut* 29: 465–472.

Basso, D. and Plebani, M. (**2004**). *H. pylori* infection: bacterial virulence factors and cytokine gene polymorphisms as determinants of infection outcome. *Crit. Rev. Clin. Lab. Sci.* 41: 313–337.

Bayerdorffer, E., Ritter, M.M., Hatz, R., Brooks, W., Ruckdeschel, G., and Stolte, M. (**1994**). Healing of protein losing hypertrophic gastropathy by eradication of *Helicobacter pylori* – is *Helicobacter pylori* a pathogenic factor in Menetrier's disease? *Gut* 35: 701–704.

Berg, D.J., Davidson, N., Kuhn, R., Muller, W., Menon, S., Holland, G., Thompson-Snipes, L., Leach, M.W., and Rennick, D. (**1996**). Enterocolitis and colon cancer in interleukin-10-deficient mice are associated with aberrant cytokine production and CD4(+) TH1-like responses. *J. Clin. Invest.* 98, 1010–1020.

Bizzozero, G. (**1893**). Über die schlauchförmigen Drüsen des Magendarmkanals und die Beziehungen ihres Epithels zu dem Oberflächenepithel der Schleimhaut. *Arch. Mikrob. Anat.* 42: 82.

Bjelakovic, G., Nikolova, D., Simonetti, R.G., and Gluud, C. (**2004**). Antioxidant supplements for prevention of gastrointestinal cancers: a systematic review and meta-analysis. *Lancet* 364: 1219–1228.

Bjorkholm, B., Sjolund, M., Falk, P.G., Berg, O.G., Engstrand, L., and Andersson, D.I. (**2001**). Mutation frequency and biological cost of antibiotic resistance in *Helicobacter pylori*. *Proc. Natl. Acad. Sci. USA* 98: 14 607–14 612.

Blaser, M.J. (**1999 a**). Hypothesis: the changing relationships of *Helicobacter pylori* and humans: implications for health and disease. *J. Infect. Dis.* 179: 1523–1530.

Blaser, M.J. (**1999 b**). In a world of black and white, *Helicobacter pylori* is gray. *Ann. Intern. Med.* 130: 695–697.

Blaser, M.J. (**2002**). Polymorphic bacteria persisting in polymorphic hosts: assessing *Helicobacter pylori*-related risks for gastric cancer. *J. Natl. Cancer Inst.* 94: 1662–1663.

Blaser, M.J., Chyou, P.H., and Nomura, A. (**1995**). Age at establishment of *Helicobacter pylori* infection and gastric carcinoma, gastric ulcer, and duodenal ulcer risk. *Cancer Res.* 55: 562–565.

Bode, G., Mauch, F., Ditschuneit, H., and Malfertheiner, P. (**1993 a**). Identification of structures containing polyphosphate in *Helicobacter pylori*. *J. Gen. Microbiol.* 139: 3029–3033.

Bode, G., Mauch, F., and Malfertheiner, P. (**1993 b**). The coccoid forms of *Helicobacter pylori*. Criteria for their viability. *Epidemiol. Infect.* 111: 483–490.

Boivin, G.P., Washington, K., Yang, K., Ward, J.M., Pretlow, T.P., Russell, R., Besselsen, D.G., Godfrey, V.L., Doetschman, T., Dove, W.F., Pitot, H.C., Halberg, R.B., Itzkowitz, S. H., Groden, J., and Coffey, R.J. (**2003**). Pathology of mouse models of intestinal cancer: consensus report and recommendations. *Gastroenterology* 124: 762–777.

Borhan-Manesh, F. and Farnum, J.B. (**1993**). Study of *Helicobacter pylori* colonization of patches of heterotopic gastric mucosa (HGM) at the upper esophagus. *Dig. Dis. Sci.* 38: 142–146.

Bottcher, I. (**1874**). *Dopater Medicinische Zeitschrift* 5: 148.

Boutin, S. R., Rogers, A.B., Shen, Z., Fry, R.C., Love, J.A., Nambiar, P.R., Suerbaum, S., and Fox, J.G. (**2004**). Hepatic temporal gene expression profiling in *Helicobacter hepaticus*-infected A/JCr mice. *Toxicol. Pathol.* 32: 678–693.

Boutin, S. R., Shen, Z., Rogers, A.B., Feng, Y., Ge, Z., Xu, S., Sterzenbach, T., Josenhans, C., Schauer, D.B., Suerbaum, S., and Fox, J.G. (**2005**). Different *Helicobacter hepaticus* strains with variable genomic content induce various degrees of hepatitis. *Infect. Immun.* 73: 8449–8452.

Bravo, L.E., van Doom, L.J., Realpe, J.L., and Correa, P. (**2002**). Virulence-associated genotypes of *Helicobacter pylori:* do they explain the African enigma? *Am. J. Gastroenterol.* 97: 2839–2842.

Brenes, F., Ruiz, B., Correa, P., Hunter, F., Rhamakrishnan, T., Fontham, E., and Shi, T.Y. (**1993**). *Helicobacter pylori* causes hyperproliferation of the gastric epithelium: pre- and post-eradication indices of proliferating cell nuclear antigen. *Am. J. Gastroenterol.* 88: 1870–1875.

Brenner, H., Berg, G., Lappus, N., Kliebsch, U., Bode, G., and Boeing, H. (**1999**). Alcohol consumption and *Helicobacter pylori* infection: results from the German National Health and Nutrition Survey. *Epidemiology* 10: 214–218.

Brenner, H., Arndt, V., Stegmaier, C., Ziegler, H., and Rothenbacher, D. (**2004**). Is *Helicobacter pylori* infection a necessary condition for noncardia gastric cancer? *Am. J. Epidemiol.* 159: 252–258.

Bronsdon, M.A. and Schoenknecht, F.D. (**1988**). *Campylobacter pylori* isolated from the stomach of the monkey, *Macaca nemestrina*. *J. Clin. Microbiol.* 26: 1725–1728.

Brown, L.M. (**2000**). *Helicobacter pylori:* epidemiology and routes of transmission. *Epidemiol. Rev.* 22: 283–297.

Brown, L.M., Thomas, T.L., Ma, J.L., Chang, Y.S., You, W.C., Liu, W.D., Zhang, L., Pee, D., and Gail, M.H. (**2002**). *Helicobacter pylori* infection in rural China: demographic, lifestyle and environmental factors. *Int. J. Epidemiol.* 31: 638–645.

Burnens, A.P., Stanley, J., Morgenstern, R., and Nicolet, J. (**1994**). Gastroenteritis associated with *Helicobacter pullorum*. *Lancet* 344: 1569–1570.

Cahill, R.J., Foltz, C.J., Fox, J.G., Dangler, C.A., Powrie, F., and Schauer, D.B. (**1997**). Inflammatory bowel disease: an immunity-mediated condition triggered by bacterial infection with *Helicobacter hepaticus*. *Infect. Immun.* 65: 3126–3131.

Cai, X., Carlson, J., Stoicov, C., Li, H., Wang, T.C., and Houghton, J. (**2005**). *Helicobacter felis* eradication restores normal architecture and inhibits gastric cancer progression in C57BL/6 mice. *Gastroenterology* 128: 1937–1952.

Calvert, R., Randerson, J., Evans, P., Cawkwell, L., Lewis, F., Dixon, M.F., Jack, A., Owen, R., Shiach, C., and Morgan, G.J. (**1995**). Genetic abnormalities during transition from *Helicobacter pylori*-associated gastritis to low-grade MALToma. *Lancet* 345: 26–27.

Canella, K.A., Diwan, B.A., Gorelick, P.L., Donovan, P.J., Sipowicz, M.A., Kasprzak, K.S., Weghorst, C.M., Snyderwine, E.G., Davis, C.D., Keefer, L.K., Kyrtopoulos, S. A., Hecht, S. S., Wang, M., Anderson, L.M., and Rice, J.M. (**1996**). Liver tumorigenesis by *Helicobacter hepaticus*: considerations of mechanism. *In Vivo* 10: 285–292.

Cavaggioni, A. and Mucignat-Caretta, C. (**2000**). Major urinary proteins, alpha(2 U)-globulins and aphrodisin. *Biochim. Biophys. Acta* 1482: 218–228.

Cave, D.R. (**1997**). How is *Helicobacter pylori* transmitted? *Gastroenterology* 113: S9–S14.

Celler, H. and Thalheimer, W. (**1916**). Bacteriological and experimental studies on gastric ulcer. *J. Exp. Med.* 23: 791–800.

Censini, S., Lange, C., Xiang, Z., Crabtree, J.E., Ghiara, P., Borodovsky, M., Rappuoli, R., and Covacci, A. (**1996**). cag, a pathogenicity island of *Helicobacter pylori*, encodes type I-specific and disease-associated virulence factors. *Proc. Natl. Acad. Sci. USA* 93: 14 648–14 653.

Chien, C.C., Taylor, N.S., Ge, Z., Schauer, D.B., Young, V.B., and Fox, J.G. (**2000**). Identification of cdtB homologues and cytolethal distending toxin activity in enterohepatic *Helicobacter* spp. *J. Med. Microbiol.* 49: 525–534.

Chow, W.H., Blaser, M.J., Blot, W.J., Gammon, M.D., Vaughan, T.L., Risch, H.A., Perez-Perez, G.I., Schoenberg, J.B., Stanford, J.L., Rotterdam, H., West, A.B., and Fraumeni, J.F., Jr. (**1998**). An inverse relation between cagA+ strains of *Helicobacter pylori* infection and risk of esophageal and gastric cardia adenocarcinoma. *Cancer Res.* 58: 588–590.

Chu, F.F., Esworthy, R.S., Chu, P.G., Longmate, J.A., Huycke, M.M., Wilczynski, S., and Doroshow, J.H. (**2004**). Bacteria-induced intestinal cancer in mice with disrupted Gpx1 and Gpx2 genes. *Cancer Res.* 64: 962–968.

Claviez, A., Meyer, U., Dominick, C., Beck, J.F., Rister, M., and Tiemann, M. (**2005**). MALT lymphoma in children: A report from the NHL-BFM study group. *Pediatr. Blood Cancer* (e-pub August 25, 2005).

Clyne, M., Dillon, P., Daly, S., O'Kennedy, R., May, F.E., Westley, B.R., and Drumm, B. (**2004**). *Helicobacter pylori* interacts with the human single-domain trefoil protein TFF1. *Proc. Natl. Acad. Sci. USA* 101: 7409–7414.

Collett, J.A., Burt, M.J., Frampton, C.M., Yeo, K.H., Chapman, T.M., Buttimore, R.C., Cook, H.B., and Chapman, B.A. (**1999**). Seroprevalence of *Helicobacter pylori* in the adult population of Christchurch: risk factors and relationship to dyspeptic symptoms and iron studies. *N. Z. Med. J.* 112: 292–295.

Correa, P. (**1992**). Human gastric carcinogenesis: a multistep and multifactorial process. First American Cancer Society Award Lecture on Cancer Epidemiology and Prevention. *Cancer Res.* 52: 6735–6740.

Correa, P. (**1995**). *Helicobacter pylori* and gastric carcinogenesis. *Am. J. Surg. Pathol.* 19 Suppl 1: S37–S43.

Correa, P., Fontham, E.T., Bravo, J.C., Bravo, L.E., Ruiz, B., Zarama, G., Realpe, J.L., Malcom, G.T., Li, D., Johnson, W.D., and Mera, R. (**2000**). Chemoprevention of gastric dysplasia: randomized trial of antioxidant supplements and anti-*Helicobacter pylori* therapy. *J. Natl. Cancer Inst.* 92: 1881–1888.

Coussens, L.M. and Werb, Z. (**2002**). Inflammation and cancer. *Nature* 420: 860–867.

Covacci, A., Censini, S., Bugnoli, M., Petracca, R., Burroni, D., Macchia, G., Massone, A., Papini, E., Xiang, Z., Figura, N., et al. (**1993**). Molecular characterization of the 128-kDa immunodominant antigen of *Helicobacter pylori* associated with cytotoxicity and duodenal ulcer. *Proc. Natl. Acad. Sci. USA* 90: 5791–5795.

Covacci, A., Telford, J.L., Del Giudice, G., Parsonnet, J., and Rappuoli, R. (**1999**). *Helicobacter pylori* virulence and genetic geography. *Science* 284: 1328–1333.

Cover, T.L. (**1996**). The vacuolating cytotoxin of *Helicobacter pylori*. *Mol. Microbiol.* 20: 241–246.

Crabtree, J.E., Farmery, S. M., Lindley, I.J., Figura, N., Peichl, P., and Tompkins, D.S. (**1994**). CagA/cytotoxic strains of *Helicobacter pylori* and interleukin-8 in gastric epithelial cell lines. *J. Clin. Pathol.* 47: 945–950.

Crabtree, J.E., Xiang, Z., Lindley, I.J., Tompkins, D.S., Rappuoli, R., and Covacci, A. (**1995**). Induction of interleukin-8 secretion from gastric epithelial cells by a cagA negative isogenic mutant of *Helicobacter pylori*. *J. Clin. Pathol.* 48: 967–969.

Cui, G., Houghton, J.M., Finkel, N., Carlson, J., and Wang, T.C. (**2003**). IFN-gamma infusion induces gastric atrophy, metaplasia and dysplasia in the absence of Helicobacter infection – a role for immune response in Helicobacter disease. *Gastroenterology* 124: 4.

Cui, G., Koh, T.J., Chen, D., Zhao, C.M., Takaishi, S., Dockray, G.J., Varro, A., Rogers, A.B., Fox, J.G., and Wang, T.C. (**2004**). Overexpression of glycine-extended gastrin inhibits parietal cell loss and atrophy in the mouse stomach. *Cancer Res.* 64: 8160–8166.

Daniel, D., Meyer-Morse, N., Bergsland, E.K., Dehne, K., Coussens, L.M., and Hanahan, D. (**2003**). Immune enhancement of skin carcinogenesis by CD4+ T cells. *J. Exp. Med.* 197: 1017–1028.

De Giacomo, C., Valdambrini, V., Lizzoli, F., Gissi, A., Palestra, M., Tinelli, C., Zagari, M., and Bazzoli, F. (**2002**). A population-based survey on gastrointestinal tract symptoms and *Helicobacter pylori* infection in children and adolescents. *Helicobacter* 7: 356–363.

de Martel, C. and Parsonnet, J. (**2006**). *Helicobacter pylori* infection and gender: a meta-analysis of population-based prevalence surveys. *Dig. Dis. Sci.* (in press).

de Martel, C., Llosa, A.E., Farr, S. M., Friedman, G.D., Vogelman, J.H., Orentreich, N., Corley, D.A., and Parsonnet, J. *Helicobacter pylori* infection and the risk of development of esophageal adenocarcinoma. *J. Infect. Dis.* 191: 761–767, **2005**.

Delchier, J.C., Lamarque, D., Levy, M., Tkoub, E.M., Copie-Bergman, C., Deforges, L., Chaumette, M.T., and Haioun, C. (**2001**). *Helicobacter pylori* and gastric lymphoma: high seroprevalence of CagA in diffuse large B-cell lymphoma but not in low-grade lymphoma of mucosa-associated lymphoid tissue type. *Am. J. Gastroenterol.* 96: 2324–2328.

Devireddy, L.R., Teodoro, J.G., Richard, F.A., and Green, M.R. (**2001**). Induction of apoptosis by a secreted lipocalin that is transcriptionally regulated by IL-3 deprivation. *Science* 293: 829–834.

Diwan, B.A., Rice, J.M., Ohshima, M., and Ward, J.M. (**1986**). Interstrain differences in susceptibility to liver carcinogenesis initiated by N-nitrosodiethylamine and its promotion by phenobarbital in C57BL/6NCr, C3H/HeNCrMTV-and DBA/2NCr mice. *Carcinogenesis* 7: 215–220.

Diwan, B.A., Ward, J.M., Ramljak, D., and Anderson, L.M. (**1997**). Promotion by *Helicobacter hepaticus*-induced hepatitis of hepatic tumors initiated by N-nitrosodimethylamine in male A/JCr mice. *Toxicol. Pathol.* 25: 597–605.

Doenges, J.L. (**1939**). Spirochetes in the gastric glands of macacus rhesus and of man without related disease. *Arch. Pathol.* 27: 469–477.

Donato, R. (**2001**). S100: a multigenic family of calcium-modulated proteins of the EF-hand type with intracellular and extracellular functional roles. *Int. J. Biochem. Cell Biol.* 33: 637–668.

Dore, M.P., Sepulveda, A.R., El-Zimaity, H., Yamaoka, Y., Osato, M.S., Mototsugu, K., Nieddu, A.M., Realdi, G., and Graham, D.Y. (**2001**). Isolation of *Helicobacter pylori* from sheep-implications for transmission to humans. *Am. J. Gastroenterol.* 96: 1396–1401.

Dore, M.P., Malaty, H.M., Graham, D.Y., Fanciulli, G., Delitala, G., and Realdi, G. (**2002a**). Risk Factors Associated with *Helicobacter pylori* Infection among children in a defined geographic area. *Clin. Infect. Dis.* 35: 240–245.

Dore, M.P., Realdi, G., Mura, D., Graham, D.Y., and Sepulveda, A.R. (**2002b**). *Helicobacter* infection in patients with HCV-related chronic hepatitis, cirrhosis, and hepatocellular carcinoma. *Dig. Dis. Sci.*47: 1638–1643.

Dowsett, S. A. and Kowolik, M.J. (**2003**). Oral *Helicobacter pylori:* can we stomach it? *Crit. Rev. Oral Biol. Med.* 14: 226–233.

Dubois, A., Fiala, N., Heman-Ackah, L.M., Drazek, E.S., Tarnawski, A., Fishbein, W.N., Perez-Perez, G.I., and Blaser, M.J. (**1994**). Natural gastric infection with *Helicobacter pylori* in monkeys: a model for spiral bacteria infection in humans. *Gastroenterology* 106: 1405–1417.

Duchmann, R., Kaiser, I., Hermann, E., Mayet, W., Ewe, K., and Meyer zum Buschenfelde, K.H. (**1995**). Tolerance exists towards resident intestinal flora but is broken in active inflammatory bowel disease (IBD). *Clin. Exp. Immunol.* 102: 448–455.

Eaton, K.A., Brooks, C.L., Morgan, D.R., and Krakowka, S. (**1991**). Essential role of urease in pathogenesis of gastritis induced by *Helicobacter pylori* in gnotobiotic piglets. *Infect. Immun.* 59: 2470–2475.

Eaton, K.A., Morgan, D.R., and Krakowka, S. (**1992**). Motility as a factor in the colonisation of gnotobiotic piglets by *Helicobacter pylori. J. Med. Microbiol.* 37: 123–127.

Eaton, K.A., Dewhirst, F.E., Radin, M.J., Fox, J.G., Paster, B.J., Krakowka, S., and Morgan, D.R. (**1993**). *Helicobacter acinonyx* sp. nov., isolated from cheetahs with gastritis. *Int. J. Syst. Bacteriol.* 43: 99–106.

Eaton, K.A., Suerbaum, S., Josenhans, C., and Krakowka, S. (**1996**). Colonization of gnotobiotic piglets by *Helicobacter pylori* deficient in two flagellin genes. *Infect. Immun.* 64: 2445–2448.

Eaton, K.A., Cover, T.L., Tummuru, M.K., Blaser, M.J., and Krakowka, S. (**1997**). Role of vacuolating cytotoxin in gastritis due to *Helicobacter pylori* in gnotobiotic piglets. *Infect. Immun.* 65: 3462–3464.

Ekstrom, A.M., Serafini, M., Nyren, O., Hansson, L.E., Ye, W., and Wolk, A. (**2000**). Dietary antioxidant intake and the risk of cardia cancer and noncardia cancer of the intestinal and diffuse types: a population-based case-control study in Sweden. *Int. J. Cancer* 87: 133–140.

Ekstrom, A.M., M. Held, L.E. Hansson, L. Engstrand, and O. Nyren. **2001**. *Helicobacter pylori* in gastric cancer established by CagA immunoblot as a marker of past infection. *Gastroenterology* 121: 784-791.

El-Omar, E.M., Carrington, M., Chow, W.H., McColl, K.E., Bream, J.H., Young, H.A., Herrera, J., Lissowska, J., Yuan, C.C., Rothman, N., Lanyon, G., Martin, M., Fraumeni, J.F., Jr., and Rabkin, C.S. (**2000**). Interleukin-1 polymorphisms associated with increased risk of gastric cancer. *Nature* 404: 398–402.

El-Omar, E.M., Rabkin, C.S., Gammon, M.D., Vaughan, T.L., Risch, H.A., Schoenberg, J.B., Stanford, J.L., Mayne, S. T., Goedert, J., Blot, W.J., Fraumeni, J.F., Jr., and Chow, W.H. (**2003**). Increased risk of noncardia gastric cancer associated with proinflammatory cytokine gene polymorphisms. *Gastroenterology* 124: 1193–1201.

Elshal, M.F., Elsayed, I.H., El Kady, I.M., Badra, G., El-Refaei, A., El-Batanony, M., and Hendy, O.M. (**2004**). Role of concurrent S. mansoni infection in *H. pylori*-associated gastritis: a flow cytometric DNA-analysis and oxyradicals correlations. *Clin. Chim. Acta* 346: 191–198.

Elwell, C., Chao, K., Patel, K., and Dreyfus, L. (**2001**). *Escherichia coli* CdtB mediates cytolethal distending toxin cell cycle arrest. *Infect. Immun.* 69: 3418–3422.

El-Zimaity, H.M., Ota, H., Graham, D.Y., Akamatsu, T., and Katsuyama, T. (**2002**). Patterns of gastric atrophy in intestinal type gastric carcinoma. *Cancer* 94: 1428–1436.

Engle, S. J., Ormsby, I., Pawlowski, S., Boivin, G.P., Croft, J., Balish, E., and Doetschman, T. (**2002**). Elimination of colon cancer in germ-free transforming growth factor beta 1-deficient mice. *Cancer Res.* 62: 6362–6366.

Enno, A., O'Rourke, J.L., Howlett, C.R., Jack, A., Dixon, M.F., and Lee, A. (**1995**). MALToma-like lesions in the murine gastric mucosa after long-term infection with *Heli-*

cobacter felis. A mouse model of *Helicobacter pylori* -induced gastric lymphoma. *Am. J. Pathol.* 147: 217–222.

Enroth, H., Kraaz, W., Engstrand, L., Nyren, O., and Rohan, T. (**2000**). *Helicobacter pylori* strain types and risk of gastric cancer: a case-control study. *Cancer Epidemiol. Biomarkers Prev.* 9: 981–985.

Erdman, S. E., Poutahidis, T., Tomczak, M., Rogers, A.B., Cormier, K., Plank, B., Horwitz, B.H., and Fox, J.G. (**2003a**). CD4+ CD25+ regulatory T lymphocytes inhibit microbially induced colon cancer in Rag2-deficient mice. *Am. J. Pathol.* 162: 691–702.

Erdman, S. E., Rao, V.P., Poutahidis, T., Ihrig, M.M., Ge, Z., Feng, Y., Tomczak, M., Rogers, A.B., Horwitz, B.H., and Fox, J.G. (**2003b**). CD4(+)CD25(+) regulatory lymphocytes require interleukin 10 to interrupt colon carcinogenesis in mice. *Cancer Res.* 63: 6042–6050.

Erdman, S. E., Sohn, J.J., Rao, V.P., Nambiar, P.R., Ge, Z., Fox, J.G., and Schauer, D.B. (**2005**). CD4+CD25+ regulatory lymphocytes induce regression of intestinal tumors in ApcMin/+ mice. *Cancer Res.* 65: 3998–4004.

Everhart, J.E., Kruszon-Moran, D., Perez-Perez, G.I., Tralka, T.S., and McQuillan, G. (**2000**). Seroprevalence and ethnic differences in *Helicobacter pylori* infection among adults in the United States. *J. Infect. Dis.* 181: 1359–1363.

Falk, P., Roth, K.A., Boren, T., Westblom, T.U., Gordon, J.I., and Normark, S. (**1993**). An in vitro adherence assay reveals that *Helicobacter pylori* exhibits cell lineage-specific tropism in the human gastric epithelium. *Proc. Natl. Acad. Sci. USA* 90: 2035–2039.

Falush, D., Wirth, T., Linz, B., Pritchard, J.K., Stephens, M., Kidd, M., Blaser, M.J., Graham, D.Y., Vacher, S., Perez-Perez, G.I., Yamaoka, Y., Megraud, F., Otto, K., Reichard, U., Katzowitsch, E., Wang, X., Achtman, M., and Suerbaum, S. (**2003**). Traces of human migrations in *Helicobacter pylori* populations. *Science* 299: 1582–1585.

Fan, X.G., Peng, X.N., Huang, Y., Yakoob, J., Wang, Z.M., and Chen, Y.P. (**2002**). *Helicobacter* species ribosomal DNA recovered from the liver tissue of Chinese patients with primary hepatocellular carcinoma. *Clin. Infect. Dis.* 35: 1555–1557.

Fennell, C.L., Totten, P.A., Quinn, T.C., Patton, D.L., Holmes, K.K., and Stamm, W.E. (**1984**). Characterization of Campylobacter-like organisms isolated from homosexual men. *J. Infect. Dis.* 149: 58–66.

Ferlay, J., Bray, F., Pisani, P., and Parkin, D.M. (**2004**). *GLOBOCAN 2002: Cancer incidence, mortality and prevalence worldwide.* IARC Press.

Ferrell, L., Theise, N., and Scheuer, P. (**2002**). Acute and chronic viral hepatitis. In: R. MacSween, A. Burt, B. Portman, K. Ishak, P. Scheuer, and P. Anthony (Eds.), *Pathology of Liver.* Churchill Livingston, London, pp. 313–362.

Figueiredo, C., Machado, J.C., Pharoah, P., Seruca, R., Sousa, S., Carvalho, R., Capelinha, A.F., Quint, W., Caldas, C., van Doorn, L.J., Carneiro, F., and Sobrinho-Simoes, M. (**2002**). *Helicobacter pylori* and interleukin 1 genotyping: an opportunity to identify high-risk individuals for gastric carcinoma. *J. Natl. Cancer Inst.* 94: 1680–1687.

Flores, B.M., Fennell, C.L., Kuller, L., Bronsdon, M.A., Morton, W.R., and Stamm, W.E. (**1990**). Experimental infection of pig-tailed macaques (*Macaca nemestrina*) with *Campylobacter cinaedi* and *Campylobacter fennelliae*. *Infect. Immun.* 58: 3947–3953.

Foley, J.E., Marks, S. L., Munson, L., Melli, A., Dewhirst, F.E., Yu, S., Shen, Z., and Fox, J.G. (**1999**). Isolation of *Helicobacter canis* from a colony of Bengal cats with endemic diarrhea. *J. Clin. Microbiol.* 37: 3271–3275.

Foltz, C.J., Fox, J.G., Yan, L., and Shames, B. (**1995**). Evaluation of antibiotic therapies for eradication of *Helicobacter hepaticus*. *Antimicrob. Agents Chemother.* 39: 1292–1294.

Foltz, C.J., Fox, J.G., Cahill, R., Murphy, J.C., Yan, L., Shames, B., and Schauer, D.B. (**1998**). Spontaneous inflammatory bowel disease in multiple mutant mouse lines: association with colonization by *Helicobacter hepaticus*. *Helicobacter* 3: 69–78.

Forman, D. (**1996**). *Helicobacter pylori* and gastric cancer. *Scand. J. Gastroenterol. Suppl.* 220: 23–26.

Forman, D., Newell, D.G., Fullerton, F., Yarnell, J.W., Stacey, A.R., Wald, N., and Sitas, F. (**1991**). Association between infection with *Helicobacter pylori* and risk of gastric cancer: evidence from a prospective investigation. *Br. Med. J.* 302: 1302–1305.

Foster, J.R. (1984). Bacterial infection of the common bile duct in chronic fascioliasis in the rat. *J. Comp. Pathol.* 94: 175–181.

Fox, J.G. (1988). *Biology and Diseases of the Ferret.* Lea & Febiger, Philadelphia.

Fox, J.G. (1997). The expanding genus of *Helicobacter*: pathogenic and zoonotic potential. *Semin. Gastrointest. Dis.* 8: 124–141.

Fox, J.G. (2002). The non-*H. pylori* helicobacters: their expanding role in gastrointestinal and systemic diseases. *Gut* 50: 273–283.

Fox, J.G. and Wang, T.C. (2001). *Helicobacter pylori* – not a good bug after all! *N. Engl. J. Med.* 345: 829–832.

Fox, J.G., Edrise, B.M., Cabot, E.B., Beaucage, C., Murphy, J.C., and Prostak, K.S. (1986). Campylobacter-like organisms isolated from gastric mucosa of ferrets. *Am. J. Vet. Res.* 47: 236–239.

Fox, J.G., Cabot, E.B., Taylor, N.S., and Laraway, R. (1988 a). Gastric colonization by *Campylobacter pylori* subsp. mustelae in ferrets. *Infect. Immun.* 56: 2994–2996.

Fox, J.G., Taylor, N.S., Edmonds, P., and Brenner, D.J. (1988 b). *Campylobacter pylori* subspecies mustelae subsp. nov. isolated from the gastric mucosa of ferrets (*Mustela putorius furo*), and an emended description of *Campylobacter pylori. Int. J. Syst. Bact.* 38: 367–370.

Fox, J.G., Chilvers, T., Goodwin, C.S., Taylor, N.S., Edmonds, P., Sly, L.I., and Brenner, D.J. (1989). *Campylobacter mustelae*, a new species resulting from the elevation of *Campylobacter pylori* subsp. mustelae to species status. *Int. J. Syst. Bact.* 39: 301–303.

Fox, J.G., Correa, P., Taylor, N.S., Lee, A., Otto, G., Murphy, J.C., and Rose, R. (1990). *Helicobacter mustelae*-associated gastritis in ferrets. An animal model of *Helicobacter pylori* gastritis in humans. *Gastroenterology* 99: 352–361.

Fox, J.G., Paster, B.J., Dewhirst, F.E., Taylor, N.S., Yan, L.L., Macuch, P.J., and Chmura, L.M. (1992). *Helicobacter mustelae* isolation from feces of ferrets: evidence to support fecal-oral transmission of a gastric *Helicobacter. Infect. Immun.* 60: 606–611.

Fox, J.G., Blanco, M.C., Yan, L., Shames, B., Polidoro, D., Dewhirst, F.E., and Paster, B.J. (1993 a). Role of gastric pH in isolation of *Helicobacter mustelae* from the feces of ferrets. *Gastroenterology* 104: 86–92.

Fox, J.G., Wishnok, J.S., Murphy, J.C., Tannenbaum, S. R., and Correa, P. (1993 b). MNNG-induced gastric carcinoma in ferrets infected with *Helicobacter mustelae. Carcinogenesis* 14: 1957–1961.

Fox, J.G., Dewhirst, F.E., Tully, J.G., Paster, B.J., Yan, L., Taylor, N.S., Collins, M.J., Jr., Gorelick, P.L., and Ward, J.M. (1994). *Helicobacter hepaticus* sp. nov., a microaerophilic bacterium isolated from livers and intestinal mucosal scrapings from mice. *J. Clin. Microbiol.* 32: 1238–1245.

Fox, J.G., Yan, L.L., Dewhirst, F.E., Paster, B.J., Shames, B., Murphy, J.C., Hayward, A., Belcher, J.C., and Mendes, E.N. (1995). *Helicobacter bilis* sp. nov., a novel *Helicobacter* species isolated from bile, livers, and intestines of aged, inbred mice. *J. Clin. Microbiol.* 33: 445–454.

Fox, J.G., Drolet, R., Higgins, R., Messier, S., Yan, L., Coleman, B.E., Paster, B.J., and Dewhirst, F.E. (1996 a). *Helicobacter canis* isolated from a dog liver with multifocal necrotizing hepatitis. *J. Clin. Microbiol.* 34: 2479–2482.

Fox, J.G., Li, X., Yan, L., Cahill, R.J., Hurley, R., Lewis, R., and Murphy, J.C. (1996 b). Chronic proliferative hepatitis in A/JCr mice associated with persistent *Helicobacter hepaticus* infection: a model of helicobacter-induced carcinogenesis. *Infect. Immun.* 64: 1548–1558.

Fox, J.G., Perkins, S., Yan, L., Shen, Z., Attardo, L., and Pappo, J. (1996 c). Local immune response in *Helicobacter pylori*-infected cats and identification of *H. pylori* in saliva, gastric fluid and faeces. *Immunology* 88: 400–406.

Fox, J.G., Yan, L., Shames, B., Campbell, J., Murphy, J.C., and Li, X. (1996 d). Persistent hepatitis and enterocolitis in germfree mice infected with *Helicobacter hepaticus. Infect. Immun.* 64: 3673–3681.

Fox, J.G., Dangler, C.A., Sager, W., Borkowski, R., and Gliatto, J.M. (1997). *Helicobacter mustelae*-associated gastric adenocarcinoma in ferrets (*Mustela putorius furo*). *Vet. Pathol.* 34: 225–229.

Fox, J.G., Dewhirst, F.E., Shen, Z., Feng, Y., Taylor, N.S., Paster, B.J., Ericson, R.L., Lau,

C.N., Correa, P., Araya, J.C., and Roa, I. (**1998**). Hepatic *Helicobacter* species identified in bile and gallbladder tissue from Chileans with chronic cholecystitis. *Gastroenterology* 114: 755–763.

Fox, J.G., Dangler, C.A., Taylor, N.S., King, A., Koh, T.J., and Wang, T.C. (**1999a**). High-salt diet induces gastric epithelial hyperplasia and parietal cell loss, and enhances *Helicobacter pylori* colonization in C57 BL/6 mice. *Cancer Res.* 59: 4823–4828.

Fox, J.G., Gorelick, P.L., Kullberg, M.C., Ge, Z., Dewhirst, F.E., and Ward, J.M. (**1999b**). A novel urease-negative *Helicobacter* species associated with colitis and typhlitis in IL-10-deficient mice. *Infect. Immun.* 67: 1757–1762.

Fox, J.G., Beck, P., Dangler, C.A., Whary, M.T., Wang, T.C., Shi, H.N., and Nagler-Anderson, C. (**2000a**). Concurrent enteric helminth infection modulates inflammation and gastric immune responses and reduces helicobacter-induced gastric atrophy. *Nat. Med.* 6: 536–542.

Fox, J.G., Chien, C.C., Dewhirst, F.E., Paster, B.J., Shen, Z., Melito, P.L., Woodward, D.L., and Rodgers, F. G. (**2000b**). *Helicobacter canadensis* sp. nov. isolated from humans with diarrhea as an example of an emerging pathogen. *J. Clin. Microbiol.* 38: 2546–2549.

Fox, J.G., Handt, L., Sheppard, B.J., Xu, S., Dewhirst, F.E., Motzel, S., and Klein, H. (**2001**). Isolation of *Helicobacter cinaedi* from the colon, liver, and mesenteric lymph node of a rhesus monkey with chronic colitis and hepatitis. *J. Clin. Microbiol.* 39: 1580–1585.

Fox, J.G., Shen, Z., Xu, S., Feng, Y., Dangler, C.A., Dewhirst, F.E., Paster, B.J., and Cullen, J.M. (**2002a**). *Helicobacter marmotae* sp. nov. isolated from livers of woodchucks and intestines of cats. *J. Clin. Microbiol.* 40: 2513–2519.

Fox, J.G., Sheppard, B.J., Dangler, C.A., Whary, M.T., Ihrig, M., and Wang, T.C. (**2002b**). Germ-line p53-targeted disruption inhibits helicobacter-induced premalignant lesions and invasive gastric carcinoma through down-regulation of Th1 proinflammatory responses. *Cancer Res.* 62: 696–702.

Fox, J.G., Rogers, A.B., Ihrig, M., Taylor, N.S., Whary, M.T., Dockray, G., Varro, A., and Wang, T.C. (**2003a**). *Helicobacter pylori*-associated gastric cancer in INS-GAS mice is gender specific. *Cancer Res.* 63: 942–950.

Fox, J.G., Wang, T.C., Rogers, A.B., Poutahidis, T., Ge, Z., Taylor, N., Dangler, C.A., Israel, D.A., Krishna, U., Gaus, K., and Peek, R.M., Jr. (**2003b**). Host and microbial constituents influence *Helicobacter pylori*-induced cancer in a murine model of hypergastrinemia. *Gastroenterology* 124: 1879–1890.

Fox, J.G., Rogers, A.B., Whary, M.T., Taylor, N.S., Xu, S., Feng, Y., and Keys, S. (**2004**). *Helicobacter bilis*-associated hepatitis in outbred mice. *Comp. Med.* 54: 571–577.

Franco, A.T., Israel, D.A., Washington, M.K., Krishna, U., Fox, J.G., Rogers, A.B., Neish, A.S., Collier-Hyams, L., Perez-Perez, G.I., Hatakeyama, M., Whitehead, R., Gaus, K., O'Brien, D.P., Romero-Gallo, J., and Peek, R.M., Jr. (**2005**). Activation of beta-catenin by carcinogenic *Helicobacter pylori*. *Proc. Natl. Acad. Sci. USA* 102: 10646–10651.

Franklin, C.L., Beckwith, C.S., Livingston, R.S., Riley, L.K., Gibson, S. V., Besch-Williford, C.L., and Hook, R.R., Jr. (**1996**). Isolation of a novel *Helicobacter* species, *Helicobacter cholecystus* sp. nov., from the gallbladders of Syrian hamsters with cholangiofibrosis and centrilobular pancreatitis. *J. Clin. Microbiol.* 34: 2952–2958.

Franklin, C.L., Riley, L.K., Livingston, R.S., Beckwith, C.S., Besch-Williford, C.L., and Hook, R.R., Jr. (**1998**). Enterohepatic lesions in SCID mice infected with *Helicobacter bilis*. *Lab. Anim. Sci.* 48: 334–339.

Franklin, C.L., Riley, L.K., Livingston, R.S., Beckwith, C.S., Hook, R.R., Jr., Besch-Williford, C.L., Hunziker, R., and Gorelick, P.L. (**1999**). Enteric lesions in SCID mice infected with "*Helicobacter typhlonicus*", a novel urease-negative *Helicobacter* species. *Lab. Anim. Sci.* 49: 496–505.

Franklin, C.L., Gorelick, P.L., Riley, L.K., Dewhirst, F.E., Livingston, R.S., Ward, J.M., Beckwith, C.S., and Fox, J.G. (**2001**). *Helicobacter typhlonicus* sp. nov., a novel murine urease-negative *Helicobacter* species. *J. Clin. Microbiol.* 39: 3920–3926.

Freedburg, A. and Barron, L. (**1940**). The presence of spirochetes in human gastric mucosa. *Am. J. Dig. Dis.* 7: 443–445.

Frommer, D.J., Carrick, J., Lee, A., and Hazell, S. L. (**1988**). Acute presentation of

Campylobacter pylori gastritis. *Am. J. Gastroenterol.* 83: 1168–1171.

Fujioka, T., Shuto, R., and Kodama, R. (**1993**). Experimental model for chronic gastritis with *Helicobacter pylori:* long term follow up study in *H. pylori*-infected Japanese macaques. *Eur. J. Gastroenterol. Hepatol.* Suppl. 1: S73–S77.

Fukuda, K., Kuroki, T., Tajima, Y., Tsuneoka, N., Kitajima, T., Matsuzaki, S., Furui, J., and Kanematsu, T. (**2002**). Comparative analysis of Helicobacter DNAs and biliary pathology in patients with and without hepatobiliary cancer. *Carcinogenesis* 23: 1927–1931.

Fukuda, Y., Yamamoto, I., and Tonokatsu, Y. (**1992**). Inoculation of rhesus monkeys with human *Helicobacter pylori:* a long term investigation on gastric mucosa by endoscopy. *Dig. Endosc.* 4: 19–30.

Furuta, T., Shirai, N., and Sugimoto, M. (**2004**). Controversy in polymorphisms of interleukin-1 beta in gastric cancer risks. *J. Gastroenterol.* 39: 501–503.

Garza-Gonzalez, E., Bosques-Padilla, F.J., Perez-Perez, G.I., Flores-Gutierrez, J.P., and Tijerina-Menchaca, R. (**2004**). Association of gastric cancer, HLA-DQA1, and infection with *Helicobacter pylori* CagA+ and VacA+ in a Mexican population. *J. Gastroenterol.* 39: 1138–1142.

Ge, Z., Doig, P., and Fox, J.G. (**2001**). Characterization of proteins in the outer membrane preparation of a murine pathogen, *Helicobacter bilis. Infect. Immun.* 69: 3502–3506.

Ge, Z., Feng, Y., Whary, M.T., Nambiar, P.R., Xu, S., Ng, V., Taylor, N.S., and Fox, J.G. (**2005**). Cytolethal distending toxin is essential for *Helicobacter hepaticus* colonization in outbred Swiss Webster mice. *Infect. Immun.* 73: 3559–3567.

Gebert, B., Fischer, W., Weiss, E., Hoffmann, R., and Haas, R. (**2003**). *Helicobacter pylori* vacuolating cytotoxin inhibits T lymphocyte activation. *Science* 301: 1099–1102.

Gebhart, C.J., Fennell, C.L., Murtaugh, M.P., and Stamm, W.E. (**1989**). *Campylobacter cinaedi* is normal intestinal flora in hamsters. *J. Clin. Microbiol.* 27: 1692–1694.

Ghiara, P., Marchetti, M., Blaser, M.J., Tummuru, M.K., Cover, T.L., Segal, E.D., Tompkins, L.S., and Rappuoli, R. (**1995**). Role of the *Helicobacter pylori* virulence factors vacuolating cytotoxin, CagA, and urease in a mouse model of disease. *Infect. Immun.* 63: 4154–4160.

Go, M.F., Kapur, V., Graham, D.Y., and Musser, J.M. (**1996**). Population genetic analysis of *Helicobacter pylori* by multilocus enzyme electrophoresis: extensive allelic diversity and recombinational population structure. *J. Bacteriol.* 178: 3934–3938.

Goddard, A.F., Logan, R.P., Atherton, J.C., Jenkins, D., and Spiller, R.C. (**1997**). Healing of duodenal ulcer after eradication of *Helicobacter heilmannii. Lancet* 349: 1815–1816.

Goh, K.L. and Parasakthi, N. (**2001**). The racial cohort phenomenon: seroepidemiology of *Helicobacter pylori* infection in a multiracial South-East Asian country. *Eur. J. Gastroenterol. Hepatol.* 13: 177–183.

Goodman, K.J., Correa, P., Tengana Aux, H.J., Ramirez, H., DeLany, J.P., Guerrero Pepinosa, O., Lopez Quinones, M., and Collazos Parra, T. (**1996**). *Helicobacter pylori* infection in the Colombian Andes: a population-based study of transmission pathways. *Am. J. Epidemiol.* 144: 290–299.

Goodwin, C., Armstrong, J.A., Chilvers, T., et al. (**1989**). Transfer of *Campylobacter pylori* and *Campylobacter mustelae* to *Helicobacter pylori* gen. nov. and *Helicobacter mustelae* comb. nov. and *Helicobacter mustelae* comb. nov., respectively. *Int. J. Syst. Bacteriol.* 39: 397–405.

Graham, D.Y., Lew, G.M., Klein, P.D., Evans, D.G., Evans, D.J., Jr., Saeed, Z.A., and Malaty, H.M. (**1992**). Effect of treatment of *Helicobacter pylori* infection on the long-term recurrence of gastric or duodenal ulcer. A randomized, controlled study. *Ann. Intern. Med.* 116: 705–708.

Greten, F.R., Eckmann, L., Greten, T.F., Park, J.M., Li, Z.W., Egan, L.J., Kagnoff, M.F., and Karin, M. (**2004**). IKKbeta links inflammation and tumorigenesis in a mouse model of colitis-associated cancer. *Cell* 118: 285–296.

Guillemin, K., Salama, N.R., Tompkins, L.S., and Falkow, S. (**2002**). Cag pathogenicity island-specific responses of gastric epithelial cells to *Helicobacter pylori* infection. *Proc. Natl. Acad. Sci. USA* 99: 15 136–15 141.

Hagemann, T., Wilson, J., Kulbe, H., Li, N.F., Leinster, D.A., Charles, K., Klemm, F.,

Pukrop, T., Binder, C., and Balkwill, F.R. (**2005**). Macrophages induce invasiveness of epithelial cancer cells via NF-kappa B and JNK. *J. Immunol.* 175: 1197–1205.

Haggerty, T.D., Perry, S., Sanchez, L., Perez-Perez, G., and Parsonnet, J. (**2005**). Significance of transiently positive enzyme-linked immunosorbent assay results in detection of *Helicobacter pylori* in stool samples from children. *J. Clin. Microbiol.* 43: 2220–2223.

Halldorsdottir, A.M., Sigurdardottrir, M., Jonasson, J.G., Oddsdottir, M., Magnusson, J., Lee, J.R., and Goldenring, J.R. (**2003**). Spasmolytic polypeptide-expressing metaplasia (SPEM) associated with gastric cancer in Iceland. *Dig. Dis. Sci.* 48: 431–441.

Handt, L.K., Fox, J.G., Dewhirst, F.E., Fraser, G.J., Paster, B.J., Yan, L.L., Rozmiarek, H., Rufo, R., and Stalis, I.H. (**1994**). *Helicobacter pylori* isolated from the domestic cat: public health implications. *Infect. Immun.* 62: 2367–2374.

Hansson, L.E., Nyren, O., Hsing, A.W., Bergstrom, R., Josefsson, S., Chow, W.H., Fraumeni, J.F., Jr., and Adami, H.O. (**1996**). The risk of stomach cancer in patients with gastric or duodenal ulcer disease. *N. Engl. J. Med.* 335: 242–249.

Harper, C.G., Feng, Y., Xu, S., Taylor, N.S., Kinsel, M., Dewhirst, F.E., Paster, B.J., Greenwell, M., Levine, G., Rogers, A., and Fox, J.G. (**2002**). *Helicobacter cetorum* sp. nov., a urease-positive *Helicobacter* species isolated from dolphins and whales. *J. Clin. Microbiol.* 40: 4536–4543.

Harper, C.G., Whary, M.T., Feng, Y., Rhinehart, H.L., Wells, R.S., Xu, S., Taylor, N.S., and Fox, J.G. (**2003**). Comparison of diagnostic techniques for *Helicobacter cetorum* infection in wild Atlantic bottlenose dolphins (*Tursiops truncatus*). *J. Clin. Microbiol.* 41: 2842–2848.

Harris, P.R., Cover, T.L., Crowe, D.R., Orenstein, J.M., Graham, M.F., Blaser, M.J., and Smith, P.D. (**1996**). *Helicobacter pylori* cytotoxin induces vacuolation of primary human mucosal epithelial cells. *Infect. Immun.* 64: 4867–4871.

Hassane, D.C., Lee, R.B., and Pickett, C.L. (**2003**). *Campylobacter jejuni* cytolethal distending toxin promotes DNA repair responses in normal human cells. *Infect. Immun.* 71: 541–545.

Heilmann, K.L. and Borchard, F. (**1991**). Gastritis due to spiral shaped bacteria other than *Helicobacter pylori*: clinical, histological, and ultrastructural findings. *Gut* 32: 137–140.

Helicobacter and Cancer Collaborative. (**2001**). Gastric cancer and *Helicobacter pylori*: A combined analysis of 12 case control studies nested within prospective cohorts. *Gut* 49: 347–353.

Hentschel, E., Brandstatter, G., Dragosics, B., Hirschl, A.M., Nemec, H., Schutze, K., Taufer, M., and Wurzer, H. (**1993**). Effect of ranitidine and amoxicillin plus metronidazole on the eradication of *Helicobacter pylori* and the recurrence of duodenal ulcer. *N. Engl. J. Med.* 328: 308–312.

Herbarth, O., Krumbiegel, P., Fritz, G.J., Richter, M., Schlink, U., Müller, D.M., and Richter, T. (**2001**). *Helicobacter pylori* prevalences and risk factors among school beginners in a German urban center and its rural county. *Environ. Health Perspect.* 109: 573–577.

Higashi, H., Tsutsumi, R., Fujita, A., Yamazaki, S., Asaka, M., Azuma, T., and Hatakeyama, M. (**2002a**). Biological activity of the Helicobacter pylori virulence factor CagA is determined by variation in the tyrosine phosphorylation sites. *Proc. Natl. Acad. Sci. USA* 99: 14428–14433.

Higashi, H., Tsutsumi, R., Muto, S., Sugiyama, T., Azuma, T., Asaka, M., and Hatakeyama, M. (**2002b**). SHP-2 tyrosine phosphatase as an intracellular target of *Helicobacter pylori* CagA protein. *Science* 295: 683–686.

Hill, P. and Rode, J. (**1998**). *Helicobacter pylori* in ectopic gastric mucosa in Meckel's diverticulum. *Pathology* 30: 7–9.

Hilzenrat, N., Lamoureux, E., Weintrub, I., Alpert, E., Lichter, M., and Alpert, L. (**1995**). *Helicobacter heilmannii*-like spiral bacteria in gastric mucosal biopsies. Prevalence and clinical significance. *Arch. Pathol. Lab. Med.* 119: 1149–1153.

Hirayama, F., Takagi, S., Kusuhara, H., Iwao, E., Yokoyama, Y., and Ikeda, Y. (**1996**). Induction of gastric ulcer and intestinal metaplasia in Mongolian gerbils infected with *Helicobacter pylori*. *J. Gastroenterol.* 31: 755–757.

Ho, S. A., Hoyle, J.A., Lewis, F.A., Secker, A.D., Cross, D., Mapstone, N.P., Dixon,

M.F., Wyatt, J.I., Tompkins, D.S., Taylor, G.R., et al. (**1991**). Direct polymerase chain reaction test for detection of *Helicobacter pylori* in humans and animals. *J. Clin. Microbiol.* 29: 2543–2549.

Hocker, M., Rosenberg, I., Xavier, R., Henihan, R.J., Wiedenmann, B., Rosewicz, S., Podolsky, D.K., and Wang, T.C. (**1998**). Oxidative stress activates the human histidine decarboxylase promoter in AGS gastric cancer cells. *J. Biol. Chem.* 273: 23 046–23 054.

Hojo, M., Miwa, H., Ohkusa, T., Ohkura, R., Kurosawa, A., and Sato, N. (**2002**). Alteration of histological gastritis after cure of *Helicobacter pylori* infection. *Aliment. Pharmacol. Ther.* 16: 1923–1932.

Honda, S., Fujioka, T., Tokieda, M., Gotoh, T., Nishizono, A., and Nasu, M. (**1998 a**). Gastric ulcer, atrophic gastritis, and intestinal metaplasia caused by *Helicobacter pylori* infection in Mongolian gerbils. *Scand. J. Gastroenterol.* 33: 454–460.

Honda, S., Fujioka, T., Tokieda, M., Satoh, R., Nishizono, A., and Nasu, M. (**1998 b**). Development of *Helicobacter pylori*-induced gastric carcinoma in Mongolian gerbils. *Cancer Res.* 58: 4255–4259.

Hopkins, R.J., Vial, P.A., Ferreccio, C., Ovalle, J., Prado, P., Sotomayor, V., Russell, R.G., Wasserman, S. S., and Morris, J.G., Jr. (**1993**). Seroprevalence of *Helicobacter pylori* in Chile: vegetables may serve as one route of transmission. *J. Infect. Dis.* 168: 222–226.

Houghton, J. and Wang, T.C. (**2005**). *Helicobacter pylori* and gastric cancer: a new paradigm for inflammation-associated epithelial cancers. *Gastroenterology* 128: 1567–1578.

Houghton, J., Macera-Bloch, L.S., Harrison, L., Kim, K.H., and Korah, R.M. (**2000 a**). Tumor necrosis factor alpha and interleukin 1 beta up-regulate gastric mucosal Fas antigen expression in *Helicobacter pylori* infection. *Infect. Immun.* 68: 1189–1195.

Houghton, J.M., Bloch, L.M., Goldstein, M., Von Hagen, S., and Korah, R.M. (**2000 b**). In vivo disruption of the fas pathway abrogates gastric growth alterations secondary to *Helicobacter* infection. *J. Infect. Dis.* 182: 856–864.

Houghton, J., Fox, J.G., and Wang, T.C. (**2002**). Gastric cancer: laboratory bench to clinic. *J. Gastroenterol. Hepatol.* 17: 495–502.

Houghton, J., Stoicov, C., Nomura, S., Rogers, A.B., Carlson, J., Li, H., Cai, X., Fox, J.G., Goldenring, J.R., and Wang, T.C. (**2004**). Gastric cancer originating from bone marrow-derived cells. *Science* 306: 1568–1571.

Howson, C.P., Hiyama, T., and Wynder, E.L. (**1986**). The decline in gastric cancer: epidemiology of an unplanned triumph. *Epidemiol. Rev.* 8: 1–27.

Huang, J.Q., Zheng, G.F., Sumanac, K., Irvine, E.J., and Hunt, R.H. (**2003**). Meta-analysis of the relationship between cagA seropositivity and gastric cancer. *Gastroenterology* 125: 1636–1644.

Hulten, K., Han, S. W., Enroth, H., Klein, P.D., Opekun, A.R., Gilman, R.H., Evans, D.G., Engstrand, L., Graham, D.Y., and El-Zaatari, F.A. (**1996**). *Helicobacter pylori* in the drinking water in Peru. *Gastroenterology* 110: 1031–1035.

Hunt, R.H. (**1996**). The role of *Helicobacter pylori* in pathogenesis: the spectrum of clinical outcomes. *Scand. J. Gastroenterol. Suppl.* 220: 3–9.

Hussell, T., Isaacson, P.G., Crabtree, J.E., and Spencer, J. (**1996**). *Helicobacter pylori*-specific tumour-infiltrating T cells provide contact dependent help for the growth of malignant B cells in low-grade gastric lymphoma of mucosa-associated lymphoid tissue. *J. Pathol.* 178: 122–127.

IARC working group on the evaluation of carcinogenic risks to humans. (**1994**). *Schistosomes, liver flukes and* Helicobacter pylori. International Agency for Research on Cancer, Lyon, France.

Ihrig, M., Schrenzel, M.D., and Fox, J.G. (**1999**). Differential susceptibility to hepatic inflammation and proliferation in AXB recombinant inbred mice chronically infected with *Helicobacter hepaticus. Am. J. Pathol.* 155: 571–582.

Ihrig, M., Whary, M.T., Dangler, C.A., and Fox, J.G. (**2005**). Gastric helicobacter infection induces a Th2 phenotype but does not elevate serum cholesterol in mice lacking inducible nitric oxide synthase. *Infect. Immun.* 73: 1664–1670.

Ilver, D., Arnqvist, A., Ogren, J., Frick, I.M., Kersulyte, D., Incecik, E.T., Berg, D.E., Covacci, A., Engstrand, L., and Boren, T. (**1998**). *Helicobacter pylori* adhesin binding fucosylated histo-blood group antigens revealed by retagging. *Science* 279: 373–377.

International Agency for Research on Cancer, a. WHO (**1994**). *Schistosomes, liver flukes and* Helicobacter pylori. Lyon, France: IARC; Geneva: Distributed for the International Agency for Research on Cancer by the Secretariat of the World Health Organization.

Israel, D.A., Salama, N., Arnold, C.N., Moss, S. F., Ando, T., Wirth, H.P., Tham, K.T., Camorlinga, M., Blaser, M.J., Falkow, S., and Peek, R.M., Jr. (**2001**). *Helicobacter pylori* strain- specific differences in genetic content, identified by microarray, influence host inflammatory responses. *J. Clin. Invest.* 107: 611–620.

Itoh, T., Wakatsuki, Y., Yoshida, M., Usui, T., Matsunaga, Y., Kaneko, S., Chiba, T., and Kita, T. (**1999**). The vast majority of gastric T cells are polarized to produce T helper 1 type cytokines upon antigenic stimulation despite the absence of *Helicobacter pylori* infection. *J. Gastroenterol.* 34: 560–570.

Jarvis, D., Luczynska, C., Chinn, S., and Burney, P. (**2004**). The association of hepatitis A and *Helicobacter pylori* with sensitization to common allergens, asthma and hay fever in a population of young British adults. *Allergy* 59: 1063–1067.

Jiang, H.Q., Kushnir, N., Thurnheer, M.C., Bos, N.A., and Cebra, J.J. (**2002**). Monoassociation of SCID mice with *Helicobacter muridarum*, but not four other enterics, provokes IBD upon receipt of T cells. *Gastroenterology* 122: 1346–1354.

Jones, D. and Curry, A. (**1990**). The genesis of coccal forms of *Helicobacter pylori*. In: P. Malfertheiner and H. Ditschuneit (Eds.), Helicobacter pylori, *Gastritis and Peptic Ulcer*. Springer, Berlin, pp. 29–37.

Judd, L.M., Alderman, B.M., Howlett, M., Shulkes, A., Dow, C., Moverley, J., Grail, D., Jenkins, B.J., Ernst, M., and Giraud, A.S. (**2004**). Gastric cancer development in mice lacking the SHP2 binding site on the IL-6 family co-receptor gp130. *Gastroenterology* 126: 196–207.

Kandasami, P., Tan, W.J., and Norain, K. (**2003**). Gastric cancer in Malaysia: the need for early diagnosis. *Med. J. Malaysia* 58: 758–762.

Kane, M. (**1995**). Global programme for control of hepatitis B infection. *Vaccine* 13 (Suppl 1): S47–S49.

Kang, W., Rathinavelu, S., Samuelson, L.C., and Merchant, J.L. (**2005**). Interferon gamma induction of gastric mucous neck cell hypertrophy. *Lab. Invest.* 85: 702–715.

Kansau, I., Raymond, J., Bingen, E., Courcoux, P., Kalach, N., Bergeret, M., Braimi, N., Dupont, C., and Labigne, A. (**1996**). Genotyping of *Helicobacter pylori* isolates by sequencing of PCR products and comparison with the RAPD technique. *Res. Microbiol.* 147: 661–669.

Karim, Q.N. and Maxwell, R.H. (**1989**). Survival of *Campylobacter pylori* in artificially contaminated milk. *J. Clin. Pathol.* 42: 778.

Kawasaki, K., Nishio, A., Nakamura, H., Uchida, K., Fukui, T., Ohana, M., Yoshizawa, H., Ohashi, S., Tamaki, H., Matsuura, M., Asada, M., Nishi, T., Nakase, H., Toyokuni, S., Liu, W., Yodoi, J., Okazaki, K., and Chiba, T. (**2005**). *Helicobacter felis*-induced gastritis was suppressed in mice overexpressing thioredoxin-1. *Lab. Invest.* 85: 1104–1117.

Keates, S., Hitti, Y.S., Upton, M., and Kelly, C.P. (**1997**). *Helicobacter pylori* infection activates NF-kappa B in gastric epithelial cells. *Gastroenterology* 113: 1099–1109.

Kelly, S. M., Pitcher, M.C., Farmery, S. M., and Gibson, G.R. (**1994**). Isolation of *Helicobacter pylori* from feces of patients with dyspepsia in the United Kingdom. *Gastroenterology* 107: 1671–1674.

Kersulyte, D., Chalkauskas, H., and Berg, D.E. (**1999**). Emergence of recombinant strains of *Helicobacter pylori* during human infection. *Mol. Microbiol.* 31: 31–43.

Kiehlbauch, J.A., Tauxe, R.V., Baker, C.N., and Wachsmuth, I.K. (**1994**). *Helicobacter cinaedi*-associated bacteremia and cellulitis in immunocompromised patients. *Ann. Intern. Med.* 121: 90–93.

Kirkbride, C.A., Gates, C.E., Collins, J.E., and Ritchie, A.E. (**1985**). Ovine abortion associated with an anaerobic bacterium. *J. Am. Vet. Med. Assoc.* 186: 789–791.

Klein, P.D., Graham, D.Y., Gaillour, A., Opekun, A.R., and Smith, E.O. (**1991**).

Water source as risk factor for *Helicobacter pylori* infection in Peruvian children. Gastrointestinal Physiology Working Group. *Lancet* 337: 1503–1506.

Koike, K., Tsutsumi, T., Fujie, H., Shintani, Y., and Kyoji, M. (**2002**). Molecular mechanism of viral hepatocarcinogenesis. *Oncology* 62 (Suppl 1): S29–S37.

Körber-Golze, B. and Scupin, E. (**1993**). *Helicobacter pylori:* studies in domestic swine. *Dtsch. Tierarztl. Wochenschr.* 100: 465–468.

Kornilovs'ka, I., Nilsson, I., Utt, M., Ljungh, A., and Wadstrom, T. (**2002**). Immunogenic proteins of *Helicobacter pullorum, Helicobacter bilis* and *Helicobacter hepaticus* identified by two-dimensional gel electrophoresis and immunoblotting. *Proteomics* 2: 775–783.

Kountouras, J., Zavos, C., and Chatzopoulos, D. (**2005**). New concepts of molecular biology on gastric carcinogenesis. *Hepatogastroenterology* 52: 1305–1312.

Kraft, C., Stack, A., Josenhans, C., Niehus, E., Dietrich, G., Correa, P., Fox, J.G., Falush, D., and Suerbaum, S. (**2006**). Genomic changes during chronic *Helicobacter pylori* infection. *J. Bacteriol.* 188: 249–254.

Krienitz, W. (**1906**). Über das Auftreten von Mageninhalt bei carcinoma ventriculi. *Dtsch. Med. Wochenschr.* 22: 872.

Kuhn, R., Lohler, J., Rennick, D., Rajewsky, K., and Muller, W. (**1993**). Interleukin-10-deficient mice develop chronic enterocolitis. *Cell* 75: 263–274.

Kuipers, E.J., Uyterlinde, A.M., Pena, A.S., Roosendaal, R., Pals, G., Nelis, G.F., Festen, H.P., and Meuwissen, S. G. (**1995**). Long-term sequelae of *Helicobacter pylori* gastritis. *Lancet* 345: 1525–1528.

Kullavanijaya, P., Tangkijvanich, P., and Poovorawan, Y. (**1999**). Current status of infection-related gastrointestinal and hepatobiliary diseases in Thailand. *Southeast Asian J. Trop. Med. Public Health* 30: 96–105.

Kullberg, M.C., Ward, J.M., Gorelick, P.L., Caspar, P., Hieny, S., Cheever, A., Jankovic, D., and Sher, A. (**1998**). *Helicobacter hepaticus* triggers colitis in specific-pathogen-free interleukin-10 (IL-10)-deficient mice through an IL-12- and gamma interferon-dependent mechanism. *Infect. Immun.* 66: 5157–5166.

Kullberg, M.C., Jankovic, D., Gorelick, P.L., Caspar, P., Letterio, J.J., Cheever, A.W., and Sher, A. (**2002**). Bacteria-triggered CD4(+) T regulatory cells suppress *Helicobacter hepaticus*-induced colitis. *J. Exp. Med.* 196: 505–515.

Kusmartsev, S. and Gabrilovich, D.I. (**2005**). STAT1 signaling regulates tumor-associated macrophage-mediated T cell deletion. *J. Immunol.* 174: 4880–4891.

Labenz, J., Blum, A.L., Bayerdorffer, E., Meining, A., Stolte, M., and Borsch, G. (**1997**). Curing *Helicobacter pylori* infection in patients with duodenal ulcer may provoke reflux esophagitis. *Gastroenterology* 112: 1442–1447.

Lane, J.A., Harvey, R.F., Murray, L.J., Harvey, I.M., Donovan, J.L., Nair, P., and Egger, M. (**2002**). A placebo-controlled randomized trial of eradication of *Helicobacter pylori* in the general population: study design and response rates of the Bristol Helicobacter Project. *Control. Clin. Trials* 23: 321–332.

Lara-Tejero, M. and Galan, J.E. (**2000**). A bacterial toxin that controls cell cycle progression as a deoxyribonuclease I-like protein. *Science* 290: 354–357.

Lara-Tejero, M. and Galan, J.E. (**2001**). CdtA, CdtB, and CdtC form a tripartite complex that is required for cytolethal distending toxin activity. *Infect. Immun.* 69: 4358–4365.

Lavelle, J.P., Landas, S., Mitros, F.A., and Conklin, J.L. (**1994**). Acute gastritis associated with spiral organisms from cats. *Dig. Dis. Sci.* 39: 744–750.

Lee, A. and O'Rourke, J. (**1993**). Gastric bacteria other than *Helicobacter pylori*. *Gastroenterol. Clin. North Am.* 22: 21–42.

Lee, A., Hazell, S. L., O'Rourke, J., and Kouprach, S. (**1988**). Isolation of a spiral-shaped bacterium from the cat stomach. *Infect. Immun.* 56: 2843–2850.

Lee, A., Fox, J.G., Otto, G., and Murphy, J. (**1990**). A small animal model of human *Helicobacter pylori* active chronic gastritis. *Gastroenterology* 99: 1315–1323.

Lee, A., Phillips, M.W., O'Rourke, J.L., Paster, B.J., Dewhirst, F.E., Fraser, G.J., Fox, J.G., Sly, L.I., Romaniuk, P.J., Trust, T.J., et al. (**1992**). *Helicobacter muridarum* sp. nov., a microaerophilic helical bacterium with a novel ultrastructure isolated from the intestinal mucosa of rodents. *Int. J. Syst. Bacteriol.* 42: 27–36.

Lee, A., Fox, J., and Hazell, S. (**1993**). Pathogenicity of *Helicobacter pylori:* a perspective. *Infect Immun* 61: 1601–1610.

Lee, A., O'Rourke, J., De Ungria, M.C., Robertson, B., Daskalopoulos, G., and Dixon, M.F. (**1997**). A standardized mouse model of *Helicobacter pylori* infection: introducing the Sydney strain. *Gastroenterology* 112: 1386–1397.

Lee, J.R., Baxter, T.M., Yamaguchi, H., Wang, T.C., Goldenring, J.R., and Anderson, M.G. (**2003**). Differential protein analysis of spasomolytic polypeptide expressing metaplasia using laser capture microdissection and two-dimensional difference gel electrophoresis. *Appl. Immunohistochem. Mol. Morphol.* 11: 188–193.

Lee, W.P., Tai, D.I., Lan, K.H., Li, A.F., Hsu, H.C., Lin, E.J., Lin, Y.P., Sheu, M.L., Li, C.P., Chang, F.Y., Chao, Y., Yen, S. H., and Lee, S. D. (**2005**). The -251T allele of the interleukin-8 promoter is associated with increased risk of gastric carcinoma featuring diffuse-type histopathology in Chinese population. *Clin. Cancer Res.* 11: 6431–6441.

Leong, R.W. and Sung, J.J. (**2002**). Review article: *Helicobacter* species and hepatobiliary diseases. *Aliment. Pharmacol. Ther.* 16: 1037–1045.

Leung, W.K., Siu, K.L., Kwok, C.K., Chan, S. Y., Sung, R., and Sung, J.J. (**1999**). Isolation of *Helicobacter pylori* from vomitus in children and its implication in gastro-oral transmission. *Am. J. Gastroenterol.*94: 2881–2884.

Leunk, R.D., Johnson, P.T., David, B.C., Kraft, W.G., and Morgan, D.R. (**1988**). Cytotoxic activity in broth-culture filtrates of *Campylobacter pylori*. *J. Med. Microbiol.* 26: 93–99.

Li, L., Sharipo, A., Chaves-Olarte, E., Masucci, M.G., Levitsky, V., Thelestam, M., and Frisan, T. (**2002**). The *Haemophilus ducreyi* cytolethal distending toxin activates sensors of DNA damage and repair complexes in proliferating and non-proliferating cells. *Cell Microbiol.* 4: 87–99.

Li, Q., Karam, S. M., and Gordon, J.I. (**1996**). Diphtheria toxin-mediated ablation of parietal cells in the stomach of transgenic mice. *J. Biol. Chem.* 271: 3671–3676.

Lin, E.Y., Nguyen, A.V., Russell, R.G., and Pollard, J.W. (**2001**). Colony-stimulating factor 1 promotes progression of mammary tumors to malignancy. *J. Exp. Med.* 193: 727–740.

Linden, S., Nordman, H., Hedenbro, J., Hurtig, M., Boren, T., and Carlstedt, I. (**2002**). Strain- and blood group-dependent binding of *Helicobacter pylori* to human gastric MUC5AC glycoforms. *Gastroenterology* 123: 1923–1930.

Lipkin, M. and Higgins, P. (**1988**). Biological markers of cell proliferation and differentiation in human gastrointestinal diseases. *Adv. Cancer Res.* 50: 1–24.

Liu, C., Russell, R.M., and Wang, X.D. (**2006**). Lycopene supplementation prevents smoke-induced changes in p53, p53 phosphorylation, cell proliferation, and apoptosis in the gastric mucosa of ferrets. *J. Nutr.* 136: 106–111.

Liu, H., Ye, H., Ruskone-Fourmestraux, A., De Jong, D., Pileri, S., Thiede, C., Lavergne, A., Boot, H., Caletti, G., Wundisch, T., Molina, T., Taal, B.G., Elena, S., Thomas, T., Zinzani, P.L., Neubauer, A., Stolte, M., Hamoudi, R.A., Dogan, A., Isaacson, P.G., and Du, M.Q. (**2002**). T(11;18) is a marker for all stage gastric MALT lymphomas that will not respond to *H. pylori* eradication. *Gastroenterology* 122: 1286–1294.

Lockard, V.G. and Boler, R.K. (**1970**). Ultrastructure of a spiraled microorganism in the gastric mucosa of dogs. *Am. J. Vet. Res.* 31: 1453–1462.

Lu, Y., Redlinger, T.E., Avitia, R., Galindo, A., and Goodman, K. (**2002**). Isolation and genotyping of *Helicobacter pylori* from untreated municipal wastewater. *Appl. Environ. Microbiol.* 68: 1436–1439.

Luperchio, S., Tamir, S., and Tannenbaum, S. R. (**1996**). No-induced oxidative stress and glutathione metabolism in rodent and human cells. *Free Radic. Biol. Med.* 21: 513–519.

Machado, J.C., Pharoah, P., Sousa, S., Carvalho, R., Oliveira, C., Figueiredo, C., Amorim, A., Seruca, R., Caldas, C., Carneiro, F., and Sobrinho-Simoes, M. (**2001**). Interleukin 1B and interleukin 1RN polymorphisms are associated with increased risk of gastric carcinoma. *Gastroenterology* 121: 823–829.

Madden, C.R., Finegold, M.J., and Slagle, B.L. (**2001**). Hepatitis B virus X protein acts as a tumor promoter in development of diethylnitrosamine-induced preneoplastic lesions. *J. Virol.* 75: 3851–3858.

Maggio-Price, L., Bielefeldt-Ohmann, H., Treuting, P., Iritani, B.M., Zeng, W., Nicks, A., Tsang, M., Shows, D., Morrissey, P., and Viney, J.L. (**2005**). Dual infection with *Helicobacter bilis* and *Helicobacter hepaticus* in p-glycoprotein-deficient mdr1 a-/- mice results in colitis that progresses to dysplasia. *Am. J. Pathol.* 166: 1793–1806.

Maggio-Price, L., Treuting, P., Zeng, W., Tsang, M., Bielefeldt-Ohmann, H., and Iritani, B. M. (**2006**). *Helicobacter* infection is required for inflammation and colon cancer in SMAD3-deficient mice. *Cancer Res.* 66: 828–838.

Mahdavi, J., Sonden, B., Hurtig, M., Olfat, F.O., Forsberg, L., Roche, N., Angstrom, J., Larsson, T., Teneberg, S., Karlsson, K.A., Altraja, S., Wadstrom, T., Kersulyte, D., Berg, D.E., Dubois, A., Petersson, C., Magnusson, K.E., Norberg, T., Lindh, F., Lundskog, B.B., Arnqvist, A., Hammarstrom, L., and Boren, T. (**2002**). *Helicobacter pylori* SabA adhesin in persistent infection and chronic inflammation. *Science* 297: 573–578.

Mai, U.E.H., Schahamat, M., and Cowell, R.R. (**1991**). Survival of *Helicobacter pylori* in the aquatic environment. In: H. Menge, M. Gregor, G.N. Tytgat, B.J. Marshall, and C. McNulty (Eds.), *Helicobacter pylori*. Springer, Berlin.

Mandell, L., Moran, A.P., Cocchiarella, A., Houghton, J., Taylor, N., Fox, J.G., Wang, T.C., and Kurt-Jones, E.A. (**2004**). Intact gram-negative *Helicobacter pylori*, *Helicobacter felis*, and *Helicobacter hepaticus* bacteria activate innate immunity via toll-like receptor 2 but not toll-like receptor 4. *Infect. Immun.* 72: 6446–6454.

Marchetti, M., Arico, B., Burroni, D., Figura, N., Rappuoli, R., and Ghiara, P. (**1995**). Development of a mouse model of *Helicobacter pylori* infection that mimics human disease. *Science* 267: 1655–1658.

Marshall, B.J. and Warren, J.R. (**1983**). Unidentified curved bacillus on gastric epithelium in active chronic gastritis. *Lancet* i: 1273–1275.

Marshall, B.J. and Warren, J.R. (**1984**). Unidentified curved bacilli in the stomach of patients with gastritis and peptic ulceration. *Lancet* i: 1311–1315.

Marshall, B.J. and Windsor, H.M. (**2005**). The relation of *Helicobacter pylori* to gastric adenocarcinoma and lymphoma: pathophysiology, epidemiology, screening, clinical presentation, treatment, and prevention. *Med. Clin. North Am.* 89: 313–344, viii.

Marshall, B.J., Armstrong, J.A., McGechie, D.B., and Glancy, R.J. (**1985**). Attempt to fulfil Koch's postulates for pyloric *Campylobacter*. *Med. J. Aust.* 142: 436–439.

Mast, E.E., Alter, M.J., and Margolis, H.S. (**1999**). Strategies to prevent and control hepatitis B and C virus infections: a global perspective. *Vaccine* 17: 1730–1733.

Matsuda, R. and Morizane, T. (**2005**). *Helicobacter pylori* infection in dental professionals: a 6-year prospective study. *Helicobacter* 10: 307–311.

Matsukura, N., Yokomuro, S., Yamada, S., Tajiri, T., Sundo, T., Hadama, T., Kamiya, S., Naito, Z., and Fox, J.G. (**2002**). Association between *Helicobacter bilis* in bile and biliary tract malignancies: *H. bilis* in bile from Japanese and Thai patients with benign and malignant diseases in the biliary tract. *Jpn. J. Cancer Res.* 93: 842–847.

Maurer, K.J., Ihrig, M.M., Rogers, A.B., Ng, V., Bouchard, G., Leonard, M.R., Carey, M.C., and Fox, J.G. (**2005**). Identification of cholelithogenic enterohepatic *Helicobacter* species and their role in murine cholesterol gallstone formation. *Gastroenterology* 128: 1023–1033.

Mayr, M., Kiechl, S., Willeit, J., Wick, G., and Xu, Q. (**2000**). Infections, immunity, and atherosclerosis: associations of antibodies to *Chlamydia pneumoniae*, *Helicobacter pylori*, and cytomegalovirus with immune reactions to heat-shock protein 60 and carotid or femoral atherosclerosis. *Circulation* 102: 833–839.

McColl, K., Murray, L., El-Omar, E., Dickson, A., El-Nujumi, A., Wirz, A., Kelman, A., Penny, C., Knill-Jones, R., and Hilditch, T. (**1998**). Symptomatic benefit from eradicating *Helicobacter pylori* infection in patients with nonulcer dyspepsia. *N. Engl. J. Med.* 339: 1869–1874.

McCracken, V.J., Martin, S. M., and Lorenz, R.G. (**2005**). The *Helicobacter felis* model of adoptive transfer gastritis. *Immunol. Res.* 33: 183–194.

Melito, P.L., Munro, C., Chipman, P.R., Woodward, D.L., Booth, T.F., and Rodgers,

F.G. (**2001**). *Helicobacter winghamensis* sp. nov., a novel *Helicobacter* sp. isolated from patients with gastroenteritis. *J. Clin. Microbiol.* 39: 2412–2417.

Menaker, R.J., Sharaf, A.A., and Jones, N.L. (**2004**). *Helicobacter pylori* infection and gastric cancer: host, bug, environment, or all three? *Curr. Gastroenterol. Rep.* 6: 429–435.

Mendall, M.A., Goggin, P.M., Molineaux, N., Levy, J., Toosy, T., Strachan, D., and Northfield, T.C. (**1992**). Childhood living conditions and *Helicobacter pylori* seropositivity in adult life. *Lancet* 339: 896–897.

Mendes, E.N., Queiroz, D.M., Dewhirst, F.E., Paster, B.J., Rocha, G.A., and Fox, J.G. (**1994**). Are pigs a reservoir host for human *Helicobacter* infection? *Am. J. Gastroenterol.* 89: 1296.

Mendes, E.N., Queiroz, D.M., Dewhirst, F.E., Paster, B.J., Moura, S. B., and Fox, J.G. (**1996**). *Helicobacter trogontum* sp. nov., isolated from the rat intestine. *Int. J. Syst. Bacteriol.* 46: 916–921.

Mera, R., Fontham, E.T., Bravo, L.E., Bravo, J.C., Piazuelo, M.B., Camargo, M.C., and Correa, P. (**2005**). Long term follow up of patients treated for *Helicobacter pylori* infection. *Gut* 54: 1536–1540.

Mitchell, H.M., Li, Y.Y., Hu, P.J., Liu, Q., Chen, M., Du, G.G., Wang, Z.J., Lee, A., and Hazell, S. L. (**1992 a**). Epidemiology of *Helicobacter pylori* in southern China: identification of early childhood as the critical period for acquisition. *J. Infect. Dis.* 166: 149–153.

Mitchell, J.D., Mitchell, H.M., and Tobias, V. (**1992 b**). Acute *Helicobacter pylori* infection in an infant, associated with gastric ulceration and serological evidence of intrafamilial transmission. *Am. J. Gastroenterol.* 87: 382–386.

Mitchell, H.M., Ally, R., Wadee, A., Wiseman, M., and Segal, I. (**2002**). Major differences in the IgG subclass response to *Helicobacter pylori* in the first and third worlds. *Scand. J. Gastroenterol.* 37: 517–522.

Moayyedi, P., Axon, A.T., Feltbower, R., Duffett, S., Crocombe, W., Braunholtz, D., Richards, I.D. Dowell, A.C., and Forman, D. (**2002**). Relation of adult lifestyle and socioeconomic factors to the prevalence of *Helicobacter pylori* infection. *Int. J. Epidemiol.* 31: 624–631.

Mobley, H.L. (**1997**). *Helicobacter pylori* factors associated with disease development. *Gastroenterology* 113: S21–S28.

Modlin, I.M., and Sachs, G. (**1998**). Acid related diseases: Biology and treatment. In: Konstanz, H. (Ed.), *Helicobacter pylori*. Schnetztor-Verlag GmbH, Germany, pp. 315–364.

Mohammadi, M., Redline, R., Nedrud, J., and Czinn, S. (**1996**). Role of the host in pathogenesis of Helicobacter-associated gastritis: *H. felis* infection of inbred and congenic mouse strains. *Infect. Immun.* 64: 238–245.

Mohammadi, M., Nedrud, J., Redline, R., Lycke, N., and Czinn, S. J. (**1997**). Murine CD4 T-cell response to *Helicobacter* infection: TH1 cells enhance gastritis and TH2 cells reduce bacterial load. *Gastroenterology* 113: 1848–1857.

Montani, A., Sasazuki, S., Inoue, M., Higuchi, K., Arakawa, T., and Tsugane, S. (**2003**). Food/nutrient intake and risk of atrophic gastritis among the *Helicobacter pylori*-infected population of northeastern Japan. *Cancer Sci.* 94: 372–377.

Morgner, A., Bayerdorffer, E., Meining, A., Stolte, M., and Kroher, G. (**1995**). *Helicobacter heilmannii* and gastric cancer. *Lancet* 346: 511–512.

Morgner, A., Lehn, N., Andersen, L.P., Thiede, C., Bennedsen, M., Trebesius, K., Neubauer, B., Neubauer, A., Stolte, M., and Bayerdorffer, E. (**2000**). *Helicobacter heilmannii*-associated primary gastric low-grade MALT lymphoma: complete remission after curing the infection. *Gastroenterology* 118: 821–828.

Morris, A. and Nicholson, G. (**1987**). Ingestion of *Campylobacter pyloridis* causes gastritis and raised fasting gastric pH. *Am. J. Gastroenterol.* 82: 192–199.

Morris, A.J., Ali, M.R., Nicholson, G.I., Perez-Perez, G.I., and Blaser, M.J. (**1991**). Long-term follow-up of voluntary ingestion of *Helicobacter pylori*. *Ann. Intern. Med.* 114: 662–663.

Moss, S. F., Calam, J., Agarwal, B., Wang, S., and Holt, P.R. (**1996**). Induction of gastric epithelial apoptosis by *Helicobacter pylori*. *Gut* 38: 498–501.

Mueller, A., O'Rourke, J., Grimm, J., Guillemin, K., Dixon, M.F., Lee, A., and Falkow, S. (**2003**). Distinct gene expression profiles characterize the histopathological

458 | *10 Helicobacter, Chronic Inflammation, and Cancer*

stages of disease in *Helicobacter*-induced mucosa-associated lymphoid tissue lymphoma. *Proc. Natl. Acad. Sci. USA* 100: 1292–1297.

Mueller, A., Merrell, D.S., Grimm, J., and Falkow, S. (**2004**). Profiling of microdissected gastric epithelial cells reveals a cell type-specific response to *Helicobacter pylori* infection. *Gastroenterology* 127: 1446–1462.

Mueller, A., Falkow, S., and Amieva, M.R. (**2005 a**). *Helicobacter pylori* and gastric cancer: what can be learned by studying the response of gastric epithelial cells to the infection? *Cancer Epidemiol. Biomarkers Prev.* 14: 1859–1864.

Mueller, A., O'Rourke, J., Chu, P., Chu, A., Dixon, M.F., Bouley, D.M., Lee, A., and Falkow, S. (**2005 b**). The role of antigenic drive and tumor-infiltrating accessory cells in the pathogenesis of *Helicobacter*-induced mucosa-associated lymphoid tissue lymphoma. *Am. J. Pathol.* 167: 797–812.

Murray, L.J., McCrum, E.E., Evans, A.E., and Bamford, K.B. (**1997**). Epidemiology of *Helicobacter pylori* infection among 4742 randomly selected subjects from Northern Ireland. *Int. J. Epidemiol.* 26: 880–887.

Nilsson, H.O., Taneera, J., Castedal, M., Glatz, E., Olsson, R., and Wadstrom, T. (**2000**). Identification of *Helicobacter pylori* and other *Helicobacter* species by PCR, hybridization, and partial DNA sequencing in human liver samples from patients with primary sclerosing cholangitis or primary biliary cirrhosis. *J. Clin. Microbiol.* 38: 1072–1076.

Nomura, A., Stemmermann, G.N., Chyou, P.H., Kato, I., Perez-Perez, G.I., and Blaser, M.J. (**1991**). *Helicobacter pylori* infection and gastric carcinoma among Japanese Americans in Hawaii. *N. Engl. J. Med.* 325: 1132–1136.

Nomura, S., Baxter, T., Yamaguchi, H., Leys, C., Vartapetian, A.B., Fox, J.G., Lee, J.R., Wang, T.C., and Goldenring, J.R. (**2004**). Spasmolytic polypeptide expressing metaplasia to preneoplasia in *H. felis*-infected mice. *Gastroenterology* 127: 582–594.

Nyska, A., Maronpot, R.R., Eldridge, S. R., Haseman, J.K., and Hailey, J.R. (**1997**). Alteration in cell kinetics in control B6C3F1 mice infected with *Helicobacter hepaticus*. *Toxicol. Pathol.* 25: 591–596.

Odenbreit, S., Puls, J., Sedlmaier, B., Gerland, E., Fischer, W., and Haas, R. (**2000**). Translocation of *Helicobacter pylori* CagA into gastric epithelial cells by type IV secretion. *Science* 287: 1497–1500.

Oh, J.D., Karam, S. M., and Gordon, J.I. (**2005**). Intracellular *Helicobacter pylori* in gastric epithelial progenitors. *Proc. Natl. Acad. Sci. USA* 102: 5186–5191.

Ohkusa, T., Takashimizu, I., Fujiki, K., Suzuki, S., Shimoi, K., Horiuchi, T., Sakurazawa, T., Ariake, K., Ishii, K., Kumagai, J., and Tanizawa, T. (**1998**). Disappearance of hyperplastic polyps in the stomach after eradication of *Helicobacter pylori*. A randomized, clinical trial. *Ann. Intern. Med.* 129: 712–715.

Ohno, S., Inagawa, H., Dhar, D.K., Fujii, T., Ueda, S., Tachibana, M., Suzuki, N., Inoue, M., Soma, G., and Nagasue, N. (**2003**). The degree of macrophage infiltration into the cancer cell nest is a significant predictor of survival in gastric cancer patients. *Anticancer Res.* 23: 5015–5022.

On, S. L. and Holmes, B. (**1995**). Classification and identification of Campylobacters and Helicobacters and allied taxanumerical analysis of phenotypic characters. *Syst. Appl. Microbiol.* 18: 374–390.

Orlicek, S. L., Welch, D.F., and Kuhls, T.L. (**1993**). Septicemia and meningitis caused by *Helicobacter cinaedi* in a neonate. *J. Clin. Microbiol.* 31: 569–571.

Osaka Cancer Registry. (**2004**). *Osaka Cancer Registry, 2004.*

Oshima, H., Oshima, M., Inaba, K., and Taketo, M.M. (**2004**). Hyperplastic gastric tumors induced by activated macrophages in COX-2/mPGES-1 transgenic mice. *EMBO J.* 23: 1669–1678.

Oshima, M., Oshima, H., Matsunaga, A., and Taketo, M.M. (**2005**). Hyperplastic gastric tumors with spasmolytic polypeptide-expressing metaplasia caused by tumor necrosis factor-alpha-dependent inflammation in cyclooxygenase-2/microsomal prostaglandin E synthase-1 transgenic mice. *Cancer Res.* 65: 9147–9151.

Otto, G., Hazell, S. H., Fox, J.G., Howlett, C.R., Murphy, J.C., O'Rourke, J.L., and Lee, A. (**1994**). Animal and public health implications of gastric colonization of cats by *Helicobacter*-like organisms. *J. Clin. Microbiol.* 32: 1043–1049.

Palli, D., Decarli, A., Cipriani, F., Sitas, F., Forman, D., Amadori, D., Avellini, C., Giacosa, A., Manca, P., Russo, A., et al. (**1993**). *Helicobacter pylori* antibodies in areas of Italy at varying gastric cancer risk. *Cancer Epidemiol. Biomarkers Prev.* 2: 37–40.

Palli, D., Saieva, C., Luzzi, I., Masala, G., Topa, S., Sera, F., Gemma, S., Zanna, I., D'Errico, M., Zini, E., Guidotti, S., Valeri, A., Fabbrucci, P., Moretti, R., Testai, E., del Giudice, G., Ottini, L., Matullo, G., Dogliotti, E., and Gomez-Miguel, M.J. (**2005**). Interleukin-1 gene polymorphisms and gastric cancer risk in a high-risk Italian population. *Am. J. Gastroenterol.* 100: 1941–1948.

Palmer, E.D. (**1954**). Investigation of the gastric spirochetes of the human. *Gastroenterology* 27: 218–220.

Parkin, D.M., Pisani, P., and Ferlay, J. (**1999**). Global cancer statistics. *CA Cancer J. Clin.* 49: 33–64.

Parkin, D.M., Bray, F.I., and Devesa, S. S. (**2001**). Cancer burden in the year **2000**. The global picture. *Eur. J. Cancer* 37 (Suppl 8): S4 –S66.

Parsonnet, J. (**1993**). *Helicobacter pylori* and gastric cancer. *Gastroenterol. Clin. North Am.* 22: 89–104.

Parsonnet, J. (**1995**). The incidence of *Helicobacter pylori* infection. *Aliment. Pharmacol. Ther.* 9 (Suppl 2): 45–51.

Parsonnet, J., Friedman, G.D., Vandersteen, D.P., Chang, Y., Vogelman, J.H., Orentreich, N., and Sibley, R.K. (**1991**). *Helicobacter pylori* infection and the risk of gastric carcinoma. *N. Engl. J. Med.* 325: 1127–1131.

Parsonnet, J., Hansen, S., Rodriguez, L., Gelb, A.B., Warnke, R.A., Jellum, E., Orentreich, N., Vogelman, J.H., and Friedman, G.D. (**1994**). *Helicobacter pylori* infection and gastric lymphoma. *N. Engl. J. Med.* 330: 1267–1271.

Parsonnet, J., Harris, R.A., Hack, H.M., and Owens, D.K. (**1996**). Modelling cost-effectiveness of *Helicobacter pylori* screening to prevent gastric cancer: a mandate for clinical trials. *Lancet* 348: 150–154.

Parsonnet, J., Friedman, G.D., Orentreich, N., and Vogelman, H. (**1997 a**). Risk for gastric cancer in people with CagA positive or CagA negative *Helicobacter pylori* infection. *Gut* 40: 297–301.

Parsonnet, J., Replogle, M., Yang, S., and Hiatt, R. (**1997 b**). Seroprevalence of CagA-positive strains among *Helicobacter pylori*-infected, healthy young adults. *J. Infect. Dis.* 175: 1240–1242.

Parsonnet, J., Shmuely, H., and Haggerty, T. (**1999**). Fecal and oral shedding of *Helicobacter pylori* from healthy infected adults. *JAMA* 282: 2240–2245.

Peek, R.M., Jr., Wirth, H.P., Moss, S. F., Yang, M., Abdalla, A.M., Tham, K.T., Zhang, T., Tang, L.H., Modlin, I.M., and Blaser, M.J. (**2000**). *Helicobacter pylori* alters gastric epithelial cell cycle events and gastrin secretion in Mongolian gerbils. *Gastroenterology* 118: 48–59.

Perez-Perez, G.I., Garza-Gonzalez, E., Portal, C., and Olivares, A.Z. (**2005**). Role of cytokine polymorphisms in the risk of distal gastric cancer development. *Cancer Epidemiol. Biomarkers Prev.* 14: 1869–1873.

Perkins, S. E., Fox, J.G., and Walsh, J.H. (**1996**). *Helicobacter mustelae*-associated hypergastrinemia in ferrets (*Mustela putorius furo*). *Am. J. Vet. Res.* 57: 147–150.

Philip, M., Rowley, D.A., and Schreiber, H. (**2004**). Inflammation as a tumor promoter in cancer induction. *Semin. Cancer Biol.* 14: 433–439.

Philpott, D.J., Belaid, D., Troubadour, P., Thiberge, J.M., Tankovic, J., Labigne, A., and Ferrero, R.L. (**2002**). Reduced activation of inflammatory responses in host cells by mouse-adapted *Helicobacter pylori* isolates. *Cell Microbiol.* 4: 285–296.

Pirog, E.C. and Collins, D.C. (**1999**). Metabolism of dihydrotestosterone in human liver: importance of 3 alpha- and 3 beta-hydroxysteroid dehydrogenase. *J. Clin. Endocrinol. Metab.* 84: 3217–3221.

Ponzetto, A., Pellicano, R., Leone, N., Cutufia, M.A., Turrini, F., Grigioni, W.F., D'Errico, A., Mortimer, P., Rizzetto, M., and Silengo, L. (**2000**). *Helicobacter* infection and cirrhosis in hepatitis C virus carriage: is it an innocent bystander or a troublemaker? *Med. Hypotheses* 54: 275–277.

Poovorawan, Y., Chatchatee, P., and Chongsrisawat, V. (**2002**). Epidemiology and prophylaxis of viral hepatitis: a global perspective. *J. Gastroenterol. Hepatol.* 17 (Suppl): S155 –S166.

Powrie, F., Mauze, S., and Coffman, R.L. (**1997**). CD4 + T-cells in the regulation of inflammatory responses in the intestine. *Res. Immunol.* 148: 576–581.

Pull, S. L., Doherty, J.M., Mills, J.C., Gordon, J.I., and Stappenbeck, T.S. (**2005**). Activated macrophages are an adaptive element of the colonic epithelial progenitor niche necessary for regenerative responses to injury. *Proc. Natl. Acad. Sci. USA* 102: 99–104.

Queiroz, D.M., Rocha, G.A., Mendes, E.N., Lage, A.P., Carvalho, A.C., and Barbosa, A.J. (**1990**). A spiral microorganism in the stomach of pigs. *Vet. Microbiol.* 24: 199–204.

Rao, V.P., Poutahidis, T., Ge, Z., Nambiar, P.R., Horwitz, B.H., Fox, J.G., and Erdman, S. E. (**2006**). Proinflammatory CD4 +CD45 RBhi lymphocytes promote mammary and intestinal carcinogenesis in ApcMin/+ mice. *Cancer Res.* 66: 57–61.

Rao, V.P., Poutahidis, T., Ge, Z., Nambiar, P.R., Boussahmain, C., Horwitz, B.H., Fox, J.G., Erdman, S. E. Innate immune inflammatory response against enteric bacterial pathogen *Helicobacter hepaticus* triggers mammary adenocarcinoma in mice. Can. Res. (in press)

Rappin, J.P. (**1948**). Contra l'étude de bacterium de la bouche a l'etat normal (1881). As quoted by Breed, R.S., Murray, E.G.D., Hitchens, AP. In: *Bergey's Manual of Determinative Bacteriology*, 6th edn. Williams & Wilkins, Co., Baltimore.

Rathinavelu, S., Zavros, Y., and Merchant, J.L. (**2003**). *Acinetobacter wolffii* infection and gastritis. *Microbes Infect.* 5: 651–657.

Regimbeau, C., Karsenti, D., Durand, V., D'Alteroche, L., Copie-Bergman, C., Metman, E. H., and Machet, M.C. (**1998**). Low-grade gastric MALT lymphoma and *Helicobacter heilmannii* (*Gastrospirillum hominis*). *Gastroenterol. Clin. Biol.* 22: 720–723.

Reindel, J.F., Fitzgerald, A.L., Breider, M.A., Gough, A.W., Yan, C., Mysore, J.V., and Dubois, A. (**1999**). An epizootic of lymphoplasmacytic gastritis attributed to *Helicobacter pylori* infection in cynomolgus monkeys (*Macaca fascicularis*). *Vet. Pathol.* 36: 1–13.

Rektorschek, M., Weeks, D., Sachs, G., and Melchers, K. (**1998**). Influence of pH on metabolism and urease activity of *Helicobacter pylori*. *Gastroenterology* 115: 628–641.

Ries, L., Eisner, M.P., Kosary, C.L., et al. (**2005**). *SEER Cancer Statistics Review, 1975–2002*. National Cancer Institute, Bethesda, MD.

Rocha, G.A., Queiroz, D.M., Mendes, E.N., Oliveira, A.M., Moura, S. B., and Silva, R.J. (**1992**). Source of *Helicobacter pylori* infection: studies in abattoir workers and pigs. *Am. J. Gastroenterol.* 87: 1525.

Rogers, A.B. and Fox, J.G. (**2004**). Inflammation and Cancer. I. Rodent models of infectious gastrointestinal and liver cancer. *Am. J. Physiol. Gastrointest. Liver Physiol.* 286: G361–G366.

Rogers, A.B., Boutin, S. R., Whary, M.T., Sundina, N., Ge, Z., Cormier, K., and Fox, J.G. (**2004**). Progression of chronic hepatitis and preneoplasia in *Helicobacter hepaticus*-infected A/JCr mice. *Toxicol. Pathol.* 32: 668–677.

Rogers, A.B., Taylor, N.S., Whary, M.T., Stefanich, E.D., Wang, T.C., and Fox, J.G. (**2005**). *Helicobacter pylori* but not high salt induces gastric intraepithelial neoplasia in B6129 mice. *Cancer Res.* 65: 10709–10715.

Roggero, E., Zucca, E., Pinotti, G., Pascarella, A., Capella, C., Savio, A., Pedrinis, E., Paterlini, A., Venco, A., and Cavalli, F. (**1995**). Eradication of *Helicobacter pylori* infection in primary low-grade gastric lymphoma of mucosa-associated lymphoid tissue. *Ann. Intern. Med.* 122: 767–769.

Rollinson, S., Levene, A.P., Mensah, F.K., Roddam, P.L., Allan, J.M., Diss, T.C., Roman, E., Jack, A., MacLennan, K., Dixon, M.F., and Morgan, G.J. (**2003**). Gastric marginal zone lymphoma is associated with polymorphisms in genes involved in inflammatory response and antioxidative capacity. *Blood* 102: 1007–1011.

Roosendaal, R., Kuipers, E.J., Buitenwerf, J., van Uffelen, C., Meuwissen, S. G., van Kamp, G.J., and Vandenbroucke-Grauls, C.M. (**1997**). *Helicobacter pylori* and the birth cohort effect: evidence of a continuous decrease of infection rates in childhood. *Am. J. Gastroenterol.* 92: 1480–1482.

Roth, K.A., Kapadia, S. B., Martin, S. M., and Lorenz, R.G. (**1999**). Cellular immune responses are essential for the development of *Helicobacter felis*-associated gastric pathology. *J. Immunol.* 163: 1490–1497.

Rothenbacher, D., Bode, G., Berg, G., Gommel, R., Gonser, T., Adler, G., and Brenner,

H. (**1998**). Prevalence and determinants of *Helicobacter pylori* infection in preschool children: a population-based study from Germany. *Int. J. Epidemiol.* 27: 135–141.

Sakagami, T., Dixon, M., O'Rourke, J., Howlett, R., Alderuccio, F., Vella, J., Shimoyama, T., and Lee, A. (**1996**). Atrophic gastric changes in both *Helicobacter felis* and *Helicobacter pylori* infected mice are host dependent and separate from antral gastritis. *Gut* 39: 639–648.

Salama, N., Guillemin, K., McDaniel, T.K., Sherlock, G., Tompkins, L., and Falkow, S. (**2000**). A whole-genome microarray reveals genetic diversity among *Helicobacter pylori* strains. *Proc. Natl. Acad. Sci. USA* 97: 14 668–14 673.

Salomon, H. (**1896**). Über das Spirillium des Säugetier-Magens und sein Verhalten zu Belegzellen. *Zentralbl. fur Bacteriologie Parasitenkunde und Infektionskrankheiten* 19: 433–442.

Sato, T. and Takeuchi, A. (**1982**). Infection by spirilla in the stomach of the rhesus monkey. *Vet. Pathol. Suppl.* 19 Suppl 7: 17–25.

Savio, A., Franzin, G., Wotherspoon, A.C., Zamboni, G., Negrini, R., Buffoli, F., Diss, T.C., Pan, L., and Isaacson, P.G. (**1996**). Diagnosis and posttreatment follow-up of *Helicobacter pylori*-positive gastric lymphoma of mucosa-associated lymphoid tissue: histology, polymerase chain reaction, or both? *Blood* 87: 1255–1260.

Sawai, N., Kita, M., Kodama, T., Tanahashi, T., Yamaoka, Y., Tagawa, Y., Iwakura, Y., and Imanishi, J. (**1999**). Role of gamma interferon in *Helicobacter pylori*-induced gastric inflammatory responses in a mouse model. *Infect. Immun.* 67: 279–285.

Schmidt, P., Lee, J., Goldenring, J.R., Wright, N., and Pousom, R. (**1998**). Association of an aberrant spasmolytic polypeptide-expressing cell lineage with gastric adenocarcinoma in humans. *Gastroenterology* 114: G2781.

Schmidt, P.H., Lee, J.R., Joshi, V., Playford, R.J., Poulsom, R., Wright, N.A., and Goldenring, J.R. (**1999**). Identification of a metaplastic cell lineage associated with human gastric adenocarcinoma. *Lab. Invest.* 79: 639–646.

Schreiber, S., Konradt, M., Groll, C., Scheid, P., Hanauer, G., Werling, H.O., Josenhans,

C., and Suerbaum, S. (**2004**). The spatial orientation of *Helicobacter pylori* in the gastric mucus. *Proc. Natl. Acad. Sci. USA* 101: 5024–5029.

Schwarz, M., Wright, A.C., Davis, D.L., Nazer, H., Bjorkhem, I., and Russell, D.W. (**2000**). The bile acid synthetic gene 3 beta-hydroxy-delta(5)-C(27)-steroid oxidoreductase is mutated in progressive intrahepatic cholestasis. *J. Clin. Invest.* 106: 1175–1184.

Segal, E.D., Lange, C., Covacci, A., Tompkins, L.S., and Falkow, S. (**1997**). Induction of host signal transduction pathways by *Helicobacter pylori*. *Proc. Natl. Acad. Sci. USA* 94: 7595–7599.

Semino-Mora, C., Doi, S. Q., Marty, A., Simko, V., Carlstedt, I., and Dubois, A. (**2003**). Intracellular and interstitial expression of *Helicobacter pylori* virulence genes in gastric precancerous intestinal metaplasia and adenocarcinoma. *J. Infect. Dis.* 187: 1165–1177.

Seo, J.K., Ko, J.S., and Choi, K.D. (**2002**). Serum ferritin and *Helicobacter pylori* infection in children: a sero-epidemiologic study in Korea. *J. Gastroenterol. Hepatol.* 17: 754–757.

Seymour, C., Lewis, R.G., Kim, M., Gagnon, D.F., Fox, J.G., Dewhirst, F.E., and Paster, B.J. (**1994**). Isolation of *Helicobacter* strains from wild bird and swine feces. *Appl. Environ. Microbiol.* 60: 1025–1028.

Shames, B., Krajden, S., Fuksa, M., Babida, C., and Penner, J.L. (**1989**). Evidence for the occurrence of the same strain of *Campylobacter pylori* in the stomach and dental plaque. *J. Clin. Microbiol.* 27: 2849–2850.

Shames, B., Fox, J.G., Dewhirst, F., Yan, L., Shen, Z., and Taylor, N.S. (**1995**). Identification of widespread *Helicobacter hepaticus* infection in feces in commercial mouse colonies by culture and PCR assay. *J. Clin. Microbiol.* 33: 2968–2972.

Sharma, S. A., Tummuru, M.K., Blaser, M.J., and Kerr, L.D. (**1998**). Activation of IL-8 gene expression by *Helicobacter pylori* is regulated by transcription factor nuclear factor-kappa B in gastric epithelial cells. *J. Immunol.* 160: 2401–2407.

Shen, Z., Fox, J.G., Dewhirst, F.E., Paster, B.J., Foltz, C.J., Yan, L., Shames, B., and Perry, L. (**1997**). *Helicobacter rodentium* sp. nov., a urease-negative *Helicobacter* species isolated from laboratory mice. *Int. J. Syst. Bacteriol.* 47:627–634.

Shen, Z., Feng, Y., Dewhirst, F.E., and Fox, J.G. (**2001**). Coinfection of enteric *Helicobacter* spp. and *Campylobacter* spp. in cats. *J. Clin. Microbiol.* 39:2166–2172.

Shibata, A., Parsonnet, J., Longacre, T.A., Garcia, M.I., Puligandla, B., Davis, R.E., Vogelman, J.H., Orentreich, N., and Habel, L.A. (**2002**). CagA status of *Helicobacter pylori* infection and p53 gene mutations in gastric adenocarcinoma. *Carcinogenesis* 23:419–424.

Shuto, R., Fujioka, T., Kubota, T., and Nasu, M. (**1993**). Experimental gastritis induced by *Helicobacter pylori* in Japanese monkeys. *Infect. Immun.* 61:933–939.

Singh, R., Leuratti, C., Josyula, S., Sipowicz, M.A., Diwan, B.A., Kasprzak, K.S., Schut, H.A., Marnett, L.J., Anderson, L.M., and Shuker, D.E. (**2001**). Lobe-specific increases in malondialdehyde DNA adduct formation in the livers of mice following infection with *Helicobacter hepaticus. Carcinogenesis* 22:1281–1287.

Sipowicz, M.A., Chomarat, P., Diwan, B.A., Anver, M.A., Awasthi, Y.C., Ward, J.M., Rice, J.M., Kasprzak, K.S., Wild, C.P., and Anderson, L.M. (**1997a**). Increased oxidative DNA damage and hepatocyte overexpression of specific cytochrome P450 isoforms in hepatitis of mice infected with *Helicobacter hepaticus. Am. J. Pathol.* 151:933–941.

Sipowicz, M.A., Weghorst, C.M., Shiao, Y.H., Buzard, G.S., Calvert, R.J., Anver, M.R., Anderson, L.M., and Rice, J.M. (**1997b**). Lack of p53 and ras mutations in *Helicobacter hepaticus*-induced liver tumors in A/JCr mice. *Carcinogenesis* 18:233–236.

Slagle, B.L., Lee, T.H., Medina, D., Finegold, M.J., and Butel, J.S. (**1996**). Increased sensitivity to the hepatocarcinogen diethylnitrosamine in transgenic mice carrying the hepatitis B virus X gene. *Mol. Carcinog.* 15:261–269.

Smoot, D.T., Resau, J.H., Earlington, M.H., Simpson, M., and Cover, T.L. (**1996**). Effects of *Helicobacter pylori* vacuolating cytotoxin on primary cultures of human gastric epithelial cells. *Gut* 39:795–799.

Smythies, L.E., Waites, K.B., Lindsey, J.R., Harris, P.R., Ghiara, P., and Smith, P.D. (**2000**). *Helicobacter pylori*-induced mucosal

inflammation is Th1 mediated and exacerbated in IL-4, but not IFN-gamma, gene-deficient mice. *J. Immunol.* 165: 1022–1029.

Solnick, J.V. and Schauer, D.B. (**2001**). Emergence of diverse *Helicobacter* species in the pathogenesis of gastric and enterohepatic diseases. *Clin. Microbiol. Rev.* 14: 59–97.

Solnick, J.V., O'Rourke, J., Lee, A., Paster, B.J., Dewhirst, F.E., and Tompkins, L.S. (**1993**). An uncultured gastric spiral organism is a newly identified *Helicobacter* in humans. *J. Infect. Dis.* 168: 379–385.

Sorlin, P., Vandamme, P., Nortier, J., Hoste, B., Rossi, C., Pavlof, S., and Struelens, M.J. (**1999**). Recurrent "*Flexispira rappini*' bacteremia in an adult patient undergoing hemodialysis: case report. *J. Clin. Microbiol.* 37: 1319–1323.

Stanley, J., Linton, D., Burnens, A.P., Dewhirst, F.E., Owen, R.J., Porter, A., On, S. L., and Costas, M. (**1993**). *Helicobacter canis* sp. nov., a new species from dogs: an integrated study of phenotype and genotype. *J. Gen. Microbiol.* 139: 2495–2504.

Stanley, J., Linton, D., Burnens, A.P., Dewhirst, F.E., On, S. L., Porter, A., Owen, R.J., and Costas, M. (**1994**). *Helicobacter pullorum* sp. nov.-genotype and phenotype of a new species isolated from poultry and from human patients with gastroenteritis. *Microbiology* 140 (Pt 12): 3441–3449.

Steer, H.W. (**1975**). Ultrastructure of cell migration through the gastric epithelium and its relationship to bacteria. *J. Clin. Pathol.* 28: 639–646.

Steer, H.W. (**1984**). Surface morphology of the gastroduodenal mucosa in duodenal ulceration. *Gut* 25: 1203–1210.

Steer, H.W. and Colin-Jones, D.G. (**1975**). Mucosal changes in gastric ulceration and their response to carbenoxolone sodium. *Gut* 16: 590–597.

Stein, M., Rappuoli, R., and Covacci, A. (**2000**). Tyrosine phosphorylation of the *Helicobacter pylori* CagA antigen after cag-driven host cell translocation. *Proc. Natl. Acad. Sci. USA* 97: 1263–1268.

Steinberg, E.B., Mendoza, C.E., Glass, R., Arana, B., Lopez, M.B., Mejia, M., Gold, B.D., Priest, J.W., Bibb, W., Monroe, S. S., Bern, C., Bell, B.P., Hoekstra, R.M., Klein, R., Mintz, E.D., and Luby, S. (**2004**). Prevalence of infection with waterborne pathogens: a seroepidemiologic study in children 6–36 months old in San Juan Sacatepequez, Guatemala. *Am. J. Trop. Med. Hyg.* 70: 83–88.

Stolte, M., Bayerdorffer, E., Morgner, A., Alpen, B., Wundisch, T., Thiede, C., and Neubauer, A. (**2002**). *Helicobacter* and gastric MALT lymphoma. *Gut* 50 (Suppl 3): III19–III24.

Stone, M.A., Patel, H., Panja, K.K., Barnett, D.B., and Mayberry, J.F. (**1998**). Results of *Helicobacter pylori* screening and eradication in a multi-ethnic community in central England. *Eur. J. Gastroenterol. Hepatol.* 10: 957–962.

Strandberg, T.E., Tilvis, R.S., Vuoristo, M., Lindroos, M., and Kosunen, T.U. (**1997**). Prospective study of *Helicobacter pylori* seropositivity and cardiovascular diseases in a general elderly population. *Br. Med. J.* 314: 1317–1318.

Suerbaum, S. and Michetti, P. (**2002**). *Helicobacter pylori* infection. *N. Engl. J. Med.* 347: 1175–1186.

Suerbaum, S., Smith, J.M., Bapumia, K., Morelli, G., Smith, N.H., Kunstmann, E., Dyrek, I., and Achtman, M. (**1998**). Free recombination within *Helicobacter pylori*. *Proc. Natl. Acad. Sci. USA* 95: 12 619–12 624.

Suerbaum, S., Josenhans, C., Sterzenbach, T., Drescher, B., Brandt, P., Bell, M., Droge, M., Fartmann, B., Fischer, H.P., Ge, Z., Horster, A., Holland, R., Klein, K., Konig, J., Macko, L., Mendz, G.L., Nyakatura, G., Schauer, D.B., Shen, Z., Weber, J., Frosch, M., and Fox, J.G. (**2003**). The complete genome sequence of the carcinogenic bacterium *Helicobacter hepaticus*. *Proc. Natl. Acad. Sci. USA* 100: 7901–7906.

Sung, J.J., Chung, S. C., Ling, T.K., Yung, M.Y., Leung, V.K., Ng, E.K., Li, M.K., Cheng, A.F., and Li, A.K. (**1995**). Antibacterial treatment of gastric ulcers associated with *Helicobacter pylori*. *N. Engl. J. Med.* 332: 139–142.

Taguchi, A., Ohmiya, N., Shirai, K., Mabuchi, N., Itoh, A., Hirooka, Y., Niwa, Y., and Goto, H. (**2005**). Interleukin-8 promoter polymorphism increases the risk of atrophic gastritis and gastric cancer in Japan. *Cancer Epidemiol. Biomarkers Prev.* 14: 2487–2493.

Takaishi, S., Cui, G., Frederick, D.M., Carlson, J.E., Houghton, J., Varro, A., Dockray, G.J., Ge, Z., Whary, M.T., Rogers, A.B., Fox, J.G., and Wang, T.C. (**2005**). Synergistic inhibitory effects of gastrin and histamine receptor antagonists on *Helicobacter*-induced gastric cancer. *Gastroenterology* 128: 1965–1983.

Talley, N.J., Vakil, N., Ballard, E.D., II, and Fennerty, M.B. (**1999**). Absence of benefit of eradicating *Helicobacter pylori* in patients with nonulcer dyspepsia. *N. Engl. J. Med.* 341: 1106–1111.

Taylor, N. S., Ge, Z., Shen, Z., Dewhirst, F.E., and Fox, J.G. (**2003**). Cytolethal distending toxin: a potential virulence factor for *Helicobacter cinaedi*. *J. Infect. Dis.* 188: 1892–1897.

Tee, W., Anderson, B.N., Ross, B.C., and Dwyer, B. (**1987**). Atypical campylobacters associated with gastroenteritis. *J. Clin. Microbiol.* 25: 1248–1252.

Teh, B.H., Lin, J.T., Pan, W.H., Lin, S. H., Wang, L.Y., Lee, T.K., and Chen, C.J. (**1994**). Seroprevalence and associated risk factors of *Helicobacter pylori* infection in Taiwan. *Anticancer Res.* 14: 1389–1392.

Telford, J.L., Ghiara, P., Dell'Orco, M., Comanducci, M., Burroni, D., Bugnoli, M., Tecce, M.F., Censini, S., Covacci, A., Xiang, Z., et al. (**1994**). Gene structure of the *Helicobacter pylori* cytotoxin and evidence of its key role in gastric disease. *J. Exp. Med.* 179: 1653–1658.

Thomas, J.E., Gibson, G.R., Darboe, M.K., Dale, A., and Weaver, L.T. (**1992**). Isolation of *Helicobacter pylori* from human faeces. *Lancet* 340: 1194–1195.

Thompson, L.J., Danon, S. J., Wilson, J.E., O'Rourke, J.L., Salama, N.R., Falkow, S., Mitchell, H., and Lee, A. (**2004**). Chronic *Helicobacter pylori* infection with Sydney strain 1 and a newly identified mouse-adapted strain (Sydney strain **2000**) in C57 BL/6 and BALB/c mice. *Infect. Immun.* 72: 4668–4679.

Thomsen, L.L., Gavin, J.B., and Tasman-Jones, C. (**1990**). Relation of *Helicobacter pylori* to the human gastric mucosa in chronic gastritis of the antrum. *Gut* 31: 1230–1236.

Tolia, V., Nilsson, H.O., Boyer, K., Wuerth, A., Al-Soud, W.A., Rabah, R., and Wadstrom, T. (**2004**). Detection of *Helicobacter gan-*

mani-like 16 S rDNA in pediatric liver tissue. *Helicobacter* 9: 460–468.

Tomb, J.F., White, O., Kerlavage, A.R., Clayton, R.A., Sutton, G.G., Fleischmann, R.D., Ketchum, K.A., Klenk, H.P., Gill, S., Dougherty, B.A., Nelson, K., Quackenbush, J., Zhou, L., Kirkness, E.F., Peterson, S., Loftus, B., Richardson, D., Dodson, R., Khalak, H.G., Glodek, A., McKenney, K., Fitzegerald, L.M., Lee, N., Adams, M.D., Hickey, E.K., Berg, D.E., Gocayne, J.D., Utterback, T.R., Peterson, J.D., Kelley, J.M., Cotton, M.D., Weidman, J.M., Fujii, C., Bowman, C., Watthey, L., Wallin, E., Hayes, W.S., Borodovsky, M., Karp, P.D., Smith, H.O., Fraser, C.M., and Venter, J.C. (**1997**). The complete genome sequence of the gastric pathogen *Helicobacter pylori*. *Nature* 388: 539–547.

Torres, J., Leal-Herrera, Y., Perez-Perez, G., Gomez, A., Camorlinga-Ponce, M., Cedillo-Rivera, R., Tapia-Conyer, R., and Munoz, O. (1998). A community-based seroepidemiologic study of *Helicobacter pylori* infection in Mexico. *J. Infect. Dis.* 178: 1089–1094.

Totten, P.A., Fennell, C.L., Tenover, F.C., Wezenberg, J.M., Perine, P.L., Stamm, W.E., and Holmes, K.K. (**1985**). *Campylobacter cinaedi* (sp. nov.) and *Campylobacter fennelliae* (sp. nov.): two new *Campylobacter* species associated with enteric disease in homosexual men. *J. Infect. Dis.* 151: 131–139.

Toyokuni, S., Okamoto, K., Yodoi, J., and Hiai, H. (**1995**). Persistent oxidative stress in cancer. *FEBS Lett.* 358: 1–3.

Trivett-Moore, N.L., Rawlinson, W.D., Yuen, M., and Gilbert, G.L. (**1997**). *Helicobacter westmeadii* sp. nov., a new species isolated from blood cultures of two AIDS patients. *J. Clin. Microbiol.* 35: 1144–1150.

Tsugane, S., Sasazuki, S., Kobayashi, M., and Sasaki, S. (**2004**). Salt and salted food intake and subsequent risk of gastric cancer among middle-aged Japanese men and women. *Br. J. Cancer* 90: 128–134.

Tsutsumi, R., Higashi, H., Higuchi, M., Okada, M., and Hatakeyama, M. (**2003**). Attenuation of Helicobacter pylori CagA x SHP-2 signaling by interaction between CagA and C-terminal Src kinase. *J. Biol. Chem.* 278: 3664–3670.

Tu, S., Cui, G., Takaishi, S., Tran, A.V., Frederick, D.M., Carlson, J.E., Kurt-Jones, E., and Wang, T.C. (**2005**). Overexpression of human interleukin-1 beta in transgenic mice results in spontaneous gastric inflammation and carcinogenesis. *Gastroenterology* 421: 4.

Tummuru, M.K., Cover, T.L., and Blaser, M.J. (**1993**). Cloning and expression of a high-molecular-mass major antigen of *Helicobacter pylori:* evidence of linkage to cytotoxin production. *Infect. Immun.* 61: 1799–1809.

Tummuru, M.K., Cover, T.L., and Blaser, M.J. (**1994**). Mutation of the cytotoxin-associated cagA gene does not affect the vacuolating cytotoxin activity of *Helicobacter pylori*. *Infect. Immun.* 62: 2609–2613.

Tummuru, M.K., Sharma, S. A., and Blaser, M.J. (**1995**). *Helicobacter pylori* picB, a homologue of the *Bordetella pertussis* toxin secretion protein, is required for induction of IL-8 in gastric epithelial cells. *Mol. Microbiol.* 18: 867–876.

U.S. Cancer Statistics Working Group. (**2005**). *United States Cancer Statistics: 1999–2002 Incidence and Mortality Web based report.* Atlanta.

Uemura, N., Mukai, T., Okamoto, S., Yamaguchi, S., Mashiba, H., Taniyama, K., Sasaki, N., Haruma, K., Sumii, K., and Kajiyama, G. (**1997**). Effect of *Helicobacter pylori* eradication on subsequent development of cancer after endoscopic resection of early gastric cancer. *Cancer Epidemiol. Biomarkers Prev.* 6: 639–642.

Uemura, N., Okamoto, S., Yamamoto, S., Matsumura, N., Yamaguchi, S., Yamakido, M., Taniyama, K., Sasaki, N., and Schlemper, R.J. (**2001**). *Helicobacter pylori* infection and the development of gastric cancer. *N. Engl. J. Med.* 345: 784–789.

Ullrich, A., Fischbach, W., and Blettner, M. (**2002**). Incidence of gastric B-cell lymphomas: a population-based study in Germany. *Ann. Oncol.* 13: 1120–1127.

Umeda, M., Kobayashi, H., Takeuchi, Y., Hayashi, J., Morotome-Hayashi, Y., Yano, K., Aoki, A., Ohkusa, T., and Ishikawa, I. (**2003**). High prevalence of *Helicobacter pylori* detected by PCR in the oral cavities of periodontitis patients. *J. Periodontol.* 74: 129–134.

Vaira, D., Ferron, P., Negrini, R., et al. (**1990**). Identification by monoclonal antibody of *Helicobacter pylori* like organisms in non primates (Abstract). *Enfermedades Digestivas* 78: 51.

Van der Hulst, R.W., Rauws, E.A., Koycu, B., Keller, J.J., Bruno, M.J., Tijssen, J.G., and Tytgat, G.N. (**1997**). Prevention of ulcer recurrence after eradication of *Helicobacter pylori:* a prospective long-term follow-up study. *Gastroenterology* 113: 1082–1086.

Van Doorn, L.J., Figueiredo, C., Megraud, F., Pena, S., Midolo, P., Queiroz, D.M., Carneiro, F., Vanderborght, B., Pegado, M.D., Sanna, R., De Boer, W., Schneeberger, P.M., Correa, P., Ng, E.K., Atherton, J., Blaser, M.J., and Quint, W.G. (**1999**). Geographic distribution of vacA allelic types of *Helicobacter pylori. Gastroenterology* 116: 823–830.

van Loon, A.J., Botterweck, A.A., Goldbohm, R.A., Brants, H.A., van Klaveren, J.D., and van den Brandt, P.A. (**1998**). Intake of nitrate and nitrite and the risk of gastric cancer: a prospective cohort study. *Br. J. Cancer* 78: 129–135.

Vandamme, P., Falsen, E., Pot, B., Kersters, K., and De Ley, J. (**1990**). Identification of *Campylobacter cinaedi* isolated from blood and feces of children and adult females. *J. Clin. Microbiol.* 28: 1016–1020.

Viala, J., Chaput, C., Boneca, I.G., Cardona, A., Girardin, S. E., Moran, A.P., Athman, R., Memet, S., Huerre, M.R., Coyle, A.J., DiStefano, P.S., Sansonetti, P.J., Labigne, A., Bertin, J., Philpott, D.J., and Ferrero, R.L. (**2004**). Nod1 responds to peptidoglycan delivered by the *Helicobacter pylori* cag pathogenicity island. *Nat. Immunol.* 5: 1166–1174.

Vicari, J.J., Peek, R.M., Falk, G.W., Goldblum, J.R., Easley, K.A., Schnell, J., Perez-Perez, G.I., Halter, S. A., Rice, T.W., Blaser, M.J., and Richter, J.E. (**1998**). The seroprevalence of cagA-positive *Helicobacter pylori* strains in the spectrum of gastroesophageal reflux disease. *Gastroenterology* 115: 50–57.

Wang, T.C. and Fox, J.G. (**1998**). *Helicobacter pylori* and gastric cancer: Koch's postulates fulfilled? *Gastroenterology* 115: 780–783.

Wang, T.C., Goldenring, J.R., Dangler, C., Ito, S., Mueller, A., Jeon, W.K., Koh, T.J., and Fox, J.G. (**1998**). Mice lacking secretory phospholipase A2 show altered apoptosis and differentiation with *Helicobacter felis* infection. *Gastroenterology* 114: 675–689.

Wang, T.C., Dangler, C.A., Chen, D., Goldenring, J.R., Koh, T., Raychowdhury, R., Coffey, R.J., Ito, S., Varro, A., Dockray, G.J., and Fox, J.G. (**2000**). Synergistic interaction between hypergastrinemia and *Helicobacter* infection in a mouse model of gastric cancer. *Gastroenterology* 118: 36–47.

Wang, X.D., Krinsky, N.I., Marini, R.P., Tang, G., Yu, J., Hurley, R., Fox, J.G., and Russell, R.M. (**1992**). Intestinal uptake and lymphatic absorption of beta-carotene in ferrets: a model for human beta-carotene metabolism. *Am. J. Physiol.* 263: G480–G486.

Ward, J.M., Anver, M.R., Haines, D.C., and Benveniste, R.E. (**1994 a**). Chronic active hepatitis in mice caused by *Helicobacter hepaticus. Am. J. Pathol.* 145: 959–968.

Ward, J.M., Fox, J.G., Anver, M.R., Haines, D.C., George, C.V., Collins, M.J., Jr., Gorelick, P.L., Nagashima, K., Gonda, M.A., Gilden, R.V., et al. (**1994 b**). Chronic active hepatitis and associated liver tumors in mice caused by a persistent bacterial infection with a novel *Helicobacter* species. *J. Natl. Cancer Inst.* 86: 1222–1227.

Watanabe, T., Tada, M., Nagai, H., Sasaki, S., and Nakao, M. (**1998**). *Helicobacter pylori* infection induces gastric cancer in Mongolian gerbils. *Gastroenterology* 115: 642–648.

Watanapa, P. and Watanapa, W.B. (**2002**). Liver fluke-associated cholangiocarcinoma. *Br. J. Surg.* 89: 962–970.

Weghorst, C.M., Pereira, M.A., and Klaunig, J.E. (**1989**). Strain differences in hepatic tumor promotion by phenobarbital in diethylnitrosamine- and dimethylnitrosamine-initiated infant male mice. *Carcinogenesis* 10: 1409–1412.

Weir, S., Cuccherini, B., Whitney, A.M., Ray, M.L., MacGregor, J.P., Steigerwalt, A., Daneshvar, M.I., Weyant, R., Wray, B., Steele, J., Strober, W., and Gill, V.J. (**1999**). Recurrent bacteremia caused by a "Flexispira'-like organism in a patient with X-linked (Bruton's) agammaglobulinemia. *J. Clin. Microbiol.* 37: 2439–2445.

West, A.P., Millar, M.R., and Tompkins, D.S. (**1990**). Survival of *Helicobacter pylori* in water and saline. *J. Clin. Pathol.* 43: 609.

Whary, M.T., Morgan, T.J., Dangler, C.A., Gaudes, K.J., Taylor, N.S., and Fox, J.G. (**1998**). Chronic active hepatitis induced by *Helicobacter hepaticus* in the A/JCr mouse is associated with a Th1 cell-mediated immune response. *Infect. Immun.* 66: 3142–3148.

Whary, M.T., Cline, J.H., King, A.E., Hewes, K.M., Chojnacky, D., Salvarrey, A., and Fox, J.G. (**2000**). Monitoring sentinel mice for *Helicobacter hepaticus, H. rodentium*, and *H. bilis* infection by use of polymerase chain reaction analysis and serologic testing. *Comp. Med.* 50: 436–443.

Whary, M.T., Sundina, N., Bravo, L.E., Correa, P., Quinones, F., Caro, F., and Fox, J.G. (**2005**). Intestinal helminthiasis in Colombian children promotes a Th2 response to *Helicobacter pylori:* possible implications for gastric carcinogenesis. *Cancer Epidemiol. Biomarkers Prev.* 14: 1464–1469.

Whitehouse, C.A., Balbo, P.B., Pesci, E.C., Cottle, D.L., Mirabito, P.M., and Pickett, C.L. (**1998**). *Campylobacter jejuni* cytolethal distending toxin causes a G2-phase cell cycle block. *Infect. Immun.* 66: 1934–1940.

Wilkinson, S. M., Uhl, J.R., Kline, B.C., and Cockerill, F.R., III. (**1998**). Assessment of invasion frequencies of cultured HEp-2 cells by clinical isolates of *Helicobacter pylori* using an acridine orange assay. *J. Clin. Pathol.* 51: 127–133.

Wirth, H.P., Beins, M.H., Yang, M., Tham, K.T., and Blaser, M.J. (**1998**). Experimental infection of Mongolian gerbils with wild-type and mutant *Helicobacter pylori* strains. *Infect. Immun.* 66: 4856–4866.

Witherell, H.L., Hansen, S., Jellum, E., Orentreich, N., Vogelman, J.H., and Parsonnet, J. (**1997**). Risk for gastric lymphoma in persons with CagA+ and CagA- *Helicobacter pylori* infection. *J. Infect. Dis.* 176: 1641–1644.

Wong, B.C., Lam, S. K., Wong, W.M., Chen, J.S., Zheng, T.T., Feng, R.E., Lai, K.C., Hu, W.H., Yuen, S. T., Leung, S. Y., Fong, D.Y., Ho, J., and Ching, C.K. (**2004**). *Helicobacter pylori* eradication to prevent gastric cancer in a high-risk region of China: a randomized controlled trial. *JAMA* 291: 187–194.

Woodward, M., Morrison, C., and McColl, K. (**2000**). An investigation into factors associated with *Helicobacter pylori* infection. *J. Clin. Epidemiol.* 53: 175–181.

World Cancer Research Fund, A. I. f. C. R. **1997**. Stomach. Washington, DC.

Wotherspoon, A.C., Ortiz-Hidalgo, C., Falzon, M.R., and Isaacson, P.G. (**1991**). *Helicobacter pylori*-associated gastritis and primary B-cell gastric lymphoma. *Lancet* 338: 1175–1176.

Wotherspoon, A.C., Doglioni, C., Diss, T.C., Pan, L., Moschini, A., de Boni, M., and Isaacson, P.G. (**1993**). Regression of primary low-grade B-cell gastric lymphoma of mucosa-associated lymphoid tissue type after eradication of *Helicobacter pylori*. *Lancet* 342: 575–577.

Wundisch, T., Thiede, C., Morgner, A., Dempfle, A., Gunther, A., Liu, H., Ye, H., Du, M. Q., Kim, T.D., Bayerdorffer, E., Stolte, M., and Neubauer, A. (**2005**). Long-term follow-up of gastric MALT lymphoma after *Helicobacter pylori* eradication. *J. Clin. Oncol.* 23: 8018–8024.

Wyckoff, J., Wang, W., Lin, E.Y., Wang, Y., Pixley, F., Stanley, E.R., Graf, T., Pollard, J.W., Segall, J., and Condeelis, J. (**2004**). A paracrine loop between tumor cells and macrophages is required for tumor cell migration in mammary tumors. *Cancer Res.* 64: 7022–7029.

Xiang, Z., Censini, S., Bayeli, P.F., Telford, J.L., Figura, N., Rappuoli, R., and Covacci, A. (**1995**). Analysis of expression of CagA and VacA virulence factors in 43 strains of *Helicobacter pylori* reveals that clinical isolates can be divided into two major types and that CagA is not necessary for expression of the vacuolating cytotoxin. *Infect. Immun.* 63: 94–98.

Xu, H., Chaturvedi, R., Cheng, Y., Bussiere, F.I., Asim, M., Yao, M.D., Potosky, D., Meltzer, S. J., Rhee, J.G., Kim, S. S., Moss, S. F., Hacker, A., Wang, Y., Casero, R.A., Jr., and Wilson, K.T. (**2004**). Spermine oxidation induced by Helicobacter pylori results in apoptosis and DNA damage: implications for gastric carcinogenesis. *Cancer Res.* 64: 8521–8525.

Xu, S. and Venge, P. (**2000**). Lipocalins as biochemical markers of disease. *Biochim. Biophys. Acta* 1482: 298–307.

Yamori, M., Yoshida, M., Watanabe, T., Shirai, Y., Iizuka, T., Kita, T., and Wakatsuki, Y. (**2004**). Antigenic activation of Th1 cells in the gastric mucosa enhances dys-regulated apoptosis and turnover of the epithelial cells. *Biochem. Biophys. Res. Commun.* 316: 1015–1021.

Yang, H., Li, X., Xu, Z., and Zhou, D. (**1995**). "*Helicobacter heilmannii*' infection in a patient with gastric cancer. *Dig. Dis. Sci.* 40: 1013–1014.

Yokota, K., Kurebayashi, Y., Takayama, Y., Hayashi, S., Isogai, H., Isogai, E., Imai, K., Yabana, T., Yachi, A., and Oguma, K. (**1991**). Colonization of *Helicobacter pylori* in the gastric mucosa of Mongolian gerbils. *Microbiol. Immunol.* 35: 475–480.

Young, V.B., Chien, C.C., Knox, K.A., Taylor, N.S., Schauer, D.B., and Fox, J.G. (**2000a**). Cytolethal distending toxin in avian and human isolates of *Helicobacter pullorum*. *J. Infect. Dis.* 182: 620–623.

Young, V.B., Knox, K.A., and Schauer, D.B. (**2000b**). Cytolethal distending toxin sequence and activity in the enterohepatic pathogen *Helicobacter hepaticus*. *Infect. Immun.* 68: 184–191.

Young, V.B., Knox, K.A., Pratt, J.S., Cortez, J.S., Mansfield, L.S., Rogers, A.B., Fox, J.G., and Schauer, D.B. (**2004**). In vitro and *in vivo* characterization of *Helicobacter hepaticus* cytolethal distending toxin mutants. *Infect. Immun.* 72: 2521–2527.

Yu, J., Russell, R.M., Salomon, R.N., Murphy, J.C., Palley, L.S., and Fox, J.G. (**1995**). Effect of *Helicobacter mustelae* infection on ferret gastric epithelial cell proliferation. *Carcinogenesis* 16: 1927–1931.

Zavros, Y., Rieder, G., Ferguson, A., Samuelson, L.C., and Merchant, J.L. (**2002**). Genetic or chemical hypochlorhydria is associated with inflammation that modulates parietal and G-cell populations in mice. *Gastroenterology* 122: 119–133.

Zavros, Y., Eaton, K.A., Kang, W., Rathinavelu, S., Katukuri, V., Kao, J.Y., Samuelson, L.C., and Merchant, J.L. (**2005**). Chronic gastritis in the hypochlorhydric gastrin-deficient mouse progresses to adenocarcinoma. *Oncogene* 24: 2354–2366.

11
Parasites and Human Cancers

11.1
Schistosoma Infections

Early suspicions that specific parasite infections play a role in human cancer development were discussed in Chapter 1. In 1905, Goebel postulated a causal association between *Schistosoma haematobium* infection and bladder cancer.

A total of five species of *Schistosoma* trematodes (Fig. 11.1) infect humans: *Schistosoma haematobium, S. mansoni, S. japonicum, S. mekongi*, and *S. intercalatum*. The first three represent the most important organisms, and have long been considered risk factors for cancers of the gastrointestinal tract and of the liver (Inaba et al., 1984; Chen and Mott, 1989).

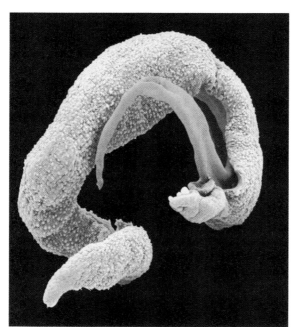

Fig. 11.1 A pair of *Schistosoma* parasites. The female is kept tightly linked within the deep ventral groove or schist of the male, where it resides permanently. (SPL / Agentur Focus.)

Infections Causing Human Cancer. Harald zur Hausen
Copyright © 2006 WILEY-VCH Verlag GmbH & Co. KGaA, Weinheim
ISBN: 3-527-31056-8

It has been estimated that 600 million people are at risk for schistosomiasis (IARC, 1994), and that within 74 countries about 200 million are currently infected (WHO, 1993). The vast majority of human infections are due to *S. mansoni* and *S. haematobium*.

The life cycle of *Schistosoma* infections is complex (Fig. 11.2). Adult worms may persist for up to 30 years in the vesical plexus of the urinary bladder (*S. haematobium*) or in mesenteric veins (von Lichtenberg, 1987). The median life span of schistosomes amounts to three to six years (Anderson, 1987). All schistosomes produce large numbers of eggs which are excreted into the urinary bladder (*S. haematobium*) or the intestines and excreted with urine or feces. Retained eggs survive for a further three weeks and cause most of the pathological manifestations (Warren, 1978). Released embryonated eggs hatch in water and liberate the miracidium larvae. In the infected snail, sporocysts are formed from which several hundred daughter sporocysts are produced. These migrate to the digestive and reproductive tract of the snail and produce cercariae, which may infect humans. Once the cercaria has penetrated the human skin, it metamorphosizes to a "schistosomulum"; this occurs as the cercaria enters a lymphatic vessel or capillary. Further morphologic changes lead to a schistosomulum, which enters the lung and subsequently the left side of the heart (Wilson, 1987). After a few recirculations, the schistosomulum reaches the portal vein system, where a further metamorphosis occurs. Here, the mature worms pair and migrate to the final sites in the vesical plexus of the bladder (*S. haematobium*) and mesenteric veins.

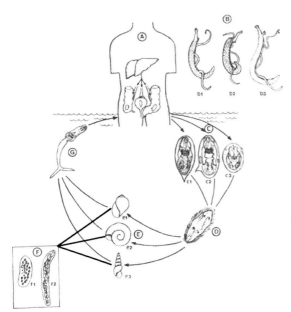

Fig. 11.2 Life cycle of *Schistosoma* infections. Illustrations b1–b3 show adult *S. haematobium*, *S. mansoni*, and *S. japonicum*, respectively. Embryonated eggs (c1–c3) of the three species, respectively, are also shown. The larvae (miracidium) infect as an intermediate host the snail species *Bulinus* sp. (*S. haematobium*), *Biomphalaria* sp. (*S. mansoni*), and *Oncomelania* sp. (*S. japonicum*), respectively. F shows the intramolluscum stage, and G a cercaria. (WHO, The Control of Schistosomiasis. Second Report of the WHO Expert Committee (WHO tech. Rep. Ser. 830), Geneva, 1993.)

11.1.1
Epidemiology

The geographic distribution of *Schistosoma* infections depends in turn on the geographic distribution of their respective intermediate snail hosts. *S. mansoni* is widely spread and occurs in 52 countries in Africa, the Eastern Mediterranean, South America, and the Caribbean (*IARC*, 1994). *S. haematobium* shares many of these areas, but does not occur in the Americas (Fig. 11.3).

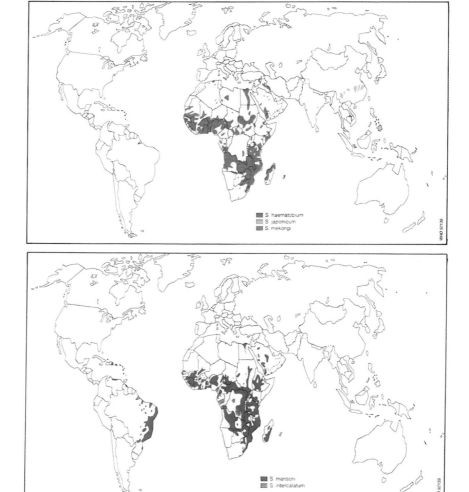

Fig. 11.3 Geographic distribution of *S. haematonium*, *S. japonicum*, and *S. mekongi* (upper panel), and of *S. mansoni* and *S. intercalatum* (lower panel). (WHO, The Control of Schistosomiasis. Second Report of the WHO Expert Committee (WHO tech. Rep. Ser. 830), Geneva, 1993.)

The main risk factor for acquiring schistosoma infections is contact with contaminated water (Jordan and Webbe, 1993), though genetic factors also seem to play a role in patient susceptibility (Abel et al., 1991). In hyperendemic regions for *S. haematobium* infection, such as lower Egypt, Zambia, and Malawi, the peak of bladder cancer incidence occurs at about the age of 45 years (El Bolkainy et al., 1981; Lucas, 1982; Elem and Purohit, 1983). In these countries cancer of the bladder is one of the most prevalent carcinomas. In non-endemic areas for schistosomiasis, bladder cancer occurs most frequently in age groups above 60 years.

A clear-cut relationship between *S. mansoni* infections and human cancer has not yet been established. Moreover, the rates of incidence for colorectal cancer in Africa do not differ significantly between endemic and non-endemic regions (Parkin, 1994).

In spite of a few positive correlations with liver cancer and cancers of the esophagus and stomach (Liu et al., 1983; Xu and Su, 1984; Chen et al., 1990; Guo et al., 1993) for areas with high rates of *S. japonicum* infections, the available data do not seem to permit firm conclusions to be made. An earlier study did not identify the reported associations (Inaba, 1984). Major problems in interpretation arise from the high prevalence of other potentially tumorigenic infections within the same areas, including *Helicobacter pylori*, hepatitis B and C, and Epstein–Barr virus.

Thus, *S. haematobium* emerges as the only well-documented infection linked to human cancer, and this will be discussed later. *S. haematobium* has been linked specifically to squamous cell carcinomas of the bladder (Lucas, 1982; Al-Fouadi and Parkin, 1984). In fact, in areas where males provide most of the agricultural labor (e.g., in the Nile Delta), the male:female ratio of bladder cancer cases may rise to 12:1 (Makhyoun et al., 1971). In other areas, where women perform the majority of agricultural tasks, the male:female ratio may fall to 1:1 or 1:2 (Keen and Fripp, 1980). In Egypt, a ratio of 70:25:5 has been reported for squamous cell carcinomas, transitional cell carcinomas, and adenocarcinomas (Khafagy et al., 1972). whereas in western countries the ratio is 5:94:1 (Mostofi, 1956).

11.1.2
Experimental Studies in Animals

A number of experimental studies with *S. haematobium* have been conducted in mice, rats, hamsters, opossums, and nonhuman primates (for a review, see IARC, 1994), though the data in relation to cancer induction are inconclusive. Among non-human primates, the exposure of capuchin monkeys to 1000–2000 cercariae resulted in papillary hyperplasia of the bladder in six of nine animals, and focal nodular hyperplasia in two animals (Kuntz et al., 1978). The infection of five baboons with 1000 cercariae, followed 2.5 years later with the chemical carcinogen *N*-butyl-*N*-(4-hydroxybutyl)nitrosamine, led to polyploidy hyperplasia of the urinary tract in four animals, and to endophytic papillary hyperplasia of the ureter in one animal (Hicks et al., 1980; Hicks, 1982). In contrast, baboons treated only with the chemical carcinogen did not develop any lesions.

In *S. japonicum* infections, the induction of cancer by known chemical carcinogens is increased (Ishii et al., 1994), though many of the relevant experiments date back more than 30 years and are the results presently difficult to interpret.

One interesting aspect has been discovered by analyzing *S. japonicum* and *S. mansoni* genomes for host cell sequences following passage in mice (Imase et al., 2003). Mouse MHC class I sequences and a type A retroviral sequence were detected in the cercarial DNA of both organisms by blot hybridization; however, this observation requires further confirmation. The presence of a larger number or retrotransposons within the *Schistosoma* genome has been noted in genomic analyses (DeMarco et al., 2005).

11.1.3
Schistosoma Eggs and Cancer

In areas of hyperendemic *S. haematobium* infections, schistosoma eggs are regularly found in bladder tumors (el-Bolkainy et al., 1981; Lucas, 1982; Al-Adnani and Saleh, 1983; Elem and Purohit, 1983). Normally, these eggs escape in the host's excretions, but if they are retained in the host tissue they elicit immunopathological reactions (Perrin and Phillips, 1988; Perrin et al., 1989), with delayed-type hypersensitivity granulomatous reactions developing. These granulomata, which may by far exceed the size of the egg, can lead to early obstructive lesions in the lower end of the ureter. Fibrotic responses may follow, resulting in obstructive changes (WHO Report, 1987).

In this respect it remains remarkable that adult worms persist in the venous system without being recognized by the immune system of the host. No inflammatory responses are detectable at the site of their persistence. Immunity against schistosomes is mainly active against invading larvae in the skin, and anti-disease immunity, which controls abnormal fibrosis in tissues invaded by schistosome eggs (Dessein et al., 2004). Interleukin (IL)-13 in the skin and interferon (IFN)-γ in the liver seem to represent the key players in protective immunity against schistosomes. These roles relate to the high anti-fibrogenic activities of IFN-γ and to the unique ability of IL-3 in Th2 priming in the skin and in the mobilization of eosinophils in tissues (Dessein et al., 2004).

Unlike the adult trematodes, however, the eggs are recognized by the host, and sensitized lymphocytes, inflammatory cells, and antibodies each contribute to the granulomatous process (King and Mahmoud, 1992). Since *Schistosoma* egg excretion is dependent on an intact host CD4 T-helper (Th) cell response to egg antigens, eggs may have evolved to be highly immunogenic and capable of inducing potent Th responses (Pearce, 2005). The egg-induced Th response is unusual in that it is highly Th2-polarized. The selective pressure on the host to mount a Th2 response against eggs is apparent in the fact that Th2 response-defective mice develop acutely lethal disease when infected with schistosomes (Pearce, 2005). Activation of Toll-like receptor 3 was recently implicated as one of the primary events responding to immunological stimulation by *Schistosoma* eggs (Aksoy et al., 2005). Activation of this receptor resulted in the activation of NF-κB and the positive regulatory domain III-I site from the IFN-β promoter.

It seems that the inflammatory responses directed against the *Schistosoma* eggs contribute in particular to bladder cancer development in *S. haematobium* infections. It remains, however, unresolved as to what extent other factors might also contribute. Interactions with additional infections or chemical carcinogens seem also to contribute.

11.1.4
Interactions of *Schistosoma* with Other Infections, and Chemical Factors

Early suspicions that *Schistosoma* infection might interact with papillomavirus infections were mainly based on an increased incidence of cancer of the cervix in regions of high rates of *Schistosoma* infections (Petry et al., 2003). However, in the case of bladder cancer no evidence was found for any interaction with human papillomavirus (HPV) (Cooper et al., 1997).

A relatively high prevalence of bacteriuria was found in young men with schistosomiasis, and low levels of *N*-nitroso compounds were present in all specimens (Hicks et al., 1982). When the groups were subdivided on the basis of the ability of their bacterial flora to reduce nitrate to nitrite, significantly higher levels of *N*-nitroso compounds were found in *S. haematobium*-infected individuals also infected with nitrate-reducing bacteria by comparison either with uninfected controls ($p < 0.0005$) or with those infected with non-nitrate-reducing bacteria ($p < 0.001$).

Significant increases in the excretion of volatile *N*-nitroso compounds were found in *S. haematobium*-infected patients, with a mean excretion of 19.2 ± 21 μg per day of *N*-nitroso-dimethylamine (NDMA). In the control group, NDMA was detected at concentrations (mean $\pm$ SD) of 0.27 ± 0.47 μg per day (Mostafa et al., 1994). These data point to the formation of potentially carcinogenic nitrosamines in *Schistosoma*-infected patients which may either arise from metabolic processes of the trematodes or from concomitant bacterial infections. Since *Escherichia coli* contains the enzyme nitrate reductase, this infection may contribute to higher nitrite levels (El-Aaser et al., 1982; Bonnefoy and Demoss, 1994; Blasco et al., 2001). An enzyme known to be involved in activating carcinogens, namely β-glucuronidase, has been detected in high concentrations in *E. coli*-infected bladders of patients with schistosomiasis (El-Aaser et al., 1982).

Inflammatory cells, such as neutrophils, macrophages, and eosinophils, are an important endogenous source of oxygen radicals. Stimulation of these cells by tumor promoters or by foreign agents (parasites, bacteria, etc.) causes the release of reactive oxygen species (ROS). Studies on ROS formation were mainly conducted in *S. mansoni* egg-induced granulomatous inflammation (Chensue et al., 1984), or in sporocyst-carrying snails (Connors et al., 1991). In granulomatous inflammations, the formation of ROS is favored, including superoxide ions, hydrogen peroxide and hydroxyl radicals, all of which may induce lipid peroxidation (Facundo et al., 2004). In snails, a high rate of production of ROS emerges as a protective mechanism against *Schistosoma* infection, and also determines the susceptibility to infection (Bender et al., 2005). Apparently, IL-4 plays a protective role by controlling the tight regulation of the generation of reactive oxygen and nitrogen intermediates in the liver (La Flamme et al., 2001).

11.1.5
Mechanism of *Schistosoma*-Induced Cancers

Mechanistic events leading to bladder cancer in *S. haematobium* infections are still poorly understood. Clearly, these parasites have an indirect impact on the induction of malignant proliferations. In all likelihood, carcinogenic metabolites produced by concomitant infections cause mutational events at the sites of granulomatous proliferations surrounding persisting *Schistosoma* eggs. Inflammatory reactions at these sites result in the production of reactive oxygen and nitrogen intermediates which add to the mutational modifications.

Although a number of genetic modifications have been noted in cellular oncogenes in *Schistosoma*-associated bladder cancers (Ramchurren et al., 1995), no characteristic genetic changes were found in these tumors.

11.1.6
Control and Therapy

Several modes for the control of schistosomiasis are possible, with health education, the provision of safe water supplies and sanitation and the avoidance of contaminated water emerging as the most clear and effective measurements. Unfortunately, chemical elimination of the snail intermediate host causes adverse effects, in almost all circumstances, for other organic forms of life within the environment.

Effective drugs are available for treatment. Praziquantel, (2-cyclohexylcarbonyl)-1,2,3,6,7,11 b-hexa-hydro-2H pyrazino[2,1a]isoquinolin-4-one, belongs to a series of very effective antischistosomal compounds (Gönnert and Andrews, 1977). The discovery of praziquantel has been a breakthrough for the treatment of patients infected with schistosomes (Chen, 2005). Praziquantel is usually administered as a single oral dose and has no or only mild and transient side effects. The drug is highly efficacious against *S. japonicum*, whether in patients with acute and chronic stages of the infection, among subjects with extensive hepatosplenic involvement, or in patients with other complicated disease forms. Chemotherapy with praziquantel also plays a role in the transmission control of schistosomiasis, although the interruption of subsequent transmissions cannot be achieved by chemotherapy alone (Chen, 2005).

Nonetheless, by using integrated control measures, the eradication or substantial reduction of *Schistosoma* infections have been achieved in several countries (for a review, see IARC, 1994).

References

Abel, L., Demenais, F., Prata, A., Souza, A.E., and Dessein, A. Evidence for the segregation of a major gene in human susceptibility/resistance to infection by *Schistosoma mansoni*. *Am. J. Hum. Genet.* 48: 959–970, **1991** .

Aksoy, E., Zouain, C.S., Vanhoutte, F., Fontaine, J., Pavelka, N., Thieblemont, N., Willems, F., Ricciardi-Castagnoli, P., Goldman, M., Capron, M., Ryffel, B., and Trottein, F. Double-stranded RNAs from the helminth parasite *Schistosoma* activate

TLR3 in dendritic cells. *J. Biol. Chem.* 280: 277–283, **2005**.

Al-Adnani, M.S. and Saleh, K.M. Extraurinary schistosomiasis in Southern Iraq. *Histopathology* 6: 747–752, **1982**.

Al-Fouadi, A. and Parkin, D.M. Cancer in Iraq: seven years' data from the Baghdad Tumour Registry. *Int. J. Cancer* 34: 207–213, **1984**.

Anderson, R.M. Determinants of infection in human schistosomiasis. In: Mahmoud, A.A.F. (Ed.), *Ballière's Clinical Tropical Medicine and Communicable Diseases. Vol. 2. Schistosomiasis.* Ballière Tindall; London, pp. 279–300, **1987**.

Bender, R.C., Broderick, E.J., Goodall, C.P., and Bayne, C.J. Respiratory burst of *Biomphalaria glabrata* hemocytes: *Schistosoma mansoni*-resistant snails produce more extracellular H_2O_2 than susceptible snails. *J. Parasitol.* 91: 275–279, **2005**.

Blasco, F., Guigliarelli, B., Magalon, A., Asso, M., Giordano, G., and Rothery, R.A. The coordination and function of the redox centres of the membrane-bound nitrate reductases. *Cell. Mol. Life Sci.* 58: 179–193, **2001**.

Bonnefoy, V. and Demoss, J.A. Nitrate reductases in *Escherichia coli*. *Antonie Van Leeuwenhoek* 66: 47–56, **1994**.

Chen, J., Campbell, T.C., Li, J., and Peto, R. *Diet, life-style, and mortality in China. A study of the characteristics of 65 Chinese counties.* Oxford University Press, Oxford, **1990**.

Chen, M.G. Use of praziquantel for clinical treatment and morbidity control of schistosomiasis japonica in China: a review of 30 years' experience. *Acta Trop.* 96: 168–176, **2005**.

Chen, M.G. and Mott, K.E. Progress in assessment of morbidity due to *Schistosoma haematobium* infection. A review of recent literature. *Trop. Dis. Bull.* 86: R2–R56, **1989**.

Chensue, S. W., Quinlan, L., Higashi, G.I., and Kunkel, S. L. Role of oxygen reactive species in *Schistosoma mansoni* egg-induced granulomatous inflammation. *Biochem. Biophys. Res. Commun.* 122: 184–190, **1984**.

Connors, V.A., Lodes, M.J., and Yoshino, T.P. Identification of a *Schistosoma mansoni* sporocyst excretory-secretory antioxidant molecule and its effect on superoxide production by *Biomphalaria glabrata* hemocytes. *J. Invertebr. Pathol.* 58: 387–395, **1991**.

Cooper, K., Haffajee, Z., and Taylor, L. Human papillomavirus and schistosomiasis associated bladder cancer. *Mol. Pathol.* 50: 145–148, **1997**.

DeMarco, R., Machado, A.A., Bisson-Filho, A.W., and Verjovski-Almeida, S. Identification of 18 new transcribed retrotransposons in *Schistosoma mansoni*. *Biochem. Biophys. Res. Commun.* 333: 230–240, **2005**.

Dessein, A., Kouriba, B., Eboumbou, C., Dessein, H., Argiro, L., Marquet, S., Elwali, N.E., Rodrigues, V., Li, Y., Doumbo, O., and Chevillard, C. Interleukin-13 in the skin and interferon-gamma in the liver are key players in immune protection in human schistosomiasis. *Immunol. Rev.* 201: 180–190, **2004**.

El-Aaser, A.A., El-Merzabani, M.M., Higgy, N.A., and El-Habet, A.E. A study on the etiological factors of bilharzial bladder cancer in Egypt. 6. The possible role of urinary bacteria. *Tumori* 68: 23–28, **1982**.

el-Bolkainy, M.N., Mokhtar, N.M., Ghoneim, M.A., and Hussein, M.H. The impact of schistosomiasis on the pathology of bladder carcinoma. *Cancer* 48: 2643–2648, **1981**.

[kape]Elem, B. and Purohit, R. Carcinoma of the urinary bladder in Zambia. A quantitative estimation of *Schistosoma haematobium* infection. *Br. J. Urol.* 55: 275–278, **1983**.

Facundo, H.T., Brandt, C.T., Owen, J.S., and Lima, V.L. Elevated levels of erythrocyte-conjugated dienes indicate increased lipid peroxidation in schistosomiasis mansoni patients. *Braz. J. Med. Biol. Res.* 37: 957–962, **2004**.

Goebel, C. Über die bei Bilharziakrankheit vorkommenden Blasentumoren mit besonderer Berücksichtigung des Carcinoms. *Zeitschr. Krebsforsch.* 3: 369–513, **1905**.

Gönnert, R. and Andrews, P. Praziquantel, a new broad-spectrum antischistosomal agent. *Z. Parasitenkd.* 52: 129–150, **1977**.

Guo, W., Zheng, W., Li, J.Y., Chen, J.S., and Blot, W.J. Correlations of colon cancer mortality with dietary factors, serum markers, and schistosomiasis in China. *Nutr. Cancer* 20: 13–20, **1993**.

Hicks, R.M. Nitrosamines as possible etiological agents in bilharzial bladder cancer. In: Magee, P.N. (Ed.), *Nitrosamines and Human Cancer*. Banburry Report No. 12, Cold Spring Harbor Laboratory Press, pp. 455–471, **1982**.

Hicks, R.M., James, C., and Webbe, G. Effect of *Schistosoma haematobium* and *N*-butyl-*N*-(4-hydroxybutyl)nitrosamine on the development of urothelial neoplasia in the baboon. *Br. J. Cancer* 42: 730–755, **1980**.

Hicks, R.M., Ismail, M.M., Walters, C.L., Beecham, P.T., Rabie, M.F., and El Alamy, M.A. Association of bacteriuria and urinary nitrosamine formation with *Schistosoma haematobium* infection in the Qalyub area of Egypt. *Trans. R. Soc. Trop. Med. Hyg.* 76: 519–527, **1982**.

IARC Monographs on the Evaluation of Carcinogenic Risks to Humans. Volume 61. *Schistosomes, Liver Flukes and* Helicobacter pylori. IARC Lyon, **1994**.

Imase, A., Matsuda, H., Irie, Y., and Iwamura, Y. Existence of host DNA sequences in schistosomes – horizontal and vertical transmission. *Parasitol. Int.* 52: 369–373, **2003**.

Inaba, Y. A cohort study on the causes of death in an endemic area of schistosomiasis japonica in Japan. *Ann. Acad. Med. Singapore* 13: 142–148, **1984**.

Inaba, Y., Maruchi, N., Matsuda, M., Yoshihara, N., and Yamamoto, S. A case-control study on liver cancer with special emphasis on the possible aetiological role of schistosomiasis. *Int. J. Epidemiol.* 13: 408–412, **1984**.

Ishii, A., Matsuoka, H., Aji, T., Ohta, N., Arimoto, S., Wataya, Y., and Hayatsu, H. Parasite infection and cancer: with special emphasis on *Schistosoma japonicum* infections (Trematoda). A review. *Mutat Res.* 305: 273–281, **1994**.

Jordan, P. and Webbe, G. In: Jordan, P., Webbe, G. and Sturrock, R.F. (Eds.), *Human Schistosomiasis. Epidemiology*. Wallingford, CAB International, pp. 87–158, **1993**.

Khafagy, M.M., el-Bolkainy, M.N., and Mansour, M.A. Carcinoma of the bilharzial urinary bladder. A study of the associated mucosal lesions in 86 cases. *Cancer* 30: 150–159, **1972**.

Keen, P. and Fripp, P.J. Bladder cancer in an endemic schistosomiasis area: geographical and sex distribution. *S. Afr. J. Sci.* 76: 228–230, **1980**.

King, C.H. and Mahmoud, A.A.F. Schistosoma and other trematodes. In: Gorbach, S. L., Bartlett, J.G., and Blacklow, N.R. (Eds.), *Infectious Diseases*. W.B. Saunders Co. Philadelphia, pp. 2015–2021, **1992**.

Kuntz, R.E., Cheever, A.W., Bryan, G.T., Moore, J.A., and Huang, T. Natural history of papillary lesions of the urinary bladder in schistosomiasis. *Cancer Res.* 38: 3836–3839, **1978**.

La Flamme, A.C., Patton, E.A., Bauman, B., and Pearce, E.J. IL-4 plays a crucial role in regulating oxidative damage in the liver during schistosomiasis. *J. Immunol.* 166: 1903–1911, **2001**.

Liu, B.C., Rong, Z.P., Sun, X.T., Wu, Y.P., and Gao, R.Q. Study of geographic correlation between colorectal cancers and schistosomiasis in China. *Acta Acad. Med. Sin.* 5: 173–177, **1983**.

Lucas, S. B. Bladder tumours in Malawi. *Br. J. Urol.* 54: 275–279, **1982**.

Makhyoun, N.A., el-Kashlan, K.M., al-Ghorab, M.M., and Mokhles, A.S. Aetiological factors in bilharzial bladder cancer. *J. Trop. Med. Hyg.* 74: 73–78, **1971**.

Mostafa, M.H., Helmi, S., Badawi, A.F., Tricker, A.R., Spiegelhalder, B., and Preussmann, R. Nitrate, nitrite and volatile N-nitroso compounds in the urine of *Schistosoma haematobium* and *Schistosoma mansoni* infected patients. *Carcinogenesis* 15: 619–625, **1994**.

Mostofi, F.K. A study of 2678 patients with initial carcinoma of the bladder. II. Survival rates in relation to therapy. *J. Urol.* 75: 492–500, **1956**.

Parkin, D.M. Cancer in developing countries. *Cancer Surv.* 19–20: 519–561, **1994**.

Pearce, E.J. Priming of the immune response by schistosome eggs. *Parasite Immunol.* 27: 265–270, **2005**.

Perrin, P.J. and Phillips, S. M. The molecular basis of granuloma formation in schistosomiasis. I. A T cell-derived suppressor effector factor. *J. Immunol.* 141: 1714–1719, **1988**.

Perrin, P.J., Prystowsky, M.B., and Phillips, S. M. The molecular basis of granuloma formation in schistosomiasis. II. Analogies of a T cell-derived suppressor effector factor to the T cell receptor. *J. Immunol.* 142: 985–991, **1989** .

Petry, K.U., Scholz, U., Hollwitz, B., Von Wasielewski, R., and Meijer, C.J.M. Human papillomavirus, coinfection with *Schistosoma hematobium*, and cervical neoplasia in rural Tanzania. *Int. J. Gynecol. Cancer* 13: 505–509, **2003**.

Ramchurren, N., Cooper, K., and Summerhayes, I.C. Molecular events underlying schistosomiasis-related bladder cancer. *Int. J. Cancer* 62: 237–244, **1995**.

von Lichtenberg, F. Consequences of infections with schistosomes. In: Rollinson, D. and Simpson, A.J.G. (Eds.), *The Biology of Schistosomes. From Genes to Latrines.* Academic Press, London, pp. 185–232, **1987**.

Warren, K.S., Siongok, T.K., Houser, H.B., Ouma, J.H., and Peters, P.A. Quantification of infection with *Schistosoma haematobium* in relation to epidemiology and selec-

tive population chemotherapy. I. Minimal number of daily egg counts in urine necessary to establish intensity of infection. *J. Infect. Dis.* 138: 849–855, **1978**.

WHO Report. *The control of Schistosomiasis.* Second Report of the WHO Expert Committee. Geneva, WHO Tech. Rep. Ser. 830, **1993**.

WHO Report. *Progress in assessment of morbidity due to Schistosoma mansoni infection: a review of recent literature.* Geneva, pp. 3–66, **1987**.

Wilson, R.A. Cercariae to liver worms: development and migration in the mammalian host. In: Rollinson, D. and Simpson, A.J.G. (Eds.), *The Biology of Schistosomes. From Genes to Latrines.* Academic Press, London, pp. 115–146, **1987**.

Xu, Z. and Su, D.L. Schistosoma japonicum and colorectal cancer: an epidemiological study in the People's Republic of China. *Int. J. Cancer* 34: 315–318, **1984**.

11.2
Infection with Liver Flukes (*Opisthorchis viverrini, O. felineus, Clonorchis sinensis*)

The three *Opisthorchis* liver flukes represent food-borne members of the Trematode family. They establish chronic infections within the smaller intrahepatic bile ducts, more rarely in the pancreas and the gall bladder of fish-eating mammals and humans (IARC, 1994).

The life cycle of these trematodes is even more complex than that of *Schistosoma* trematodes. Infection occurs by consumption of raw or undercooked fish. The metacercaria evade from the cyst in the duodenum, enter the ampulla of Vateri, and finally reach the smaller bile ducts of the liver. They can also be found in pancreatic ducts and exceptionally within the gall bladder (Hou, 1955; Sithithaworn et al., 1991). After about one month, the adult worms have matured and produce large quantities of eggs, which are released via the bile duct into the feces. The average life span of the worm is about 10 years, but occasionally more than 25 years may be reached (Attwood and Chou, 1978). The life cycle of these trematodes is depicted in Figure 11.4. Although only a small number of snails as the first immediate host become infected in a water pond or stream, commonly 100% of the local fish subsequently carry the metacercaria (Brockelman et al., 1986). More than 80 species of Cyprinidae fish and 13 species of other fish families may serve as second intermediate hosts (Komiya, 1966; Vichasri et al., 1982; Rim, 1986; Joo, 1988).

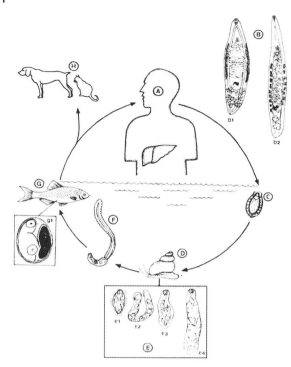

Fig. 11.4 The life cycle of liver flukes. Adult liver flukes in the bile duct (b1 = *Clonorchis sinensis*; b2 = *Opisthorchis viverrini*). C represents an embryonated egg. D is the first intermediate host, *Bithyria* sp. E represents the intramolluscan stages (miracidium e1, sporocyst e2, mother redia e3, daughter redia e4). F shows a cercaria and G the second intermediate host (cyprinoid fish). From the fish muscle (when eaten), the metacercaria (g1) reaches the final host (dog, cat, or human). (IARC Monographs on the Evaluation of Carcinogenic Risks to Humans, Volume 61 (Schistosomes, liver flukes and Helicobacter pylori). Lyon, France: IARC, 1994.)

11.2.1
Epidemiology

The worldwide distribution of the three liver fluke species is illustrated in Figure 11.5. Infections are mainly found in China, Korea, Laos, Thailand, Vietnam, Russia, Ukraine, and parts of Eastern Europe. In 1994, the World Health Organization (WHO) estimated that about 17 million people were infected by these trematodes. Of these subjects, seven million are thought to be infected by *Clonorchis sinensis*, nine million by *O. viverrini*, and 1.5 million by *O. felineus*.

Opisthorchis viverrini infections are most prevalent in North-East and those northern provinces of Thailand that border Laos (Jongsuksuntigul and Imsomboon, 1997). It is also common in the low lands of Laos (Giboda et al., 1991; Pholsena et al., 1991), although the total number of infected persons is difficult to estimate. *Opisthorchis felineus* is mainly found in Western Siberia and also along the Volga-Kama river basin (Iarotski and Be'er, 1993). Infections are also noted in the Ukraine and Kazakhstan.

Clonorchis infections are distributed throughout China, notably in regions where raw or undercooked fish is consumed (Chen et al., 1994). The infection is also frequent in Hong Kong and Taiwan (Hou et al., 1989; Chen, 1991), but it has been largely eliminated in Japan (Chen et al., 1994). Northern Vietnam and the Amur River basin in Russia also represent regions with a high rate of infections.

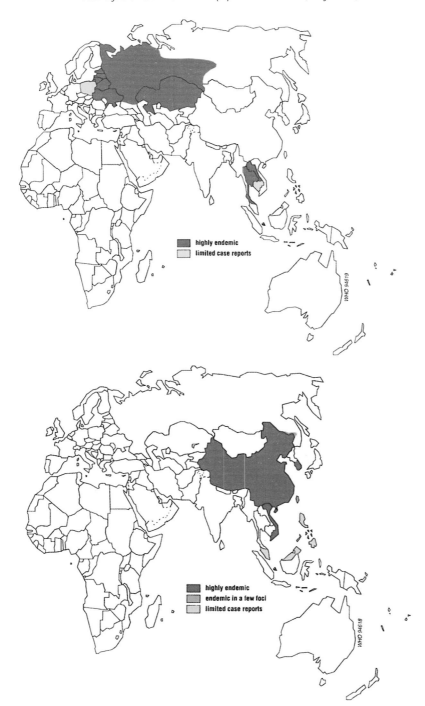

Fig. 11.5 Worldwide distribution of *Opisthorchis viverrini* and *O. felineus* (upper panel), and of *Clonorchis sinensis* (lower panel). (WHO, Control of Foodborne Nematode Infections (WHO Tech. Rep. Ser.), Geneva, 1994.)

The sole risk factor for these three infections is the consumption of raw or incompletely cooked fish, sometimes moderately or completely fermented, smoked or salted fish (IARC, 1994). Infection may occur in young children, but peaks among late teenage groups (Upatham et al., 1982; Sithithaworn et al., 1991).

11.2.2
Immune Response

A significant degree of humoral and cell-mediated immune responses to the parasite can be detected both in patients as well as in animal models (Wongratanacheewin et al., 2003). The patients' IgG levels appear to correlate with the *Opisthorchis* egg count, and decrease after treatment. A number of antigens of *Clonorchis* and *Opisthorchis* have been defined (Choi et al., 2003); the frequency and intensity of immunoblot reactions against these antigens were positively correlated with the intensity of the liver fluke infection. Even egg-negative residents of an opisthorchiasis-endemic area possess high levels of anti-*Opisthorchis* antibodies (Akai et al., 1995 a). A serological crossreactivity exists with antigens of other parasitic trematodes and possibly a broader spectrum of parasites (Sakolvaree et al., 1997). Serum antibodies persist for prolonged periods of time, even after successful chemotherapy of the fluke infections (Akai et al., 1995 b).

The immune response does not seem to influence the worm burden or the egg output, since T-cell-deprived *Opisthorchis*-infected animals produced the same egg counts as immunocompetent controls (Flavell and Flavell, 1986). The parasites survive high levels of parasite-specific immunoglobulins in both, serum and bile (Wongratanacheewin et al., 1988). The reasons for the escape of these trematodes from immunosurveillance in spite of an active immune response against parasite-specific antigens presently remain unclear.

High levels of antibodies have been observed in *Opisthorchis*-infected individuals with hepatobiliary disease and cholangiocarcinoma (Poopyruchpong et al., 1990; Haswell-Elkins et al., 1991; Mairiang et al., 1992).

11.2.3
Role of Liver Flukes in Human Cancer, and Studies in Animals

The geographic coincidence of *Opisthorchis* and *Clonorchis* infections and cholangiocarcinomas is striking. In hyperendemic regions of Thailand, the incidence rate of these tumors may reach 84.6 and 36.8 per 100 000 per year in men and women, respectively (Srivatanakul et al., 1991 a; Parkin et al., 1993). Outside of Thailand, the incidence of choriocarcinomas varies only to a limited degree (0.1 to 4.8 per 100 000 per year).

The infection of Syrian golden hamsters with metacercariae of *O. viverrini* results in acute inflammatory reactions, but usually not in cholangiocarcinomas (Flavell and Lucas, 1982, 1983). Only exceptionally were such tumors noted (Thamavit et al., 1993). The concomitant or subsequent administration of specific chemical carcinogens resulted, however, more frequently in cholangiocarcinomas. Treatment of *O.*

viverrini-infected hamsters with *N*-nitrosodimethlyamine resulted in cholangio-carcinoma induction within 23 weeks, whereas the animals receiving exclusively the chemical carcinogen did not develop tumors (Thamavit et al., 1978). Similar obser-vations were made in other studies with the same compound (Flavell and Lucas, 1983; Thamavit et al., 1988) and with *N*-nitrosodiethylamine (Thamavit et al., 1987).

Increased endogenous nitrosation was reported in *O. viverrini*-infected patients (Srivatanakul et al., 1991 b; Haswell-Elkins et al., 1994; Satarug et al., 1996, 1998), as well as in infected hamsters (Oshima et al., 1994). It is presently unclear whether these data were the direct result of the parasitic infection, or that they originated from concomitant bacterial infections.

Cholangiocarcinomas have also been noted in *Clonorchis sinensis*-infected cats (Hou, 1964), and in a C. sinensis-infected dog (Hou, 1965).

11.2.4
Mechanism of Carcinogenicity

Opisthorchis viverrini infection induces inflammation in and around the bile duct, leading to cholangiocarcinoma in humans. In cells of the RAW 264.7 macrophage line treated with an extract of *O. viverrini* antigen, the expression of Toll-like receptor 2 (TLR-2) was induced (Pinlaor et al., 2005). This treatment also resulted in a dose-dependent induction of NF-κB, inducible nitric oxide synthase (iNOS) and cyclooxy-genase-2 (COX-2). These results suggest that *O. viverrini* induces inflammatory re-sponse through the TLR2-mediated pathway, leading to NF-κB-mediated expression of iNOS and COX-2 (Pinlaor et al., 2005).

As discussed in Section 11.1 for *Schistosoma*-linked carcinogenesis, liver flukes in all likelihood also act as indirect carcinogens. The trematode-induced inflammation with concomitant induction of reactive NOS might be sufficient to induce mu-tational events which eventually lead to the outgrowth of a malignant cell clone (for reviews, see Gentile and Gentile, 1994; Oshima and Bartsch, 1994). Moreover, the available experimental data obtained from infected animals stress the syncarcino-genic potential of other carcinogens, in particular of nitrosamines.

11.2.5
Control and Therapy

Improved sanitation and health education, and persuading people not to eat raw fish, can prevent infection and reinfection (Sornmani et al., 1984; Saowakontha et al., 1993).

As in *Schistosoma* infection, a single dose of praziquantel is effective in killing the trematodes in over 90% of cases (Vivatanasesth et al., 1982; Chen et al., 1983; Viravan et al., 1986). Cured patients are, however, immediately thereafter suscep-tible to reinfection (Upatham et al., 1988), since they fail to develop an immune re-sponse.

References

Akai, P.S., Pungpak, S., Kitikoon, V., Bunnag, D., and Befus, D. Egg-negative residents of an Opisthorchiasis-endemic area possess high levels of anti-*Opisthorchis* antibodies. *Adv. Exp. Med. Biol.* 371B: 983–986, **1995a**.

Akai, P.S., Pungpak, S., Chaicumpa, W., Kitikoon, V., Ruangkunaporn, Y., Bunnag, D., and Befus, A.D. Serum antibody responses in opisthorchiasis. *Int. J. Parasitol.* 25: 971–973, **1995b**.

Attwood, H.D. and Chou, S. T. The longevity of *Clonorchis sinensis*. *Pathology* 10: 153–156, **1978**.

Brockelman, W.Y., Upatham, E.S., Viyanant, V., Ardsungnoen, S., and Chantanawat, R. Field studies on the transmission of the human liver fluke, *Opisthorchis viverrini*, in northeast Thailand: population changes of the snail intermediate host. *Int. J. Parasitol.* 16: 545–552, **1986**.

Chen, E.R. Clonorchiasis in Taiwan. *S. E. Asian J. Trop. Med. Public Health* 22 (Suppl.): 184–185, **1991**.

Chen, M.G., Hua, X.J., Wan, Z.R., Weng, Y.Q., Wang, M.J., Zhu, P.J., He, B.Z., and Xu. M.Y. Praziquantel in 237 cases of clonorchiasis sinensis. *Chin. Med. J.* 96: 935–940, **1983**.

Chen, M.G., Lu, Y., Hua, X.J., and Mott. K.E. Progress in assessment of morbidity due to *Clonorchis sinensis* infection: a review of recent literature. *Trop. Dis. Bull.* 91: R7–R65, **1994**.

Choi, M.H., Ryu, J.S., Lee, M., Li, S., Chung, B.S., Chai, J.Y., Sithithaworn, P., Tesana, S., and Hong, S. T. Specific and common antigens of *Clonorchis sinensis* and *Opisthorchis viverrini* (Opisthorchidae, Trematoda). *Korean J. Parasitol.* 41: 155–163, **2003**.

Flavell, D.J. and Lucas, S. B. Potentiation by the human liver fluke, *Opisthorchis viverrini*, of the carcinogenic action of N-nitrosodimethylamine upon the biliary epithelium of the hamster. *Br. J. Cancer* 46: 985–989, **1982**.

Flavell, D.J. and Lucas, S. B. Promotion of N-nitrosodimethylamine-initiated bile duct carcinogenesis in the hamster by the human liver fluke, *Opisthorchis viverrini*. *Carcinogenesis* 4: 927–930, **1983**.

Flavell, D.J. and Flavell, S. U. *Opisthorchis viverrini*: pathogenesis of infection in immunodeprived hamsters. *Parasite Immunol.* 8: 455–466, **1986**.

Gentile, J.M. and Gentile, G.J. Implications for the involvement of the immune system in parasite-associated cancers. *Mutat. Res.* 305: 315–320, **1994**.

Giboda, M., Ditrich, O., Scholz, T., Viengsay, T., and Bouaphanh, S. Human *Opisthorchis* and *Haplorchis* infections in Laos. *Trans. R. Soc. Trop. Med. Hyg.* 85: 538–540, **1991**.

Haswell-Elkins, M.R., Sithithaworn, P., Mairiang, E., Elkins, D.B., Wongratanacheewin, S., Kaewkes, S., and Mairiang, P. Immune responsiveness and parasite-specific antibody levels in human hepatobiliary disease associated with *Opisthorchis viverrini* infection. *Clin. Exp. Immunol.* 84: 213–218, **1991**.

Haswell-Elkins, M.R., Satarug, S., Tsuda, M., Mairiang, E., Esumi, H., Sithithaworn, P., Mairiang, P., Saitoh, M., Yongvanit, P., and Elkins, D.B. Liver fluke infection and cholangiocarcinoma: model of endogenous nitric oxide and extragastric nitrosation in human carcinogenesis. *Mutat. Res.* 305: 241–252, **1994**.

Hou, P.C. The pathology of *Clonorchis sinensis* infestation of the liver. *J. Pathol. Bacteriol.* 70: 53–64, **1955**.

Hou, P.C. Primary carcinoma of bile duct of the liver of the cat (*Felis catus*) infested with *Clonorchis sinensis*. *J. Pathol. Bacteriol.* 87: 239–244, **1964**.

Hou, P.C. Hepatic clonorchiasis and carcinoma of the bile duct in a dog. *J. Pathol. Bacteriol.* 89: 365–367, **1965**.

Hou, M.F., Ker, C.G., Sheen, P.C., and Chen, E.R. The ultrasound survey of gallstone diseases of patients infected with *Clonorchis sinensis* in southern Taiwan. *J. Trop. Med. Hyg.* 92: 108–111, **1989**.

IARC Monographs on the Evaluation of Carcinogenic Risks to Humans. Volume 61. *Schistosomes, Liver Flukes and* Helicobacter pylori. IARC Lyon, **1994**.

Iarotski, L.S. and Be'er, S. A. *Epidemiology and control of Opisthorchiasis in the former USSR*. WHO, Geneva, 1993.

Jongsuksuntigul, P. and Imsomboon, T. The impact of a decade long opisthorchiasis control program in northeastern Thailand. *Southeast Asian J. Trop. Med. Public Health* 28: 551–557, **1997**.

Joo, C.Y. Changing patterns of infection with digenetic larval trematodes from freshwater fish in river Taewha, Kyongnam province. *Kisaengchunghak Chapchi* 26: 263–274, **1988**.

Komiya, Y. *Clonorchis* and clonorchiasis. *Adv. Parasitol.* 4: 53–106, **1966**.

Mairiang, E., Elkins, D.B., Mairiang, P., Chaiyakum, J., Chamadol, N., Loapaiboon, V., Posri, S., Sithithaworn, P., and Haswell-Elkins, M. Relationship between intensity of *Opisthorchis viverrini* infection and hepatobiliary disease detected by ultrasonography. *J. Gastroenterol. Hepatol.* 7: 17–21, **1992**.

Ohshima, H. and Bartsch, H. Chronic infections and inflammatory processes as cancer risk factors: possible role of nitric oxide in carcinogenesis. *Mutat. Res.* 305: 253–264, **1994**.

Ohshima, H., Bandaletova, T.Y., Brouet, I., Bartsch, H., Kirby, G., Ogunbiyi, F., Vatanasapt, V., and Pipitgool, V. Increased nitrosamine and nitrate biosynthesis mediated by nitric oxide synthase induced in hamsters infected with liver fluke (*Opisthorchis viverrini*). *Carcinogenesis* 15: 271–275, **1994**.

Parkin, D.M., Ohshima, H., Srivatanakul, P., and Vatanasapt. V. Cholangiocarcinoma: epidemiology, mechanisms of carcinogenesis and prevention. *Cancer Epidemiol. Biomarkers Prev.* 2: 537–544, **1993**.

Pinlaor, S., Tada-Oikawa, S., Hiraku, Y., Pinlaor, P., Ma, N., Sithithaworn, P., and Kawanishi, S. *Opisthorchis viverrini* antigen induces the expression of Toll-like receptor 2 in macrophage RAW cell line. *Int. J. Parasitol.* 35: 591–596, **2005**.

Pholsena, K., Sayaseng, B., Hongvanthong, B., and Vanisaveth, V. The prevalence of helminth infection in Ban Nanin, Laos. *Southeast Asian J. Trop. Med. Public Health* 22: 137–138, **1991**.

Poopyruchpong, N., Viyanant, V., Upatham, E.S., and Srivatanakul, P. Diagnosis of opisthorchiasis by enzyme-linked immunosorbent assay using partially purified antigens. *Asian Pac. J. Allergy Immunol.* 8: 27–31, **1990**.

Rim, H.J. The current pathobiology and chemotherapy of clonorchiasis. *Kisaengchunghak Chapchi*. 24 (Suppl): 1–141, **1986**.

Sakolvaree, Y., Ybanez, L., and Chaicumpa, W. Parasites elicited cross-reacting antibodies to *Opisthorchis viverrini*. *Asian Pac. J. Allergy Immunol.* 15: 115–122, **1997**.

Saowakontha, S., Pipitgool, V., Pariyanonda, S., Tesana, S., Rojsathaporn, K., and Intarakhao, C. Field trials in the control of *Opisthorchis viverrini* with an integrated programme in endemic areas of northeast Thailand. *Parasitology* 106: 283–288, **1993**.

Satarug, S., Haswell-Elkins, M.R., Tsuda, M., Mairiang, P., Sithithaworn, P., Mairiang, E., Esumi, H., Sukprasert, S., Yongvanit, P., and Elkins, D.B. Thiocyanate-independent nitrosation in humans with carcinogenic parasite infection. *Carcinogenesis* 17: 1075–1081, **1996**.

Satarug, S., Haswell-Elkins, M.R., Sithithaworn, P., Bartsch, H., Ohshima, H., Tsuda, M., Mairiang, P., Mairiang, E., Yongvanit, P., Esumi, H., Elkins, D.B. Relationships between the synthesis of *N*-nitrosodimethylamine and immune responses to chronic infection with the carcinogenic parasite, *Opisthorchis viverrini*, in men. *Carcinogenesis* 19: 485–491, **1998**.

Sithithaworn, P., Tesana, S., Pipitgool, V., Kaewkes, S., Thaiklar, K., Pairojkul, C., Sripa, B., Paupairoj, A., Sanpitak, P., and Aranyanat, C. Quantitative post-mortem study of *Opisthorchis viverrini* in man in north-east Thailand. *Trans. R. Soc. Trop. Med. Hyg.* 85: 765–768, **1991**.

Sornmani, S., Vivatanasesth, P., Impand, P., Phatihatakorn, W., Sitabutra, P., Schelp, F.P. Infection and re-infection rates of opisthorchiasis in the water resource development area of Nam Pong project, Khon Kaen Province, northeast Thailand. *Ann. Trop. Med. Parasitol.* 78: 649–656, **1984**.

Srivatanakul, P., Parkin, D.M., Jiang, Y.Z., Khlat, M., Kao-Ian, U.T., Sontipong, S., and Wild, C. The role of infection by *Opisthorchis viverrini*, hepatitis B virus, and aflatoxin exposure in the etiology of liver cancer in Thailand. A correlation study. *Cancer* 68: 2411–2417, **1991 a**.

Srivatanakul, P., Ohshima, H., Khlat, M., Parkin, M., Sukaryodhin, S., Brouet, I., and Bartsch, H. *Opisthorchis viverrini* infestation and endogenous nitrosamines as risk factors for cholangiocarcinoma in Thailand. *Int. J. Cancer* 48: 821–825, **1991 b**.

Thamavit, W., Bhamarapravati, N., Sahaphong, S., Vajrasthira, S., and Angsubhakorn, S. Effects of dimethylnitrosamine on induction of cholangiocarcinoma in *Opisthorchis viverrini*-infected Syrian golden hamsters. *Cancer Res.* 38: 4634–4639, **1978**.

Thamavit, W., Ngamying, M., Boonpucknavig, V., Boonpucknavig, S., and Moore, M.A. Enhancement of DEN-induced hepatocellular nodule development by *Opisthorchis viverrini* infection in Syrian golden hamsters. *Carcinogenesis* 8: 1351–1353, **1987**.

Thamavit, W., Moore, M.A., Hiasa, Y., and Ito, N. Enhancement of DHPN induced hepatocellular, cholangiocellular and pancreatic carcinogenesis by *Opisthorchis viverrini* infestation in Syrian golden hamsters. *Carcinogenesis* 9: 1095–1098, **1988**.

Thamavit, W., Pairojkul, C., Tiwawech, D., Itoh, M., Shirai, T., and Ito, N. Promotion of cholangiocarcinogenesis in the hamster liver by bile duct ligation after dimethylnitrosamine initiation. *Carcinogenesis* 14: 2415–2417, **1993** .

Upatham, E.S., Viyanant, V., Kurathong, S., Brockelman, W.Y., Menaruchi, A., Saowakontha, S., Intarakhao, C., Vajrasthira, S., and Warren, K.S. Morbidity in relation to intensity of infection in opisthorchiasis viverrini: study of a community in Khon Kaen, Thailand. *Am. J. Trop. Med. Hyg.* 31: 1156–1163, **1982**.

Upatham, E.S., Viyanant, V., Brockelman, W.Y., Kurathong, S., Lee, P., and Kraengraeng, R. Rate of re-infection by *Opisthorchis viverrini* in an endemic northeast Thai community after chemotherapy. *Int. J. Parasitol.* 18: 643–649, **1988**.

Vichasri, S., Viyanant, V., and Upatham, E.S. Opisthorchis viverrini: intensity and rates of infection in cyprinoid fish from an endemic focus in Northeast Thailand. *Southeast Asian J. Med. Public Health* 13: 138–141, **1982**.

Viravan, C., Bunnag, D., Harinasuta, T., Upatham, S., Kurathong, S., and Viyanant, V. Clinical field trial of praziquantel in opisthorchiasis in Nong Rangya Village, Khon Kaen Province, Thailand. *Southeast Asian J. Trop. Med. Public Health* 17: 63–66, **1986**.

Vivatanasesth, P., Sornmani, S., Schelp, F.P., Impand, P., Sitabutra, P., Preuksaraj, S., and Harinasuta, C. Mass treatment of opisthorchiasis in Northeast Thailand. *Southeast Asian J. Trop. Med. Public Health* 13: 609–613, **1982**.

Wongratanacheewin, S., Bunnag, D., Vaeusorn, N., and Sirisinha, S. Characterization of humoral immune response in the serum and bile of patients with opisthorchiasis and its application in immunodiagnosis. *Am. J. Trop. Med. Hyg.* 38: 356–362, **1988**.

Wongratanacheewin, S., Sermswan, R.W., and Sirisinha, S. Immunology and molecular biology of *Opisthorchis viverrini* infection. *Acta Trop.* 88: 195–207, **2003**.

12
Cancers with a Possible Infectious Etiology

12.1
Leukemias and Lymphomas

An increased risk for leukemias for persons exposed for prolonged periods to X-irradiation or exposure to radioactive irradiation is well established. A broad spectrum of additional risk factors has been reported for non-Hodgkin lymphoma (NHL) (reviewed by Fisher and Fisher, 2004), and most of these seem also to account for acute lymphoblastic leukemias and Hodgkin's disease. Yet, the etiology of spontaneously occurring human leukemias and lymphomas remains presently poorly understood. In the past, some hints have pointed to a possible involvement of infectious agents, particularly in childhood leukemias and lymphomas. In the United States, these two malignancies constitute approximately 41% of childhood cancers; the distribution of childhood cancers in the United States is shown in graphically Figure 12.1.

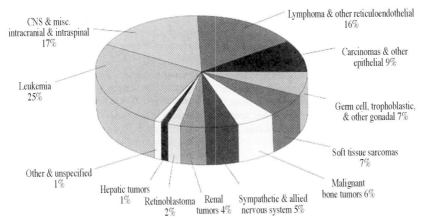

Source: *Pediatric Monograph* 1999, Surveillance, Epidemiology, and End Results Program, Division of Cancer Control and Population Sciences, National Cancer Institute.

Fig. 12.1 Distribution of childhood cancers within the United States (ages 0–19 years). (Pediatric Monograph 1999, Surveillance, Epidemiology, and End Results Program, Division of Cancer Control and Population Sciences, National Cancer Institute.)

Infections Causing Human Cancer. Harald zur Hausen
Copyright © 2006 WILEY-VCH Verlag GmbH & Co. KGaA, Weinheim
ISBN: 3-527-31056-8

A number of specific chromosomal translocations have been identified in various types of human leukemias and lymphomas (for a review, see Greaves and Wiemels, 2003), commonly involving transcription factors. Their induction, together with several epidemiological observations published during the past three to four decades, still require an explanation. Infectious agents have been repeatedly suspected to be involved in the etiology of leukemias and lymphomas, yet specific infectious agents have been identified in only a relatively small percentage of these neoplasias. Epstein-Barr virus (EBV) occurs in approximately 50% of B-cell lymphomas arising under immunosuppressive conditions, preferentially also in the endemic form of Burkitt's lymphomas and in a small subset of T-cell lymphomas. As outlined in previous chapters, human herpesvirus type 8 contributes to rare primary effusion lymphomas, and HTLV-1, a retrovirus, is responsible for adult T-cell leukemias occurring in endemic in coastal regions of Southern Japan. Indirect evidence points to a role of a bacterial infection (i.e., *Helicobacter pylori*) in specific gastric lymphomas, the MALT-tumors.

Thus, although some causative agents have been identified, there is still no explanation available for the majority of these malignant proliferations. Indeed, for certain of the virus-positive tumors, such as EBV-positive Burkitt's lymphoma within the African tumor belt, an explanation of the epidemiological pattern poses substantial problems.

12.1.1
Epidemiological Data

Epidemiological data are based on changes in cancer incidence, case/control and prospective studies, as well as on space-time clustering of leukemias and lymphomas. A general decline in cancer incidence has been noted in the United States, most likely related to a reduction in smoking. In contrast to the general trend, the incidence of NHL, and also of melanomas, non-melanoma skin and liver cancers, has increased substantially between 1991 and 1995 (McKean-Cowdin et al., 2000). In fact, the SEER statistics reveal approximately twice as many cases of NHL in the year 2000 when compared to 1973 (SEER, 2003) A slight increase was also noted within the same period for acute lymphoblastic leukemia (Figs. 12.2 and 12.3). The rate of other leukemias and of Hodgkin lymphomas remained more or less constant during that period.

The dramatic increase in NHL incidence has mainly been observed in developed parts of the world, although the AIDS epidemic resulted in a sharp rise of these lymphomas also in developing countries (Devessa and Fears, 1992). In the United States, the incidence in Caucasians was approximately 30% higher than in African Americans up to the year 2000 (Fig. 12.2). The rate of all other leukemias and lymphomas, with the exception of chronic myelogenous leukemia, was lower in socially less privileged populations than in affluent societies (SEER, 2003).

A larger number of publications appeared during the past 25 years, describing space-time clustering of childhood leukemias and lymphomas. In 1981, Hamadeh et al. analyzed a possible clustering of leukemias, Hodgkin's disease and other lymphomas in Bahrein by comparing 125 cases with matched controls. These authors found a trend for some clustering of cases in urban areas. Districts far away from large urban centers of higher socioeconomic status revealed an excess risk of childhood acute lymphoblastic leukemia (ALL) (Alexander et al., 1990; Pearce et al., 2004). A larger number of these studies were conducted in Great Britain (Alexander, 1992; Alexander et al., 1993; Knox, 1994; Gilman and Knox, 1995; Gilman et al., 1999; Birch et al., 2000; McNally et al. 2002), showing evidence for space-time clustering of ALL and Hodgkin's lymphoma. Similar data were also reported from Sweden (Gustafsson and Carstensen, 2000), Greece (Petridou et al., 1996), Italy (Magnani et al., 2003), from the EUROLOCUS project carried out in 17 defined geographic regions of Europe (Alexander et al., 1998), from Israel (Chen et al., 1997), from San Francisco (Philippe, 1999), and from Hong Kong (Alexander et al., 1997; Chan et al., 2002). Spatial clustering was found particularly for childhood leukemias in children aged up to 4 years (Petridou et al., 1996; Alexander et al., 1997). Local increases in areas of high population mixing have also been described (Kinlen et al., 1993; Kinlen, 1995). Negative results for time-space distribution of childhood leukemia was reported in two small studies from the Netherlands (van Steensel-Moll et al., 1983) and from New Zealand (Dockerty et al., 1999).

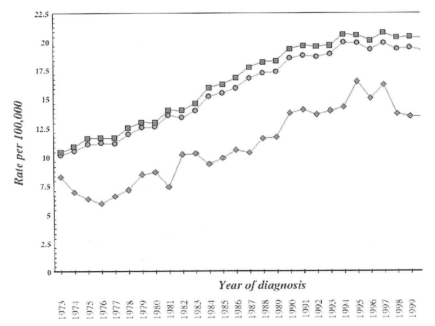

Fig. 12.2 SEER statistics for 1973–1999 for non-Hodgkin lymphoma. Red line: all races. Blue line: white. Green line: black. (National Cancer Institute, SEER Program. Statistics for 1973–1999. http://can-ques.seer.cancer.gov/)

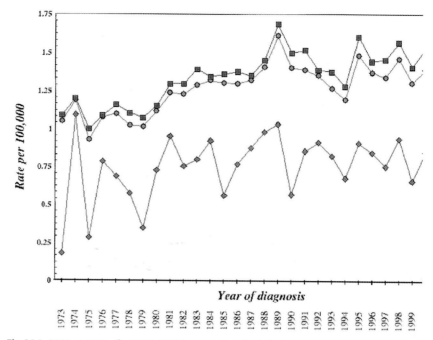

Fig. 12.3 SEER statistics for 1973–1999 for acute lymphatic leukemias.
Red line: all races. Blue line: white. Green line: black. (National Cancer
Institute, SEER Program. Statistics for 1973–1999. http://can-
ques.seer.cancer.gov/)

The vast majority of all the reports observing space-time clustering of childhood
ALL interpret these findings as indirect evidence for a transmissible agent (Alexander, 1992; MacMahon, 1992), and that such transmissible agents may share some
of the epidemiological characteristics of herpesviruses (Alexander, 1993). There
exist additional observations which have been interpreted as indirect evidence pointing in the same direction. This concerns several risk factors that have been identified, linked particularly with ALL and NHL. These involve agricultural occupations
(Milham, 1971; Blair et al., 1985; Saftlas et al., 1987; La Vecchia et al., 1989; Eriksson
and Karlsson, 1992; MacMahon, 1992) and contact with cattle (Pearce et al., 1986 a,b;
Assenato et al., 1995; Metayer et al., 1998; Fritschi et al., 2002; Becker et al., 2004).
Several authors also report an elevated risk for these neoplasms in butchers, abattoir
workers and meat cutters (Johnson et al., 1986; Pearce et al., 1988; Metayer et al.,
1998). Recently, a case-control study involving 5900 subjects from seven European
countries, after adjusting for smoking, revealed an increased risk for lung cancer
after exposure to meat aerosols and even more so after exposure to live animals
(Durusoy et al., 2006). An increased risk for colon cancer after red meat consumption was attributed to the formation of DNA adducts of O6-carboxymethyl guanine
(Lewin et al., 2006). Since exposure to live animals reveals an even higher risk, at
least for lung cancer, this interpretation does not seem to hold up for this malig-

nancy and has been interpreted in favor of an infectious agent (Durusoy et al., 2006). Additional incriminated factors were occupational exposure to pesticides, industrial paints, and solvents, hair dyes, the leather industry (Scherr et al., 1992; Pearce and Bethwaite, 1992), and forestry work (Feychting et al., 2001). The latter study failed to confirm pesticides and paints as risk factors for leukemias. There are no clear-cut data available pointing to a significant effect of specific paternal occupations and subsequent development of childhood leukemias. Increased birth weight seems to represent another risk factor for developing acute lymphoblastic leukemia during the first four years of life, as shown in several publications (Kaye et al., 1991; Murray et al., 2002; Ou et al., 2002; Hjalgrim et al., 2004). The risk for ALL was also higher among children of older mothers and fathers (Dockerty et al., 2001).

Interestingly, a number of protective factors have been reported to reduce the risk for these hematological malignancies. Several epidemiological studies demonstrate a protective effect of whole-day care of children in the age group 0 to 4 years, and of intermittent infections in this time period for leukemias (van Steensel-Moll et al., 1986; Greaves and Alexander, 1993; Petridou et al., 1993; McKinney et al., 1999; Infante-Rivard et al., 2000; Perrillat et al., 2002; Jordan-Da Silva et al., 2004), lymphomas (McKinney et al., 1987), Hodgkin's disease (Pfaffenbarger et al., 1977; Chang et al., 2004), and neuroblastomas (Menegaux et al., 2004). Other studies, unable to confirm this directly, quoted significant effects of other socioeconomic parameters increasing the risk for the respective diseases, such as parameters suggestive of a protected environment in early childhood in the case of leukemias (Roman et al., 1997; Smith et al., 1998; Pearce et al., 2004), or a higher level of education in Hodgkin's lymphoma (Serraino et al., 1991). Two reports could not find any association with day care and early infections (Neglia et al., 2000; Rosenbaum et al., 2000). A marked inverse association of leukemia risk with birth order was first noted in 1966 (Stark and Mantel, 1966; Shaw et al., 1984; Dockerty et al., 2001; Hjalgrim et al., 2004). Correspondingly, children living in more crowded households had a substantially lower risk than children born into less crowded homes (Murray et al., 2002). Three reports also found an inverse association between alcohol intake and NHL risk (Nelson et al., 1997; Chiu et al., 1999; Morton et al., 2005). Very recently, a case-control study involving 6305 children (aged 2–14 years) without cancer and 3140 children with cancer (diagnosed in the United Kingdom, 1991–1996), of whom 1286 had ALL, showed that increasing levels of social activity were associated with consistent reductions in risk of ALL (Gilham et al., 2005). Interestingly, even children with non-ALL malignancies (mainly central nervous system tumors, other leukemias, NHL and Hodgkin's lymphoma) revealed a similar pattern. The greatest reduction for risk of ALL was seen in children who attended formal day care during the first three months of life. The established risk, as well as protective factors, are summarized in Figures 12.4 and 12.5.

It has been argued that there exists a biological heterogeneity of childhood leukemia, and that a family of related malignancies is derived from different stem cells in the hematopoietic hierarchy (Greaves, 1999). This would render it *a priori* unlikely that even a well-defined hematologic subtype has an exclusive etiology (Greaves, 2000). This seems to account for environmental chemical and physical

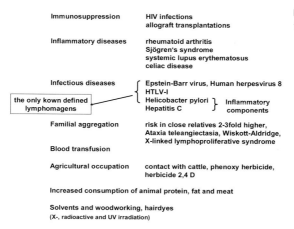

Fig. 12.4 Reported risk factors for non-Hodgkin lymphoma.

- **Multiple infections in early childhood**

- whole-day care

- underprivileged social state

- low level of education

- crowded household, many siblings

- inverse risk with birth order

- (alcohol consumption)

Fig. 12.5 Reported protective factors against childhood leukemias, lymphomas, and Hodgkin's disease.

carcinogenic factors. Among infectious agents, EBV is an excellent example to demonstrate that the same agent is able to infect and transform cells at different stages of differentiation (see Chapter 4, Section 4.3.1).

The observed protective effects of early infections and whole-day care and the observations on space-time clustering of childhood leukemias and lymphomas stimulated speculations arguing for an infectious etiology of childhood hematopoietic malignancies (Greaves, 1988, 1997; Alexander, 1992, 1993; Greaves and Alexander, 1993; Kinlen et al., 1993; Kinlen, 1995; Alexander et al., 1998; Smith et al., 1998; Pearce et al., 2004). Two hypotheses have been developed along these lines: Greaves (1988, 1997; Greaves and Alexander, 1993) speculated that delayed exposure to common infections results in an increased risk for childhood leukemia, especially of the pre-B acute lymphoblastic leukemia. According to Greaves' view, a first step takes place during pregnancy, where the occurrence of a specific chromosomal translocation leads to the appearance of a rearranged B-cell precursor clone (Greaves and Wiemels, 2003). As a second event, Greaves postulated an unspecified common infection and labeled it the "delayed infection hypothesis" (Greaves, 2000). According to this hypothesis, the pattern and timing of infection in early life would be of critical importance in relation to the developmental programming of the immune system. Early infections educate the immune system and result in an expansion and elimination or suppression of T-cell subsets or clones. In the absence of early exposures, the immune system may remain un-modulated and un-educated. Later infections may result in abnormal immunological responses that increase the risk for leukemia.

Kinlen developed a different interpretation: he hypothesized that mixing of a population of low exposure to a putative leukemogenic agent (anticipated for rural residences with low population density) with another population originating from urban areas previously highly exposed to the incriminated agent, could promote an epidemic of the relevant infection (Kinlen et al., 1993, Kinlen, 1995). Examples would be represented by oil drilling or industrial plant development in rural areas with a sudden influx of people from urban areas. Kinlen noted under these circumstances a higher than expected incidence of childhood leukemias. The lack of an increase in childhood leukemias in the context of massive evacuations of mothers and children during the Second World War (MacMahon, 1992) could, however, argue against these considerations.

An additional hypothesis speculating on an infectious origin of childhood leukemias and lymphomas was developed based on some virologic data (zur Hausen and de Villiers, 2005). This was triggered by the analysis of a possible role of a recently discovered virus family, the so-called TT viruses (Nishizawa et al., 1997), in human malignant proliferations. This virus group reveals a remarkable heterogeneity of genotypes (Okamoto et al., 2002; Peng et al., 2002) varying in genome size between 2100 and 3800 nucleotides in a single-stranded circular genome (Takahashi et al., 2000; Okamoto et al., 2002). A substantial variation also exists in the amino acid composition of putative proteins derived from the various open reading frames (ORFs) of the virus. TT viruses are widely spread among all human populations (Abe et al., 1999; Itoh et al., 1999; Jelcic et al., 2004). They replicate preferentially in bone marrow cells (Okamoto et al., 2000), and cells of the hematopoietic system act as a reservoir for these viruses (Takahashi et al., 2002).

Initial attempts to detect TT viruses resulted in a high rate of detection of viral DNA in human cancers, particularly in gastrointestinal tumors, in breast and lung cancer, as well as in leukemias and multiple myelomas (de Villiers et al., 2002). However, these experiments could not exclude a contamination of the tumor material with TT virus-positive cells of lymphatic origin. In addition, it was disturbing that TT virus-DNA was not detected in tissue culture lines derived from tumor types with a high TT virus presence.

Surprisingly, the analysis of a single heavily infiltrated spleen biopsy from a patient with Hodgkin's lymphoma showed 24 different TT virus genotypes (Jelcic et al., 2004). The cloned viral DNA revealed a remarkable heterogeneity, particularly within two viral clades: one contained substantial variations within three regions of the long ORF, whereas several clones of the second clade had stop codons within the same ORF, resulting in the formation of new ORFs. The variation in genotypes points to a remarkable heterogeneity and instability of TT virus genomes.

Recently, a short stretch of TT-like viral DNA was found in several cell lines of lymphatic origin and derived from other tumors: EBV-negative lines derived from Hodgkin's lymphoma and of other leukemic and lymphatic origin were found to contain this DNA (zur Hausen and de Villiers, 2005; E.-M. de Villiers et al., unpub-

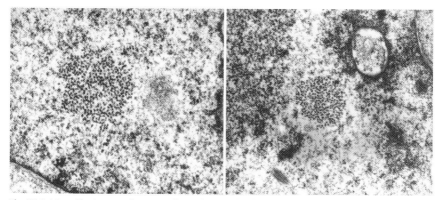

Fig. 12.6 Virus-like intranuclear particles within a cell of the Hodgkin's lymphoma line L1236 (left) and a Jurkat cell (right).

lished results). This sequence was cloned with the aid of consensus primers and identified to represent the most highly conserved region of the TT virus genome (Peng et al., 2002). Several of these cell lines contained nuclear virus-like particles in very rare occasional single cells, which corresponded in size with TT viruses (Fig. 12.6). Some of the structures revealed also tubular forms, suggesting cylindrical structures or an abnormal aggregation of proteins to specific areas of cellular chromatin (Fig. 12.6) (H. zur Hausen and R. Schmidt, unpublished data). It is not clear whether these particles have indeed a viral origin or may represent nuclear speckles (Huang and Spector, 1992).

The use of primers to amplify the newly identified TT virus-like sequences occasionally resulted in the amplification of sequences involved in translocation events (e.g., *TEL-AML*) or of sequences of the dgl tumorsuppressor gene coding for a protein which interacts with the APC protein (Makino et al., 1997). These results formed the basis for a hypothesis which proposed a novel mechanism for the possible involvement of infectious events in the etiology of hematopoietic malignancies, and for a novel role of specific viruses in human carcinogenesis (zur Hausen and de Villiers, 2005).

12.1.2
The Target Cell Conditioning Model

According to this model, the initial event potentially leading to leukemia and lymphoma development is triggered by a ubiquitous virus infection acquired either prenatally or perinatally. Transplacental or perinatal infection results in virus persistence, as observed in previous studies for established TT virus genotypes (Saback et al., 1999; Goto et al., 2000; Matsubara et al., 2001). The expansion of latently infected cells during the course of a newborn child's development in the first year of life (Peng et al., 2002) should result in an increasing number of infected cells and, correspondingly, to a steadily increasing viral load. For TT viruses it has been reported that viral concentrations increase with age (Saback et al., 1999). Existing partial homologies of this viral DNA with host cell genes frequently engaged in translocations of leukemic or lymphoma cells should increase the risk for specific translocations during the course of viral and cellular DNA replication proportional to the number of viral genome-positive cells. Occasionally, such translocations are also found in healthy individuals, as for example described for the lymphoma-associated translocation t(14;18) (Limpens et al., 1995). Intermittent infections by other viruses (e.g., influenza, measles, rubella, mumps or other respiratory or gastrointestinal infections) result in interferon synthesis, blocking the production of persisting agent and thus reducing the respective viral load. Interferon treatment indeed reduces for instance the TT virus level, as described by Akahane et al. (1999). Frequent infections in early childhood consequently lead to a low load of the incriminated agent and to a reduced level of virus persistence in hematopoietic cells. This in turn should reduce the risk for specific translocations. Absence or a low number of early childhood infections should have the opposite effect and increase the respective risks; this is outlined schematically in Figure 12.7.

Second events, caused either by further translocations or by infection with specific viruses (possibly as yet unknown herpesviruses) mediate the conversion to a malignant phenotype. This is exemplified in the case of EBV-positive cases of Hodgkin's disease, where expression of EBNA-1, LMP-1 and LMP-2 of EBV seems to provide the "second hit". The infection of previously "conditioned target cells", conditioned by the induction of specific translocations, provides here the basis for malignant conversion. It seems to be an interesting footnote that reported roseola and/or fever and rash during the first year of life reduced the risk for ALL (OR = 0.33 [95% CI 0.16, 0.68]), whereas tonsillitis during the period 3–12 months before the reference date increased the risk (OR = 2.56 [95% CI 1.22, 5.38] (Chan et al., 2002). Infectious mononucleosis and apparently also some HHV-8 infections frequently start with tonsillitis-like symptoms (Veltri et al., 1975; Ryan et al., 2004; Chen et al., 2004).

This model does not necessarily relate to TT viruses of TT-related agents. Endogenous retroviruses, activated during the prenatal or perinatal period, would also fit into this model. It readily explains the protective effect of intermittent infections in early childhood occurring at higher frequency in whole-day care conditions. Thus, a highly protective environment during this time period in affluent societies emerges

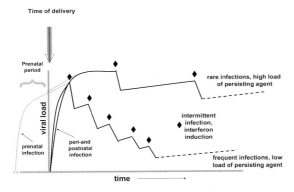

Fig. 12.7 Scheme of the target cell conditioning model hypothesis.

as a risk factor for hematological malignancies and could explain (and even predict) the observed increase in those malignant conditions in such populations.

Another aspect originates from the observed higher risk of agricultural occupations and exposure to cattle. It is possible that at least some genotypes of TTV-like agents found in human malignancies or tumorviruses of bovine origin are shed by cattle or are transmitted to humans by beef products (dairy products, meat, leather materials or close contact with cattle) (zur Hausen, 2001). They may also establish persistent infections in humans. For example, TT virus sequences have been reported in 25% of the cows analyzed (Leary et al., 1999).

Remarkable differences exist in the epidemiology of individual types of lymphomas and leukemias; this is most pronounced for the pattern of Burkitt's lymphomas. These tumors occur as an early childhood disease within the African equatorial "tumor belt" and are mainly EBV-positive. Outside of this region, Burkitt's lymphoma is rare and the majority of tumors are EBV-negative. It could be postulated that a specific agent endemic in these high-risk Burkitt's lymphoma regions is involved in preferentially inducing the c-*myc*/immunoglobulin gene rearrangements. At least in theory, it could be transmitted from wild animals (e.g., wild buffalos, specific antelopes) to cattle, sheep or goats in common grazing areas where Burkitt's lymphoma is endemic. Persistent infections of humans with such agents, followed by severe EBV infections, would lead to malignant conversion of modified cell clones. Indeed, emerging evidence points to a role for specific EBV genes in the maintenance of the malignant phenotype of EBV-positive Burkitt's lymphoma cells (Kennedy et al., 2003; Sheng et al., 2003). Outside the high-risk regions, similar translocations may be mediated by related agents at a much lower frequency. Support for this speculation could be derived from differences in the breakpoint of the c-*myc* gene at chromosome 8 q24 between endemic and sporadic cases of Burkitt's lymphoma (Shirimizu et al., 1991; Ambinder and Griffin, 1991). A previously discussed alternative interpretation implying holo-endemic *Plasmodium falciparum* malaria as the first triggering event (Burkitt, 1962; Magrath, 1990) is difficult to reconcile with the existence of regions with a high prevalence of malaria and low Burkitt's lymphoma incidence in south-east Asia.

Although the model presented here is a hypothesis, it could explain some of the epidemiological characteristics of various hematological malignancies which have been poorly understood until now. Moreover, it provides a model for a novel mechanism by which persistent infections may contribute to the development of human cancers. It could support previous speculations on a possible role of transmission of tumor-inducing agents from farm animals and pets to humans (zur Hausen, 2001). Models should stimulate further experimentation and hopefully promote a better understanding of the etiology of these frequently fatal childhood malignancies. The numerous epidemiologic data quoted before demand an explanation. They are suggestive for a role of infectious events in these malignancies.

References

Abe, K., Inami T., Asano K., Miyoshi C., Masaka N., Hayashi S., Ishikawa K., Takebe Y., Win K.M., El-Zayadi A.R., Han, K.H., and Zhang, D.Y. TT virus infection is widespread in the general populations from different geographic regions. *J. Clin. Microbiol.* 37 : 2703–2705, **1999**.

Akahane, Y., Sakamoto, M., Miyazaki, Y., Okada, S., Inoue, T., Ukita, M., Okamoto, H., Miyakawa, Y., and Mayumi, M. Effect of interferon on a nonenveloped DNA virus (TT virus) associated with acute and chronic hepatitis of unknown etiology. *J. Med. Virol.* 58: 196–200, **1999**.

Alexander, F.E., Ricketts, T.J., McKinney, P.A., and Cartwright, R.A. Community lifestyle characteristics and risk of acute lymphoblastic leukaemia in children. *Lancet* 336: 1461–1465, **1990**.

Alexander, F.E. Space-time clustering of childhood acute lymphoblastic leukaemia: indirect evidence for a transmissible agent. *Br. J. Cancer* 65: 589–592, **1992**.

Alexander, F.E. Viruses, clusters and clustering of childhood leukaemia: a new perspective? *Eur. J. Cancer* 29 A: 1424–1443, **1993**.

Alexander, F.E., McKinney, P.M., and Cartwright, R.A. Migration patterns of children with leukaemia and non-Hodgkin's lymphoma in three areas of northern England. *J. Public Health Med.* 15: 9–15, **1993**.

Alexander, F.E., Chan, L.C., Lam, T.H., Yuen, P., Leung, N.K., Ha, S. Y., Yuen, H.L., Li, C.K., Li, C.K., Lau, Y.L., and Greaves, M.F. Clustering of childhood leukaemia in Hong Kong: association with the childhood peak and common acute lymphoblastic leukaemia and with population mixing. *Br. J. Cancer* 75: 457–463, **1997**.

Alexander, F.E., Boyle, P., Carli, P.M., Coebergh, J.H., Draper, G.J., Ekbom, A., Levi, F., McKinney, P.A., McWhirter, W., Magnani, C., Michaelis, J., Olsen, J.H., Peris-Bonet, R., Petridou, E., Pukkala, E., and Vatten, L. Spatial temporal patterns in childhood leukaemia: further evidence for an infectious origin. EUROLOCUS project. *Br. J. Cancer* 77: 812–817, **1998**.

Ambinder, R.F. and Griffin, C.A. Biology of the lymphomas: cytogenetics, molecular biology, and virology. *Curr. Opin. Oncol.* 3: 806–812, **1991**.

Assennato, G., Ferri, G.M., Tria, G., Porro, A., Macinagrossa, L., Ruggirei, M [Tumors of the hemolymphopoietic tract and employment in agriculture: a case-control study carried out in an epidemiologic area in southern Italy] Article in Italian. *G. Ital. Med. Lav.* 17: 91–97, **1995**.

Becker, N., Deeg, E., and Nieters, A. Population-based study of lymphoma in Germany: rationale, design and first results. *Leuk. Res.* 28: 713–724, **2004**.

Birch, J.M., Alexander, F.E., Blair, V., Eden, O.B., Taylor, G.M., and McNally, R.J. Space-time clustering patterns in childhood leukaemia support a role for infection. *Br. J. Cancer* 82: 1571–1576, **2000**.

Blair, A., Malker, H., Cantor, K.P., Burmeister, L., and Wiklund, K. Cancer among farmers. A review. *Scand. J. Work. Environ. Health* 11: 397–407, **1985**.

Burkitt, D. A children's cancer dependent upon climatic factors. *Nature* 194: 232–234, **1962**.

Chan, L.C., Lam, T.H., Li, C.K., Lau, Y.L., Li, C.K., Yuen, H.L., Lee, C.W., Ha, S. Y., Yuen, P.M., Leung, N.K., Patheal, S. L., Greaves, M.F., and Alexander, F.E. Is the timing of exposure to infection a major determinant of acute lymphoblastic leukaemia in Hong Kong? *Paediatr. Perinat. Epidemiol.* 16: 154–165, **2002**.

Chang, E.T., Zheng, T., Weir, E.G., Borowitz, M., Mann, R.B., Spiegelman, D., and Mueller, N.E. Childhood social environment and Hodgkin s lymphoma: new findings from a population-based case-control study. *Cancer Epidemiol. Biomarkers Prev .* 13: 1361–1370, **2004**.

Chen, R., Iscovich, J., and Goldbourt, U. Clustering of leukaemia cases in a city in Israel. *Stat. Med.* 16: 1873–1887, **1997**.

Chen, R.L., Lin, J.C., Wang, P.J., Lee, C.P., and Hsu, Y.H. Human herpesvirus 8-related childhood mononucleosis: a series of three cases. *Pediatr. Infect. Dis. J.* 23: 671–674, **2004**.

Chiu, B.C.H., Cerhan, J.R., Gapstur, S. M., Sellers, T.A., Zheng, W., Lutz, C.T., Wallace, R.B., and Potter, J.D. Alcohol consumption and non-Hogkin lymphoma in a cohort of older women. *Br. J. Cancer* 80: 1476–1482, **1999**.

Devessa, S. S. and Fears, T. Non-Hodgkin's lymphoma time trends: United States and international data. *Cancer Res.* 52: 5432s–5440s, **1992**.

de Villiers, E.-M., Schmidt, R., Delius, H., and zur Hausen, H. Heterogeneity of TT virus-like sequences isolated from human tumour biopsies. *J. Mol. Med.* 80: 44–50, **2002**.

Dockerty, J.D., Sharples, K.J., and Borman, B. An assessment of spatial clustering of leukaemias and lymphomas among young people in New Zealand. *J. Epidemiol. Community Health* 53: 154–158, **1999**.

Dockerty, J.D., Draper, G., Vincent, T., Rowan, S. D., and Bunch, K.J. Case-control study of parental age, parity and socioeconomic level in relation to childhood cancers. *Int. J. Epidemiol.* 30: 1428–1437, **2001**.

Durusoy, R., Boffetta, P., Mannetje, A., Zaridze, D., Szeszenia-Dabrowska, N., Rudnai, P., Lissowska, J., Fabiánová, E., Cassidy, A., Mates, D., Bencko, V., Salajka, F., Janout, V., Fevotte, J., Fletcher, T., and Brennan, P. Lung cancer risk and occupational exposure to meat and live animals. *Int. J. Cancer* 118: 2543–2547, **2006**.

Eriksson, M. and Karlsson, M. Occupational and other environmental factors and multiple myeloma: a population-based case-control study. *Br. J. Ind. Med.* 49: 95–103, **1992**.

Feychting, M., Plato, N., Nise, G., and Ahlbom, A. Paternal occupational exposures and childhood cancer. *Environ. Health Perspect.* 109: 193–196, **2001**.

Fisher, S. G. and Fisher, R.I. The epidemiology of non-Hodgkin's lymphoma. *Oncogene* 23: 6524–6534, **2004**.

Fritschi, L., Johnson, K.C., Kliewer, E.V., Fry, R., and Canadian Cancer Registries Epidemiology Research Group. Animal-related occupations and the risk of leukaemia, myeloma, and non-Hodgkin's lymphoma in Canada. *Cancer Causes Control* 13: 563–571, **2002**.

Gilham, C., Peto, J., Simpson, J., Roman, E., Eden, T.O.B., Greaves, M.F., and Alexander, F.E. UKCCS Investigators. Day care in infancy and risk of childhood acute lymphoblastic leukaemia: findings from UK case-control study. *Br. Med. J.* 330: 1294, **2005**.

Gilman, E.A. and Knox, E.G. Childhood cancers: space-time distribution in Britain. *J. Epidemiol. Community Health* 49: 158–163, **1995**.

Gilman, E.A., McNally, R.J., and Cartwright, R.A. Space-time clustering in acute lymphoblastic leukaemia in parts of the U.K. (1984–1993). *Eur. J. Cancer* 35: 91–96, **1999**.

Goto, K., Sugiyama, K., Ando, T., Mizutani, F., Terabe, K., Tanaka, K., Nishiyama, M., and Wade, Y. Detection rates of TT virus DNA in serum of umbilical cord blood, breast milk and saliva. *Tohoku J. Exp. Med.* 191: 203–207, **2000** .

Greaves, M.F. Speculations on the cause of childhood acute lymphoblastic leukaemia. *Leukaemia* 2: 120–125, **1988**.

Greaves, M.F. Aetiology of acute leukaemia. *Lancet* 349: 344–349, **1997**.

Greaves, M.F. Molecular genetics, natural history and the demise of childhood leukemia. *Eur. J. Cancer* 35: 173–185, **1999**.

Greaves, M.F. Does childhood acute lymphoblastic leukemia have an infectious origin? In: Goedert, J.J. (Ed.), *Infectious Causes of Cancer*. Humana Press, Totowa, N.J., pp. 451–460, **2000**.

Greaves, M.F. and Alexander, F.E. An infectious etiology for common lymphatic leukaemia in childhood? *Leukemia* 7: 349–360, **1993**.

Greaves, M.F. and Wiemels, J. Origins of chromosome translocations in childhood leukaemias. *Nat. Rev. Cancer* 3: 639–649, **2003**.

Gustafsson, B. and Carstensen, J. Space-time clustering of childhood lymphatic leukaemias and non-Hodgkin lymphomas in Sweden. *Eur. J. Epidemiol.* 16: 1111–1116, **2000**.

Hamadeh, R.R., Armenian, H.K., and Zurayk, H.C. A study of clustering of cases of leukemia, Hodgkin's disease and other lymphomas in Bahrein. *Trop. Geogr. Med.* 33: 42–48, **1981**.

Hjalgrim, L.L., Rostgaard, K., Hjalgrim, H., Westergaard, T., Thomassen, H., Forestier, E., Gustafsson, G., Kristinsson, J., Melbye, M., and Schmiegelow, K. Birth weight and risk for childhood leukaemia in Denmark, Sweden, Norway, and Iceland. *J. Natl. Cancer Inst.* 96: 1549–1556, **2004**.

Huang, S. and Spector, D.L. U1 and U2 small nuclear RNAs are present in nuclear speckles. *Proc. Natl. Acad. Sci. USA* 89: 305–308, **1992**

Infante-Rivard, C., Fotier, I., and Olson, E. Markers of infection, breast-feeding and childhood acute lymphoblastic leukaemia. *Br. J. Cancer* 83: 1559–1564, **2000**.

Itoh, K., Takahashi, M., Ukita, M., Nishizawa, T., and Okamoto, H. Influence of primers on the detection of TT virus DNA by polymerase chain reaction. *J. Infect. Dis.* 180: 1750–1751, **1999**.

Jelcic, I., Hotz-Wagenblatt, A., Hunzicker, A., zur Hausen, H., and de Villiers, E.-M. Isolation of multiple TT virus genotypes from spleen biopsy tissue from a Hodgkin's disease patient: genome reorganization and diversity in the hypervariable region. *J. Virol.* 78: 7498–7507 **2004**.

Johnson, E.S., Fishmann, H.R., Matanoski, G.M., and Diamond, E. Occurrence of Cancer in women in the meat industry. *Br. J. Ind. Med.* 43, 597–604, **1986**.

Jordan-Da Silva, N., Perel, Y., Méchinaud, F., Plouvier, E., Gandemer, V., Lutz, P., Vannier, J.P., Lamagnére, J.L., Margueritte, G., Boutard, P., Robert, A., Armari, C., Munzer, M., Millot, F., de Lumley, L., Berthou, C., Rialland, X., Pautard, B., Hémon, D., and Clavel, J. Infectious diseases in the first year of life, perinatal characteristics and childhood acute leukaemia. *Br. J. Cancer* 90: 139–145, **2004**.

Kaye, S. A., Robison, L.L., Smithson, W.A., Gunderson, P., King, F.L., and Neglia, J.P. Maternal reproductive history and birth characteristics in childhood acute lymphoblastic leukaemia. *Cancer* 68: 1351–1355, **1991**.

Kennedy, G., Kamano, J., and Sugden, B. Epstein-Barr virus provides a survival factor to Burkitt's lymphomas. *Proc. Natl. Acad. Sci. USA* 100: 14 269–14 274, **2003**.

Kinlen, M.J., O'Brian, F., Clarke, K., Balkwill, A., and Matthews, F. Rural population mixing and childhood leukaemia: effects of the North Sea oil industry in Scotland, including the area near Dounreay nuclear site. *Br. Med. J.* 306: 743–748, **1993**.

Kinlen, M.J. Epidemiological evidence of an infectious basis for childhood leukaemia. *Br. J. Cancer* 71: 1–5, **1995**.

Knox, E.G. Leukaemia clusters in childhood: geographical analysis in Britain. *J. Epidemiol. Community Health* 48: 369–376, **1994**.

La Vecchia, C., Negri, E., D'Avanzo, B., and Franceschi, S. Occupation and lymphoid neoplasms. *Br. J. Cancer* 60: 385–388, **1989**.

Leary, T.P., Erker, J.C., Chalmers, M.L., Desai, S. M., and Mushahwar, I.K. Improved detection systems for TT virus reveal high prevalence in humans, non-human primates and farm animals. *J. Gen. Virol.* 80: 2115–2120, **1999**.

Lewin, M.H., Bailey, N., Bandeletova, T., Bowman, R., Cross, A.J., Pollock, J., Shuker, D.E., and Bingham, S. A. Red meat enhances colonic formation of the DNA adduct o-6-carboxymethyl guanine: implications for colorectal cancer risk. *Cancer Res* . 66: 1859–1865, **2006**.

Limpens, J., Stad, R., Vos, C., de Vlaam, C., de Jong, D., van Ommen, G.J., Schuuring, E., and Kluin, P.M. Lymphoma-associated translocation t(14;18) in blood B cells of normal individuals. *Blood* 85: 2528–2536, **1995**.

MacMahon, B. Is acute lymphoblastic leukaemia in children virus-related? *Am. J. Epidemiol.* 136: 916–924, **1992**.

Magnani, C., Dalmsso, P., Pastore, G., Terracini, B., Martucci, M., Mosso, M.L., and Merletti, F. Increasing incidence of childhood leukemia in Northwest Italy 1975–1998. *Int. J. Cancer* 105: 552–557, **2003**.

Magrath, I. The pathogenesis of Burkitt's lymphoma. Adv. Cancer Res. 55: 133–269, **1990**.

Makino, K., Kuwahara, H., Masuko, N., Nishiyama, Y., Morisaki, T., Sasaki, J., Nakao, M., Kuwano, A., Nakata, M., and Saya, H. Cloning and characterization of NE-dlg: a novel human homolog of the *Drosophila* disc large (dlg) tumor suppressor protein interacts with the APC protein. *Oncogene* 14: 2425–2433, **1997**.

Matsubara, H., Michitaka, K., Horiike, N., Kihana, T., Yano, M., Mori, T., and Onji, M. Existence of TT virus DNA and TTV-like mini virus DNA in infant cord blood: mother-to neonatal transmission. *Hepatol. Res.* 21: 280–287, **2001** .

McKean-Cowdin, R., Feigelson, H.S., Ross, R.K., Pike, M.C., and Henderson, B.E. Declining cancer rates in the 1990s. *J. Clin. Oncol.* 18: 2258–2268, **2000**.

McKinney, P.A., Cartwright, R.A., Saiu, J.M., Mann, J.R., Stiller, C.A., Draper, C.W., Hartley, A.L., Hopton, P.A., Birch, J.M., and Waterhouse, J.A. The inter-regional epidemiological study of childhood cancer (IRESCC): a case control study of aetiological factors in leukaemia and lymphoma. *Arch. Dis. Child.* 62: 279–287, **1987**.

McKinney, P.A., Juszszak, E., Findey, E., Smith, K., and Thompson, C.S. Pre- and perinatal risk factors for childhood leukaemia and other malignancies: a Scottish case control study. *Br. J. Cancer* 80: 1844–1851, **1999**.

McNally, R.J., Alexander, F.E., and Birch, J.M. Space-time clustering analyses of childhood acute lymphoblastic leukaemia by immunophenotype. *Br. J. Cancer* 87: 513–515, **2002**.

Menegaux, F., Olshan, A.F., Neglia, J.P., Pollock, B.H., and Bondy, M.L. Day care, childhood infections, and risk of neuroblastoma. *Am. J. Epidemiol.* 159: 843–851, **2004**.

Metayer, C., Johnson, E.S., and Rice, J.C. Nested case-control study of tumors of the hemopoietic system among workers in the meat industry. *Am. J. Epidemiol.* 147: 727–738, **1998**.

Milham, S., Jr. Leukemia and multiple myeloma in farmers. *Am. J. Epidemiol.* 94: 507–510, **1971**.

Morton, L.M., Zheng, T., Holford, T.R., Hol-Chin, B.C., Constantini, A.S., Stagnaro, E., Willett, E.V., Dal Maso, L., Serraino, D., Chang, E.T., Cozen, W., Davis, S., Severson, R.K., Bernstein, L., Mayne, S. T., Dee, F.R., Cerhan, J.R., Hartge, P. and Interlymph Consortium. Alcohol consumption and risk of non-Hodgkin lymphoma: a pooled analysis. *Lancet Oncol.* 6: 469–476, **2005**.

Murray, L., McCarran, P., Baillie, K., Middleton, R., Dave Smith, G. , Dempsey, S., McCarthy, A., and Gavin, A. Association of early life factors and acute lymphoblastic leukaemia in childhood: historical cohort study. *Br. J. Cancer* 86: 356–361, **2002**.

Neglia, J.P., Linnet, M.S., Shun, X.O., Severson, R.K., Potter, J.D., Martens, A.C., Went , W., Kersey, J.H., and Robison L.L. Patterns of infection and day care utilization and risk of childhood acute lymphoblastic leukaemia. *Br. J. Cancer* 82: 234–240, **2000**.

Nelson, R.A., Levine, A.M., Marks, G., and Bernstein, L. Alcohol, tobacco, and recreational drugs use and the risk of non-Hodgkin's lymphoma. *Br. J. Cancer* 76: 1532–1537, **1997**.

Nishizawa, T., Okamoto, H., Konishi, K., Yoshizawa, H., Miyakawa, Y., and Mayumi, M. A novel DNA virus (TTV) associated with elevated transaminase levels in post-transfusion hepatitis of unknown etiology. *Biochem. Biophys. Res. Commun.* 241: 92–97, **1997**.

Okamoto, H., Nishizawa, T., Tawara, A., Takahashi, M., Kishimoto, J., Sai, T., and Sugai, Y. TT virus mRNAs detected in the bone marrow cells from an infected individual. *Biochem. Biophys. Res. Commun.* 279: 700–707, **2000**.

Okamoto, H., Takahashi, M., Nishizawa, T., Tawara, A., Fukai, K., Muramatsu, U., Maito, Y., and Yoshikawa, A. Genomic characterization of TT viruses (TTVs) in pigs, cats and dogs and their relatedness with species-specific TTVs in primates and tupaias. *J. Gen. Virol.* 83: 1291–1297, **2002**.

Ou, S. X., Han, D., Severson, R.K., Chen, Z., Neglia, J.P., Reaman, G.H., Buckley, R.D., and Robison, L.L. Birth characteristics, maternal reproductive history, hormone use during pregnancy, and risk of childhood acute lymphocytic leukemia by immunophenotype (United States). *Cancer Causes Control* 13: 15–25, **2002**.

Pearce, N.E., Smith, A.H., Howard, J.K., Sheppard, RA., Giles, H.J., and Teague, C.A. Case-control study of multiple myeloma and farming. *Br. J. Cancer* 54: 493–500, **1986 a**.

Pearce, N.E., Smith, A.H., Howard, J.K., Sheppard, R.A., Giles, T.H., and Teague, C.A. Non-Hodgkin's lymphoma and exposure to phenoxyherbicide chlorophenols, fencing work, and meat works employment: a case-control study. *Br. J. Ind. Med.* 43: 75–83, **1986 b**.

Pearce, N.E., Smith, A.H., and Reif, J.S. Increased risks of soft tissue sarcoma, malignant lymphoma, and acute myeloid leukaemia in abattoir workers. *Am. J. Ind. Med.* 14, 63–72, **1988**.

Pearce, N. and Bethwaite, P. Increasing incidence of non-Hodgkin lymphoma: occupation and environmental factors. *Cancer Res.* 52: 5496s–5500s, **1992**.

Pearce, M.S., Cotterill, S. J., and Parker, L. Fathers' occupational contacts and risk of childhood leukemia and non-Hodgkin lymphoma. *Epidemiology* 15: 352–356, **2004**.

Peng, Y.H., Nishizawa, T., Takahashi, M., Ishikawa T., Yoshikawa, A., and Okamoto, H. Analysis of the entire genomes of thirteen TT virus variants classifiable into the fourth and fifth genetic groups, isolated from viremic infants. *Arch. Virol* . 147: 21–41, **2002**.

Perrillat, F., Clavel, J., Auclerc, M.F., Baruchel, A., Leverger, G., Nelken, B., Philippe, N., Schaison, G., Sommelet, D., Vilner, E., and Hémon, D. Day-care, early common infections and childhood acute leukaemia: a multicentre French case-control study. *Br. J. Cancer* 86: 1064–1069, **2002**.

Petridou, E., Kassimos, D., Calmanti, M., Kosmidis, H., Haidas, S., Flytzani, V. Tong, D., and Trichopoulos, D. Age of exposure to infections and risk of childhood leukaemias. *Br. Med. J.* 307: 774, **1993**.

Petridou, E., Revinthi, K., Alexander, F.E., Haidas, S., Koliouskas, D., Kosmidis, H., Piperopoulou, F., Tzortzutou, F., and Trichopoulos, D. Space-time clustering of childhood leukaemia in Greece: evidence supporting a viral aetiology. *Br. J. Cancer* 73: 1278–1283, **1996**.

Pfaffenbarger, R.S., Jr., Wing, A.L., and Hyde, R.T. Characteristics in youth indicative of adult-onset Hodgkin's disease. *J. Natl. Cancer Inst.* 58: 1489–1491, **1977**.

Philippe, P. The scale-invariant spatial clustering of leukemia in San Francisco. *J. Theor. Biol.* 199: 371–381, **1999**.

Roman, E., Ansell, P., and Bull, D. Leukaemia and non-Hodgkin's lymphoma in children and young adults: are prenatal and neonatal factors important determinants of disease? *Br. J. Cancer* 76: 406–415, **1997**.

Rosenbaum, P.F., Buck, G.M., and Brecher, M.L. Early child-care and preschool experiences and the risk of childhood acute lymphoblastic leukaemia. *Am. J. Epidemiol.* 152: 1136–144, **2000**.

Ryan, C., Dutta, C., and Simo, R. Role of screening for infectious mononucleosis in patients admitted with isolated, unilateral peritonsillar abscess. *J. Laryngol. Otol.* 118: 362–365, **2004**.

Saback, F.L., Gomes, S. A., de Paula, V.S., da Silva, R.R., Lewis-Ximenez, L.L., and Niel, C. Age-specific prevalence and transmission of TT virus. *J. Med. Virol.* 59: 318–322, **1999**.

Saftlas, A.F., Blair, A., Cantor, K.P., Hanrahan, L., and Anderson, H.A. Cancer and other causes of death among Wisconsin farmers. *Am. J. Ind. Med.* 11: 119–129, **1987**.

Scherr, P.A., Hutchison, G.B., and Neiman, R.S. Non-Hodgkin's lymphoma and occupational exposure. *Cancer Res.* 52: 5503s–5509s, **1992**.

SEER. Surveillance, epidemiology and end results program public use data 1973–2000, National Cancer Institute, DCCPS, Surveillance Research Program, Cancer Statistics Branch, **2003**.

Serraino, D., Franceschi, S., Salamini, R., Barra, S., Negri, E., Carbone, A., La Vecchia, C. Socio-economic indicators, infectious diseases and Hodgkin's disease. *Int. J. Cancer* 47: 352–357, **1991**.

Shaw, G., Lavey, R., Jackson, R., and Austin, D. Association of childhood leukemia with maternal age, birth order, and paternal occupation. A case-control study. *Am. J. Epidemiol.* 119: 788–795, **1984**.

Sheng, W., Decaussin, G., Ligout, A., Takada, K., and Ooka, T. Malignant transformation of Epstein-Barr virus-negative Akata cells by introduction of the BARF1 gene carried by Epstein-Barr virus. *J. Virol.* 77: 3859–3865, **2003**.

Shirimizu, B., Barriga, F., Neequaye, J., Jafri, A., Dalla-Favera, R., Neri, A., Guttierez, M., Levine, P., and Magrath, I. Patterns of chromosomal breakpoint locations in Burkitt's lymphoma: relevance to geography and Epstein-Barr virus association. *Blood* 77: 1516–1526, **1991**.

Smith, M.A., Simon, R., Strickler, H.D., McQuillan, G., Ries, L.A., and Linet, M.S. Evidence that childhood acute lymphoblastic leukaemia is associated with an infectious agent linked to hygiene conditions. *Cancer Causes Control* 9: 285–298, **1998**.

Stark, C.R. and Mantel, N. Effects of maternal age and birth order on the risk of mongolism and leukaemia. *J. Natl. Cancer Inst.* 37: 687–698, **1966**.

Takahashi, K., Hijikata, M., Samokhvalov, E.I., and Mishiro, S. Full or near full-length nucleotides sequence of TT virus variants (types SANBAN and YONBAN) and the TT virus-like mini virus. *Intervirology* 43: 119–123, **2000**.

Takahashi, M., Asabe, S., Gotanda, Y., Kisihimoto J., Tsuda, F., and Okamoto, H. TT virus distributed in various leukocyte sub-populations at distinct levels, with the highest viral load in granulocytes. *Biochem. Biophys. Res. Commun.* 290: 242–248, **2002**.

van Steensel-Moll, H.A., Valkenburg, H.A., Vandenbroucke, J.P., and van Zanen, G.E. Time space distribution of childhood leukaemia in the Netherlands. *J. Epidemiol. Community Health* 37: 145–148, **1983**.

van Steensel-Moll, H.A., Valkenburg, H.A., and van Zanen, G.E. Childhood leukemia and infectious diseases in the first year of life: a register-based case-control study. *Am. J. Epidemiol.* 124: 590–594, **1986**.

Veltri, R.W., Sprinkle, P.M., and McClung, J.E. Epstein-Barr virus associated with episodes of recurrent tonsillitis. *Arch. Otolaryngol.* 101: 552–556, **1975**.

zur Hausen, H. Proliferation-inducing viruses in non-permissive systems as possible causes of human cancers. *Lancet* 357: 381–384, **2001**.

zur Hausen, H. and de Villiers, E.-M. Virus target cell conditioning model to explain some epidemiologic characteristics of childhood leukemias and lymphomas. *Int. J. Cancer* 115: 1–5, **2005**.

12.2
Human Breast Cancer

A number of viruses have been reported to be involved in human breast cancer, among them Epstein–Barr virus, cytomegalovirus, and various papillomavirus types. The published data have not been confirmed in other studies and, thus, remain difficult to interpret.

For more than 30 years reports have been appearing which claiming the presence of an agent which is closely related to mouse mammary tumor virus (MMTV) in human breast cancer patients and in high-risk populations for breast cancer. The non-Mendelian maternal inheritance of mammary cancer in high-incidence laboratory strains of mice suggested, at an early stage, the involvement of an extrachromosomal agent in the etiology of this cancer (Staff of the Roscoe B. Jackson Memorial Laboratory, 1933). Bittner (1936) subsequently showed that an agent was passed from the mother to offspring with the milk. Offspring from low-incidence mothers foster-nursed on high-incidence mothers developed mammary cancer at a higher rate (DeOme, 1940). A detailed electron microscopic description of the virus particles followed in 1948 (Porter and Thompson), and the virus was later identified as a member of the retrovirus family.

One interesting aspect which came out of MMTV research was that its horizontal transmission via milk was accompanied by germline Mendelian inheritance (Bentvelzen, 1975). Viral genomes persist as endogenous DNA in more than 25 copies per mouse genome (Kozak et al., 1987). Another interesting observation was the detection of preferred sites for MMTV integration in the genomes of mammary tumors after exogenous infection (Nusse and Varmus, 1982). Direct stimulation of MMTV expression by hormones was suggested by a high number of MMTV particles in mammary tumors from late pregnant and lactating infected mice when compared to tumors from nonlactating infected mice (Hairstone et al., 1964). Subsequently, multiple glucocorticoid response elements were discovered within the long terminal repeat (LTR) promoter regions of MMTV (Chandler et al., 1983; Payvar et al., 1983).

The pathway of MMTV from the infected gut to the mammary glands has been clarified during the past two decades. Manifestation of the infection in B lymphocytes of intestinal Peyer's patches leads to transfer of the virus to T lymphocytes which eventually transfer the virus to mammary epithelial cells (Tsubara et al., 1988). The MMTV 3' LTR sequence encodes a superantigen that orchestrates the multiplication of T and B lymphocytes, resulting in an amplification of virus-producing cells capable of delivering the infection to the mammary gland (for reviews, see Matzuzawa et al., 1995; Ross, 1998). Immunosuppression thus, as the most interesting consequence of these observations, does not facilitate MMTV-mediated mammary carcinogenesis but has a slight protective function (Fig. 12.8). This is in remarkable contrast to most other virus-caused cancers, the emergence of which is commonly enhanced under conditions of immunosuppression (see Chapters 4, 5, and 7). Since the incidence of human breast cancer is also under hormonal control and is not increased under immunosuppression, these data might suggest an analogous mechanism in the development of the human malignancy.

During the late 1960s and the 1970s, a number of reports appeared claiming the detection of MMTV-like particles in women from families with a history of breast cancer and in ethnic groups with a high breast cancer incidence (Moore et al., 1969, 1971; Chopra et al., 1973). A simultaneous detection test permitting the demonstration of reverse transcriptase activity linked to supposedly viral 60–70 S RNA genomes was also reported to be positive for specific fractions of human milk and breast tumors (Schlom et al., 1971, 1972; Axel et al., 1972; McGrath et al., 1974). Subsequent studies produced conflicting results (Wooding, 1972; Calafat and Hageman, 1973), while one epidemiologic survey did not reveal any differences in breast cancer rates between breast- or bottle-fed babies (Henderson, 1974). For a few years no additional data were obtained in support of an exogenous virus hypothesis in human breast cancer.

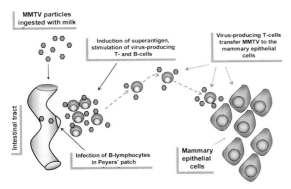

Fig. 12.8 Schematic outline of mouse mammary tumor virus (MMTV) transfer to the mammary gland epithelial cells, which may be transformed after specific integration of the viral genome.

Since MMTV persists as an endogenous agent, and endogenous human retroviruses were discovered which belonged to the same retrovirus subfamily as MMTV (HERV-K) and also possessed a glucocorticoid-responsive element in the LTR region, interest in a possible role for these genomes in human breast cancer was resurrected during the late 1980s. Particles containing HERV-K-related sequences are released from a human breast cancer cell line T47-D (Ono et al., 1987; Patience et al., 1996; Seifarth et al., 1995, 1998), their production is up-regulated by glucocorticoids, the sequences in the particles are highly defective, and the *env* gene is not transcribed. Serologic studies provided ambiguous data with HERV-K antigens (Vogetseder et al., 1993; Boller et al., 1997), although one report referred to MMTV-related antigen in particularly aggressive breast cancers of Tunisian women (Levine et al., 1984). Thus, a relationship between endogenous retrovirus expression and human breast cancer is far from being established.

In recent years there have been several reports of bona fide MMTV sequences in a high percentage of human breast cancers (Wang et al., 1995, 1998). Initially, a 660-bp sequence with 98% homology to the MMTV *env* gene was amplified from 40% of breast cancer biopsies, but from only 2% of normal donors. In 66% of positive samples the env sequence was also transcribed (Pogo et al., 1999; Liu et al., 2001; Ford et al., 2003; Faedo et al., 2004). Even a MMTV-like superantigen coded for by the MMTV-like LTR was described in human breast cancer (Wang et al., 2004). Infection of human mammary cells by MMTV has been demonstrated in tissue culture studies (Katz et al., 2005; Indik et al., 2005). Other groups have been unable to confirm the presence of MMTV-like sequences in human breast cancer (Zangen et al., 2002; Mant et al., 2004).

Although the evidence linking human breast cancer to infectious events remains scarce, it should be re-emphasized here that there exists in one other aspect a striking similarity to MMTV-linked mammary carcinoma development in mice: this is the remarkable absence of increased breast cancer incidence under conditions of immunosuppression. One report has even described a protective effect for breast cancer development in organ xenograft recipient women maintained under long-term immunosuppression (*Stewart et al.*, 1995). The reason is well established for the MMTV system, where immunosuppression reveals a protective effect. For humans, however, further studies should establish similar effects in human breast cancer.

12.3
Other Human Cancers Possibly Linked to Infectious Events

Several cancers develop on the basis of chronic inflammation; these seem to include prostate cancer, thyroid cancer, cancers developing in chronic skin ulcerations, and many others. The evidence for specific events in the development of these tumors is presently non-existent, and so will not be discussed here. One possible exception is that cutaneous lymphomas rarely develop at sites of chronic *Borrelia burgdorferi* infections (for reviews, see Grange et al., 2002; Bogle et al., 2005). In view of the frequency of *Borrelia* infections these complications must be exceedingly rare, while the possible mechanism is poorly understood.

Research into infectious causes of human cancer has been more than rewarding during the past 40 years. Nonetheless, it would be very surprising if further links between specific infectious agents and human malignancies were not identified during the next few years.

References

Axel, R., Schlom, J., and Spiegelman, S. Presence in human breast cancer of RNA homologous to mouse mammary tumour virus RNA. *Nature* 235: 32–36, **1972**.

Bentvelzen, P. Endogenous mammary tumor viruses in mice. *Cold Spring Harbor Symp. Quant. Biol.* 39 Pt. 2: 1145–1150, **1975**.

Bittner, J.J. Some possible effects of nursing on the mammary tumor incidence in mice. *Science* 84: 162–169, **1936**.

Bogle, M.A., Riddle, C.C., Triana, E.M., Jones, D., and Duvic, M. Primary cutaneous B-cell lymphoma. *J. Am. Acad. Dermatol.* 53: 479–484, **2005**.

Boller, K., Janssen, O., Schuldes, H., Tönjes, R.R., and Kurth, R. Characterization of the antibody response specific for the human endogenous retrovirus HTDV/HERV-K. *J. Virol.* 71: 4581–4588, **1997**.

Calafat, J. and Hageman, P.C. Remarks on virus-like particles in human breast cancer. *Nature* 242: 260–262, **1973**.

Chandler, V.L., Maier, B.A., and Yamamoto, K.R. DNA sequences bound specifically by glucocorticoid receptor in vitro render a heterologous promoter hormone responsive in vivo. *Cell* 33: 489–499, **1983**.

Chopra, H., Ebert, P., Woodside, N., Kvedar, J., Albert, S., and Brennan, M. Electron microscopic detection of simian-type virus particles in human milk. *Nature New Biol.* 243: 159–160, **1973**.

DeOme, K.B. The incidence of mammary tumors among low-tumor strain C57 BLK mice when foster-nursed by high tumor strain A females. *Am. J. Cancer* 40: 231–234, **1940**.

Faedo, M., Ford, C.E., Mehta, R., Blazek, K., and Rawlinson, W.D. Mouse mammary tumor-like virus is associated with p53 nuclear accumulation and progesterone receptor positivity but not estrogen positivity in human female breast cancer. *Clin. Cancer Res.* 10: 4417–4419, **2004**.

Ford, C.E., Tran, D., Deng, Y., Ta, V.T., Rawlinson, W.D., and Lawson, J.S. Mouse mammary tumor virus-like gene sequences in breast tumors of Australian and Vietnamese women. *Clin. Cancer Res.* 9: 1118–1120, **2003**.

Grange, F., Wechsler, J., Guillaume, J.C., Tortel, J., Tortel, M.C., Audhuy, B., Jaulhac, B., and Cerroni, L. *Borrelia burgdorferi*-associated lymphocytoma cutis simulating a primary cutaneous large B-cell lymphoma. *J. Am. Acad. Dermatol.* 47: 530–534, **2002**.

Hairstone, M.A., Sheffield, J.B., and Moore, D.H. Studies of B particles in the mammary tumors of different mouse strains. *J. Natl. Cancer Inst.* 33: 825–836, **1964**.

Henderson, B.E. Type B virus and human breast cancer. *Cancer* 34 (Suppl.): 1386–1389, **1974**.

Indik, S., Gunzburg, W.H., Salmons, B., and Rouault, F. Mouse mammary tumor virus infects human cells. *Cancer Res.* 65: 6651–6659, **2005**

Katz, E., Lareef, M.H., Rassa, J.C., Grande, S.M., King, L.B., Russo, J., Ross, S.R., and Monroe, J.G.. MMTV Env encodes an ITAM responsible for transformation of mammary epithelial cells in three-dimensional culture. *J. Exp. Med.* 201: 431–439, **2005**.

Kozak, C., Peters, G., Pauley, R., Morris, V., Michalides, R., Dudley, J., Green, M., Davisson, M., Prakash, O., Vaidya, A., et al. A standard nomenclature for endogenous mammary tumor virus. *J. Virol.* 61: 1631–1654, **1987**.

Levine, P.H., Mesa-Tejeda, R., Keydar, I., Tabbane, F., Spiegelman, S., and Mourali, N. Increased incidence of mouse mammary tumor virus-related antigen in Tunisian patients with breast cancer. *Int. J. Cancer* 33: 305–308, **1984**.

Liu, B., Wang, Y., Melana, S. M., Pelisson, I., Najfeld, V., Holland, J.F., and Pogo, B.G. Identification of a proviral structure in human breast cancer. *Cancer Res.* 61: 1754–1759, **2001**.

Mant, C., Gillett, C., D'Arrigo, C., and Cason, J. Human murine mammary tumour virus-like agents are genetically distinct from endogenous retroviruses and are not detectable in breast cancer cell lines or biopsies. *Virology* 318: 393–404, **2004**.

Matsuzawa, A., Nakano, H., Yoshimoto, T., and Sayama, K. Biology of mouse mammary tumor virus (MMTV). *Cancer Lett.* 90: 3–11, **1995**.

McGrath, C.M., Grant, P.M., Soule, H.D., Glancy, T., and Rich, M.A. Replication of oncornavirus-like particles in human breast carcinoma cell line, MCF-7. *Nature* 252: 247–250. **1974**.

Moore, D.M., Sarkar, N.H., Kelly, C.E., Pillsbury, N., and Charney, J. Type B particles in human milk. *Texas Rep. Biol. Med.* 27: 1027–1039, **1969**.

Moore, D.M., Charney, J., Kramarsky, B., Lasfargues, E.Y., Sarkar, N.H., Brennan, M.J., Burrows, J.H., Sirsat, S. M., Paymaster, J.C., and Vaidya, A.B. Search for a human breast cancer virus. *Nature* 229: 611–614, **1971**.

Nusse, R. and Varmus, H.E. Many tumors induced by the mouse mammary tumor virus contain provirus integrated in the same region of the host genome. *Cell* 31: 99–109, **1982**.

Ono, M., Kawakami, M., and Ushikobo, H. Stimulation of expression of the human endogenous retrovirus genome by female steroid hormones in human breast cancer cell line T47 D. *J. Virol.* 61: 2059–2062, **1987**.

Patience, C., Simpson, G.R., Colletta, A.A., Welch, H.M., Weiss, R.A., and Boyd, M.T. Human endogenous retrovirus expression and reverse transcriptase activity in the T47 D mammary carcinoma cell line. *J. Virol.* 70: 2654–2657, **1996**.

Payvar, F., DeFranco, D., Firestone, G.L., Edgar, B., Wrange, Ö., Okret, S., Gustafsson, J.A., and Yamamoto, K.R. Sequence-specific binding of the glucocorticoid receptor to MTV DNA at sites within and upstream of the transcribed region. *Cell* 35: 381–392, **1983**.

Pogo, B.G., Melana, S. M., Holland, J.F., Mandeli, J.F., Pilotti, S., Casalini, P., and Menard, S. Sequences homologous to the mouse mammary tumor virus env gene in human breast carcinoma correlate with overexpression of laminin receptor. *Clin. Cancer Res.* 5: 2108–2111, **1999**.

Porter, K.R. and Thompson, H.P. A particulate body associated with epithelial cells cultured from mammary carcinomas of mice of a milk-factor strain. *J. Exp. Med.* 88: 15–23, **1948**.

Ross, S. R. Mouse mammary tumor virus and its interaction with the immune system. *Immunol. Res.* 17: 209–216, **1998**.

Schlom, J., Spiegelman, S., and Moore, D.H. RNA-dependent DNA polymerase activity in virus-like particles isolated from human milk. *Nature* 231: 97–102, **1971**.

Schlom, J., Spiegelman, S., and Moore, D.H. Reverse transcriptase and high molecular weight RNA in particles from mouse and human milk. *J. Natl. Cancer Inst.* 48: 1197–1203, **1972**.

Seifarth, W., Skladny, H., Krieg-Schneider, F., Reichert, A., Hehlmann, R., and Leib-Mösch, C., retrovirus-like particles released from the human breast cancer cell line T47-D display type B- and C-related endogenous retroviral sequences. *J. Virol .* 69: 6408–6416, **1995**.

Seifarth, W., Baust, C., Murr, A., Skladny, H., Krieg-Schneider, F., Blusch, J., Werner, T., Hehlmann, R., and Leib-Mösch, C. Proviral structure, chromosomal location, and expression of HERV-K-T47 D, a novel human endogenous retrovirus derived from T47 D particles. *J. Virol.* 72: 8384–8391, **1998**.

Staff of the Roscoe B. Jackson Memorial Laboratory. The existence of nonchromosomal influence in the incidence of mammary tumors in mice. *Science* 78: 465, **1933**.

Stewart, T., Tsai, S. C., Grayson, H., Henderson, R., and Opelz, G. Incidence of de-novo breast cancer in women chronically immunosuppressed after organ transplantation. *Lancet* 346: 796–798, **1995**.

Tsubura, A., Inaba, M., Imai, S., Murakami, A., Oyaizu, N., Yasumizu, R., Ohnishi, Y.,

Tanaka, H., Morii, S., and Ikehara, S. Intervention of T-cells in transportation of mouse mammary tumor virus (milk factor) to mammary gland cells in vivo. *Cancer Res.* 48: 6555–6559, **1988**.

Vogetseder, W., Dumfarth, A., Mayersbach, P., Schonitze, D., and Dierich, M.P. Antibodies to human sera recognizing a recombinant outer membrane protein encoded by the envelop gene of the human endogenous retrovirus K. *AIDS Res. Hum. Retroviruses* 9: 687–694, **1993**.

Wang, Y., Holland, J.F., Bleiweiss, I.J., Melana, S., Liu, X., Pelisson, I., Cantarella, A., Stellrecht, K., Mani, S., and Pogo, B.G. Detection of mammary tumor virus-like env gene sequences in human breast cancer. *Cancer Res.* 55: 5173–5179, **1995**.

Wang, Y., Go, V., Holland, J.F., Melana, S. M., and Pogo, B.G. Expression of mouse mammary tumor virus-like env gene sequences in human breast cancer. *Clin. Cancer Res.* 4: 2565–2568, **1998**.

Wang, Y., Jiang, J.D., Xu, D., Li, Y., Qu, C., Holland, J.F., and Pogo, B.G. A mouse mammary tumor virus-like long terminal repeat superantigen in human breast cancer. *Cancer Res.* 64: 4105–4111, **2004**.

Wooding, R.B.P. Milk microsomes, viruses, and the milk fat globule membrane. *Experientia* 28: 1077–1079, **1972**.

Zangen, R., Harden, S., Cohen, D., Parrella, P., and Sidransky, D. Mouse mammary tumor-like env gene as a molecular marker for breast cancer? *Int. J. Cancer*. 102: 304–307, **2002**.

Index

Infections Causing Human Cancer. Harald zur Hausen
Copyright © 2006 WILEY-VCH Verlag GmbH & Co. KGaA, Weinheim
ISBN: 3-527-31056-8